Nutrition Education

Nutrition Education

Linking Research, Theory, and Practice

Second Edition

Isobel R. Contento, PhD

Mary Swartz Rose Professor of Nutrition Education

Teachers College Columbia University

JONES AND BARTLETT PUBLISHERS

Sudbury, Massachusetts

BOSTON   TORONTO   LONDON   SINGAPORE

World Headquarters

Jones and Bartlett Publishers
40 Tall Pine Drive
Sudbury, MA 01776
978-443-5000
info@jbpub.com
www.jbpub.com

Jones and Bartlett Publishers Canada
6339 Ormindale Way
Mississauga, Ontario L5V 1J2
Canada

Jones and Bartlett Publishers International
Barb House, Barb Mews
London W6 7PA
United Kingdom

Jones and Bartlett's books and products are available through most bookstores and online booksellers. To contact Jones and Bartlett Publishers directly, call 800-832-0034, fax 978-443-8000, or visit our website, www.jbpub.com.

Substantial discounts on bulk quantities of Jones and Bartlett's publications are available to corporations, professional associations, and other qualified organizations. For details and specific discount information, contact the special sales department at Jones and Bartlett via the above contact information or send an email to specialsales@jbpub.com.

Production Credits

Publisher, Higher Education: Cathleen Sether
Acquisitions Editor: Shoshanna Goldberg
Senior Associate Editor: Amy L. Bloom
Senior Editorial Assistant: Kyle Hoover
Production Manager: Julie Champagne Bolduc
Associate Production Editor: Jessica Steele Newfell
Associate Marketing Manager: Jody Sullivan
V.P., Manufacturing and Inventory Control: Therese Connell
Composition: Publishers' Design and Production Services, Inc.
Cover Design: Scott Moden
Photo and Permissions Associate: Emily Howard
Cover and Title Page Image: © Elana Elisseeva/ShutterStock, Inc.
Printing and Binding: Courier Westford
Cover Printing: Courier Westford

Library of Congress Cataloging-in-Publication Data

Contento, Isobel R.
  Nutrition education : linking research, theory, and practice / Isobel R. Contento. — 2nd ed.
       p. ; cm.
  Includes bibliographical references and index.
  ISBN 978-0-7637-7508-7 (pbk. : alk. paper)
 1. Nutrition—Study and teaching. I. Title.
 [DNLM: 1. Dietetics—education. 2. Health Education—methods. 3. Food Habits.   WB 18 C759n 2011]
  TX364.C685 2011
  613.2—dc22

                                                                                          2009052356

6048

Printed in the United States of America
14 13 12 11 10   10 9 8 7 6 5 4 3 2

Brief Contents

Contents

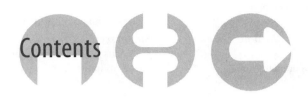

Preface

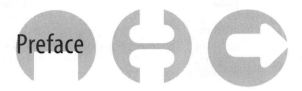

Nutrition education is defined in this text as any combination of educational strategies, accompanied by environmental supports, designed to facilitate the voluntary adoption of food choices and other food- and nutrition-related behaviors conducive to health and well-being. It is delivered through multiple venues and involves activities at the individual, institutional, community, and policy levels.

Nutrition education ranks high on the public agenda, and interest in food and nutrition is widespread. This is an exciting time: The explosion of research in nutrition education and behavioral nutrition; an increased awareness of nutrition education in schools, worksites, and communities; and policy initiatives in institutions and government over the past few years have made it important to update this text. In all of these activities, it is clear that nutrition education must be grounded in theory and evidence to be effective. We now have a better understanding of why people eat what they do and how they change as well as how nutrition education can increase the motivation of, skills for, and opportunities for people to engage in health-promoting actions.

In the foundational chapters of Part I, this *Second Edition* provides a clearly organized description of each of the key theories that can be used in nutrition education interventions to address potential determinants or mediators of action and behavior change as well as updated evidence for their use. The chapters also describe how each of the theories can be translated into practical nutrition education activities. Case examples have been added to complement the examples found in the Nutrition Education in Action features to further clarify the use of theory in educational activities in practical settings.

There also is increased appreciation that our food choices are influenced by social and environmental contexts. Nutrition education needs to address the numerous personal, environmental, and policy influences on food choices and dietary behaviors to assist individuals and communities in practicing healthy behaviors. A larger scope for nutrition education thus has evolved. While group sessions remain primary, nutrition educators also work in collaboration with others on activities such as school and community gardens, cooking with children and adults, farm-to-school programs, school and community wellness policies, and initiatives to improve policy, social structures, and systems. The chapter on environmental supports for action has been completely revised in the *Second Edition* to reflect this new emphasis, using a social ecological model.

This text focuses on how to *design*, *deliver*, and *evaluate* the types of educational interventions and programs that the vast majority of nutrition educators conduct on an ongoing basis in their places of work. It

is designed for upper division and graduate nutrition students who are taking their first course in nutrition education as well as for those already working in nutrition education who want a comprehensive resource for planning and delivering effective programs to their audiences.

The centerpiece of this text is a stepwise procedural model, described in Part II, to make it easier for students and nutrition educators to design effective nutrition education. Using a six-step process, this procedural model shows how *behavioral theory* is translated into *educational objectives and theory-based strategies* and then into *practical ways* to implement these strategies. It integrates theory, research, and practice at every step, providing guidance on designing, implementing, and evaluating theory-based nutrition education. At the end of each chapter in this part, the procedure is illustrated by a case study and worksheets are provided for readers to use. In the *Second Edition*, the case studies and worksheets have been completely revised and reformatted based on feedback from both faculty members and students who have used this text, making them easier for all to use. The worksheets also are available on the book's website (http://nutrition.jbpub.com/education/2e), further increasing the ease of use.

In sum, the basic structure in the *Second Edition* remains the same, but each chapter has been fully updated with new research findings; the text has been streamlined; the theories are clearly organized with application examples; the stepwise procedural model is reformatted; and the trim size of the book is enlarged. We believe these changes will make the book easy to read and use.

This book is divided into three parts. Part I provides background of useful theories for nutrition education and the research evidence for effective practice with four theories described in Chapter 4 and another four described in Chapter 5. These theories include the health belief model, precaution adoption process model, theory of planned behavior, self-determination theory, social cognitive theory, the health action process model, the transtheoretical model, and qualitative grounded theory. For each theory, a *leader* orients the student to the theory, and a *take-home message* summarizes it. Each theory is followed by a description of how to implement the theory in practice and a *case example* of its use. In each chapter, the theories and fundamental concepts also are illustrated in the Nutrition Education in Action features, where examples are taken from current programs.

Part II describes the six-step process for translating theory and evidence into *educational plans*, for program components directed at groups involving educational objectives, theory-based educational strategies, and practical activities to enhance motivation and build skills, and *environmental support plans*, for changes in policy, social structures, and systems to increase opportunities for action. It also provides guidance on how to link *evaluation* to theory and intervention objectives.

Part III describes the nuts and bolts of implementing nutrition education with diverse groups ranging from preschool children to older adults to low-literacy and low-income audiences through a variety of venues, including group sessions, written and visual materials, new technologies, and social marketing.

Nutrition Education: Linking Research, Theory, and Practice, Second Edition, includes a variety of features to prepare students to provide effective nutrition education to specific groups and foster environmental supports for action:

- At the beginning of each chapter, an overview and outline help students anticipate what will be covered. Learning objectives improve retention of the material presented.
- Nutrition Education in Action boxes highlight concepts discussed in the chapter through examples of best practices and research.
- Key theories used in nutrition education are described in the foundational chapters along with evidence from research and interventions.
- Tables, boxes, and case examples in the foundational chapters illustrate the use of each specific theory in practice.

- A logic model approach is used in the stepwise procedure, with the tasks and products of each step clearly stated.
- A flowchart is provided in each chapter to make following the steps easier.
- The case study introduced in Chapter 7 and followed throughout Part II illustrates each step of the stepwise procedure for designing nutrition education.
- The worksheets in Part II allow students and nutrition educators to develop their own programs using the stepwise procedure system.
- At the end of each chapter, review questions reinforce key concepts and references provide an opportunity for further study.

Students also are encouraged to visit this text's companion website, http://nutrition.jbpub.com/education/2e, for additional resources to enhance their learning, including downloadable PDFs of the worksheets from the main text, lesson plans, practice quizzes, web links, and additional nutrition resources. An Instructor's Manual, TestBank, and Power-Point Presentations are available for instructors to download.

The public needs and wants what nutrition education can offer. This text is designed to help students and nutrition educators gain the knowledge and skills needed to provide that nutrition education effectively.

Acknowledgments

The field of nutrition education has grown rapidly over the past few years, and I have had the privilege of being a part of this exciting development. Many people have influenced my thinking and contributed to my understanding of the field, and I thank them all. They include colleagues across the country, members of the Society for Nutrition Education, publishers of research, presenters at professional meetings, members of committees I have been on, practitioners in community sites, and many others with whom I have worked. In particular, I want to thank a few I have worked with more closely: Joan Gussow first introduced me to the field of nutrition education, and her insights and forward-thinking have always challenged me to dig deeper. She encouraged me to write this book and has been supportive throughout. Pamela Koch has been an essential partner in this effort. She is a gifted nutrition educator with whom I have worked for the past decade. She spent many hours helping make this book more readable and the diagrams more visually appealing. Kathleen Porter provided valuable assistance with the references, diagrams, worksheets, and ancilliary materials for this edition.

The many reviewers of the manuscript for both editions provided extremely valuable feedback from their vantage points as faculty members who teach nutrition education or community nutrition courses in a wide variety of colleges and universities. This book has benefited from their insights. A special thank you to:

- Jennifer Anderson, PhD, RD, Colorado State University
- Marilyn Townsend, PhD, University of California, Davis
- Marci K. Campbell, PhD, University of North Carolina, Chapel Hill
- Deborah I. Myers, EdD, RD, Bluffton University
- Martine I. Scannavino, DHSc, RD, LDN, Cedar Crest College
- Jeffrey S. Hampl, PhD, RD, Arizona State University
- Teri L. Burgess–Champoux, PhD, RD, LD, University of Wisconsin–Stout
- Cynthia Blanton, PhD, RD, Idaho State University
- Tawni Holmes, PhD, RD, LD, University of Central Oklahoma
- Paula DN Dworatzek, PhD, RD, Brescia University College
- Bonita Manson, PhD, CFCS, CFLE, South Carolina State University

Equally important are the numerous students who road-tested the many versions of this book in a decade of my nutrition education courses. Their reactions, feedback, and suggestions have provided reality checks on using this book in the classroom.

I also want to thank the people at Jones and Bartlett for their support for this project: Jacqueline Geraci, who was willing to take the risk to publish a first-ever textbook on nutrition education, and Shoshanna Goldberg, acquisitions editor, who has been a delight to work with. Kyle Hoover, senior editorial assistant, and Jess Newfell, associate production editor, have been wonderfully helpful and supportive.

And last, but definitely not least, I thank my husband Robert Clark for his many years of unwavering support. Having worked in the textbook business himself, he understands the effort that writing a textbook requires.

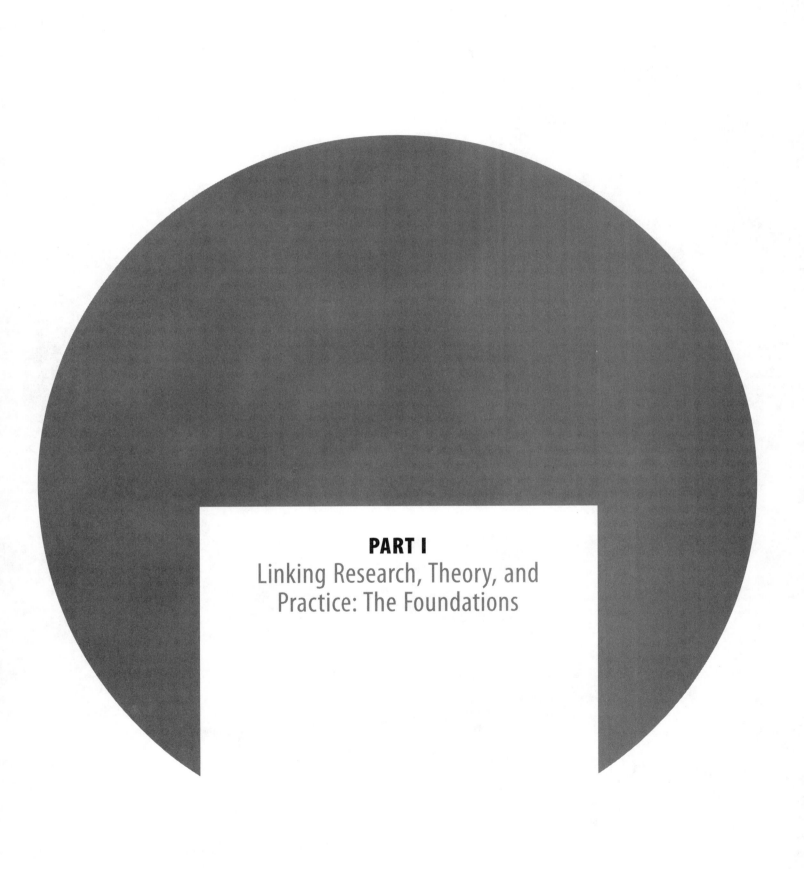

PART I
Linking Research, Theory, and
Practice: The Foundations

Issues in Nutrition Education: An Introduction

OVERVIEW This chapter introduces the reader to the field of nutrition education, its history and its aims. It provides the definition of nutrition education that is used throughout this book as well as an overview of the book.

CHAPTER OUTLINE
- Introduction
- Why is nutrition education needed?
- The challenge of educating people about eating well
- What is nutrition education?
- Is nutrition education effective?
- What do nutrition educators do?
- Nutrition education, public health nutrition, and health promotion
- The purpose of this book

LEARNING OBJECTIVES At the end of the chapter, you will be able to:
- State why nutrition education is both important and difficult to do
- Describe whether nutrition education is effective
- Evaluate differing points of view about the purposes and scope of nutrition education
- Define nutrition education
- Describe what nutrition educators do

■ INTRODUCTION

This is an exciting time for the field of nutrition education. Everyone seems to be interested in food and nutrition. Most newspapers have weekly sections on food. Restaurant guides have proliferated, and chefs are now celebrities. Cooking shows are popular on television, and in some areas entire television channels are devoted to food. The cookbook and food sections of bookstores have grown, and diet books abound. Nutrition and health issues are discussed on the nightly news and the Internet has exploded with information. Annual surveys of supermarket shoppers show that nutrition is increasingly important as a factor in people's shopping decisions (Food Marketing Institute 2004).

Food companies and food service providers, recognizing that *nutrition* is a buzzword that sells products, also are getting in on the act. They have created fat-free baked goods, low-fat yogurt, and a host of other products to satisfy one set of enthusiasms as well as low-carbohydrate products in response to another set of enthusiasms. Reduced-sodium products sit side by side with their original, higher-salt versions. The fruit and vegetables sections of many supermarkets have doubled and tripled in size. Farmers' markets and farm stands are mushrooming, and buying "local" or "organic" has gone mainstream, with even large supermarkets identifying such items for consumers. Although "sustainable food systems" is not yet a household phrase, more people understand what that means, and CSAs (community-supported agriculture) no longer seem esoteric. Many communities are requiring fast food chains to provide calorie information on their boards.

Food also is an important topic of conversation. As you have probably experienced, mentioning that you are in the field of nutrition means that people immediately have questions for you. In addition, food is not just a necessity but also one of life's great pleasures. Almost 200 years ago, Brillat-Savarin pointed out in a book on the physiology of taste that "the pleasure of eating . . . occurs necessarily at least once a day, and may be repeated without inconvenience two or three times in this space of time; . . . it can be combined with all our other pleasures, and even console us for their absence" (Brillat-Savarin 1825).

■ WHY IS NUTRITION EDUCATION NEEDED?

It would appear, then, that eating well should be getting easier for everyone. If the news media are providing information, and healthful foods abound in food supermarkets, why is nutrition education needed? But first, a clarification about the term *nutrition education*.

Nutrition is the word used to talk about the way in which food nourishes people. Good nutrition is essential for growth and development in children, and for health and well-being in people of all ages, and the relationship between nutrition and health involves many dietary components. Nutrition education is thus education about nutrition. However, people eat foods, not nutrients. Education about food is sometimes referred to as *food education*. Generally, and in this book, the term *nutri-*

tion education includes education about foods as well as about nutrition. Many nutrition education programs address physical activity as well.

Our Health Needs Improvement

Current eating patterns are associated with 4 of the 10 leading causes of death in developed countries such as the United States: coronary heart disease, some types of cancer, stroke, and type 2 diabetes (Ogden 1999; National Center for Health Statistics 2003). Dietary factors are also associated with osteoporosis, a major underlying cause of bone fractures in older persons (Frazao 1999). Obesity is on the rise, carrying with it an increased risk of various chronic diseases (Ogden et al. 2006; Hill et al. 2003; Hedley et al. 2004). (See **Figure 1-1**.) The rate of obesity has jumped in every state. In 1990, obesity rates in most states were below 14%; now most states have an obesity rate of 20% or more. Indeed, it has been estimated that diet and other social and behavioral factors such as smoking, sedentary lifestyles, alcohol use, and accidents account for about half of all the causes of death in the United States (Institutes of Medicine 2000).

The fact that many chronic diseases are to some extent the result of individual and social patterns of behavior (Food and Nutrition Board 1989; Institutes of Medicine 2000; U.S. Department of Health and Human Services 1988, 2000) means that positive changes in individual dietary behaviors, community conditions of living, social structures, and food- and physical activity–related policies may lead to reduction in risk of disease. Prevention becomes a possibility. In addition, people

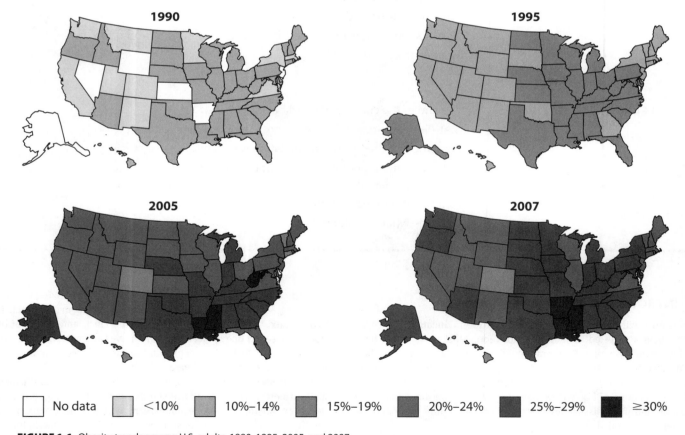

| | No data | | <10% | | 10%–14% | | 15%–19% | | 20%–24% | | 25%–29% | | ≥30% |

FIGURE 1-1 Obesity trends among U.S. adults, 1990, 1995, 2005, and 2007.

Source: Centers for Disease Control and Prevention. Behavioral Risk Factor Surveillance Systems (BRFSS). http://www.cdc.gov/bfrss.

are becoming increasingly interested not just in preventing disease but also in enhancing their health. Better health provides people a better quality of life and enhanced functioning so that they are able to do the many things in life they value. By exercising control over modifiable behavioral and socioenvironmental factors that affect health, people can live more healthfully as well as longer. Consequently, recommendations have been made for implementing national strategies to improve health and reduce disease risk (U.S. Department of Health and Human Services 2000; Institutes of Medicine 2000).

Dietary and Physical Activity Patterns Are Not Optimal

Despite the abundance of food and food products, dietary intakes for many are not optimal. Survey trends show that the average per person intakes of various foods and food products in the United States over the years have improved in some categories but are not as healthful as they could be in others. For example, Americans today consume a little less fresh fruit than 100 years ago and a lot more processed fruit, particularly orange juice; vegetable consumption has increased in the past 25 years, but it is about the same as it was 100 years ago when home-produced vegetables were the major source. Moreover, about 50% of vegetable consumption is white potatoes, much of which is in the form of french fries or potato chips. Average milk intakes have declined in the past 50 years and intakes of soda have increased over the same period, from 10 gallons per person per year to about 55 gallons. Meat consumption is high, as is the quantity of total added fats and sugars. Finally, survey data show that about 74% of American adults have eating patterns that "need improvement" and another 16% have diets that are "poor" as measured by the Healthy Eating Index (Bastiosis et al. 2004). Young children start out well, with one third having "good" diets, but by age 9, only 12% have good diets, nearly the same as for adults (Center for Nutrition Policy and Promotion 2001).

These eating patterns can be compared to the U.S. government's dietary guidance graphic, MyPyramid, which depicts a healthful eating pattern based on scientific evidence. This graphic, shown in **Figure 1-2**, indicates the amount that people should eat, on average, from each of several basic food groups. The width of each group in the graphic rep-resents how much individuals should eat from each group: more from grains and vegetables, for example, than from milk or meat. The food groups are presented in the shape of a pyramid to convey the concept that *within* each group, individuals should eat *more* lower-fat or higher-fiber foods in that group, which are shown in the bottom of the figure, and *fewer* highly processed, higher-fat, or lower-fiber foods within that group, which are in the tip of the pyramid and are not shown.

National data show that Americans are not eating in the way recommended by this pyramid (Bastiosis et al. 2004; Cook & Friday 2004). These data are shown in **Table 1-1**. Indeed, only about 1 of 10 Americans meets all the recommended intakes from all the basic food groups. **Figure 1-3** shows that American eating patterns are like an inverted pyramid: narrower at the base and broader at the top. People are eating more from the highly processed, higher-fat, or lower-fiber foods within each group than from the lower-fat, higher-fiber foods within each group. At the same time, Americans as a nation eat on average 43% of their daily calories from the "other foods" category.

Physical activity patterns are likewise far from optimal. Regular physical activity reduces the risk of many health conditions and promotes health. The percentage of Americans who are meeting physical activity guidelines has increased somewhat in the past few years, but in 2005, fewer than half of the adult U.S. population engaged in recommended levels of physical activity, based on self-reports (Centers for Disease Control and Prevention 2008).

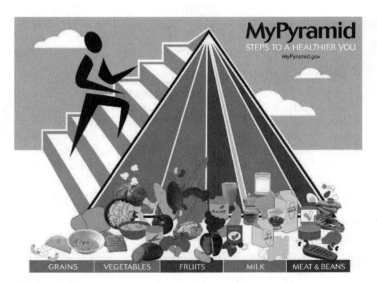

FIGURE 1-2 MyPyramid.
Source: U.S. Department of Agriculture. http://www.MyPyramid.gov.

TABLE 1-1   We Are Not Watching What We Eat

Americans are doing fairly well at watching cholesterol intake. But we are not eating nearly enough fruit and vegetables, and only about 40% of us are taking it easy on the fat and about one third on the salt.

	Daily Recommended Amounts	Percentages of People Meeting Daily Recommendations
Grains	6–11 servings	51% (34% for calories)
Vegetables	3–5 servings	42% (34% for calories)
Fruits	2–4 servings	30% (24% for calories)
Milk	2–3 servings	33% (26% for age)
Meat	2–3 servings	44% (38% for calories)
Total fat	30% of calories	38%
Saturated fat	Less than 10% of calories	41%
Cholesterol	300 milligrams or less	69%
Sodium	2,400 milligrams or less	32%
Variety	Eight or more different items in a day	55%

Sources: Cook, A.J., and J.E. Friday. 2004. *Pyramid servings intakes in the United States 1999–2002, 1 day* (CNRG Table Set 3.0). Beltsville, MD: U.S. Department of Agriculture, Agricultural Research Service, Community Nutrition Research Group. http://www.ba.ars.usda.gov/cnrg; and Basiotis, P.P., A. Carlson, S.A. Gerrior, W.Y. Juan, and M. Lino. 2004. The Healthy Eating Index 1999–2000: Charting dietary patterns of Americans. *Family Economics and Nutrition Review* 16(1):39–48.

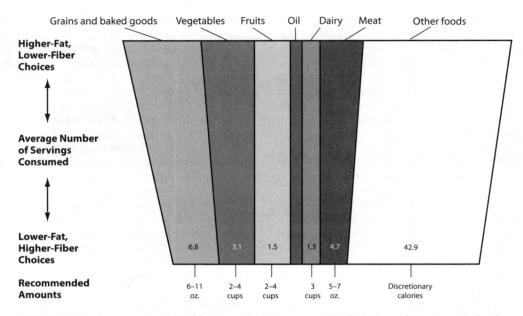

FIGURE 1-3 Food consumption pyramid: Average servings consumed by the U.S. population compared with MyPyramid recommendations.

Source: Community Nutrition Research Group, Agriculture Research Service. 2000, October. *Pyramid servings intakes by U.S. children and adults 1994–1996, 1998.* Beltsville, MD: U.S. Department of Agriculture.

Complex Food Choice Environment

Another reason why people need help making dietary choices is that the food environment has become increasingly complex. People in previous centuries lived on several hundred different foods, mostly locally grown. In 1928, large supermarkets in the United States stocked about 900 items. By the 1980s, a typical supermarket stocked approximately 12,000 food items, taken from an available supply of 60,000 items (Moliter 1980). Even more dramatic increases have occurred during the past two decades as a growing food industry converts basic foods into an ever-expanding array of food products through increasingly complex technologies. Some 50,000 different brand-name processed food items now perch on many supermarket shelves, from an available supply of 320,000 in the marketplace (Gallo 1998; Lipton, Edmondson, & Manchester 1998). In addition, the food preparation that was once done by a family member is now frequently in the hands of a stranger because 40% of all foods consumed are eaten away from home. Even food that is eaten in the home often has been prepared, purchased, and brought in from elsewhere.

Consumers must make choices among these options. The criteria for food choice also have expanded. Many consumers make choices on the basis of environmental concerns as well as health. For example, most food items come highly packaged, and many have traveled long distances. Many consumers and professionals note that the way food is grown, processed, packaged, distributed, and consumed has serious consequences for the sustainability of our food systems, and believe that it is important to consider these consequences in making food choices (Gussow & Clancy 1986; Clancy 1999; Gussow 1999, 2006). Others are interested in social justice concerns and want to choose foods that were produced using fair labor practices. For all these reasons, individual and community food choices have become very complex.

Complex Information Environment

The complexity of the foods available in the marketplace makes wise selection even harder. Our ancestors readily knew the foods they were eating just by looking at them, or could learn about them from family or cultural traditions. Most of the 50,000 items in today's supermarket bear little resemblance to the simple foodstuffs previously eaten by humans. Foods with artificial sweeteners in them are being joined by foods made with artificial fats. Some 10,000 "new" food-related items are being introduced by food processors in the United States every year (or about 30 a day). Knowledge about these items cannot possibly be derived from simply looking at them, and neither can their composition and effects on the body be learned by stories and attitudes passed down through the generations. People must learn about foods through other means.

The increasing complexity of this food environment demands consumers who are nutritionally literate. Yet nutritional literacy does not come easily. For packaged foods, nutritional labels are very important. Although 80% of consumers report that they attempt to read food labels, most admit that they don't always understand what they mean (Levy et al. 2000). Some labels on products are actually misleading—lean frozen dinners labeled as "95% fat free" can contain 30% of calories as fat, and 2% "low-fat" milk also has 30% of its calories as fat. Nutrition educators ask people to "eat no more than 30% to 35% of calories from fat," yet it is almost impossible for consumers to know what that means in terms of food. Moreover, diet books highlight low-fat diets as the ideal one year and low-carbohydrate diets the next year.

Consumer Bewilderment and Concern

No wonder, then, that consumers are bewildered. Although many Americans are concerned about their health and are indeed eating more healthful foods than they were a decade or so ago, the average person's diet is getting better and worse at the same time. For instance, mothers may buy skim milk for their families along with high-fat premium "home-style" ice cream, the latter because of its perceived superior quality.

These contradictory behaviors often derive from genuine confusion about what is good to eat. Although food manufacturers have responded to consumer concern about healthful food, they have introduced at least as many less healthful items as they have more healthful ones. There is considerable confusion in developing countries as well: many people exchange locally grown whole foods for imported, processed items, believing the latter to be better for health. Well-off people in such countries are thus developing the same chronic diseases as are the people in more affluent countries and are experiencing increased obesity rates at the same time that those who are poor are suffering from malnutrition (Monteiro, Conde, & Popkin 2004).

All these facts suggest that people need education about food and nutrition.

■ THE CHALLENGE OF EDUCATING PEOPLE ABOUT EATING WELL: WHY IS THIS BOOK NEEDED?

Our analysis so far would suggest that what consumers need is information on food composition, label reading skills, and skills in preparing foods in a healthy fashion. However, if practical information of this sort is all people need to eat more healthfully, then a book such as this one would not be needed. If nutrition education were simply *telling* people a variety of needed information, then what would be needed is a book devoted to describing interesting ways to translate the findings of nutrition science for different audiences.

However, research provides evidence that even if everyone became more knowledgeable about food and nutrition, and food companies produced more healthful food products, consumers would still need help making nutritious food choices. There is more to good nutrition than knowing which foods to eat and having those foods available. Information is not enough. The potent influences of biological factors, cultural and social preferences, and emotional and psychological factors make the job of assisting people to eat well demanding. Understanding these and addressing them are the major tasks of nutrition education.

Biological Influences: Is There Such a Thing as Body Wisdom?

Some have argued that people have an innate "body wisdom" that guides them to select healthful foods naturally, thus implying that nutrition education is not needed. Much of this line of thought grew out of the work of Clara Davis (1928), who studied the spontaneous food choices of infants. The infants, ages 6 to 11 months, were weaned by allowing them to self-select their entire diets from a total of 34 foods, without added salt or sugar, which were rotated—a few at a time—at each meal. Davis reported that after several months of such "spontaneous" food selection, the children's nutritional status and health were excellent. However, one should note that the 34 foods were all simply prepared, minimally processed, and nutritious whole foods, such as steamed vegetables, fruit juice, milk, meat, and oatmeal. There were no poisons, and nothing was allowed to influence the children's food choices except their own appetites: the food items were offered by caretakers who were trained to provide no encouragements or discouragements while the children ate. It comes as no surprise that the infants' health was superb. Whether infants would demonstrate a similar "instinct" if they

were offered tasty, energy-dense, low-nutrient food items has not been examined, but such an outcome seems unlikely given experiments in which rats exposed to such diets became obese. Neither do conditions of freedom from all outside influences exist in real-world settings.

Sensory-Specific Satiety

Although there is no evidence that any sort of innate body wisdom could function in an environment in which exposure to negative influences of all kinds seems almost inescapable, humans appear to have a built-in mechanism that helps ensure that they eat a variety of foods. Through the centuries, people obtained their needed nutrients mostly by getting enough calories. The key was in getting a varied diet. Yudkin (1978) argues that in the past, people could get what they *needed* simply by eating what they *wanted*. As people eat more of a particular food in the course of a short time period such as a meal, they come to like its taste less, but the desire for other foods offered remains relatively unchanged (Rolls 2000). You know this phenomenon: when you are so full as not to be able to eat another mouthful of the entrée, you find yourself quite able to eat dessert! Although the experience of hunger ensures that people will eat, their enjoyment of tasty foods combined with this *sensory-specific satiety* mechanism, as it is called, would have ensured—in a "primitive" environment—that they move from one food to another and thus select a balanced diet over the long term. Interestingly, a varied diet also appears to make people eat more, a fact that may have helped our ancestors but that, in a food-rich environment, may now work against us.

Our Bodies and Today's Food

Technology has made it possible to manipulate foods' sensory properties to make them sweeter or saltier or richer tasting or more colorful at will (Gussow & Contento 1984). Thus, technology has fully separated the tastiness of foods from their nutritional worth. In addition, current technology creates notorious hazards for energy perception. The fat content of many processed foods is not clearly evident from either the appearance of the food, its feel and taste, or from the packaging and shape of the item. The energy content of a variety of similar-tasting foods can vary considerably. And the array of such processed food products, made tasty by the addition of fat, sugar, and salt, is vast. This means that by following their food preferences—eating a variety of tasty foods—people are no longer assured that they will get a nutritionally adequate diet. Indeed, such behavior increases the likelihood of overconsumption of high-fat, low-fiber diets that may place people at greater risk for a number of chronic diseases. There appears to be no set point for the amount of fat or sugar people will eat. Taken together, people's desire to eat foods that are tasty and marketers' desire to put into the marketplace foods that cater to people's biological attraction to sugar, fat, and salt make the task of educating for a healthful diet a difficult one.

Cultural and Social Preferences
Cultural Context

Whatever biological predispositions humans possess operate in the context of food availability, and as Rozin (1982) notes, what is available to eat is determined not only by what is available geographically and economically but also by what a culture dictates is appropriate to eat. Although humans as a worldwide group eat just about everything edible, any particular group of people uses only a small proportion of the possible sources of nutrients around them. Consequently, Rozin says that "the best predictor of the food preferences, habits and attitudes of any particular human would be information about his/her ethnic group (and hence, native cuisine) rather than any biological measure one might imagine" (Rozin 1982).

Indeed, anthropologist Margaret Mead years ago argued that traditionally, in all known societies, it was not biological mechanisms but transmission of culturally imposed eating patterns that kept humans alive. Each such eating pattern was derived from the group's experience with foods, and this experience was transmitted through the culture. These traditional food patterns were not necessarily optimal but were nutritionally viable and enabled people to survive at least through the reproductive years (Gussow & Contento 1984). Biological preference and cultural influences are thus intertwined. What is made available by a culture comes to taste good: people may eat what they like, but they also come to like what they eat.

Social Preferences

Today, what is available to eat in the United States is determined largely by what is mass produced by food companies and available in the supermarket. These products are highly promoted by the communication instruments of mass culture (e.g., television, advertising), leading to consumer demand. Because so many of today's food products are neither biologically or culturally familiar, culturally transmitted traditional "craft skills" are most often no longer useful (Gussow & Contento 1984; Leiss 1976).

Studies show that taste and availability are closely followed by convenience in influencing food selection. Modern culture emphasizes convenience or quickness in preparing or obtaining foods, to fit in with today's hectic lifestyles. Many people today think of a food as available only if it can be purchased already prepared or can be prepared quickly without much effort. Away-from-home foods account for 32% of calories (up from 18% in the 1970s) and about half of total food expenditures (Stewart, Blisard, & Jolliffe 2006). Yet quick and convenient foods that are readily available commercially are not always the most healthful, and neither are they produced, transported, or packaged in the most environmentally sound manner. All these cultural and social influences can make educating about foods, nutrition, and dietary change difficult.

Family and Psychological Factors

People have many expectations about the food they eat: it should taste good, it should look good, it should impress friends when they serve it to them, it should be healthful, it should help them stay thin, and it should remind them of the warmth of family. They have many beliefs and attitudes relating to food in general and to specific foods in particular. The opinions of family or important others as well as moral and religious values also influence food choices.

Within the constraints of biology and culture, people as they grow up also develop individual food preferences and patterns of eating because any given individual amasses a unique set of experiences with respect to food (Rozin 1982). This uniqueness stems partly from the fact that an individual's exposure to the culture is filtered through the family's interpretation of culture. For example, there is evidence that one of the major influences on the acquisition of eating patterns by children is familiarity with given foods (Birch 1999). Such familiarity is determined by what the family serves, which in turn reflects the family's cultural and other beliefs about food.

Thus, eating patterns and dietary behaviors are influenced by many familial and psychological factors, as well as by cultural and social ones.

People learn very early that the foods they eat or don't eat will elicit reactions from parents, teachers, and friends ("If we push away our vegetables, Mommy may get cross at us"). During adolescence, peer pressure dominates what people choose to eat. Even as adults, few business lunches pass without a few mental nutritional notes ("Joe Davis was the only one who ordered red meat during lunch").

Eating is clearly deeply embedded in the early development of individuals and continues to be tied in with many other aspects of life. Consequently, any changes in eating behaviors may involve many other changes as well, such as family traditions, social and professional occasions that involve food, making time in busy schedules for eating well, or changing how one handles stress (for example, by exercising instead of eating). A person must be motivated to make changes and to maintain them.

Sense of Empowerment: Individual and Community

Even if a person is motivated, the sheer number of food products available makes decision making a daunting task for the consumer. It is also a daunting task for the nutrition educator because the consumer needs a great deal of complex information, yet in an information-overloaded society, the consumer wants or can handle only simple messages. So, the challenge to the nutrition educator is how to convert complex information into simple but accurate messages that consumers will attend to and act on.

At the same time, to understand some of the choices they have to make, people need to be able to analyze and evaluate complex information in the midst of conflicting claims. For example, are calories the most important item on a food label? Is a breakfast cereal that is high in sugar but low in fat a better choice for children? Which food preservation methods are safe? Does it make a difference whether one chooses organically produced foods or foods produced by more conventional agriculture? And what are the differences based on—impact of food on personal health, or impact of food production methods on the long-term sustainability of the food system? What about genetically engineered foods—should they be labeled? Thus, eaters need critical thinking skills. In addition, they need affective skills such as assertiveness, self-management, and negotiation skills that enhance their sense of competence and control over their own food choices. People also need skills in preparing healthful foods quickly and conveniently. Finally, for community as well as personal empowerment, people need to have the skills and opportunity to identify food- and nutrition-related issues facing their communities and work with others to address these issues appropriately.

Material Resources and the Environmental Context

Cost of Food

No amount of motivation and skills, however, will put healthful food on the table if material resources are inadequate for people to purchase (or grow) and prepare the food. Material resources include not only money but also time, labor, and fuel. Affordability of healthful food, as well as food availability, is crucial, particularly for low-income audiences. Having in one's neighborhood only convenience stores that charge high prices and carry limited supplies of healthful foods makes eating well extremely difficult. Whole-grain products and fruits and vegetables are not as available in fast food outlets, workplace cafeterias, or other places convenient to people's out-of-home activities as are more highly processed food items, and the whole food items often cost more (Drewnowski, Darmon, & Briend 2004).

Marketing, Social Structures, and Policy

Neither can the best of intentions be implemented and behaviors maintained if social structures, food marketing practices, food policies, and other aspects of the food (and activity) environment are not conducive to health. Fast foods that tend to be higher in fat, sugar, and salt are everywhere—convenient, tasty, and inexpensive—and their portion sizes are often large. Surveys have found that almost 60% of Americans eat away from home on any given day and are thus exposed to such foods (Agricultural Research Service U.S. Department of Agriculture 2000).

In addition, the dietary pattern emphasized by marketers, shown in **Figure 1-4**, is very different from the dietary pattern recommended by the MyPyramid (refer to Figure 1-2) as likely to enhance nutritional health—one high in whole grains, fruits, and vegetables; adequate in dairy and meat; and sparing in foods that are high in fat and sugar. More marketing and advertising dollars are spent promoting food products in the "other foods/discretionary calories" category than are spent on foods in the basic food groups, as we have seen, resulting in increased consumption and demand. Finally, people of all ages, particularly children, have become more sedentary in the last 30 years. People use more labor-saving devices and cars, and spend more time watching TV and using computers. People have hectic jobs and work long hours, leaving less time for physical activity. Thus, people cannot eat as many calories as they once could to meet their other nutrient needs. The issues that demand attention from nutrition educators, then, are not only individual food-related behaviors and personal choice but also external environmental factors such as material resources, social structures, food policies, and marketing practices.

■ WHAT IS NUTRITION EDUCATION?

So far, we have seen that nutrition education is both necessary and challenging to do. What exactly is nutrition education, and what should it

seek to accomplish? But first, a brief history of dietary guidance through nutrition education.

Dietary Guidance History in Brief

Food Guides

Although families and cultures have been educating about food since the dawn of human history, the formal field of nutrition education can be considered to have had its start when governments began publishing dietary guidance recommendations for the public based on the findings of nutrition science and taking into account cultural eating patterns. In the United States, the first food guide was published by the U.S. Department of Agriculture in 1917 as a teaching tool with the goal of improving the health of the nation's people. A basic understanding of the need for carbohydrates, proteins, and fats had emerged in the late 1800s. The need for other "protective substances" for human health became apparent with the discovery and characterization of the first vitamins in the early 1900s. The importance of minerals in food for human health also became known—for example, the importance of milk as a source of calcium for bone health. With continuing research and identification of vitamins and minerals needed for good health, sufficient information had emerged by 1917 to provide guidance to the public. In this first food guide, foods were placed into groups based on their nutrient composition, and people were provided with recommendations as to how many foods to eat from each group to be healthy. The concern was for nutritional adequacy—that is, the purpose of the food guides was to ensure that people ate the right foods in sufficient amounts to provide all the nutrients that they needed for growth and health. The early guides were directed at entire families, as shown in **Figure 1-5**. Later food guides were directed at individuals.

The number of groups, as well as which foods were categorized into which groups, has changed from time to time over the past century in these teaching tools, based on the findings of nutrition science, cultural

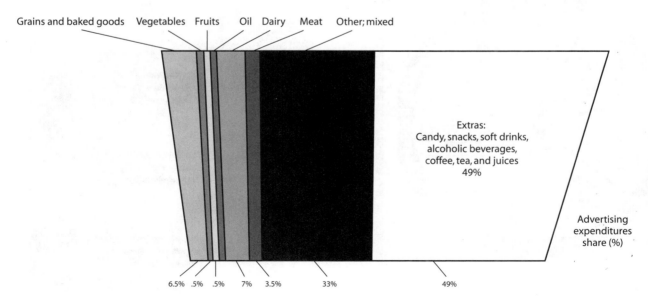

FIGURE 1-4 Food marketing pyramid: Advertising expenditures by food manufacturers.

Source: Gallo, A. 1999. Food advertising in the United States. In *America's eating habits: Changes and consequences* (Agricultural Information Bulletin No. 750), edited by E. Frazão. Washington, DC: U.S. Department of Agriculture.

FIGURE 1-5 Family-oriented food guidelines, 1921.

Source: U.S. Department of Agriculture. http://www.nal.usda.gov/fnic/history/early.htm.

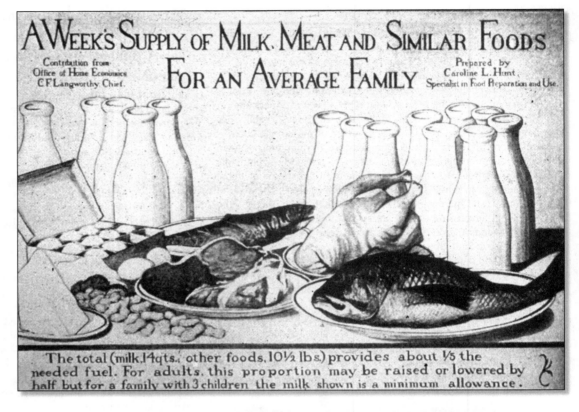

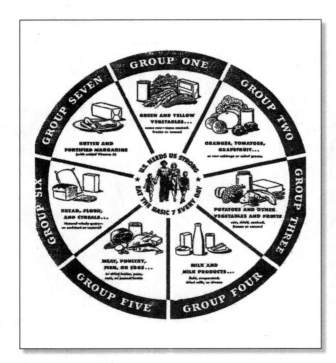

FIGURE 1-6 Food guide, 1944: The basic seven food groups.

Source: U.S. Department of Agriculture. http://www.nal.usda.gov/fnic/history/basic7.htm.

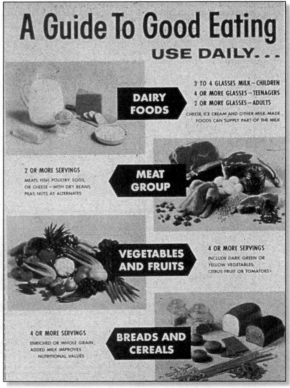

FIGURE 1-7 Food guide, 1950s: The basic four.

Source: U.S. Department of Agriculture. http://www.nal.usda.gov/fnic/history/basic4.htm.

food patterns, the interests of food producers, and other factors. Different graphics have been used over the decades to communicate this dietary guidance and make the message understandable and useful to consumers. **Figure 1-6** shows a graphic used in the 1930s in which recommended foods were placed into seven food groups, and **Figure 1-7** shows what was commonly called "the Basic Four," in use in the 1950s and 1960s.

Dietary and Physical Activity Guidelines

By the early 1970s, there was increasing recognition that the major dietary concerns for a majority of Americans were no longer related to nutrient-deficiency diseases but to the risk of chronic diseases such as heart disease, diabetes, cancer, and overweight. Consequently, the nature of the dietary advice changed. As nutrition researcher Hegsted (1979) noted at the time, "In the past, the message was, in essence, to eat more of everything. Now we are faced with the more difficult problem of teaching the public to be more discriminating. Increasingly, the message will be to eat less." After considerable discussion and debate among health professionals, the U.S. Congress, federal government agencies, and the food industry, a set of dietary guidelines, called the *Dietary Guidelines for Americans*, was adopted in 1980. The dietary guidelines were published jointly by the U.S. Department of Agriculture (USDA) and the Department of Health and Human Services (DHHS). They were designed to assist the public in making food choices that would provide for sufficient amounts of all the essential nutrients as well as reduce the risk of chronic disease and maintain a healthy weight, although they did not specifically recommend that people eat less. These guidelines are revised every 5 years to ensure that they incorporate the latest nutrition science research findings and food policy considerations (see http://www.health.gov/dietaryguidelines). DHHS also has developed physical activity guidelines that provide "science-based guidance to help Americans aged 6 and older to improve their health through appropriate physical activity" (see http://www.health.gov/paguidelines).

Recent Graphics

The graphic for the food guide as an educational tool itself was changed dramatically to account for this new advice. After careful work on the part of nutritionists working in government, considerable debate by nutrition professionals, lobbying by the food industry, and extensive consumer research, the graphic in the United States was changed from a series of equal-sized boxes representing each of the food groups, as in the Basic Four, to a pyramid shape and was called the Food Guide Pyramid (**Figure 1-8**). The pyramid shape was intended to better convey to the public the fact that the number of servings from each of the food groups differs according to group; that is, it emphasized the notion of proportionality. For example, the largest number of daily servings should come from the grain group (the bottom of the pyramid). The next largest number of daily servings should come from the fruits and vegetables groups, followed by the dairy and meat groups. The quantities shown for each of the pyramid groups were the basics recommended for good health. Foods high in sugar and fat were placed in the tip of the pyramid and were to be eaten sparingly.

The Food Guide Pyramid was modified in 2005 and is now called MyPyramid (refer to Figure 1-2). MyPyramid is a graphic that is linked to information on the Web (http://www.MyPyramid.gov), where people

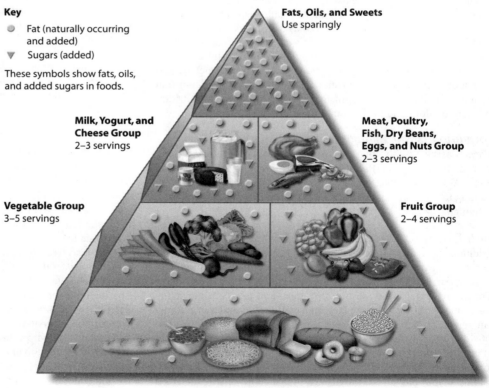

FIGURE 1-8 Food guide pyramid, 1980s.
Source: U.S. Department of Agriculture. 1992, August. (Revised 1996, October.) *The Food Guide Pyramid*. Home and Garden Bulletin (No. 252).

Key

Fat (naturally occurring and added)

▼ Sugars (added)

These symbols show fats, oils, and added sugars in foods.

Fats, Oils, and Sweets
Use sparingly

Milk, Yogurt, and Cheese Group
2–3 servings

Meat, Poultry, Fish, Dry Beans, Eggs, and Nuts Group
2–3 servings

Vegetable Group
3–5 servings

Fruit Group
2–4 servings

Bread, Cereal, Rice, and Pasta Group
6–11 servings

can download the graphic as well as information on how to personalize the recommendations for their own needs. Because of the recognition of the importance of physical activity for health, the graphic also shows a person being physically active. The information also is linked to the *Dietary Guidelines* document, which provides the basis of the pyramid recommendations. Foods higher in fiber and lower in fat and sugar within each food group should be eaten more often. Foods high in fats and sugars that were predominant in an "others" group that was at the tip of the Food Guide Pyramid and labeled "eat sparingly" are no longer shown in the MyPyramid graphic. Instead, people who have "discretionary calories" (between 100 and 300 calories for most people) can spend them on "other foods" or additional foods from the "basic five" food groups. However, as noted before, in actuality foods from this "discretionary calories" group contribute substantially to individuals' intakes (refer to Figure 1-3) and account for about half the advertising expenditures by food companies for food items (refer to Figure 1-4).

Different Views of Nutrition Education

What, then, is nutrition education? There are many definitions of nutrition education, based on different views about its purpose. These differing views are explored in this section. After that, we will arrive at a definition to be used in this book.

The Information Dissemination Approach

The information dissemination approach sees nutrition education as limited to the dissemination of nutrition science–based information only to various audiences using methods from the fields of education and communication. In this approach, the goal of nutrition education is simply—and only—to provide consumers with the information about food and nutrients needed to make decisions about what to eat, rejecting the notion that nutrition professionals should also *actively promote* healthful choices. Consumers are viewed as being savvy and not liking to be told what to do. Effectiveness in this approach can be gauged by the extent to which consumers know the needed information.

Although freedom of choice is a major value in this society, and information about foods and nutrition is a central element of nutrition education, there are criticisms of this approach that limits nutrition education to information dissemination only.

Information Is Not Enough

Surveys consistently show that most Americans believe that they are well informed about nutrition (Balzer 1997; IFIC Foundation 1999; American Dietetic Association 2002). The finding that they are also not eating according to recommendations argues that information alone is clearly not enough.

Can Information Dissemination Be Neutral?

In addition, given the nature, volume, and complexity of the information necessary for true informed choice, an approach limited to information dissemination is not really possible in practice (Contento 1980; Gussow & Contento 1984). That is, all nutrition education programs inevitably have to make choices about what information and skills to address in any given situation. For example, no usable food product label can carry information on all 60 or so nutrients essential for good health. Just leaving out data on some nutrients and including others biases the information. Neither can a single educational session or even a several-session program provide all the needed information for true informed choice on all food and nutritional matters. In making a choice of which issues to emphasize and what content to cover, the nutrition educator

must make a judgment because there is not enough time to give "all the facts" about everything. Even in group settings involving open-ended discussion and mutual dialogue, only certain issues can be explored at any given time. Choices regarding program content always have to be made. Thus, it is impossible for nutrition education to be value free even if it wanted to be.

Finally, some critics point out that nutrition education should not be value free even if it could be. For example, nutritionist Jean Mayer (1986) notes that "Nutritionists, unlike biochemists and physiologists, but like cardiologists and pediatricians, have to see their science as one whose goal is to benefit people."

Facilitating Behaviors Conducive to Health and Well-Being

A second approach to nutrition education is based on the premise that given that a major goal of nutrition education is to improve the health of the nation's people and that people's health conditions are to some extent the result of individual and social patterns of behavior, it is appropriate for nutrition education to facilitate the adoption or maintenance of individual behaviors and community practices that are conducive to long-term health. As noted earlier, consumers believe they are well informed. In addition, research evidence suggests that knowledge may be a necessary, but not a sufficient, condition for reaching the goal of improved health. Food behaviors and eating practices are influenced by many powerful psychosocial and other factors in addition to knowledge.

In this view, then, nutrition education involves much more than simply imparting food and nutrition information in the most attractive and effective way. Nutrition education facilitates behaviors that are conducive to health by focusing on the personal motivations and competence, interpersonal interactions, and environmental factors that influence individual and community patterns of behavior. In this approach, nutrition education is seen as a "form of planned change that involves the deliberate effort to improve nutritional well-being by providing information or other types of educational/behavioral interventions" (Sims 1987). The term *educational intervention* often is used, and in this approach the role of the nutrition educator moves from that of an "information dispatcher" to a "facilitator of change" of individuals and communities.

A specific example can illustrate this point. A nutrition educator was interested in increasing the rate of breastfeeding, as recommended by health professionals, among a group of low-income women in a food assistance program. She had planned to discuss the nutritional benefits of breastfeeding and teach the women how to do it successfully. However, when she went to talk with the women ahead of the scheduled time, she found that the women knew all about breastfeeding and its numerous benefits, and many had attempted it before, but that they were embarrassed to do it. That is, they had the knowledge, but the difficulty lay in the emotional and cultural barriers to breastfeeding. So, she changed her session to discuss the barriers to breastfeeding, including embarrassment, and potential ways to overcome these barriers to facilitate the adoption of this behavior rather than focusing on nutrition content alone.

Programs based on this approach use evidence-based strategies to facilitate the adoption of healthful individual behaviors and community practices. Such an approach has been the focus of many research studies and community projects in the food and nutrition education arena in the past two decades. Evaluation in this approach is measured by improvements in the food and nutrition behaviors (and physical activity patterns where appropriate) and health outcomes of individuals and communities.

Is Facilitating Behavior Change the Answer?

However, the approach of focusing on facilitating behavior change has also been criticized. It is based on the assumption that individuals have a great deal of influence over their personal decisions and actions and that changes in these personal behaviors can significantly change health outcomes. However, precisely because the individual behavior change approach helps people to acquire the motivation and competence to take increased control over their own food choices and health, people are held personally accountable for the state of their health. It can be a quick step from this personal responsibility approach to blaming the victim when individuals become ill (Allegrante & Green 1981; Green & Kreuter 2004). That is, this approach can result in "person blame" rather than "system blame." It becomes easy to ignore the fact that there are genetic factors affecting health, as well as powerful institutional and social conditions that shape and reinforce behavior. Furthermore, in this approach the behavior or practices to be addressed often are identified as needs or problems not by the groups or communities themselves but by governmental or professional groups familiar with scientific evidence. Thus, it can be paternalistic and not responsive to the specific needs or desires of communities.

To overcome these criticisms, an active, participatory approach to change can be used in which people are actively involved in all stages of nutrition education and participants identify issues of interest to them, which may not always involve dietary or physical activity changes but rather a variety of other issues, such as food accessibility, family cohesiveness, or other values in life (Kent 1988; Rody 1988; Arnold et al. 2001; Buchanan 2004). Such an approach is likely to increase effectiveness in the long run. In this approach, building capacity to take action, self-reliance, and empowerment are the focus, with dietary behavior changes self-selected.

A Focus on Environmental Change

A focus on environmental change is the third approach to nutrition education. It has become increasingly clear that environmental factors are a major influence on food choices and nutrition-related practices. Indeed, behavior and environment have a reciprocal relationship with each other (Bandura 1986). Dietary change is more likely when the physical environmental and social structures are health promoting so that personal decisions and motivations are supported and reinforced—that is, when healthful foods are available and accessible in the workplace, in schools, and in communities. Consequently, many nutrition education interventions now also address the environmental context, for example, by working in collaboration with decision makers to increase the healthy options offered in school meal programs and in workplace cafeterias, or to increase the availability of neighborhood farmers' markets and parks. The environmental component can include changes in the social environment, such as providing social support for healthful eating or in the policy and systems arena such as labeling the calorie content of foods served in restaurants or in schools.

Some health professionals have gone so far as to argue that many of our behaviors are caused in part by economic, organizational, and political factors in society that actually *encourage* at-risk behaviors (McKinley 1974).

Upstream Versus Downstream Activities

A story, attributed to sociologist Irving Zola, tells of a physician trying to explain the dilemmas of the modern practice of medicine:

"You know," he said, "sometimes it feels like this. There I am standing by the shore of a swiftly flowing river and I hear the cry of a drowning man. So I jump into the river, put my arms around him, pull him to shore and apply artificial respiration. Just when he begins to breathe, there is another cry for help. So I jump into the river, reach him, pull him to shore, apply artificial respiration, and just as he begins to breathe, another cry for help. So back in the river again, reaching, pulling; applying artificial respiration and then another yell. Again and again without end goes the sequence. You know, I am so busy jumping in, pulling them to shore, applying artificial respiration, that I have no time to see who the hell is upstream pushing all of them in."

Some thus contend that health professionals devote too many resources and attention to "downstream activities" that are short term and ultimately futile (McKinley 1974). Health practitioners should instead be devoting more attention "upstream" to the "manufacturers of illness," whose activities "foster and habituate certain at-risk behaviors."

These considerations have led to some debate in the health promotion field about the relative importance of facilitating individual behavior change versus broader institutional and social approaches to health, behavioral versus environmental strategies, and blaming the victim versus blaming the manufacturers of illness (Green & Kreuter 2004). Ultimately, all agree that attention to both individual and environmental factors is important.

In the health promotion field, *health education* has been described as any combination of learning experiences designed to facilitate voluntary actions conducive to health. *Health promotion* takes into consideration the environment as well and is thus defined as the combination of educational and ecological supports for actions and conditions of living conducive to health (Green & Kreuter 2004). In practice, there is obviously a continuum between health education and health promotion and the terms are often used interchangeably.

What Can We Conclude About Nutrition Education?

Information Environment

Some would see nutrition education as about knowledge and skills for informed decision making, not facilitation of behavior change. Clearly, enhancement of knowledge and decision-making skills for informed choice is vital in nutrition education. The public needs accurate science-based information on foods and on the relationships among food, nutrition, and health. Given that there are some 50,000 food items in the average U.S. supermarket, consumers also need to know how to select foods for optimal health from the vast array of available products. Indeed, they need to know more than just which nutrients are present in which of today's food products. The public also needs to know "how to be discriminating about dietary advice that comes, sought and unsought, from a variety of unequally reliable sources such as popular books, advertising, packaging labels, newspapers, and materials from food industry sources or 'health' food stores" (Contento 1980). There may also be concerns about where food comes from.

Food Choice, Free Choice?

It is also clear that people make choices in light of their life situations and values. For example, for a mother of several children, eating together as a family may be more important than the quality of what they eat. Balancing these myriad food choice criteria requires considerable analytical and evaluative skills on the part of consumers as well as the ability to construct conceptual frameworks and develop "personal food policies." Therefore, nutrition education needs also to enhance people's critical thinking skills. Youth in particular need information and opportunities to practice skills.

At the same time, although nutrition professionals acknowledge that eating behavior—healthful or otherwise—is voluntarily chosen by people in light of their own life situations, they also recognize that implicit in the national goal to improve the health of the nation's people is the value-laden goal of enhancing the nutritional well-being of individuals and populations. This means that nutrition education also involves promoting health by helping people see the value of health for themselves, and facilitating people's self-chosen attempts to eat healthfully and live more actively. The U.S. government has at times embarked on national campaigns to improve the nation's health, for example, by encouraging people, through mass media campaigns, to check their serum cholesterols with the message "Know Your Number" and to eat more fruit and vegetables with the message "Five a Day for Better Health!" or, more recently, "Fruits and Veggies: More Matters."

Food Marketing Environment

Many nutrition professionals are concerned that using health-promoting activities or persuasive communications as part of nutrition education may be coercive. Yet, the food industry (food manufacturers, the food service sector, and retailers) spent $26 billion in 2000 on advertising and promotions, with about $15 billion in 2002 directed at children (McNeal 1992; Center for Science in the Public Interest 2003) and $150 million a year for candy bars, $580 million for soft drinks, and more than $1.5 billion for fast food (Leading Advertisers 2001; Elitzak 2001). People are exposed to 3 hours of food advertising every week, all year. In contrast, government health-related campaigns may amount to only a few million dollars a year (e.g., $4 million for the National Cancer Institute's 5 A Day program, $34 million for the CDC's Division of Nutrition and Physical Activity, $10 million for USDA's Team Nutrition), and people may never attend a nutrition education program or see a nutritionist during their entire lives. In addition, escalators and elevators are ubiquitous, and attractive, safe walking trails and walkable streets and parks are hard to find in all settings—urban, suburban, and rural. Such a situation cannot result in genuinely free, informed choice.

Thus, nutrition educators have an obligation to bring health concerns to the attention of individuals to guarantee fully free choices. Indeed, as Gillespie (1987) points out:

> Persuasive communication is consistent with our democratic educational values if the attempts to change attitudes or behavior explain the reasons why recommended behaviors are desirable and indicate the strength of scientific evidence supporting such recommendations. Participants should be involved in decisions to change their food behavior not only as an ingredient in program success but also to guard against manipulation.

Defining Nutrition Education

Taking into account these considerations and various definitions of nutrition education and health education, for the purposes of this book *nutrition education* is defined as any combination of educational strategies, accompanied by environmental supports, designed to facilitate voluntary adoption of food choices and other food- and nutrition-related behaviors conducive to health and well-being and delivered through multiple venues, involving activities at the individual, institutional, community,

and policy levels (Contento et al. 1995; Society for Nutrition Education 1995, 2009; American Dietetic Association 2003).

Combination of educational strategies. The phrase "combination of educational strategies" emphasizes that because many factors influence behavior, nutrition education needs to employ a variety of educational strategies and learning experiences that are appropriately directed at these multiple influences on, or determinants of, food choice and dietary behavior to facilitate dietary change. Nutrition education focuses on enhancing health and facilitating solutions.

Education is *not* synonymous with information dissemination, although the public and many in the nutrition science, biomedical, public health, and policy fields think it is. The word comes from the Latin *educare*, meaning to bring up or lead out, and can be seen as a process that not only provides knowledge, information, and skills but also fosters development, growth, and change. These educational strategies are at the heart of this book and are described in great detail in the remaining chapters. They are content-free processes that can be used to address the many issues that are of concern or of interest to the public, to professionals, or to the nation at large.

Designed means that nutrition education is a systematically planned set of activities. Such systematically planned nutrition education can occur through multiple venues, such as schools, communities, workplaces, and clinics, and through the mass media. A step-wise procedural model for systematically designing nutrition education is described later in this book. Such systematically planned nutrition education should be distinguished from incidental nutrition education that is carried out by other institutions in society such as families, businesses, newspapers, magazines, and radio and television stations. The latter type of education is labeled as *informal* nutrition education. Television food commercials, claims on food product packages, newspaper articles, and popular diet books are all examples of informal nutrition education.

Facilitate is used to emphasize the fact that educators can only *assist* people to make diet-related changes: people make changes when they see the need and want to do so. Motivations ultimately come from within individuals themselves, and actions with respect to food are voluntarily chosen in the light of individuals' values and larger life goals and situations. Education about foods and nutrition, and, where appropriate, physical activity, then, is about increasing awareness, promoting active contemplation, and enhancing people's motivations through self-understanding and deliberation. It is also about facilitating the ability to take action through acquisition of knowledge and skills related to food and nutrition and through self-regulation and self-directed behavior or sense of personal agency and empowerment. Finally, it is also about engaging in coalitions with others to promote supportive food and activity environments, systems, and policies where appropriate and possible.

Voluntary means recognizing and respecting that human beings have agency and free will and make choices in light of their own personal goals and values (Bandura 1997, 2001; Rothschild 1999; Deci & Ryan 2000, 2008; Buchanan 2004). It means the program is conducted without coercion and with the full understanding of the participants about the purpose of the nutrition education activities. Individuals are both "the changers" and "the changed." *Voluntary* does not mean that the only appropriate approach is one limited to information dissemination. Health psychologist Leventhal (1973) noted some years ago that "the decision to avoid coercion does not free one of the obligation to state facts, warn, and argue skillfully."

Indeed, it can be argued that truly informed choice can be made by consumers *only* when they have the benefit of understanding arguments from all sides. Without the benefit of health communications from nutrition educators, consumers would receive only the arguments of all the other forces in society, such as food advertising and promotion activities, that are providing messages urging people to choose foods for reasons other than nutrition and health. Thus, nutrition educators have an important role in bringing food and health concerns to the attention of individuals and to make a case for these concerns while at the same time respecting individuals' right to choose whether and how to take action. Making the case is not limited to verbal discussions of benefits. It can also involve providing food tastings that demonstrate that healthful foods taste good, organizing a tour to show that shopping at a farmers' market can be convenient, or organizing a company "fun run" to show that exercise can be enjoyable. In addition, it can build on assets that people bring to the issue, such as personal and cultural practices that are already health-promoting or community structures that are supportive. In other words, nutrition education strategies can be designed in such a way as to integrate the health-promoting role of nutrition educators with the notion of free will and personal agency and empowerment on the part of individuals.

Behaviors are the food choices and other food- and nutrition-related actions that people undertake to achieve an intended effect of their own choosing and are the direct focus of nutrition education. Eating fruits and vegetables, a lower-fat diet, or calcium-rich foods or breastfeeding can be referred to as behaviors. Sometimes behaviors are defined broadly, such as "healthy eating and active living." The term *actions* is most often used synonymously with *behaviors*, although the former term can also refer to specific actions or sub-behaviors that constitute *behaviors*. Thus, the behavior of eating more fruits and vegetables may involve the specific actions of shopping for fruits and vegetables, adding orange juice at breakfast, including a vegetable at lunch, and so forth. The word *practices* is also used interchangeably with *behaviors* and *actions*, although the term *practices* tends to refer to more general and continuing behaviors, such as food-related parenting practices, eating balanced meals, being physically active, or buying foods at farmers' markets.

Environmental supports refer to the food, physical, social structure, informational, and policy environments external to a person that are relevant to the behavior or practices at issue. Taking action and maintaining a behavioral change is much more likely if the relevant environment is supportive. Promoting supportive environments usually requires nutrition educators to educate a different audience—providers of food and services, key decision makers, and others with influence—and to work in coalition with them to achieve food and nutrition goals (and physical activity goals, where relevant). These individuals and organizations might include community leaders and organizations, food service personnel, school principals, workplace managers, and policy makers at local, state, and national levels, as well as the media, government agencies, and nongovernmental or private voluntary organizations.

Health and well-being refer to both the nutritional health of individuals and an overall sense of well-being; both absence of disease and possession of positive attributes of being healthy, such as optimal functioning or high-level wellness. For some nutrition educators, the concept of health and well-being extends to include the health and sustainability of the food systems on which people depend.

Multiple venues refer to the fact that systematically planned nutrition education can be delivered through multiple channels, such as group sessions and other in-person activities, newsletters, printed materials, and visuals in formal settings such as schools and colleges or in nonformal settings such as community centers, food banks, workplaces, supermarkets, food stamp offices, Women, Infants, and Children (WIC) clinics, or outpatient clinics, and through mass media, billboards, and social marketing approaches. Activities at the institutional, community, and policy levels can promote environments supportive of healthful food choices and diet- and physical activity–related behaviors.

Summary of Nutrition Education

In sum, people and their environment are closely interrelated. In some cases, people have the needed resources and the knowledge, skills, and confidence in their ability to effect change in themselves and in the environment, but they do not have a desire to do so. In other cases, people may be motivated to eat foods that will improve their own health or the health of their community or promote a sustainable food system, but they do not have the environmental supports to act on their motivation.

Motivation

Motivation is so important in diet-related behaviors that its role in nutrition education must be specifically recognized and addressed. Individuals are more likely to take action or change a practice if they understand the factors, environmental as well as personal, that have sustained or even encouraged their current way of living. They are also more likely to take action if they have had an opportunity to examine and talk about food and health issues in relation to their own larger life goals (Deci & Ryan 2000, 2008; Buchanan 2004). Change grows out of a person's understanding of "the problems behind the problems." It also grows out of people's interest in their own well-being, health related or otherwise.

Environment

Nutrition education can help people understand that diet is related to their health and can provide information on what foods to eat for health, but it can go further: it can assist people to consider their food choices in relation to more fundamental issues in their *near environments*, such as personal relationships, home and work situations, economic and time pressures on decision making, and community structures, the built environment, and other conditions of living. It can also help them understand the influences on their diet-related practices of elements of the *far environment*, such as grocery store or food industry practices, government policy, food and beverage advertising, the general economic climate, and agricultural and trade practices. It can help people understand that the way food is grown, marketed, and consumed has an impact on the food system and has social consequences as well as nutritional ones on individuals and communities. Finally, it can also assist people to take action on the environment through enhancing capacity, coalition building, empowerment, and collective action.

Theory to Guide Nutrition Education

Nutrition education needs theory to guide its work. Theory provides nutrition educators with a mental map derived from research evidence that helps them design strategies that are likely to be effective.

Vision of the Professional Associations

The view of nutrition education described here is in keeping with the vision of the foremost nutrition education professional organization, the Society of Nutrition Education (SNE), which states that its *vision* is to "promote healthy communities through nutrition education and advocacy" and its *mission* is to "promote effective nutrition education and communication to support and improve healthful behaviors" (Society for Nutrition Education 2009) (**Box 1-1**). It also is in keeping with the position statements of the American Dietetic Association (ADA), which is "committed to improving the nation's health and advancing the profession of dietetics through research, education and advocacy." ADA's *vision* is to "optimize the nation's health through food and nutrition," and its *mission* is to "empower members to be the nation's food and nutrition leaders" (American Dietetic Association 2009).

Box 1-1 Society for Nutrition Education: Mission and Identity Statements

Mission

The Society for Nutrition Education (SNE) promotes effective nutrition education and communication to support and improve healthful behaviors.

Identity Statement

SNE is an international organization of nutrition education professionals who are dedicated to promoting effective nutrition education and communication to support and improve healthful behaviors with a vision of healthy communities through nutrition education and advocacy. Our members conduct research in education, behavior, and communication; develop and disseminate innovative nutrition education strategies; and communicate information on food, nutrition, and health issues to students, professionals, policy makers, and the public. SNE members share ideas and resources through our journal, newsletter, annual conference, and the members-only listserv. Our Divisions offer networking opportunities for members with similar interests and expertise.

About

The Society for Nutrition Education (SNE) is composed of nutrition education professionals who are dedicated to promoting effective nutrition education and communication to support and improve healthful behaviors with a vision of healthy communities through nutrition education and advocacy. Our members conduct research in education, behavior, and communication; develop and disseminate innovative nutrition education strategies; and communicate information on food, nutrition, and health issues to students, professionals, policy makers, and the public. Publications describing this work can be found in the SNE peer-reviewed *Journal of Nutrition Education and Behavior*, the leading research periodical devoted to nutrition education and promotion.

Source: Courtesy of the Society for Nutrition Education.

■ IS NUTRITION EDUCATION EFFECTIVE?

A number of reviews have been conducted to examine the question of whether nutrition education is effective, based on the preceding view of nutrition education. One such review used the statistical method of meta-analysis to examine 303 studies conducted over a 70-year period from 1910 to 1984 that included a total of 4,108 separate findings (Johnson & Johnson 1985). The meta-analysis found that, overall, nutrition education increased knowledge by 33 percentiles, attitudes by 14 percentiles, and behaviors by 19 percentiles. Some other findings are as follows.

Interventions in Diverse Age and Population Groups

A review by Contento and colleagues of 217 well-designed nutrition education intervention studies conducted with major population groups between 1980 and 1995 found that nutrition education was a significant factor in improving dietary practices when behavioral change was set as the goal and when the educational strategies employed were designed with that as a purpose (Contento et al. 1995). In the studies reviewed, interventions did not always achieve across-the-board success on all criteria used to judge effectiveness, and often intervention effects were not large. In addition, where many components were involved, nutrition education often achieved positive results in some components and not in others. Nevertheless, overall, nutrition education did contribute significantly to change in a variety of food- and nutrition-related behaviors. Reviews focused on school-based studies also found positive effects of nutrition education (Lytle & Achterberg 1995; McArthur 1998).

Interventions to Increase Fruit and Vegetable Intakes

The efficacy of interventions to modify dietary behaviors related to cancer risk in adults was examined by reviewing well-designed and controlled studies conducted from 1975 to 2000 (Ammerman et al. 2002). The review found positive effects of interventions to reduce fat intake and to increase intake of fruits and vegetables. There was a modest increase in both the average number of fruits and vegetables eaten each day and the percentage of people who met the goal of eating five or more servings of fruits and vegetables a day. Media campaigns and randomized trials in children and adults to increase fruit and vegetable consumption were evaluated in another study, providing some evidence of changes in intake that could be attributed to the interventions (Potter et al. 2000). A review of interventions conducted worldwide to increase fruit and vegetable consumption in adults found that significant increases were achieved through a variety of venues: face-to-face education, counseling, telephone motivational interviewing, computer-tailored information, and community-based multicomponent programs (Pomerleau et al. 2005). A review of carefully controlled studies designed to increase fruit and vegetable intakes in youth found many to be effective (Stables et al. 2005; Howerton et al. 2007).

Environmental Interventions

Interventions that focus on changing the school environment show potential for positively affecting fruit and vegetable consumption among youth (French & Stables 2003). Use of gardens in schools and communities as a venue for nutrition education has been gaining in popularity and has shown some effectiveness in increasing fruit and vegetable intakes (Robinson-O'Brien, Story, & Heim 2009). How exactly the environment affects changes in diet and physical activity is being actively investigated (Kremers et al. 2006; Kremers et al. 2007).

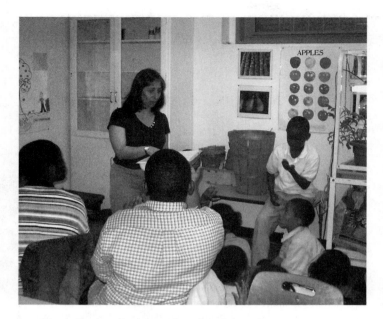

Learning about where food comes from: Examining soil.

Obesity Prevention in Youth

Recent studies have sought to prevent excessive weight gain in children. Many have resulted in improvements in one weight-related measure or another, such as body mass index or skinfold measures (Summerbell et al. 2005; Gonzalez-Suarez et al. 2009). For example, one review of studies found that 17 of 25 were effective in improving weight-related parameters (Doak et al. 2006) and another review found that 40 out of 51 interventions were effective in some parameter or another (Shaya et al. 2008). Other reviews, however, have noted that effectiveness across all outcome measures has been hard to achieve given the many factors that contribute to obesity in children and the difficulty of developing good study designs (Kropski, Keckley, & Jensen 2008; Doak et al. 2009; Zensen & Kridli 2009). Research is on-going.

Breastfeeding Interventions

Reviews of breastfeeding education show that prenatal education in small groups, often using multiple learning modes such as videos and practice, is effective in increasing breastfeeding initiation rates. In-hospital coaching and postpartum support are also important (Schlickau & Wilson 2005; Shealy et al. 2005; Dyson, McCormick, & Renfrew 2005; Mushtaq, Skaggs, & Thompson 2008; Hill 2009).

Cost–Benefit Analyses

Cost–benefit analyses have also been conducted for nutrition education programs. This type of analysis compares the economic benefits of a nutrition education program for participants to the actual costs of delivering the program. It was found in one program that for every dollar in costs, the mean benefit to participants was about $10, ranging from about $3 to $17 (Rajopal et al. 2003). In another, for each dollar in costs, the mean benefit was about $3.60 (Schuster et al. 2003). A third study found that a nutrition education program improved "quality of life years" (QALY), which suggests there might be lower health care costs in the future (Dollahite, Kenkel, & Thompson 2008). A review of studies in the physical activity area found that community-wide public health interventions similarly found cost-effectiveness ratios that ranged between $14,000 and $69,000 per QALY gained, relative to no intervention (Roux et al. 2008).

Thus, the evidence from these reviews and cost-benefit analyses of intervention studies demonstrates that nutrition education programs can make a significant contribution to improving dietary practices when they use appropriate strategies.

Nutrition Education as Translational Research and Practice

These intervention studies suggest that nutrition education can be seen as contributing to translational research and practice. Just as research in medicine is being conducted to see how best to translate laboratory research into clinical practice and then into daily practice by physicians—from "Bench to Bedside"—so nutrition education research is helping to translate nutrition science research into dietary guidelines and then to behavior—from "Bench to Behavior" (Serrano, Anderson, & Chapman-Novakofski 2007).

■ WHAT DO NUTRITION EDUCATORS DO?: SETTINGS, AUDIENCES, AND SCOPE FOR NUTRITION EDUCATION

As we have seen, the rise in chronic disease and obesity has led to an increased interest in nutrition among consumers in recent decades. In addition, interest in local and organic food and foods perceived to be high quality has upsurged. Because nutrition can be seen as the link between agriculture and health, intentional education about food and nutrition covers a wide range of issues and takes place in a variety of settings, with different audiences.

Settings: Where Is Nutrition Education Provided?

Nutrition education is provided in many settings. Some of them are described in the following sections. More examples are given throughout this book and in **Nutrition Education in Action 1-1**.

Communities

Nutrition education for the public at large occurs in communities through programs provided by many organizations, particularly those sponsored by the USDA, such as Cooperative Extension programs. Each county in the United States is served by a Cooperative Extension office funded jointly by federal, state, and county monies. The Cooperative Extension Service provides nutrition education activities to adults, families, and children to assist them to eat healthfully, through programs such as the Expanded Food and Nutrition Education Program (EFNEP). Special emphasis in recent years has been placed on assisting low-income individuals to eat more healthfully through the Supplemental Nutrition Assistance Program Education (SNAP-Ed). Most states have developed extensive nutrition education programs for SNAP participants. USDA's Women, Infants, and Children (WIC) program provides nutrition education to its participants in addition to providing food. The Head Start program provides both food and nutrition education to preschool children. The Administration on Aging provides meals to low-resources older adults in a group setting and serves most communities in the nation. Nutrition education is a required component of the program.

Many other agencies and private voluntary and nonprofit organizations, such as heart associations, cancer societies, and food banks, also provide nutrition education. Social marketing campaigns focusing on nutrition and physical activity have become more common within communities.

NUTRITION EDUCATION IN ACTION **1-1**

Nutrition Education Programs in Different Settings

Fruits and Veggies: More Matters Campaign for Healthier Eating

More Matters is a campaign to assist Americans to eat more fruits and vegetables with a simple and direct call to action: when it comes to fruits and vegetables, eating more makes a difference—it matters. The campaign is primarily Web-based, with numerous motivational messages and useful nutrition information and tips and links to other resources. It also involves print ads, school cafeteria posters, and programs in stores to highlight fruits and vegetables. The website is http://www.fruitsandveggiesmorematters.org.

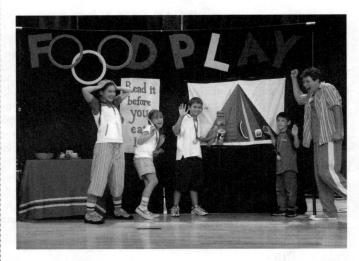

Nutrition education using live theater performances.

Theater for Kids

FOODPLAY, a live theater performance for school assemblies, conferences, and special events, was developed by a nutrition educator and has been presented all over the United States. FOODPLAY performances feature captivating characters, motivating health messages, juggling, music, magic, and audience participation to help kids take charge of growing up healthy, happy, and fit. The program uses the power of live theater to motivate kids to say YES! to healthy eating and exercise habits, seeing through media messages, and building self-esteem from the inside out. FOODPLAY performances come with extensive Follow-Up School Resource Kits providing materials for students, teachers, school food service, and health staff to continue nutrition education lessons in the classroom, integrate nutrition into core curriculum areas, and help schools improve their health environments and wellness policies. It has won an Emmy Award and has been shown to be effective. The website is http://www.foodplay.com.

Community Gardens

Can community gardens thrive in a large city? The members of many low-income communities in large cities have decided that growing their own gardens is an important way to improve the quality of fresh foods available to them, fight hunger, and promote community-based entrepreneurship and economic opportunity. With names such as Garden of Happiness, Garden of Union, and New Perspectives Community Garden, these inner-city farms produce food not only for those who work in them but also to sell at farmers' markets and other fairs and to donate to soup kitchens and related organizations. Nutrition education is provided at many of these sites. The website for one such program can be found at http://www.justfood.org.

Food- and Food System–Related Community and Advocacy Organizations

Community nutritionists work in emergency food organizations such as food pantries and soup kitchens, providing needed education to low-resources audiences. Community nutritionists also work in organizations that seek to enhance the availability and accessibility of affordable, nutritious food to individuals and communities by linking food producers to consumers through such programs as farmers' markets, community-supported agriculture, and farm-to-institution programs. Most of these programs include special outreach efforts to low-income communities. Nutrition educators provide educational sessions in these settings, take people on tours of farmers' markets and farms, and work with community policy makers.

Schools

Nutrition education is taught as a part of school health education in many states. In these instances, classroom teachers deliver the nutrition educa-tion. The role of the nutrition educator is to develop good curricular materials, provide professional development to teachers, and help teachers provide nutrition education, usually through specific funded projects. In addition, school food service personnel often provide informal nutrition education through posters and food-related activities in the lunchroom. Numerous school-based nutrition education research interventions have been conducted in schools in recent decades with funding from federal agencies such the National Institutes of Health and the USDA.

Workplaces

In recent decades, workplace health promotion has grown considerably, usually incorporating nutrition education, weight control, and physical activity along with other health education efforts to reduce the risk of chronic disease, such as cardiovascular disease and cancer. These efforts have been directed at both the general population of employees and high-risk individuals. Nutrition educators often assist in designing the programs and delivering them.

Health Care Settings

Although one-on-one nutrition counseling is the norm in health care settings, many medical centers provide outpatient nutrition education to at-risk individuals served by the center. Health maintenance organizations and health insurance plans often provide nutrition education to their membership. Nutrition educators also work in physician practices, weight control programs, and eating disorders clinics.

Audiences for Nutrition Education

Nutrition education is provided to a wide range of audiences who differ on many counts, including age, life stage, socioeconomic status, cultural background, and other characteristics.

Life Stage Groups

Nutrition education programs have been developed and delivered to people throughout the entire life span: preschool children and their caregivers; school-aged children through school curricula, after-school activities, or family-based programs; college students through nutrition or health courses, cafeteria interventions, and student health center activities; adults through community or workplace programs; pregnant and lactating women through WIC and other programs; and older adults through a variety of specifically targeted programs.

Diverse Cultural Groups

Some nutrition education programs are developed specifically for different cultural groups, such as programs for African American churches, Latino/Latina groups, or recent immigrants speaking a variety of languages.

Socioeconomic Backgrounds

Socioeconomic status (SES) has been linked to health status, with those of low SES experiencing more health problems and greater premature death than those of higher SES. Many government programs are designed to reduce these health disparities through food assistance activities such as the Supplemental Nutrition Assistance Program (SNAP) and Women, Infants, and Children (WIC) programs or public health programs. Head Start seeks to reduce educational inequities by providing free schooling to eligible preschoolers. Nutrition education is an important component of all these programs, assisting low-income participants to eat more healthfully.

Gatekeepers: Decision Makers and Policy Makers

Traditionally, the term *gatekeepers* referred to those in the family (usually the mother) who purchased and prepared the food because such people controlled what the family ate. However, the term can be used more broadly. Today, individuals receive food from a variety of sources. Gatekeepers include individuals or organizations that provide food or services or have some policy-making role in the accessibility and availability of food- or nutrition-related services in organizations, communities, and local and national government. Gatekeepers may also be those who influence social and informational environments, such as the mass media. Given the important role of the environment in facilitating healthy eating and active living, nutrition educators can educate not just individual consumers but policy makers, the mass media, the food industry, and those in the economic, agricultural, and political spheres who make decisions that affect dietary and physical activity practices. Nutrition educators can educate these gatekeepers about current food

and nutrition conditions (e.g., anemia, food insecurity, obesity) and make the case for the relevance of nutrition education and policy alternatives so as to encourage policy makers to take actions that are more supportive of healthful eating, active living, and sustainable food systems.

Scope of Nutrition Education

The major function of nutrition education activities is to assist people to eat and enjoy healthful food by increasing awareness, enhancing people's motivations, facilitating the ability to take action, and improving environmental supports for action. But nutrition education can expand its scope not only in terms of appropriate audiences but also in terms of the content to be addressed and the nature of the strategies to be used.

Wide Range of Content

Nutrition education can address an extremely wide range of content issues related to food and nutrition. The primary content issues are, of course, related to personal health, such as the relationship between diet and health, healthful eating as recommended by the *Dietary Guidelines* and MyPyramid, how to get the best nutrition within one's budget, food safety, breastfeeding, how to get ones' children to eat more healthfully, eating breakfast, balancing eating and physical activity, reducing diet-related chronic disease, and so forth. Indeed, any given nutrition education program can address any issue of concern or interest.

Food Safety and Food Systems

In recent years, there has been an increase in interest among consumers about food safety, spurred by concerns about the increasing incidence of foodborne illness, or about genetically engineered food, bovine growth hormone in milk, and so forth. Nutrition educators need to be prepared to assist consumers to evaluate these issues so that consumers can make informed decisions. Other consumers—and nutrition professionals— have become interested in issues related to how and where food is produced, believing that eating fresh and local food is good for personal health, for farmers, and for the environment (Gussow 2006). Farmers' markets have emerged in many communities. To increase the accessibility and affordability of local foods to low-resources individuals, the USDA has made it possible for such individuals to use Supplemental Nutrition Assistance Program electronic benefits transfer (EBT) cards at farmers' markets. Various community organizations have also worked to link food banks and soup kitchens to local farmers. Nutrition professional organizations have also suggested that nutrition education in schools be linked with work in school gardens and other strategies to help children develop a deeper appreciation for the environment and food systems (American Dietetic Association 2003).

Social Justice and Sustainability

Some consumers are interested in what are called social justice and sustainability issues related to food (**Table 1-2**). Indeed, the *Wall Street Journal* and the *New York Times* have noted that some surveys suggest that about one third of consumers are motivated in their purchases by concern for the environment as well as for their health, and mainstream food producers are beginning to cater to this segment (McLaughlin 2004; Burros 2006). Consequently, the scope of nutrition education can be expanded to address these content issues as well. Numerous other issues of interest and concern will no doubt emerge that can be addressed by nutrition educators.

TABLE 1-2	**Are Your Groceries Sustainable and Fairly Traded?**

Food product labels can now help consumers who wish to include considerations of social justice and sustainability in their grocery shopping practices. A variety of labels exist. Here are some of the commonly seen terms and what they mean.

Term	What It Is	What It Means
Sustainable	An unofficial, uncertified term	Food is produced in a way that is environmentally sound, beneficial to local communities, and profitable.
Certified sustainable	Certification licensed by various nonprofit organizations	Food production practices aim to protect the environment, treat workers well, and benefit local communities.
Local	An unofficial, uncertified term	Food was grown nearby—no distance specified.
Fair trade certified	Products that comply with standards set by Transfair USA the Fair Trade Labeling Organization International	Farm inspections required. Growers are guaranteed above-commodity prices; men and women are paid equal wages; no child labor is used. Some environmental protections.
Rainforest Alliance certified	A term licensed by Rainforest Alliance, a New York-based nonprofit organization dedicated to protecting biodiversity	Farm inspections performed. Farming practices are environmentally sound and fair to workers.

Source: McLaughlin, K. 2004, February 17. Food world's new buzzword is "sustainable" products; fair trade certified mangos. *Wall Street Journal* CCXLIII(32):D1–2. Reprinted with permission.

Physical Activity and Nutrition

Nutrition educators can address physical activity as well as nutrition to encourage both active living and healthful eating. Given the increasing recognition that being less sedentary and more physically active decreases the risk of chronic disease and obesity and improves health, many nutrition education programs now address physical activity in tandem with individual and community nutrition education–related behaviors and practices.

A Variety of Approaches

Nutrition educators can embark on a wider variety of activities beyond mass media campaigns, lectures, group discussions, workshops, health fairs, newsletters, videos, brochures, and other print and audiovisual materials.

Empowerment Approaches

Nutrition education can use a critical consciousness–raising approach, originally proposed by Freire (1970), in which people participate in a process involving a careful analysis of the causes of the food or health issue facing the group and of the structure of power in their communities, and then plan ways to organize to take action. This approach has been used in nutrition education to assist low-resources groups identify the causes of their problems of access to food and to take political and economic actions to reduce nutritional inequities (Travers 1997).

Nutrition educators can also use a growth-centered educational approach, which seeks to foster self-reliance by building on the abilities and assets of the participants and providing opportunities for self-directed learning and activities and building social support (Arnold et al. 2001). Both of these approaches are related to an empowerment process through which individuals, communities, and organizations gain mastery over their lives (Kent 1988; Rody 1988; Israel et al. 1994; Minkler & Wallerstein 2002). And indeed, an aim of nutrition education is for nutrition programs to assist individuals to become more able to take control of their own food choices and practices and to take collective action regarding their environments to make them more supportive—in short, to become more empowered.

Collaboration

Nutrition educators can also work in coalitions with other professionals, organizations, and governmental agencies to increase the accessibility and affordability of foods for low-income audiences; promote environments at the institutional and community levels that foster attitudes and behaviors conducive to health; encourage the development of social networks and social support; build food and nutrition programs that involve genuine community participation and control; and promote policies at local, state, and national levels that are supportive of food- and nutrition-related health.

Summary of the Settings, Audiences, and Scope

Nutrition education can encompass a wide range of content, issues, and activities, ranging from group sessions about heart disease risk reduction to assisting low-income audiences to eat better, and from helping schools and community groups to grow vegetable gardens to fostering school, worksite, and community food policy councils. It also includes educating and building coalitions with decision makers and policy makers to increase opportunities for all people, but particularly low-resources audiences, to take action about food and nutrition issues (**Figure 1-9**).

■ NUTRITION EDUCATION, PUBLIC HEALTH NUTRITION, AND HEALTH PROMOTION: THE ROLES AND CONTEXT OF NUTRITION EDUCATION

Nutrition education that addresses both environmental and personal factors and includes expanded audiences and strategies begins to overlap public health nutrition and health promotion efforts. To make the situation even more complex, we should note that dietary interventions are often integrated with interventions directed at other health-related behaviors. Many cardiovascular disease risk reduction programs involve

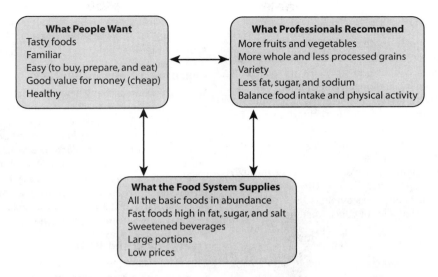

FIGURE 1-9 Nutrition education is exciting and challenging.

interventions directed not only at dietary changes but also at smoking cessation, blood pressure control, and increased physical activity. Within the context of today's emphasis on health promotion and disease prevention, the roles of nutrition education, public health nutrition, health education, and health promotion are indeed overlapping and intertwined.

At the same time, the scope of nutrition education is broader than educating about nutrition in relation to personal health. Nutrition has often been defined as the link between agriculture and health. Some nutrition educators are concerned about the agriculture-to-nutrition component of the link as well as the nutrition-to-health component. Thus, nutrition education can address such concerns as food safety and how to ensure the availability and accessibility of nutritious and wholesome food for all, poor and rich alike. As we have seen, for some nutrition educators and consumers, considerations about how and where food is produced are also important. Nutrition education can thus be visualized as including the overlapping portion of several intersecting circles (see **Figure 1-10**).

Clearly, nutrition education by itself cannot accomplish everything needed for improved nutritional well-being for all people. It must be conducted in conjunction with many other related strategies, some not educational in nature. Facilitating individual behavior change and bringing about change in the environment are both important and interactive. Nutrition education is directed primarily at individual and group behaviors through activities that enhance motivations, knowledge and skills, and social support. However, it also includes nutrition education activities conducted with decision makers and policy makers so as to promote specific environmental supports that make it easier for the public to engage in healthy behaviors. Public health nutrition efforts and food assistance programs, on the other hand, are directed primarily at environmental, systemic, and policy factors such as the availability and accessibility of food, access to nutritional services within the health care system, community structures that enable active living, policy, and legislation and secondarily at personal, behavioral factors. In addition, those in nutrition education, public health nutrition, and health promotion share an interest in fostering collective efficacy and capacity

building in communities so that communities can become empowered to act on their own food, nutrition, and physical activity issues for the long term.

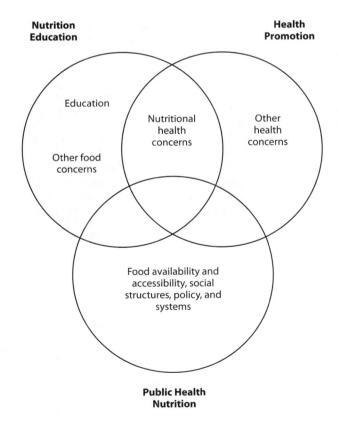

FIGURE 1-10 The overlapping roles of nutrition education, public health nutrition, and health promotion.

▪ PURPOSE OF THIS BOOK

This book is intended to be a guide to designing and implementing effective, evidence-based nutrition education interventions and dietary change strategies. Effective interventions and strategies are those that enhance people's motivation, ability, and opportunities to eat well and live actively. The book presents a systematic, stepwise procedure for designing, implementing, and evaluating nutrition education that focuses on personal behaviors and community practices, accompanied by environmental supports, is evidence based, and is grounded in the integration of theory, research, and practice.

We have seen that nutrition education can be delivered through multiple venues and that its scope is very broad. One book cannot cover all aspects of nutrition education. Consequently, this text focuses on designing and implementing the types of educational interventions and programs that the vast majority of nutrition educators offer on an ongoing basis in their places of work:

- *Providing site-based, in-person educational activities with groups* in a variety of settings, such as communities, outpatient clinics, health maintenance organizations, fitness centers, schools, workplaces, or private nonprofit organizations
- *Developing accompanying materials and activities*, such as printed materials, visual media, Internet activities, mass media and social marketing activities, or health fairs
- *Engaging in activities and coalitions* to promote environments, social structures, and policies that are supportive of the public's ability to eat healthfully

Many factors in the larger society, such as public policy, systems, and structural changes, have important impacts on food- and nutrition-related behaviors and practices. Designing interventions to change these larger environmental forces operating at the community and national levels is the subject of many available health promotion planning and social marketing books and discussion of such design in detail is beyond the scope of this book. At the same time, these books are not designed to provide information on the specifics of how to actually design educational intervention activities that are specifically based on theory and evidence. The focus of this book is thus on how to design and implement the actual educational programs that can be conducted within, or in collaboration with, these larger programs. Specifically, this book provides a systematic stepwise procedure for planning nutrition education programs *and* shows how to translate theory and incorporate evidence into each step of the planning process. At the other end of the spectrum, working with individuals one on one, as in nutrition counseling, is also the subject of available texts and will thus not be addressed in this book.

Learning a New Vocabulary

You will encounter many new terms and ideas. Indeed, you will learn a new vocabulary. Just as when you took your first course in biochemistry or nutrition you had to learn new terms such as *metabolism, glycolysis, Kreb's cycle, lipogenesis, nitrogen excretion,* and *electrolyte balance,* so you will learn new terms such as *outcome expectations* (beliefs about outcomes of behavior), *self-efficacy* (confidence in being able to perform a behavior), *attitudes, perceived social norm, personal agency,* and so forth. The terms are explained as you encounter them. You will soon be comfortable using this new vocabulary and speaking the language of behavioral nutrition and nutrition education.

Overview of the Book

This is an exciting time in the field of nutrition education. The public is interested in food and nutrition. Research is very active, drawing investigators from a variety of fields. Such research has generated evidence about effective approaches to nutrition education and has produced usable theories to guide practice. The remainder of this book is devoted to discussing theories, emerging nutrition education research evidence, and practical techniques for increasing awareness and enhancing motivation, facilitating the ability to take action, and promoting supportive environments so as to assist people to adopt and maintain food- and nutrition-related practices conducive to long-term health.

To design effective nutrition education, we need first to understand more fully the many influences on food choices and nutrition-related behaviors and the dietary change process.

- Part I of this book provides the background in behavioral nutrition and nutrition education research and theory for understanding the determinants of food choices and the processes and mediators of dietary behavior change, as well as an overview of how research and theory can enhance nutrition education practice.
- Part II presents a six-step process—a systematic stepwise procedure, a translational model—for designing practical nutrition education strategies that are based on theory and research evidence.
- Part III describes the nuts and bolts of implementing nutrition education and making theory and research practical.

Questions and Activities

1. State five reasons why nutrition education for the public is needed.
2. Describe three reasons why it is difficult for people to eat healthfully, despite the abundance of choices and extensive media coverage of diet and health.
3. Social and behavioral factors are implicated in a broad range of diseases in the United States. What are the implications for nutrition education?
4. Three approaches to nutrition education are described in this chapter: information dissemination only, facilitating behavior change, and focusing on environmental change. Describe briefly the central tenets and criticisms of each approach. What do you think about each? Discuss.
5. What is "upstream" and "downstream" nutrition education?
6. If someone now asks you to explain what nutrition education is, what would you say?
7. As you review the audiences and settings for nutrition, where do you see yourself as a nutrition educator? What would you like to do?

References

Agricultural Research Service U.S. Department of Agriculture. 2000. *Continuing food intake by individuals 1994–1996 (CSFII 1994–1996)*. Washington, DC: Author.

Allegrante, J. P., and L. W. Green. 1981. Sounding board. When health policy becomes victim blaming. *New England Journal of Medicine* 305(25):1528–1529.

American Dietetic Association. 2002. Knowledge, attitudes, beliefs, behaviors: findings of American Dietetic Association's public opinion survey. *Nutrition and You: Trends 2002*. Chicago: Author.

———. 2003. Nutrition services: An essential component of comprehensive health programs. *Journal of the American Dietetic Association* 103:505–514.

———. 2009. ADA: Who we are, what we do. http://www.eatright.org/cps/rde/xchg/ada/hs.xsl/home_404_ENU_HTML.htm.

Ammerman, A. S., C. H. Lindquist, K. N. Lohr, and J. Hersey. 2002. The efficacy of behavioral interventions to modify dietary fat and fruit and vegetable intake: A review of the evidence. *Preventive Medicine* 35(1):25–41.

Arnold, C. G., P. Ladipo, C. H. Nguyen, P. Nkinda-Chaiban, and M. Olson. 2001. New concepts for nutrition education in an era of welfare reform. *Journal of Nutrition Education* 33:341–346.

Balzer, H. 1997. *The NPD Group's 11th annual report on eating patterns in America: National eating trends tracking*. Port Washington, NY: NPD Group.

Bandura, A. 1986. *Foundations of thought and action: A social cognitive theory*. Englewood Cliffs, NJ: Prentice Hall.

———. 1997. *Self efficacy: The exercise of control*. New York: WH Freeman.

———. 2001. Social cognitive theory: An agentic perspective. *Annual Review of Psychology* 51:1–26.

Bastiosis, P. P., A. Carlson, S. A. Gerrior, W. Y. Juan, and M. Lino. 2004. The Healthy Eating Index, 1999–2000: Charting dietary patterns of Americans. *Family Economics and Nutrition Review* 16(1):39–48.

Birch, L. L. 1999. Development of food preferences. *Annual Review of Nutrition* 19:41–62.

Brillat-Savarin, A. S. 1825. *The physiology of taste: Mediations on transcendental gastronomy*, translated by M. F. K. Fisher. Reprint. Washington, DC: Counterpoint Press, 2000.

Buchanan, D. 2004. Two models for defining the relationship between theory and practice in nutrition education: Is the scientific method meeting our needs? *Journal of Nutrition Education and Behavior* 36(3):146–154.

Burros, M. 2006. Idealism for breakfast: Serving good intentions by the bowl full. *New York Times*, January 11.

Center for Nutrition Policy and Promotion, U.S. Department of Agriculture. 2001. Report card on the diet quality of children ages 2 to 9. In *Nutrition Insights* 25. Alexandria, VA: Author.

Center for Science in the Public Interest. 2003. *Pestering parents: How food companies market obesity to children*. Washington, DC: Author.

Centers for Disease Control and Prevention. 2008. Prevalence of regular physical activity among adults—United States, 2001 and 2005: Morbidity and mortality weekly report. *Journal of the American Medical Association* 299(1):30–32.

Clancy, K. 1999. Reclaiming the social and environmental roots of nutrition education. *Journal of Nutrition Education* 31(4):190–193.

Contento, I. 1980. Thinking about nutrition education: What to teach, how to teach it, and what to measure. *Teachers College Record* 81(4):422–424.

Contento, I., G. I. Balch, Y. L. Bronner, et al. 1995. The effectiveness of nutrition education and implications for nutrition education policy, programs, and research: A review of research. *Journal of Nutrition Education* 27(6):279–418.

Cook, A. J., and J. E. Friday. 2004. *Pyramid servings intakes in the United States 1999–2002, 1 day* (CNRG Table Set 3.0). Washington, DC: U.S. Department of Agriculture. Agricultural Research Service, Community Nutrition Research Group. http://www.ba.ars.usda.gov/cnrg.

Davis, C. M. 1928. Self selection of diet by newly weaned infants. *American Journal of Diseases of Children* 36:651–679.

Deci, E. L., and E. M. Ryan. 2000. The "what" and "why" of goal pursuits: Human needs and the self-determination of behavior. *Psychological Inquiry* 11(4):227–268.

———. 2008. Facilitating optimal motivation and psychological well-being across life's domains. *Canadian Psychology* 49:14–23.

Doak, C. M., T. L. Visscher, C. M. Renders, and J. C. Seidell. 2006. The prevention of overweight and obesity in children and adolescents: A review of interventions and programmes. *Obesity Reviews* 7(1):111–136.

Doak, C. M., B. L. Heitmann, C. Summerbell, and L. Lissner. 2009. Prevention of childhood obesity: What type of evidence should we consider relevant? *Obesity Reviews* 10(3):350–356.

Dollahite, J., D. Kenkel, and C. S. Thompson. 2008. An economic evaluation of the expanded food and nutrition education program. *Journal of Nutrition Education and Behavior* 40(3):134–143.

Drewnowski, A., N. Darmon, and A. Briend. 2004. Replacing fats and sweets with vegetables and fruit: A question of cost. *American Journal of Public Health* 94:1555–1559.

Dyson, L., F. McCormick, and M. J. Renfrew. 2005. Interventions for promoting the initiation of breastfeeding. *Cochrane Database Systematic Reviews* (2):CD001688.

Elitzak, H. 2001. Food marketing costs at a glance. *Food Review* 24(3):47–48.

Food and Nutrition Board, National Research Council. 1989. *Diet and health: Implications for reducing chronic disease risk*. Washington, DC: National Academies Press.

Food Marketing Institute. 2004. *Supermarket facts: Industry overview 2003*. Washington, DC: Author.

Frazao, E. 1999. High costs of poor eating patterns in the United States. In *America's eating habits: Changes and consequences*, edited by E. Frazao. Washington, DC: U.S. Department of Agriculture.

French, S. A., and G. Stables. 2003. Environmental interventions to promote vegetable and fruit consumption among youth in school settings. *Preventive Medicine* 37(6 Pt 1):593–610.

Freire, P. 1970. *Pedagogy of the oppressed*. New York: Continuum.

Gallo, A. E. 1998. The food marketing system in 1996. In *Agricultural Bulletin No AIB743*. Washington, DC: U.S. Department of Agriculture, Economic Research Service.

Gillespie, A. H. 1987. Communication theory as a basis for nutrition education. *Journal of the American Dietetic Association* 87(9 Suppl):S44–52.

Gonzalez-Suarez, C., A. Worley, K. Grimmer-Somers, and V. Dones. 2009. School-based interventions on childhood obesity: a meta-analysis. *American Journal of Preventive Medicine* 37:418–427.

Green, L. W., and M. W. Kreuter. 2004. *Health promotion planning: An educational and ecological approach.* 4th ed. New York: McGraw-Hill.

Gussow, J. D. 1999. Dietary guidelines for sustainability: Twelve years later. *Journal of Nutrition Education* 31(4):194–200.

———. 2006. Reflections on nutritional health and the environment: The journey to sustainability. *Journal of Hunger and Environmental Nutrition* 1(1):3–25.

Gussow, J. D., and K. Clancy. 1986. Dietary guidelines for sustainability. *Journal of Nutrition Education* 18(1):1–4.

Gussow, J. D., and I. Contento. 1984. Nutrition education in a changing world. A conceptualization and selective review. *World Review of Nutrition and Diet* 44:1–56.

Hedley, A. A., C. L. Ogden, C. L. Johnson, M. D. Carroll, L. R. Curtin, and K. M. Flegal. 2004. Prevalence of overweight and obesity among US children, adolescents, and adults, 1999–2002. *Journal of the American Medical Association* 291(23):2847–2850.

Hegsted, M. 1979. Interview quoted in: Anders, H. J. Nutrition and health. *Chemical and Engineering News*, March 26:27.

Hill, J. A. 2009. Evidence for excellence: Systematic review of breastfeeding education benefits. *American Journal of Nursing* 109(4):26–27.

Hill, J. O., H. R. Wyatt, G. W. Reed, and J. C. Peters. 2003. Obesity and the environment: Where do we go from here? *Science* 299(5608):853–855.

Howerton, M. W., B. S. Bell, K. W. Dodd, D. Berrigan, R. Stolzenberg-Solomon, and L. Nebeling. 2007. School-based nutrition programs produced a moderate increase in fruit and vegetable consumption: Meta and pooling analyses from 7 studies. *Journal of Nutrition Education and Behavior* 39(4):186–196.

International Food Information Council (IFIC) Foundation. 1999. Are you listening? What consumers tell us about dietary recommendations. *Food insight: Current topics in food safety and nutrition.* Washington, DC: Author.

Institutes of Medicine. 2000. *Promoting health: Intervention strategies from social and behavioral research,* edited by B. D. Smedley and S. L. Syme. Washington, DC: Division of Health Promotion and Disease Prevention, Institute of Medicine.

Israel, B. A., B. Checkoway, A. Schulz, and M. Zimmerman. 1994. Health education and community empowerment: Conceptualizing and measuring perceptions of individual, organizational, and community control. *Health Education Quarterly* 21(2):149–170.

Johnson, D. W., and R. T. Johnson. 1985. Nutrition education: A model for effectiveness, a synthesis of research. *Journal of Nutrition Education* 17(Suppl.):S1–S44.

Kent, G. 1988. Nutrition education as an instrument of empowerment. *Journal of Nutrition Education* 20:193–195.

Kropski, J. A., P. H. Keckley, and G. L. Jensen. 2008. School-based obesity prevention programs: An evidence-based review. *Obesity (Silver Spring)* 16(5):1009–1018.

Leading Advertisers. 2001, September 24. 100 leading advertisers. *Ad Age,* p. 1–36.

Leiss, W. 1976. *Limits to satisfaction: An essay on the problem of needs and commodities.* Toronto: University of Toronto Press.

Leventhal, H. 1973. Changing attitudes and habits to reduce risk factors in chronic disease. *American Journal of Cardiology* 31(5):571–580.

Levy, L., R. E. Patterson, A. R. Kristal, and S. S. Li. 2000. How well do consumers understand percentage daily value on food labels? *American Journal of Health Promotion* 14(3):157–160, ii.

Lipton, K. L., W. Edmondson, and A. Manchester. 1998. *The food and fiber system: Contributing to the U.S. and world economies.* Washington, DC: Economic Research Service, U.S. Department of Agriculture.

Lytle, L., and C. Achterberg. 1995. Changing the diet of America's children: What works and why. *Journal of Nutrition Education* 27:250–260.

Mayer, J. 1986. Social responsibilities of nutritionists. *Journal of Nutrition Education* 16:714–717.

McArthur, D. B. 1998. Heart healthy eating behaviors of children following a school-based intervention: A meta-analysis. *Issues Comprehensive Pediatric Nursing* 21(1):35–48.

McKinley, J. B. 1974. A case for refocusing upstream—the political economy of illness. In *Applying behavioral science to cardiovascular risk,* edited by A. J. Enelow and J. B. Henderson. Seattle, WA: American Heart Association.

McLaughlin, K. 2004, February 17. Food world's new buzzword is "sustainable" products; fair trade certified mangos. *Wall Street Journal* CCXLIII(32):D1–2.

McNeal, J. U. 1992. *Kids as consumers: A handbook of marketing to children.* New York: Lexington Books.

Minkler, M., and N. B. Wallerstein. 2002. Improving health through community organization and community building. In *Health education and health behavior: Theory research and practice,* edited by K. Glanz, B. K. Rimer, and F. M. Lewis. San Francisco: Jossey-Bass.

Moliter, G. T. T. 1980. The food system in the 1980s. *Journal of Nutrition Education* 12(Suppl):103–111.

Monteiro, C. A., W. L. Conde, and B. M. Popkin. 2004. The burden of disease from undernutrition and overnutrition in countries undergoing rapid nutrition transition: A view from Brazil. *American Journal of Public Health* 94(3):433–434.

Mushtaq, N., V. J. Skaggs, and D. M. Thompson. 2008. Effect of breastfeeding education and support on promoting breastfeeding: A literature review. *Journal of the Oklahoma State Medical Association* 101(10):231–236.

National Center for Health Statistics. 2003. Deaths: Final data for 2001. In *National vital statistics reports.* Hyattsville, MD: National Center for Health Statistics, Division of Vital Statistics.

Ogden, C. L., D. M., Carroll, L. R. Curtin, M. A. McDowell, C. J. Tabak, and K. M. Flegal. 2006. Prevalance of overweight and obesity in the United States, 1999–2004. *Journal of the American Medical Association* 295(13):1549–1555.

Pomerleau, J., K. Lock, C. Knai, and M. McKee. 2005. Interventions designed to increase adult fruit and vegetable intake can be effective: A systematic review of the literature. *Journal of Nutrition* 135(10):2486–2495.

Potter, J. D., J. R. Finnegan, J. X. Guinard, et al. 2000. 5 A Day for Better Health program evaluation. Bethesda, MD: National Institutes of Health, National Cancer Institute.

Robinson-O'Brien R., M. Story, and S. Heim. 2009. Impact of garden-based youth nutrition intervention programs: A review. *Journal of the American Dietetic Association* 109:273–280.

Rajopal, R., R. H. Cox, M. Lambur, and E. C. Lewis. 2003. Cost-benefit analysis indicates the positive economic benefits of the Expanded Food and Nutrition Education Program related to chronic disease prevention. *Journal of Nutrition Education and Behavior* 34:26–37.

Rody, N. 1988. Empowerment as organizational policy in nutrition intervention programs: A case study from the Pacific Islands. *Journal of Nutrition Education* 20:133–141.

Rolls, B. 2000. Sensory-specific satiety and variety in the meal. In *Dimensions of the meal: The science, culture, business, and art of eating,* edited by H. L. Meiselman. Gaithersburg, MD: Aspen Publishers.

Rothschild, M. L. 1999. Carrots, sticks, and promises: A conceptual framework for the management of public health and social issues behaviors. *Journal of Marketing* 63:24–37.

Roux, L., M. Pratt, T. O. Tengs, et al. 2008. Cost effectiveness of community-based physical activity interventions. *American Journal of Preventive Medicine* 35(6):578–588.

Rozin, P. 1982. Human food selection: The interaction of biology, culture, and individual experience. In *The psychobiology of human food selection,* edited by L. M. Barker. Westport, CT: Avi Publishing Company.

Schlickau, J. M., and M. E. Wilson. 2005. Breastfeeding as health-promoting behaviour for Hispanic women: Literature review. *Journal of Advanced Nursing* 52(2):200–210.

Schuster, E., Z. L. Zimmerman, M. Engle, J. Smiley, E. Syversen, and J. Murray. 2003. Investing in Oregon's expanded food and nutrition education program (EFNEP): Documenting costs and benefits. *Journal of Nutrition Education and Behavior* 35(4):200–206.

Serrano, E., J. Anderson, and K. Chapman-Novakofski. 2007. Not lost in translation: Nutrition education, a critical component of translational research. *Journal of Nutrition Education and Behavior* 39:164–170.

Shaya, F. T., D. Flores, C. M. Gbarayor, and J. Wang. 2008. School-based obesity interventions: A literature review. *Journal of School Health* 78(4):189–196.

Shealy, K. R., R. Li, S. Benton-Davis, and L. M. Grummer-Strawn. 2005. *The CDC guide to breastfeeding interventions.* Atlanta, GA: U.S. Department of Health and Human Services, Centers for Disease Control and Prevention.

Sims, L. S. 1987. Nutrition education research: Reaching toward the leading edge. *Journal of the American Dietetic Association* 87(9 Suppl):S10–18.

Society for Nutrition Education. 1995. Joint position of Society of Nutrition Education, the American Dietetic Association, and the American School Food Service Association: School-based nutrition programs and services. *Journal of Nutrition Education* 27(2):58–61.

———. 2009. Society for Nutrition Education mission and identity statement. http://www.sne.org.

Stables, G. J., E. M. Young, M. W. Howerton, et al. 2005. Small school-based effectiveness trials increase vegetable and fruit consumption among youth. *Journal of the American Dietetic Association* 105(2):252–256.

Stewart, H., N. Blisard, and D. Jolliffe. 2006. Let's eat out: Americans weigh taste, convenience, and nutrition. *Economic Information Bulletin* No. EIB-19.

Summerbell, C. D., E. Waters, L. D. Edmunds, S. Kelly, T. Brown, and K. J. Campbell. 2005. Interventions for preventing obesity in children. *Cochrane Database Systematic Reviews* (3):CD001871.

Travers, K. D. 1997. Reducing inequities through participatory research and community empowerment. *Health Education and Behavior* 24(3):344–356.

U.S. Department of Health and Human Services. 1988. *The surgeon general's report on nutrition and health.* Washington, DC: Author.

———. 2000. *Healthy People 2010: Understanding and improving health.* Washington, DC: Government Printing Office.

Yudkin, J. 1978. *The diet of man: Needs and wants.* London: Elsevier Science.

Overview of Determinants of Food Choice and Dietary Change: Implications for Nutrition Education

OVERVIEW

This chapter provides readers with an overview of the numerous influences on food choice and dietary practices and their implications for nutrition education. It also provides a description of the desired competencies outlined by professional nutrition societies for nutrition educators.

CHAPTER OUTLINE

- Introduction
- Determinants of food choice and dietary behavior
- Food-related determinants
- Person-related determinants
- Social and environmental determinants
- Economic determinants
- Information environment
- Implications for nutrition education
- Implications for competencies and skills for nutrition educators
- Summary

LEARNING OBJECTIVES

At the end of the chapter, you will be able to:

- Describe the research evidence for the influences of biological predispositions, experience with food, personal factors, and environmental factors on human food choice and dietary behaviors
- Understand the key role of intra- and interpersonal processes in food choice and dietary behaviors
- Appreciate the importance of these understandings for nutrition educators
- State the competencies needed to be an effective nutrition educator

---

■ INTRODUCTION: KNOWLEDGE IS NOT ENOUGH

You have known a person like Alicia: she knows a lot about nutrition, and, in particular, she knows that she should eat more fruits and vegetables. She just can't seem to do it. Or Ray, who wants to lose weight and knows what he is supposed to do, but just can't seem to get to it. Or maybe it is yourself—there is some eating habit you want to change but don't.

Nutrition education often is seen as the process of translating the findings of nutrition science to various audiences using methods from the fields of education and communication. If only the public knew all that we did, nutrition educators think, surely they would eat better. Thus, nutrition educators believe that their task is to provide the public with information to eat well. They plan sessions on MyPyramid and food label reading. They provide lists of high-fat or high-fiber foods, or food sources of nutrients such as calcium or vitamins. They discuss managing food budgets. However, studies show that simply providing this kind of knowledge is not enough. People often know to eat well but do not—just like Alicia and Ray.

A survey by a consumer research group has found that whereas about one quarter of the public consider nutrition to be very important and are very careful about what they eat, the rest fall almost equally into two groups that either don't want to be bothered or that know what they ought to do but will not or cannot do it (Balzer 1997). A U.S. Department of Agriculture (USDA) analysis found that 40% of the people surveyed said their diet needed no improvement. Of the remaining 60%, 23% were interested in improving their diet, whereas 37% were not (U.S. Department of Agriculture 2000). Similarly, another survey found that 7 of 10 consumers said their diet needed some improvement. Guilt, worry, fear, helplessness, and anger were the primary emotions expressed about their diets. However, they said they knew enough about nutrition: "Don't tell us more" (IFIC Foundation 1999). Clearly, then, although many Americans say their diets need improvement, they also indicate that they are knowledgeable about nutrition and are just unable to change or are uninterested in changing. Thus, many other factors besides knowledge must influence their food choices and diet-related behaviors.

This is not to say that knowledge is not important: knowledge in some form is a prerequisite for intentional healthful eating. However, food is more than nutrients, and eating is about more than health. Eating is a source of pleasure and is related to many of life's social functions. Eating behaviors are acquired over a lifetime, and changing them requires alterations in these behaviors for the long term—indeed, permanently. Unlike other health-related behaviors such as smoking, eating is not optional. People have to eat, and any changes they make are undertaken with a great deal of ambivalence. They want to eat to satisfy physical hunger and psychological desires and yet want to be healthy, which may require adopting eating patterns that conflict with these desires.

Nutrition education ultimately has to be about food and eating. Understanding people, their behavior, and the context of their behavior is one of the keys to effective nutrition education programs. Thus, it is very important for nutrition educators to understand the various forces that influence an individual's or a community's decision to eat in a particular way. This chapter provides a brief overview of the factors influencing food choice and dietary behaviors for the purpose of helping nutrition educators design more effective nutrition education programs.

■ DETERMINANTS OF FOOD CHOICE AND DIET-RELATED BEHAVIOR: AN OVERVIEW

People make decisions about food several times a day: when to eat, what to eat, with whom, and how much. Whether the act of eating is a meal or a snack, the decisions are complex and the influences many. Biologically determined behavioral predispositions such as liking of specific tastes are, of course, important influences. However, these can be modified by experience with food as well as by various intrapersonal and interpersonal factors. In addition, the environment either facilitates or impedes the ability of people to act on their biological predispositions, preferences, or personal imperatives. The influences are so numerous as to be overwhelming to try to understand! This chapter simplifies matters by examining these influences in three categories that are commonly used in studying food choice: factors related to food, to the individuals making the choices, and to the external physical and social environment—factors related to food, person, and environment (Shepherd 1999).

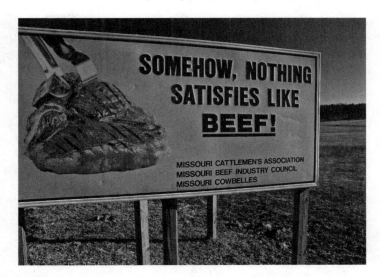

The number of influences on our diet choices is endless.

Many factors within each of these categories influence our eating. These influences are explored in greater detail in the following sections.

■ FOOD-RELATED DETERMINANTS: BIOLOGY AND EXPERIENCE

When asked, most people say their food choices are largely determined by "taste" (Glanz et al. 1998; Clark 1998; Food Marketing Institute 2002). By *taste*, they mean *flavor*, which includes smell and the oral perception of food texture as well (Small & Prescott 2005). Sensory-affective responses to the taste, smell, sight, and texture of food are a major influence on food preferences and food choices. What are people born with and what is learned?

Biologically Determined Behavioral Predispositions

The Basic Tastes

Humans are born with unlearned biological predispositions toward liking the sweet taste and rejecting sour and bitter tastes (Desor, Mahler, & Greene 1977; Mennella & Beauchamp 1996). The liking for the sweet taste remains throughout life and appears to be universal to all cultures (Pepino & Mennella 2005). The liking for salt seems to develop several months after birth, when infants have matured somewhat (Bernstein 1990). It has been suggested that these predispositions may have had adaptive value: the liking for the sweet taste because it signals a safe carbohydrate source of calories, and the rejection of bitterness because it may signal potential poisons (**Box 2-1**).

Preference for fat appears early in infancy or childhood. Fat is less a flavor than a contributor to texture (Mattes 2009). It imparts different textures to different foods: it makes dairy products such as ice cream seem creamy, meat juicy and tender, pastries flaky, and cakes moist. Many high-fat foods are those in which fat is paired with sugar (desserts) or salt (potato chips), enhancing their palatability. Foods containing fat are more varied, rich tasting, and higher in energy density than are nonfat foods and hence are more appealing.

A fifth taste has been identified: *umami*, a Japanese word for deliciousness, which is associated with the brothiness of soup or the meati-

Box **2-1 Meditation on Taste: A Nineteenth-Century Viewpoint**

Taste, such as Nature has given to us, is yet one of our senses (among others such as hearing and sight) that, all things considered, procures to us the greatest of enjoyments:

1. Because the pleasure of eating is the only one that, taken in moderation, is never followed by fatigue.
2. Because it belongs to all times, all ages, and all conditions.
3. Because it occurs necessarily at least once a day, and may be repeated without inconvenience two or three times in this space of time.
4. Because it can be combined with all our other pleasures, and even console us for their absence.
5. Because the impressions it receives are at the same time more durable and more dependent on our will.
6. Finally, because in eating we receive a certain indefinable and special comfort, which arises from the intuitive consciousness that we repair our losses and prolong our existence by the food we eat.

Source: Brillat-Savarin, A. S. 1825. *The physiology of taste: Meditations on transcendental gastronomy.* Reprinted 1949. Translated by M. F. K. Fisher. New York: Heritage Press. Reprinted 2000. Washington, DC: Counterpoint Press.

ness in mushrooms. It seems to be related to glutamate, an amino acid, and captures what is described as the taste of protein in food (de Araujo et al. 2003). In addition, because some taste buds are surrounded by free nerve endings of the trigeminal nerve, people are able to experience the burn from hot peppers and the coolness of menthol (Mela & Mattes 1988).

Individual Differences: Nontasters and Supertasters

Some genetic differences in sensitivity to tastes exist between individuals. Research shows that people differ in their responses to two bitter compounds called phenylthiocarbamide (PTC) and 6-*n*-propylthiouracil (PROP). When given PTC-impregnated paper or PROP in liquid form, some people cannot taste it and are labeled nontasters, others are medium tasters, and still others are supertasters. These individuals differ in the number of fungiform taste buds they have, with supertasters having the most taste buds and nontasters the least (Tepper & Nurse 1997). Such differences between individuals may be related to differences in being able to discriminate between different foods and may result in differences in liking for certain foods, such as some bitter vegetables, alcohol, citrus fruit, and fatty or sugary foods (Tepper & Nurse 1997; Duffy & Bartoshuk 2000; Kaminski, Henderson, & Drewnowski 2000). It has been suggested that such differences in responses to food may be related to food intake patterns and body weight variation (Tepper 1998, 2008; Keller & Tepper 2004).

Hunger and Satiety

Many genetic and biological mechanisms control hunger and satiety, ensuring that people will eat enough to meet their energy needs (de Castro 1999). Throughout most of human history, getting enough food was the primary challenge. The human body developed to function in an environment where food was scarce and high levels of physical activity were mandatory for survival. This situation resulted in the development of various physiological mechanisms that encourage the body to deposit energy (i.e., fat) and defend against energy loss (Neel 1962; Eaton, Eaton, & Konner 1997; Lowe 2003; Chakravarthy & Booth 2004). Today's environment, however, is one in which food is widely available, inexpensive, and often high in energy density, while minimal physical activity is required for daily living. Researchers have proposed that the "modern environment has taken body weight control from an instinctual (unconscious) process to one that requires substantial cognitive effort. In the current environment, people who are not devoting substantial conscious effort to managing body weight are probably gaining weight" (Peters et al. 2002). This means that nutrition education has an important role.

Sensory-Specific Satiety

Humans also appear to have a built-in biologically determined sensory-specific satiety mechanism whereby they get tired of one taste and move on to another one over a short time span, such as while eating a meal (Rolls 2000). Such a mechanism probably had adaptive value for humans because it ensures that people eat a variety of different-tasting foods and thus obtain all the nutrients they need from these foods. Studies also reveal that for adults, the variety of foods available influences meal size, with greater variety stimulating greater intake. Again, this mechanism might have been very useful in a situation of scarce food supply. However, in today's food environment, the variety possible in meals because of the wide array of foods available may contribute to overweight.

These biologically determined predispositions contribute to some degree to preference and to food intake, particularly in children, and are shown in **Figure 2-1**. However, as you shall see in the next section,

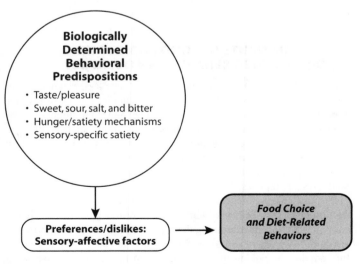

FIGURE 2-1 Our biologically determined behavioral predispositions that influence food choices and dietary behaviors.

most preferences are learned or conditioned—which is good news for nutrition educators because that means they can be modified.

Experience with Food

Research in this area suggests that people's liking for specific foods and food acceptance patterns are largely learned (Birch 1999; Mennella, Griffin, & Beauchamp 2004; Mennella & Beauchamp 2005; Beauchamp & Mennella 2009). Thus, what humans seem to inherit primarily is the innate capacity to learn about the consequences of eating particular foods. *Learning*, in this context, does not mean cognitive learning, but rather physiological learning or conditioning arising from the positive or negative consequences that people experience from repeated exposure to a food.

Pre- and Postnatal Experience

Such learning begins early, possibly even prenatally. Flavors such as garlic and alcohol have been detected in mothers' milk, possibly familiarizing infants with these flavors (Beauchamp & Mennella 2009). In one study, breastfed infants whose mothers were fed carrot juice during pregnancy or during lactation showed increased acceptance of carrot flavor in their cereal at weaning (Mennella, Jagnow, & Beauchamp 2001). In another study, infants who were fed a formula made of an unpleasant-tasting, sour and bitter protein hydrosylate from birth (from necessity because they did not tolerate milk) drank it well when tested with the hydrosylate formula at 7 months, whereas those fed milk formula rejected it (Mennella et al. 2004). Infants fed hydrosylate liked sour tastes into early childhood (Liem & Mennella 2002).

Learning from the Physiological Consequences of Eating: Preferences and Aversions

How humans feel physiologically after eating a food can have a powerful impact on food preferences. If eating is followed by negative effects, such as a feeling of nausea, a conditioned aversion follows. Conditioned aversions can be quite powerful. A one-time experience of illness following eating a food can turn individuals off that food for decades. On the other hand, liking for foods usually develops more slowly through a process of *learned* or *conditioned preference*, whereby repeated eating of a food, or familiarity, is followed by pleasant consequences such as a feeling of fullness or satiety.

Conditioning of food preferences continues throughout a person's life, but early experience with food and eating is especially crucial in the development of eating patterns, in terms of both the kinds of food the person comes to like and the amount he or she eats. Experience with food influences the development of eating patterns of children and adults in several ways.

Exposure, Familiarity, and Learning to Accept New Foods

Humans, like other omnivores, experience the "omnivore's dilemma": they need to seek variety in their diets to meet nutritional requirements, but ingesting new substances can be potentially dangerous (Rozin 1988). This dilemma can be resolved through familiarity and conditioning as described in the following sections.

Neophobia and Picky/Fussy Eating

Although food neophobia, or negative reactions to new foods, is minimal in infants, it increases through early childhood so that 2- to 5-year-olds, like other young omnivores, demonstrate neophobia (Birch 1999). This would have adaptive value because infants are fed by adults, but toddlers are beginning to explore their world and have not learned yet what

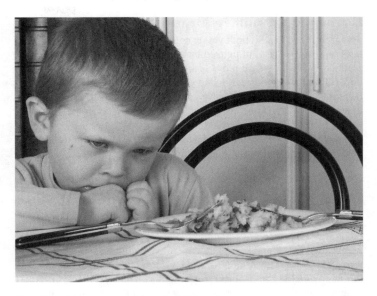

Neophobia increases through early childhood.

is safe to eat and what is not. However, neophobia can be reduced by repeated opportunities to sample new foods, sometimes requiring 12 to 15 exposures (Birch & Marlin 1982; Birch 1998, 1999), probably through a "learned safety mechanism." That is, when eating a food is not followed by negative consequences, increased food acceptance results. Once the foods are familiar, the preferences tend to persist (Skinner et al. 2002). In addition, tasting or actual ingestion has been found to be necessary—not just looking at or smelling the food (Birch, McPhee, Shoba, Pirok et al. 1987). Picky or fussy eating is somewhat different— it is the rejection of a large proportion of familiar (as well as novel) foods, tending to result in a diet that is lower in variety (Dovey et al. 2008). This quality tends to persist, even into adulthood, and may have a genetic component. Here, even more frequent food exposures may be necessary for acceptance to occur, presenting a challenge to parents and nutrition educators alike.

In sum, with repeated consumption, preference for initially novel foods tends to increase. Thus, if children are exposed to many high-sugar, high-fat, and high-salt foods at home, at school, and in other settings, then these foods will become more familiar and will become preferred over those that remain relatively unfamiliar, such as vegetables or whole grains.

Experience and the Basic Tastes

Biologically determined behavioral propensities can be modified by experience in adults as well (Pliner, Pelchat, & Grabski 1993; Pelchat & Pliner 1995). For example, those who eat lower-salt diets come to like them more (Beauchamp, Bertino, & Engelman 1983; Mattes 1997). The dislike for bitterness can be overcome, as shown by the infant study described earlier and by the fact that people come to like a variety of bitter tastes, such as coffee, dark chocolate, or bitter vegetables such as broccoli. Sour tastes, such as vinegar and grapefruit, can also become liked. Likewise the liking for dietary fat can be modified. Studies have found that those who switched from a high-fat diet to naturally low-fat foods such as grains and vegetables (Mattes 1993) or to reduced-fat foods (Ledikwe et al. 2007) came to like the fat taste less. Maintaining these changed preferences involved continuing to eat these new foods.

Learning What Fullness Means: Conditioned Satiety

Research shows that in both young children and adults, a feeling of fullness or satiety is also influenced by associative conditioning (Johnson, McPhee, & Birch 1991; Birch & Fisher 1995). The ability to learn about how full familiar foods can make you feel may explain how meals can be terminated before people have yet experienced the physiological cues that signal satiety. Thus, as a result of repeatedly consuming familiar foods, people learn about the "filling" and the "fattening" quality of familiar foods and normally make adjustments in what they eat in anticipation of the end of the meal (Stunkard 1975).

Our Preference for Calorie-Dense Foods

Humans seem to prefer calorie-dense foods over calorie-dilute versions of the same foods (Birch, McPhee, Shoba, Steinberg et al. 1987; Birch 1992). The biological mechanism that assists people to like calorie-dense foods was very adaptive when food, and especially calorie-dense food, was scarce and probably explains the universal liking for calorie-dense foods in adults. The finding that tasty high-fat and high-sugar foods induce overeating and obesity in animals (Sclafani & Ackroff 2004) suggests that this feature is less adaptive for humans in today's environment, where calorie-dense foods are widely available.

Learning from Social-Affective Context: Social Conditioning

The social-affective environment also has a powerful impact on food preferences and on the regulation of how much people eat. Food is eaten many times a day, providing opportunities for individuals' emotional responses to the social context of eating to become associated with the specific foods being eaten. This is particularly true in children.

Social Modeling

Children learn about food not only from direct experience of eating but also from observing the behaviors of peers and adults (Birch 1999). Familiar adults have been found to be more effective than unfamiliar ones, and having the adults themselves eat the same foods is more effective than when adults offer the foods without eating the foods themselves (Harper & Sanders 1975; Addessi et al. 2005). Food preferences also increase when adults offer the foods in a friendly way (Birch 1999).

Parenting Practices

Parenting practices related to food are strategies used to provide for the nourishment of children. The practices of parents, family, and other caregivers can encourage healthful eating or modify and interfere with the child's ability to respond to food appropriately. Parents and caregivers who offer healthful foods in appropriate portion sizes and enjoy the foods themselves are likely to facilitate healthful eating in their children. For example, children who are led to pay attention to their internal cues (feelings of hunger and being full) are more likely to be able to eat the appropriate amount of food than are those who are asked to focus on externally oriented cues such as the time of day or the amount of food remaining on the plate (Birch, McPhee, Shoba, Steinberg et al. 1987; Birch 1999). Children at age 3 eat about the same amount regardless of the portion size of the food offered. However, by age 5, children eat more when they are offered more (Rolls, Engell, & Birch 2000).

Rewards

The use of rewards has complex consequences (Birch 1999; Savage, Fisher, & Birch 2007; Ventura & Birch 2008). If a food is given as a reward, there is a significant *increase* in preference: "You did a good job cleaning up the toys. Here, have some peanuts." The opposite is true if the child is asked to eat a food to obtain a reward: "If you eat your spinach, you can watch TV." In particular, requiring eating of a less-liked food to obtain a better-liked food ("You can have dessert if you eat your spinach") can *decrease* even further the liking for the initially less-liked food because children reason (as do adults) that the food must taste bad if they have to be bribed to eat it. In addition, because the foods used as rewards are typically those high in sugar, fat, and salt (e.g., desserts and salty snacks), such a practice may enhance even further the preference for these items.

The Way Parents Offer Foods

Pressure to eat has been associated with lower levels of children's intake and weight and higher levels of pickiness. It could be the other way around also: that parents of picky eaters and thin children may apply pressure to eat (Ventura & Birch 2008). *Excessive restriction* of foods can make the restricted foods more attractive. Thus, highly restrictive parental controls limit the opportunities for children to practice self-regulation and maintain a healthy weight (Birch, Fisher, & Davison 2003; Faith et al. 2004). This can also result in overeating in the absence of hunger when given free access to an array of tasty snacks (Birch et al. 2003). However, in some populations, mothers' own flexible restraint can result in more healthful food choices for themselves and their children (Robinson et al. 2001; Contento, Zybert, & Williams 2005), this control being interpreted as expressing parental responsibility and caring (Lin & Liang 2005). At the same time, parents' own practices in terms of eating more fruits and vegetables highly influence what their daughters eat (Fisher et al. 2002). It has been concluded that the best practice is for adults to offer an array of *healthful* foods and for children to choose which of them to eat (Satter 2000). Thus, the practices of parents, child-care centers, and nutrition educators who work with young children can have important influences on the children's body weight and eating habits (Birch & Fisher 2000). Many of these same findings apply to adults as well and can inform the work of nutrition educators (Pliner et al. 1993).

Summary of Our Experience with Food

Biologically determined behavioral propensities, physiological mechanisms, and conditioning through experience with food all influence people's sensory experience of food and food preferences. These influences are summarized in **Figure 2-2**. Given that energy-dense, high-fat, high-sugar foods are widely available in the environment, tend to be used as rewards, are most often offered in positive social contexts such as celebrations and holidays, are liked by other family members, satisfy biological predispositions, and produce positive feelings of being full, it is not surprising that they become highly preferred by adults and children alike. On the other hand, fewer opportunities are provided for people to learn to like whole grains, fruits, and vegetables in similar social contexts.

Food preferences have a very direct impact on children's intakes because children tend to eat the foods they like and reject the foods they do not like in terms of taste, smell, or texture. The relationship between taste preferences and food choices is more indirect in older children and adults because experience with food and beliefs about the impact of food on weight, appearance, health, or other valued outcomes can modify their propensity to act on their preferences for high-fat and high-sugar foods. These considerations may lead individuals to eat more healthful diets even if these are not the most appealing, as we discuss in the next section.

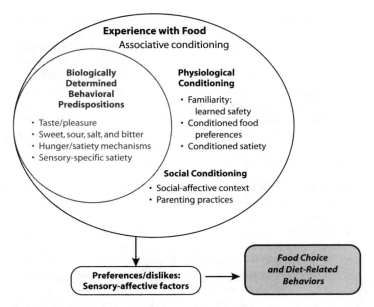

FIGURE 2-2 Our experiences with food that influence food choices and dietary behaviors.

■ PERSON-RELATED DETERMINANTS

Biology and personal experiences with food are not the only influences on individuals' food intake. People also develop perceptions, expectations, and feelings about foods. These perceptions, attitudes, beliefs, values, emotions, and personal meanings are all powerful determinants of food choice and dietary behavior, as are people's interactions with others in their social environment. These influences or determinants are shown in **Figure 2-3**.

Intrapersonal Determinants

Perceptions, Beliefs, Attitudes, and Motivations

Our food choices and dietary practices are influenced by a variety of personal factors, such as our beliefs about what we will get from these choices. We want our foods to be tasty, convenient, affordable, filling, familiar, or comforting. Our food choices may be determined by the personal meanings we give to certain foods or practices, such as chicken soup when we are ill, or chocolate when we feel self-indulgent. We may also be motivated by how the food will contribute to how we look, such as whether it will be fattening or, in contrast, good for our complexion. Our food- and nutrition-related behaviors are also determined by our attitudes toward them—for example, our attitudes toward breastfeeding or certain food safety practices. Our identity in relation to food may also influence our behaviors. For example, some teenagers may see themselves as health conscious, but many others may see themselves as part of the junk-food-eating set. We may see that there are health benefits to eating more healthfully but may consider the barriers, such as high cost or the effort required to prepare the foods in healthful ways, just too great to take action. Or perhaps we lack confidence in preparing foods in ways that are tasty and healthful. Or again, we may have specific culturally related health beliefs that influence what we eat. For example, although the concepts of balance and moderation are common among many cultures, individuals may come from cultures in which foods are believed to have hot and cold qualities and must be eaten in such a way as to balance cold and hot body conditions. These cultural beliefs can have a major influence on food choices.

We come to value some aspects of food over others. In the United States, the major values in choosing foods are taste, convenience, and cost (Glanz et al. 1998). In Europe, the major values are quality/freshness, price, nutritional value, and family preferences, in that order (Lennernas et al. 1997).

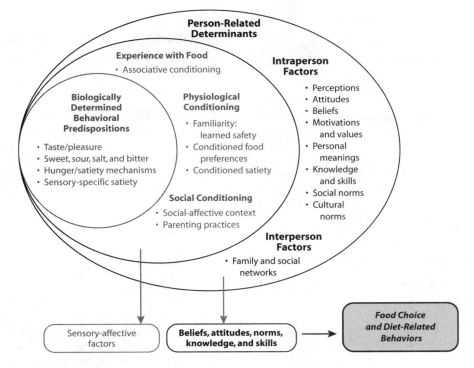

FIGURE 2-3 Intra- and interpersonal factors that influence food choices and dietary behaviors.

Food rejections are also highly influenced by psychological processes, based on both previous experience and beliefs. Rozin and Fallon (1987) place the motivations for rejecting foods into three main categories: (1) sensory-affective beliefs (e.g., the food will smell or taste bad) that lead to *distaste*, (2) anticipated consequences or beliefs about the possible harmful outcomes of eating certain foods (e.g., vomiting, disease, social disapproval), leading to *danger*, and (3) ideation or ideas about the origin or nature of foods, leading to *disgust*.

Knowledge regarding all these numerous person-related factors is crucial for nutrition educators so that we can better understand and assist our audiences to eat more healthfully.

The Process of Choosing Foods

Environmental Stimuli

Our thoughts and feelings interact with what we experience in the environment. For example, we you may see a news story on the role of fruits and vegetables in reducing cancer risk, or a friend of ours develops colon cancer (external stimuli). We process such environmental stimuli or external events both cognitively and emotionally. These stimuli are filtered through a host of internal personal reactions of the kind listed previously, such as our perceptions, beliefs, values, expectations, or emotions, and together these filters determine what actions we will take. For example, we may process the idea of eating more fruits and vegetables in terms of taste, convenience, expected benefits, perceived barriers, or what our friends and relatives do, in addition to our concerns about getting cancer. Consequently, our decisions about whether to eat more fruits and vegetables to reduce cancer risk are based on our beliefs and knowledge about *expected consequences* (of eating fruits and vegetables), our motivations and values about *desired consequences* (reduced risk of cancer), and our *personal meanings and values* (with respect to developing cancer).

Trade-Offs

In the food choice process, most times we will also need to make trade-offs among various criteria or reasons for food choice, such as among health considerations, taste, and cultural expectations. People may also trade off between items within a meal or between meals. For example, individuals may choose an item for its fillingness (e.g., a donut) but then balance it with something perceived as more healthful (e.g., orange juice). Or individuals may choose a "healthy" dinner to balance what they consider to have been a less than healthful lunch (Contento et al. 2006).

Knowledge and Skills

People's food-related knowledge and skills also influence what they eat. In particular, their misconceptions may play an important role. For example, a national survey found that about one third of individuals thought that the recommended number of servings of fruit and vegetables per day was one, and another third thought it was two; only 8% thought it was five (Krebs-Smith et al. 1995). Many consumers have major misconceptions about the amounts of fat and energy in many common foods and in their own diets (Mertz et al. 1991; Mela 1993; Brug, Glanz, & Kok 1997). Lack of skills in preparing foods also influences what individuals eat.

Social and Cultural Norms

Humans are social creatures. We all live in a social and cultural context and experience social norms and cultural expectations, which can be extraordinarily powerful. We feel compelled to subscribe to these norms and expectations to varying degrees. For example, teenagers may feel pressure to eat less-nutritious fast food items in a choice situation with peers (e.g., after school), or individuals may experience family members' expectations that they will eat in a certain way. Whether to breast-feed may be influenced very much by the desires of a woman's family. Our perceptions of our status and roles in our communities are also important. The food choices and eating patterns of celebrities create social expectations for us all. What others in our community think are appropriate foods to eat in various situations may also create social pressures. Thus, our choice of foods may be heavily influenced by our perceptions of the *social and cultural expectations* of those around us.

Interpersonal Determinants

Within societies, we all participate in a network of social relationships, the extensiveness and density of which vary among individuals. These networks involve family, peers, coworkers, and those in various organizations to which we belong. For example, in one study, food choices were 94% similar between spouses, 76% to 87% similar between adolescents and their parents, and 19% similar between adolescents and their peers (Feunekes et al. 1998). Food choices and eating patterns are also influenced by the need to negotiate with others in the family about what to buy or eat (Connors et al. 2001; Contento et al. 2006). Relationships with peers and those with whom we work also have an impact on our day-to-day choices (Devine et al. 2003).

Indeed, eating contexts and the management of social relationships in these numerous contexts play a major role in what people eat. For example, if a woman becomes motivated to reduce her fat intake by using nonfat milk instead of whole milk, she may find that other family members like whole milk and do not want to switch. She must decide whether to go along with family wishes or to buy low-fat milk separately for herself. She also must consider whether she has the space in the refrigerator to keep both types of milk, which then becomes a barrier to change.

■ SOCIAL AND ENVIRONMENTAL DETERMINANTS

Social and environmental factors are powerful influences on food choice and nutrition-related behaviors and must be considered by nutrition educators in planning programs.

Physical/Built Environment

The built environment includes all aspects of the environment that are modified by humans, including food outlets (e.g., grocery stores), homes, schools, workplaces, parks, industrial areas, and highways. There is a growing body of evidence that the built environments in relation to food and physical activity have important impacts on health (Sallis & Glanz 2009).

Food Availability and Accessibility

In developed countries and increasingly in less developed countries, food and processed food products are available in an ever-widening array of choices. More than 50,000 food items are available in U.S. supermarkets, and about 9,000 new brand-name processed food products are introduced each year (Gallo 1998; Lipton, Edmondson, & Manchester 1998). The typical shopper averages 2.2 trips to the supermarket each week (Food Marketing Institute 2005). Overall *availability* may be described as the array of food options that are present in the food system that are acceptable and affordable. *Accessibility* may be thought of as "immediate" availability, referring to the readiness and convenience of a food—whether the food requires little or no cooking, is packaged in a convenient way so that it can be eaten anywhere, or whether it can be stored for some time without spoilage.

Markets

Studies have shown that the availability of more healthful options in neighborhood grocery stores, such as fruits and vegetables or low-fat milk, is correlated with these foods being more available in the homes, which in turn is related to a higher quality of food choices and intakes (Cheadle et al. 1991; Morland, Wing, & Diez Roux 2002). Thus, what is available in the community influences what is purchased and consumed. The availability and accessibility of fruits and vegetables at home and school enable their consumption by children (Hearn et al. 1998). A study of data from 28,050 zip codes and the 2000 census found that low-income neighborhoods had only 75% as many chain supermarkets as middle-class neighborhoods and that African American neighborhoods had only 52% and Hispanic neighborhoods 32% as many chain supermarkets as in white neighborhoods (Powell et al. 2007). There is now discussion of "food deserts" in neighborhoods.

Accessibility also is dependent on where sources of food are physically located. Supermarkets, where a wide range of foods is available, may require transportation to reach, limiting the accessibility of food for many people, such as older people who are no longer able to drive or lower-income people without cars. The types of foods that are readily available in the local grocery stores, small corner stores, and restaurants within a given community depend on potential profits, consumer demand, and adequate storage and refrigeration facilities. The foods served or products stocked in them thus tend to be those that sell well, which are not always the most nutritious. Farmers' markets provide fresh, local foods but may require transportation to reach and are often only seasonal. Hence, some foods that are very important for health, such as fruits and vegetables, may not be readily accessible or are available only at a higher cost.

Workplaces, Schools, and Homes

Foods available at or near workplaces also tend to be those that are convenient, low in cost, and that sell well. In most schools, food is available and accessible. The National School Lunch Program provides meals that conform to federal guidelines that specify nutritional standards to be met. Increasingly, however, à la carte offerings, vending machines, and school stores compete for student participation; the foods available from these sources are not subject to these guidelines. Participation in the School Lunch Program declines with age so that by high school two thirds of students are obtaining their lunch from other sources. The majority of competitive foods in these other venues have been found to be high-fat and high-sugar items, including snack chips, candy, and soft drinks. It has been shown that what is available in school environments affects the dietary behaviors of children (Briefel et al. 2009). Within the home, accessibility means that a vegetable is not just available in the refrigerator but is already cut up and ready to eat, or fruit has been washed and is sitting on the counter ready to eat. The limited accessibility of healthful, convenient foods in many settings may narrow good choices and make it difficult to eat healthfully.

Built Environment and Physical Activity

The role of environmental determinants of physical activity has also been studied. The walk-ability of neighborhoods as well as the availability and accessibility of neighborhood safe parks, green spaces, and physical activity facilities have been shown to have some impact on physical activity or obesity of residents in those neighborhoods (Ferreira et al. 2007; Wendel-Vos et al. 2007).

Social Structures and Cultural Environment

Social environments and cultural contexts are no less important than the physical environment. Social influences and cultural practices all influence food choice and dietary behavior (Rozin 1996).

Social Relations

Society has been described as a group of people interacting in a common territory who have shared institutions, characteristic relationships, and a common culture. Most eating occurs in the presence of other people. The effect can be positive or negative in terms of healthful eating, in part because family and friends serve as models as well as sources of peer pressure. For example, there is evidence that eating with others can lead to eating more food compared with eating alone, especially when the others are familiar people (de Castro 1995, 2000). Spending more time at a meal eating with others also increases intake. Eating with others can result in pressure to eat higher-fat foods. On the other hand, eating with others can also result in pressure to try new foods that are healthy (MacIntosh 1996). Parents' own eating patterns likely influence that of their children (Fisher et al. 2002; Contento et al. 2005), and it has been shown that children and adolescents who eat with their families most days each week have better-quality diets than those who eat with their families less frequently (Gillman et al. 2000).

Cultural Practices and Family of Origin

Culture has been described as the knowledge, traditions, beliefs, values, and behavioral patterns that are developed, learned, shared, and transmitted by members of a group. It is a worldview that a group shares, and hence it influences perceptions about food and health. Cultural practices and family of origin have an important impact on food choices and eating practices even in modern, multiethnic societies where many different types of cuisine are available. Those from different regions of the country may have different practices. For example, for those from the American South a home-style meal is chicken-fried steak, mashed potatoes, corn bread, and bacon- and onion-laden green beans, with pie for dessert, whereas those who live in Texas may expect to eat barbecue

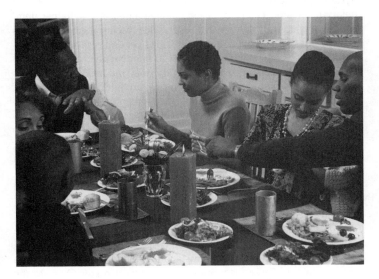

Families who eat together generally have better-quality diets.

or Tex-Mex foods that are hot and spicy. Those who have immigrated from different countries from around the world maintain some of their cultural practices in varying degrees, and these traditions influence eating patterns.

Cultural rules often specify which foods are considered acceptable and preferable, and the amount and combination of various categories of foods that are appropriate for various occasions. The cultural practices of family and friends, especially at times of special celebrations and holidays, provide occasions to eat culturally or ethnically determined foods and reinforce the importance of these foods. If dietary recommendations based on health considerations conflict with family and cultural traditions, individuals wanting to make dietary changes may find themselves having to think about and integrate their cultural expectations with their concern about their personal health. All of these considerations influence individuals' willingness and ability to make changes in their diets. These beliefs and practices must be carefully understood so that nutrition educators can become culturally competent and can design culturally sensitive nutrition education programs.

Social Structures and Policy

The organizations to which we belong can have a profound effect on our eating patterns. Some are voluntary organizations, such as religious, social, or community organizations; others include schools, our places of work, and professional associations to which we must belong. The influence of these organizations comes from their social norms as well as their policies and practices. Local, state, and national government policy can govern and determine the availability and accessibility of opportunities for healthy eating and active living.

■ ECONOMIC DETERMINANTS

Many factors in the economic environment influence food choices and dietary practices, among them price of food, income, time, and formal education. Nutrition educators must consider these factors when designing nutrition education programs.

Price

Economic theory assumes that relative differences in prices can partially explain differences among individuals in terms of their food choices and dietary behaviors. The price of food as purchased is usually per item, by unit weight, or by volume. However, price can also be considered in terms of the amount of food energy obtained per dollar. Processed foods with added fats and sugar are cheaper to manufacture, transport, and store than are perishable meats, dairy products, and fresh produce. This is partly because sugar and fat on their own are both very inexpensive, resulting in part from government agricultural policies. A diet made up of refined grains and processed foods with added sugar and fats can be quite inexpensive (a day's worth of calories for one to two dollars). Beans cost about the same, but animal protein sources may cost 5 to 10 times more per calorie, and fruits and vegetables (except potatoes and bananas) can cost some 50 to 100 times more per calorie than high-fat, high-sugar, mass-produced food products (Drewnowski & Barrett-Fornell 2004). When freely chosen diets were studied, it was found that adding fats and sweets was associated with a 5% to 40% decrease in overall food costs, whereas adding fruits and vegetables was associated with a 20% to 30% increase in overall food costs (Drewnowski, Darmon, & Briend 2004). Not surprisingly, low-income individuals eat fewer fruits and vegetables. These disparities in cost may also contribute to the higher prevalence of obesity in those of lower socioeconomic status.

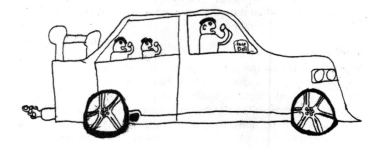

This child was asked to draw a picture of her family eating their favorite meal together.

Income

People in the United States spend only about 10% of their disposable income on food prepared and consumed at home, compared with 15% in Europe and Japan, 35% in middle-income countries, and 53% in low-income countries (Seale, Regmi, & Bernstein 2003). However, this is an average. The amount of money spent on food depends on income level. Upper-income individuals in the United States spend more money on food, but it is a smaller proportion of their income—about 8%. Lower-income households economize by buying more discounted items and generic brands and thus spend less on food; despite this, food accounts for 20% to 35% of their income (Putnam & Allhouse 1999). Compared with other economic variables, income has the strongest marginal impact (i.e., additional effect) on diet behavior: those with higher incomes eat a higher-quality diet (Macino, Lin, & Ballenger 2004).

In this context, statistics show that about 11% to 12% of American households are *food insecure*, meaning that they do not have access, at all times, to enough food for an active, healthy life for all household members. The prevalence of food insecurity with hunger is about 3% to 4%, hunger being defined as the uneasy or painful sensation caused by lack of food (Food Research and Action Council 2005).

Time Use and Household Structure

Surveys and time use diaries show that the amount of time people spend on food-related activity in the home depends on many factors, including whether men or women are employed outside the home and whether they have children (Robinson & Godbey 1999; National Pork Producers Council 2002; Cutler & Glaeser 2003).

Time is scarce for all households, regardless of income. Many people with whom nutrition educators work today say they are too busy to prepare healthful foods or to cook at all. This is particularly true of low-income families who often work long hours. For some households, time constraints may limit personal investments in healthier behaviors. For example, it has been found that men and women who are married with children have a higher-quality diet than single parents, probably because they are better able to attend to their own health (Macino et al. 2004). Nutrition educators need to consider these time constraints in the development of nutrition education interventions.

Education

In general, more highly educated individuals eat a higher-quality diet and are less sedentary partly because of watching less TV (Macino et al. 2004). People with more education may be better able to obtain,

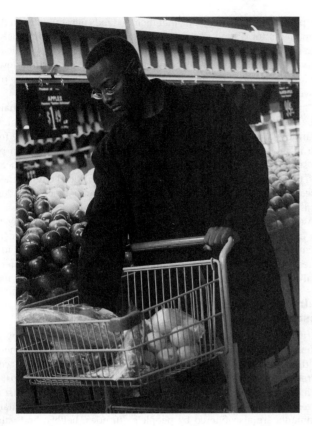

Consumers are inundated with food choices at the supermarket.

these various media is high: children ages 2 to 4 years are exposed to about 4 hours a day of various media. This increases to 8 hours a day in middle school, in consideration of the fact that adolescents often use several media simultaneously. Television viewing is dominant and increases to 25 hours per week through childhood, and then declines somewhat in adolescence to 19 hours a week as music becomes more important. Adults spend about 15 to 17 hours a week on television viewing. The media are the main source of information about food and nutrition for many people, making them collectively a major source of informal nutrition education. Information about food and nutrition is now widely covered in newspaper articles, magazines, and television programs. Many magazines are devoted to health and nutrition, and entire channels on TV are devoted to food-related shows. As **Nutrition Education in Action 2-1** shows, media and other influences also affect the decisions mothers make with regard to their children.

Advertising

The media have demonstrated a powerful capacity to persuade and the U.S. food system is the economy's largest advertiser (Gallo 1995). The food industry spends about $26 billion per year on marketing and advertising (Elitzak 2001), with $15 billion aimed at children. Most of this is spent by companies that produce high-fat and/or high-sugar products that are highly processed and packaged; examples include $150 million for candy bars, $580 million for soft drinks, and more than $1.5 billion for fast foods (Center for Science in the Public Interest 2003). Information on the impact of marketing on sales of food products is not easily available because it is considered proprietary information. However, there is evidence that these marketing activities influence food choices (Taras et al. 2000; Borzekowski & Robinson 2001; Story & French 2004; Institutes of Medicine 2006). In addition, federally sponsored promotions of commodities such as milk, cheese, grapefruit juice, and orange juice resulted in greater sales (Gallo 1996). Just for comparison, the National Cancer Institute's budget for its program to promote fruit and vegetable intake is about $4 million. The ubiquity of advertising, together with the amount of time people spend watching television and are exposed to marketing, makes these influences considerable. The environmental influences on food choice and dietary behavior are summarized in **Figure 2-4**.

process, interpret, and apply information that can make them more able to eat healthfully. They also may be more forward looking and optimistic about their future and thus willing to seek health information and make greater investments in their health (Macino et al. 2004).

Grocery Shopping Trends

The influences described earlier affect how people shop for food. Surveys of grocery shoppers have found that about one third of shoppers are *economizers*, who are budget conscious and usually come from lower-income households. They plan weekly menus, check for sales, and use coupons. Another third are *carefree spenders*, who are the least price conscious and least likely to compare prices and use coupons. The final third are *time-challenged* shoppers who are obsessed with convenience because of their hectic, multitasking lifestyles. They have the largest households and are most likely to have preteen children (Food Marketing Institute 2002).

■ INFORMATION ENVIRONMENT

Knowing the information context of the audience is important for nutrition educators to design messages and programs that are appropriate.

Media

The current media-saturated environment has undergone revolutionary changes in the past two decades, resulting in the availability to individuals and households of numerous television channels, radio stations, websites, and other emerging communication routes. Time spent on

■ IMPLICATIONS FOR NUTRITION EDUCATION

In Figure 2-4, a series of concentric circles schematically represents the ways in which biological, experiential, personal, social, and environmental determinants influence food choice and diet-related practices. No factor is independent of any other, but they are all related, each larger circle encompassing the influences of the smaller circles. These concentric circles reflect levels of influence or overlapping spheres of influence.

Addressing Food-Related Determinants

Addressing food-related determinants is very important in nutrition education. Food is a powerful primary reinforcer that produces instant gratification in taste and a sense of satisfaction and fullness. Because taste or preference is also shaped by repeated experience with foods and eating, nutrition educators working with any age group need to create opportunities to offer nutritious and healthy foods such as fruits and vegetables frequently in a positive social-affective context so that individuals will come to like nutritious foods. Similarly, interventions to decrease the intake of food components such as fat or salt should

NUTRITION EDUCATION IN ACTION **2-1**

Multiple Influences on Breastfeeding: A Study of Low-Income Mothers

Media influences: TV shows and print media foster the perception that formula feeding is the norm whereas breastfeeding is not. Instead, women's breasts are used to advertise lingerie, perfume, or alcohol: these images influence personal beliefs.

Policy influences: There is legislation that supports breastfeeding in the work setting. Legislation also requires low-income mothers to work, thus making breastfeeding difficult.

Community and organizational factors: Workplaces can be supportive or not. Baby-friendly hospitals can encourage breastfeeding, whereas free infant formula packages on discharge do not. Returning to work predicts quitting breastfeeding after having initiated it in the hospital.

Interpersonal factors: The father of the baby can be a major influence, followed by the mother's mother. Cultural beliefs are also a factor, such as the belief that women may not have enough milk, particularly when babies are "greedy."

Personal factors: Beliefs, knowledge, and skills. The study found that cultural beliefs positive to breastfeeding were often outweighed by personal beliefs or anticipation that breastfeeding would be painful. There also were concerns about the appropriateness of feeding in public settings because of sexual images in the media or the disapproval of the baby's father.

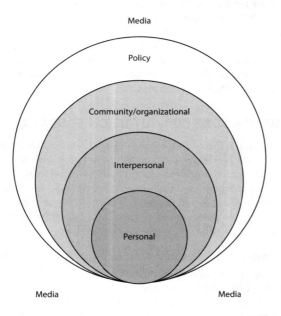

Source: Bentley, M. E., D. L. Dee, and J. L. Jensen. 2003. Breastfeeding among low-income, African-American women: Power, beliefs and decision-making. *Journal of Nutrition* 133:305S–309S. Used with permission of the American Society for Nutrition and the authors.

help people adopt eating plans that include foods naturally low in these components for a long enough time that people can become used to them and come to like them. Indeed, in a long-term nutrition education intervention with women, those who were able to stay with a low-fat diet for 2 years or more were those who came to dislike the taste of fat (Bowen et al. 1994).

The use of foods in positive contexts as rewards or treats enhances liking for those foods, whereas having people eat a food to obtain a reward likely produces a decline in liking for that food. Because foods high in fat, sugar, and salt are widely available, particularly in positive social-affective contexts such as celebrations, nutrition educators need to help people recognize the impact of such social environmental forces on their eating patterns and acquire the competencies to address them.

Although these mechanisms influence eating behaviors directly, they also exert their influence through psychological processes that can be perhaps even more powerful. Individuals develop attitudes toward foods, values, beliefs, and personal meanings, and these intra- and interpersonal determinants also influence food choices and eating patterns.

Addressing Environmental Determinants and Personal Perception

Nutrition education needs to address environmental factors by promoting the increased availability and accessibility of wholesome and healthful foods and active living options and by taking into account the resources people have, their social networks and relationships, and the influence of media and advertising. Nutrition education must also address social structures and policy. However, these environmental determinants are also filtered by people's attitudes, beliefs, and values, which in turn influence food choices and dietary behavior.

Availability: Reality and Perception

Availability, for example, means different things to different people. Recent immigrants may consider familiar food products "available" even if a long car or subway ride is needed to get to stores where the food is stocked. For others, a food is not available if it cannot be cooked in the microwave and ready to eat in 5 minutes. Such differences in the interpretation of availability influence individuals' food choices.

Economic Environment: Reality and Perception

Likewise, the economic environment is based on the analyses, values, and interpretations of individuals, all of which have an impact on dietary choices. Economics is a behavioral science based on the fundamental notion that human wants are infinitely expansible, whereas the means to satisfy them are finite. Human wants always exceed the means to satisfy them, and there is, therefore, scarcity. (This has been simplified to the statement that human greed is infinite whereas the means to satisfy that greed is finite.) Economics is the study of people's reaction to the fact of scarcity—how people make choices when they must choose among alternatives to satisfy their wants. Economics is concerned with desired *scarce* goods, not free goods, such as air in natural settings, because free goods do not present a problem of choice. Cost can be seen as the sacrifice, or what needs to be exchanged, to obtain what is desired. In this context, the full price of a food or dietary practice is not just its monetary price but includes all the costs or sacrifices individuals make, such as travel costs, time, or child-care costs while shopping. For example, a person may be willing to exchange money for time by purchasing a food that is already prepared. Nutrition educators need to learn about the sacrifices individuals are willing to make to engage in

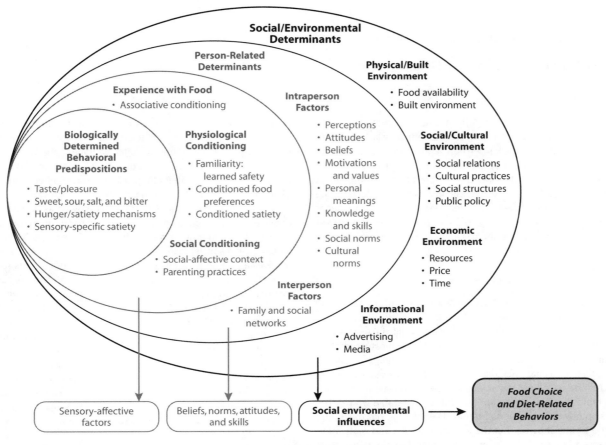

FIGURE 2-4 Social and environmental factors that influence food choices and dietary behaviors.

a healthy behavior. How willing are they to sacrifice convenience for more healthful meals?

Time: Reality and Perception

In the same way, time is both an objective feature of life and a perception. The time for food-related tasks such as cooking or eating can be easily quantified in hours and minutes. However, the *perception* of time and its worth to individuals for different tasks varies considerably. For example, the time required to make decisions about food has increased because information became more complex. There are about 50,000 items in a supermarket and about 9,000 new food items introduced each year that people must learn about. No longer do people choose from three or four types of cold breakfast cereal, but from whole supermarket aisles of cereals. This takes time.

In addition, people have become more avid consumers, and consumption takes time: it takes time to use all the gadgets and objects that people have acquired, particularly electronic devices such as cell phones, music players, and televisions. To overcome the scarcity of time, people do more than one thing at once, multitasking. Add to that the economic necessity of two jobs for many and it is not surprising that the perception is that there is not just scarcity of time, but a time famine. This has impacts that are important for nutrition educators. For example, low-wage employed parents find there is spillover from working long hours into family food-related tasks (Devine et al. 2006). There is stress and fatigue; parents reduce the time and effort spent on family meals,

they make trade-offs with other family needs, and they have to develop various time management strategies to cope. Nutrition educators need to be mindful of people's real and perceived economic and time constraints and how they make choices in light of these constraints. **Nutrition Education in Action 2-2** showcases programs that were created to work with economic and time constraints.

The Importance of Personal Perception

The point that is important for nutrition educators to understand is that although food-related factors and environmental context have significant independent influences on diet, they also influence the development of beliefs, attitudes, interpretations, feelings, and meanings, which in turn influence behavior. It becomes clear, then, that perceptions, attitudes, beliefs, and meanings play a central role in food-related behaviors. As Epictetus said many hundreds of years ago, "We are troubled not so much by events themselves but by the views we take of them." This is good news for nutrition educators because these perceptions, attitudes, and beliefs are to some extent modifiable through education.

Indeed, these perceptions and attitudes form a central focus of much of nutrition education. Thus, nutrition education can be seen as the process of addressing all the major categories of determinants as shown in **Figure 2-5**, with personal perception interacting with all of them. How these determinants of food choice and dietary behaviors can be effectively addressed through nutrition education activities is described in the remaining chapters in this book.

NUTRITION EDUCATION IN ACTION **2-2**

Programs to Accommodate Economic and Time Restraints

Barbershop Nutrition Education

Prostate cancer is twice as high in African American men as in white men. Eating fruits and vegetables may help to reduce risk. A novel site for nutrition education was the barbershop. A program was delivered to African American men while they were waiting for service. A set of five true or false statements was developed about the rate of prostate cancer in men and the role of fruits and vegetables in cancer risk reduction. The men were asked to answer them, and then the nutrition educator went over the answers. The men could keep the statements and the answer sheet. This simple intervention increased awareness of both prostate cancer and ways to reduce risk.

People at Work: 5-a-Day Tailgate Sessions

Because many people working in factories and other similar locations do not have time to go to a different site for nutrition education sessions, the nutrition educator can go to them. At one sawmill, the workers ate their lunches from coolers in their cars. The nutrition educator therefore met them in the parking lot and provided monthly tailgate sessions over the course of a year (including through the midwestern winter), providing a food each time that involved interesting ways to use fruits and vegetables (such as baked apples, chili, or vegetable wraps). The focus was on how to incorporate fruits and vegetables into meals and snacks. The results showed that the workers' interest and motivation were enhanced, as were skills in incorporating more fruits and vegetables in their diets.

Operation Frontline

Share Our Strength's Operation Frontline is a nationwide nutrition education program developed to address the root causes of hunger in the United States. Operation Frontline enables chefs, nutritionists, and dieticians to share their strengths by teaching interactive 6-week classes on nutrition and food budgeting to adults and children who are at risk of hunger. Operation Frontline classes make a concrete difference in the lives of program participants. The impact may be as basic as learning how to get a child to eat vegetables or how to cut up a chicken, or can be as profound as providing a starting point for a career in the culinary industry. One special feature is that after each class, each participant receives a bag of groceries containing all the ingredients needed to make that class's meal at home. Class participants then report to the instructors during the next class session on their success with making a meal at home and their families' reactions. Since its inception in 1993, more than 31,000 people have participated in Operation Frontline classes and an additional 89,000 have received nutrition information through nutrition fairs and events.

Sources: Magnus, M. H. 2004. Barbershop nutrition education. *Journal of Nutrition Education and Behavior* 36:45–46; Benepe, C. 2003. People at work: 5-a-Day tailgate sessions. Presentation, Annual Meeting of the Society for Nutrition Education, July 26, Philadelphia, PA; and Share Our Strength. n.d. What we do. http://www.strength.org/what/operationfrontline.

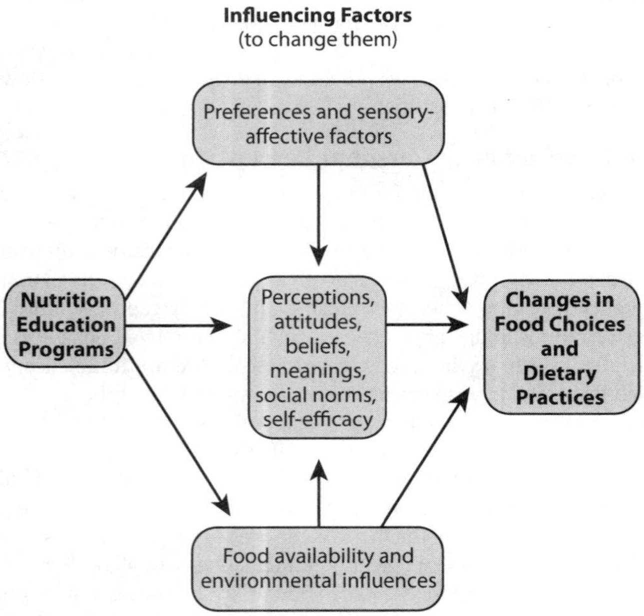

Influencing Factors
(to change them)

FIGURE 2-5 The process of nutrition education.

■ **IMPLICATIONS FOR COMPETENCIES AND SKILLS FOR NUTRITION EDUCATORS**

Nutritionists and dietitians are well grounded in nutrition science and clinical nutrition and are anxious to transmit what they know to a variety of audiences in exciting ways. They are less well grounded in the social sciences, particularly the behavioral sciences and the field of communications. Yet as we have seen, food choices and dietary behaviors are determined by a multitude of factors. Understanding behavior and its context is crucial for effective nutrition education. One approach might be for nutrition educators to deliver nutrition education through the use of teams, in which nutritionists focus only on providing the nutrition science content and behavioral specialists actually design and deliver the educational sessions. However, that is neither practical nor desirable. What the field needs is nutritionists who are sufficiently conversant with the relevant fields of behavioral science and communications to be able to design effective nutrition education programs. This book aims to help nutritionists develop these competencies.

The Society for Nutrition Education's Competencies for Nutrition Education Specialists

The Society for Nutrition Education (SNE) has adopted a list of the competencies that nutrition education specialists should have (Society for Nutrition Education 1987). The society believes that nutrition education specialists should be competent in the following five areas:

1. *Food and nutrition content:* Understanding the fundamentals of nutrition science, food science, and clinical nutrition; having the ability to accurately assess nutritional status of individuals and groups; applying appropriate dietary guidelines in making dietary recommendations
2. *Eating behavior:* Understanding the complexities of food supply systems and their effects on food selection; understanding the physiological, psychological, and environmental (social, cultural, and economic) determinants of eating behavior
3. *Behavioral and educational theory:* Ability to apply learning theory, instructional theory, and behavior change theories in nutrition education; in particular, use of theories and techniques from the behavioral sciences for modifying food behavior
4. *Research methods and program evaluation:* Ability to analyze and evaluate both popular and scientific literature, and to use appropriate designs and methods to conduct research and program evaluations in nutrition education
5. *Design and delivery of nutrition education:* Designing nutrition education programs, curricula, and materials; delivering nutrition education programs, including the ability to communicate with individuals, small groups, organizations, and mass audiences, to write clearly, and to use supplemental materials appropriately; implementing and administering nutrition education programs

American Dietetic Association's Competencies

The American Dietetic Association's standards for the education of entry-level dietitians (American Dietetic Association 2002) include some competencies that are relevant for nutrition education as well:

1. *Communications:* Graduates will have *knowledge of* negotiation techniques, lay and technical writing, media presentations, interpersonal communication skills, counseling theory and methods, interviewing techniques, educational theory and techniques, concepts of human and group dynamics, public speaking, and educational materials development. Also, graduates will have *demonstrated the ability* to use oral and written communications in presenting an educational session for a group, counsel individuals on nutrition, document appropriately a variety of activities, explain a public policy position regarding dietetics, use current information technologies, and work effectively as a team member.
2. *Social sciences:* Graduates will have *knowledge of* public policy development, psychology, and the health behaviors and educational needs of diverse populations.

3. *Nutrition:* Graduates will have *knowledge of* health promotion and disease prevention theories and guidelines.

■ SUMMARY

People's food choices and nutrition-related practices are determined by many factors. This has consequences for nutrition education.

Biology and Personal Experience with Food

Humans are born with biological predispositions toward liking the sweet and salt tastes and umami and rejecting sour and bitter tastes. Some genetic differences exist between individuals in sensitivity to tastes, and these may influence food choices. However, individuals' preferences for specific foods and food acceptance patterns are largely learned from familiarity with these foods. People's liking for foods thus can be modified by repeated exposure to them. Sense of fullness is also learned.

Person-Related Determinants

People acquire knowledge and develop perceptions, expectations, and feelings about foods. These perceptions, attitudes, beliefs, values, emotions, and personal meanings are all powerful determinants of food choice and dietary behavior. Families and social networks also influence food choices.

Social/Environmental Determinants

The *physical/built environment* influences the foods that are available and accessible as well venues for active living such as walkable streets and attractive parks. *Cultural practices* as well as *social structures and policy* make it easier or harder to be healthy. The *economic determinants* of behavior include price of food, income, time, and education. The *information environment*, including the media, is very powerful in influencing people's food choices.

Knowledge Is Not Enough

Consequently, knowledge is not enough for people to eat healthfully and live actively. Nutrition education must address all these determinants of behavior if it is to be effective.

Consequences for the Skills of Nutrition Educators

These considerations make it clear that nutrition educators need a set of skills in addition to their knowledge of food and nutrition. We need to develop the skills to understand people, their behavior, and the context of their behavior.

Questions and Activities

1. List at least five biological predispositions people are born with, and describe each in a sentence or so. Are they modifiable? If so, provide the evidence. How can the information be useful to nutrition educators?

2. One often hears parents say that their child will just not eat certain healthful foods, such as vegetables. They believe that such dislikes cannot be changed. Based on the evidence, what would you say to such a parent?

3. How can nutrition educators help young children learn to self-regulate the amount of food they eat?

4. "You can have dessert if you eat your spinach." Is this a strategy you would recommend to parents and child-care personnel to use to get children to like spinach? Why or why not?

5. Influences on dietary behavior arising from within the person have been stated to be central to his or her food choices and dietary practices. Why is this so? Describe three of these influences in a sentence or two, and indicate why they are so important. How might understandings of these personal factors help people make dietary changes?

6. People live within social networks and may experience cultural expectations about how and what they eat. Because these can't be changed by nutrition education, why should nutrition educators be interested in such information about their intended audience?

7. Distinguish between food availability and food accessibility. How can they influence food choice? How might nutrition educators address these issues?

8. Describe four environmental factors that influence people's food choices and dietary practices. What can nutrition educators do with such information?

9. Think about the influences on your eating and physical activity behaviors and list them. Compare them to the categories of influences described in this chapter. Into which categories do the items on your list fall? Are there some surprises? How would you describe the motivations for your eating patterns?

10. As stated earlier, in terms of healthy eating and active living, "knowledge is not enough." In your view, is that true? Why do you say so? Give evidence for your view.

11. In reviewing the competencies suggested by the Society for Nutrition Education for a nutrition educator, which competencies do you believe that you already possess? Which ones would you like to develop further? Keep these in mind as you read the remainder of this book.

References

Addessi, E., A. T. Galloway, E. Visalberghi, and L. L. Birch. 2005. Specific social influences on the acceptance of novel foods in 2–5-year-old children. *Appetite* 45(3):264–271.

American Dietetic Association. 2002. *CADE accreditation handbook*. Chicago: American Dietetic Association, Commission on Accreditation for Dietetics Education.

Balzer, H. 1997. *The NPD Group's 11th annual report on eating patterns in America: National eating trends tracking*. Port Washington, NY: NPD Group.

Beauchamp, G. K., M. Bertino, and K. Engelman. 1983. Modification of salt taste. *Annals of Internal Medicine* 98(5 Pt 2):763–769.

Beauchamp, G. K., and J. A. Mennella. 2009. Early flavor learning and its impact on later feeding behavior. *Journal of Pediatric Gastroenterology and Nutrition* 48(Suppl 1):S25–S30.

Bernstein, I. 1990. Salt preference and development. *Developmental Psychology* 2(4):552–554.

Birch, L. L. 1992. Children's preferences for high-fat foods. *Nutrition Reviews* 50(9):249–255.

———. 1998. Psychological influences on the childhood diet. *Journal of Nutrition* 128(2 Suppl):407S–410S.

———. 1999. Development of food preferences. *Annual Review of Nutrition* 19:41–62.

Birch, L. L., and J. A. Fisher. 1995. Appetite and eating behavior in children. *Pediatric Clinics of North America* 42(4):931–953.

Birch, L. L., and J. O. Fisher. 2000. Mothers' child-feeding practices influence daughters' eating and weight. *American Journal of Clinical Nutrition* 71(5):1054–1061.

Birch, L. L., J. O. Fisher, and K. K. Davison. 2003. Learning to overeat: Maternal use of restrictive feeding practices promotes girls' eating in the absence of hunger. *American Journal of Clinical Nutrition* 78(2):215–220.

Birch, L. L., and D. W. Marlin. 1982. I don't like it; I never tried it: Effects of exposure on two-year-old children's food preferences. *Appetite* 3(4):353–360.

Birch, L. L., L. McPhee, B. C. Shoba, E. Pirok, and L. Steinberg. 1987. What kind of exposure reduces children's food neophobia? Looking vs. tasting. *Appetite* 9(3):171–178.

Birch, L. L., L. McPhee, B. C. Shoba, L. Steinberg, and R. Krehbiel. 1987. Clean up your plate: Effects of child feeding practices on the conditioning of meal size. *Learning and Motivation* 18:301–317.

Borzekowski, D. L., and T. N. Robinson. 2001. The 30-second effect: An experiment revealing the impact of television commercials on food preferences of preschoolers. *Journal of the American Dietetic Association* 101(1):42–46.

Bowen, D. J., M. M. Henderson, D. Iverson, E. Burrows, H. Henry, and J. Foreyt. 1994. Reducing dietary fat: Understanding the successes of the Women's Health Trial. *Cancer Prevention International* 1:21–30.

Briefel, R. R., M. K. Crepinsek, C. Cabili, A. Wilson, and P. M. Gleason. 2009. School food environments and practices affect dietary behaviors of US public school children. *Journal of the American Dietetic Association* 109(2 Suppl):S91–S107.

Brug, J., K. Glanz, and G. Kok. 1997. The relationship between self-efficacy, attitudes, intake compared to others, consumption, and stages of change related to fruit and vegetables. *American Journal of Health Promotion* 12(1):25–30.

Center for Science in the Public Interest. 2003. *Pestering parents: How food companies market obesity to children*. Washington, DC: Author.

Chakravarthy, M. V., and F. W. Booth. 2004. Eating, exercise, and "thrifty" genotypes: Connecting the dots toward an evolutionary understanding of modern chronic diseases. *Journal of Applied Physiology* 96(1):3–10.

Cheadle, A., B. M. Psaty, S. Curry, E. Wagner, P. Diehr, T. Koepsell, and A. Kristal. 1991. Community-level comparisons between the grocery store environment and individual dietary practices. *Preventive Medicine* 20(2):250–261.

Clark, J. E. 1998. Taste and flavour: Their importance in food choice and acceptance. *Proceedings of the Nutrition Society* 57(4):639–643.

Connors, M., C. A. Bisogni, J. Sobal, and C. M. Devine. 2001. Managing values in personal food systems. *Appetite* 36(3):189–200.

Contento, I. R., S. S. Williams, J. L. Michela, and A. B. Franklin. 2006. Understanding the food choice process of adolescents in the context of family and friends. *Journal of Adolescent Health* 38(5):575–582.

Contento, I. R., P. Zybert, and S. S. Williams. 2005. Relationship of cognitive restraint of eating and disinhibition to the quality of food choices of Latina women and their young children. *Preventive Medicine* 40(3):326–336.

Cutler, D. M., and E. L. Glaeser. 2003. *Why have Americans become more obese?* Cambridge, MA: Harvard Institute of Economic Research, Harvard University.

de Araujo, I. E., M. L. Kringelbach, E. T. Rolls, and P. Hobden. 2003. Representation of umami taste in the human brain. *Journal of Neurophysiology* 90(1):313–319.

de Castro, J. M. 1995. The relationship of cognitive restraint to the spontaneous food and fluid intake of free living humans. *Physiology and Behavior* 57:287–295.

———. 1999. Behavioral genetics of food intake regulation in free-living humans. *Journal of Nutrition* 7(8):550–554.

———. 2000. Eating behavior: Lessons learned from the real world of humans. *Nutrition* 16:800–813.

Desor, J. A., O. Mahler, and L. S. Greene. 1977. Preference for sweet in humans: Infants, children, and adults. In *Taste and the development of the genesis for the sweet preference*, edited by J. Weiffenbach. Bethesda, MD: U.S. Department of Health, Education, and Welfare.

Devine, C. M., M. M. Connors, J. Sobal, and C. A. Bisogni. 2003. Sandwiching it in: Spillover of work onto food choices and family roles in low- and moderate-income urban households. *Social Science Medicine* 56(3):617–630.

Devine, C. M., M. Jastran, J. Jabs, E. Wethington, T. J. Farell, and C. A. Bisogni. 2006. "A lot of sacrifices": Work–family spillover and the food choice coping strategies of low-wage employed parents. *Social Science Medicine* 63(10):2591–2603.

Dovey, T. M., P. A. Staples, E. L. Gibson, and J. C. Halford. 2008. Food neophobia and "picky/fussy" eating in children: A review. *Appetite* 50(2–3):181–193.

Drewnowski, A., and A. Barrett-Fornell. 2004. Do healthier diets cost more? *Nutrition Today* 39:161–168.

Drewnowski, A., N. Darmon, and A. Briend. 2004. Replacing fats and sweets with vegetables and fruits—a question of cost. *American Journal of Public Health* 94(9):1555–1559.

Duffy, V. B., and L. M. Bartoshuk. 2000. Food acceptance and genetic variation in taste. *Journal of the American Dietetic Association* 100(6):647–655.

Eaton, S. B., S. B. Eaton III, and M. J. Konner. 1997. Paleolithic nutrition revisited: A twelve-year retrospective on its nature and implications. *European Journal of Clinical Nutrition* 51(4):207–216.

Elitzak, H. 2001. Food marketing costs at a glance. *Food Review* 24(3):47–48.

Faith, M. S., K. S. Scanlon, L. L. Birch, L. A. Francis, and B. Sherry. 2004. Parent–child feeding strategies and their relationships to child eating and weight status. *Obesity Research* 12(11):1711–1722.

Ferreira, I., K. van der Horst, W. Wendel-Vos, S. Kremers, F. J. van Lenthe, and J. Brug. 2007. Environmental correlates of physical activity in youth—a review and update. *Obesity Reviews* 8(2):129–154.

Feunekes, G. I., C. de Graaf, S. Meyboom, and W. A. van Staveren. 1998. Food choice and fat intake of adolescents and adults: Associations of intakes within social networks. *Preventive Medicine* 27(5 Pt 1):645–656.

Fisher, J. O., D. C. Mitchell, H. Smiciklas-Wright, and L. L. Birch. 2002. Parental influences on young girls' fruit and vegetable, micronutrient, and fat intakes. *Journal of the American Dietetic Association* 102(1):58–64.

Food Marketing Institute. 2002. *Shopping for health 2002*. Washington, DC: Author.

———. 2005. *Supermarket facts: Industry overview 2004*. Washington, DC: Author.

Food Research and Action Council. 2005. *Hunger in the U.S.* http://frac.org/html/federal_food_programs/federal_index.html.

Gallo, A. E. 1995. The food marketing system in 1994. In *Agricultural Information Bulletin No. 717*. Washington, DC: U.S. Department of Agriculture.

———. 1996. The food marketing system in 1995. In *Agricultural Information Bulletin No. 717*. Washington, DC: U.S. Department of Agriculture.

———. 1998. The food marketing system in 1996. In *Agricultural Bulletin No AIB743*. Washington, DC: U.S. Department of Agriculture, Economic Research Service.

Gillman, M. W., S. L. Rifas-Shiman, A. L. Frazier, et al. 2000. Family dinner and diet quality among older children and adolescents. *Archives of Family Medicine* 9(3):235–240.

Glanz, K., M. Basil, E. Maibach, J. Goldberg, and D. Snyder. 1998. Why Americans eat what they do: Taste, nutrition, cost, convenience, and weight control concerns as influences on food consumption. *Journal of the American Dietetic Association* 98(10):1118–1126.

Harper, L. V., and K. M. Sanders. 1975. The effects of adults' eating on young children's acceptance of unfamiliar foods. *Journal of Experimental Child Psychology* 20:206–214.

Hearn, M. D., T. Baranowski, J. Baranowski, et al. 1998. Environmental influences on dietary behavior among children: Availability and accessibility of fruits and vegetables enable consumption. *Journal of Health Education* 19:26–32.

International Food Information Council (IFIC) Foundation. 1999. Are you listening? What consumers tell us about dietary recommendations. *Food insight: Current topics in food safety and nutrition*. Washington, DC: Author.

Institutes of Medicine. 2006. *Food marketing to children and youth: Threat or opportunity*. Washington, DC: Institute of Medicine, National Academies Press.

Johnson, S. L., L. McPhee, and L. L. Birch. 1991. Conditioned preferences: Young children prefer flavors associated with high dietary fat. *Physiology and Behavior* 50(6):1245–1251.

Kaminski, L. C., S. A. Henderson, and A. Drewnowski. 2000. Young women's food preferences and taste responsiveness to 6-*n*-propylthiouracil (PROP). *Physiology and Behavior* 68(5):691–697.

Keller, K. L., and B. J. Tepper. 2004. Inherited taste sensitivity to 6-*n*-propylthiouracil in diet and body weight in children. *Obesity Research* 12(6):904–912.

Krebs-Smith, S. M., J. Heimendinger, B. H. Patterson, A. F. Subar, R. Kessler, and E. Pivonka. 1995. Psychosocial factors associated with fruit and vegetable consumption. *American Journal of Health Promotion* 10(2):98–104.

Ledikwe, J. H., J. Ello-Martin, C. L. Pelkman, L. L. Birch, M. L. Mannino, and B. J. Rolls. 2007. A reliable, valid questionnaire indicates that preference for dietary fat declines when following a reduced-fat diet. *Appetite* 49(1):74–83.

Lennernas, M., C. Fjellstrom, W. Becker, et al. 1997. Influences on food choice perceived to be important by nationally-representative samples of adults in the European Union. *European Journal of Clinical Nutrition* 51(Suppl 2):S8–S15.

Liem, D. G., and J. A. Mennella. 2002. Sweet and sour preferences during childhood: Role of early experiences. *Development Psychobiology* 41(4):388–395.

Lin, W., and I. S. Liang. 2005. Family dining environment, parenting practices, and preschoolers' food acceptance. *Journal of Nutrition Education and Behavior* 37(Suppl1):P47.

Lipton, K. L., W. Edmondson, and A. Manchester. 1998. *The food and fiber system: Contributing to the U.S. and world economies*. Washington, DC: Economic Research Service, U.S. Department of Agriculture.

Lowe, M. R. 2003. Self-regulation of energy intake in the prevention and treatment of obesity: Is it feasible? *Obesity Research* 11(Suppl):44S–59S.

Macino, L., B. H. Lin, and N. Ballenger. 2004. The role of economics in eating choices and weight outcomes. In *Agricultural Information Bulletin No 791*. Washington, DC: U.S. Department of Agriculture, Economic Research Service.

MacIntosh, W. A. 1996. *Sociologies of food and nutrition*. New York: Plenum Press.

Mattes, R. D. 1993. Fat preference and adherence to a reduced-fat diet. *American Journal of Clinical Nutrition* 57(3):373–381.

———. 1997. The taste for salt in humans. *American Journal of Clinical Nutrition* 65(2 Suppl):692S–697S.

———. 2009. Is there a fatty acid taste? *Annual Review of Nutrition* 29:305–327.

Mela, D. 1993. Consumer estimates of the percentage energy from fat in common foods. *European Journal of Clinical Nutrition* 47:735–740.

Mela, D. J., and R. D. Mattes. 1988. The chemical senses and nutrition: Part 1. *Nutrition Today* 23(March/April):4–9.

Mennella, J. A., and G. K. Beauchamp. 1996. The early development of human flavor preferences. In *Why we eat what we eat*, edited by E. D. Capaldi. Washington, DC: American Psychological Association.

Mennella, J. A., and G. K. Beauchamp. 2005. Understanding the origin of flavor preferences. *Chemical Senses* 30(Suppl 1):i242–i243.

Mennella, J. A., C. E. Griffin, and G. K. Beauchamp. 2004. Flavor programming during infancy. *Pediatrics* 113(4):840–845.

Mennella, J. A., C. P. Jagnow, and G. K. Beauchamp. 2001. Prenatal and postnatal flavor learning by human infants. *Pediatrics* 107(6):E88.

Mertz, W., J. C. Tsui, J. T. Judd, et al. 1991. What are people really eating? The relation between energy intake derived from estimated diet records and intake determined to maintain body weight. *American Journal of Clinical Nutrition* 54(2):291–295.

Morland, K., S. Wing, and A. Diez Roux. 2002. The contextual effect of the local food environment on residents' diets: The atherosclerosis risk in communities study. *American Journal of Public Health* 92(11):1761–1767.

National Pork Producers Council. 2002. The kitchen survey. In *The kitchen report*. Urbandale, IA: Author.

Neel, J. V. 1962. Diabetes mellitus: A "thrifty" genotype rendered detrimental by "progress"? *American Journal of Human Genetics* 14:353–362.

Pelchat, M. L., and P. Pliner. 1995. "Try it. You'll like it." Effects of information on willingness to try novel foods. *Appetite* 24(2):153–165.

Pepino, M. Y., and J. A. Mennella. 2005. Factors contributing to individual differences in sucrose preference. *Chemical Senses* 30(Suppl 1):i319–i320.

Peters, J. C., H. R. Wyatt, W. T. Donahoo, and J. O. Hill. 2002. From instinct to intellect: The challenge of maintaining healthy weight in the modern world. *Obesity Reviews* 3(2):69–74.

Pliner, P., M. Pelchat, and M. Grabski. 1993. Reduction of neophobia in humans by exposure to novel foods. *Appetite* 20(2):111–123.

Powell, L. M., S. Slater, D. Mirtcheva, Y. Bao, and F. J. Chaloupka. 2007. Food store availability and neighborhood characteristics in the United States. *Preventive Medicine* 44(3):189–195.

Putnam, J. J., and J. E. Allhouse. 1999. *Food consumption, prices, and expenditures, 1970–97 (Statistical Bulletin No. 965)*. Washington, DC: U.S. Department of Agriculture, Food and Rural Economics Division, Economic Research Service.

Robinson, J. P., and G. Godbey. 1999. *Time for life: The surprising ways Americans use their time*. 2nd ed. University Park: Pennsylvania State University Press.

Robinson, T. N., M. Kiernan, D. M. Matheson, and K. F. Haydel. 2001. Is parental control over children's eating associated with childhood obesity? Results from a population-based sample of third graders. *Obesity Research* 9(5):306–312.

Rolls, B. 2000. Sensory-specific satiety and variety in the meal. In *Dimensions of the meal: The science, culture, business, and art of eating*, edited by H. L. Meiselman. Gaithersburg, MD: Aspen Publishers.

Rolls, B. J., D. Engell, and L. L. Birch. 2000. Serving portion size influences 5-year-old but not 3-year-old children's food intakes. *Journal of the American Dietetic Association* 100(2):232–234.

Rozin, P. 1988. Social learning about food by humans. In *Social learning: Psychological and biological perspectives*, edited by T. R. Zengall and G. G. Bennett. Hillsdale, NJ: Lawrence Erlbaum.

———. 1996. Sociocultural influences on human food selection. In *Why we eat what we eat: The psychology of eating*, edited by E. D. Capaldi. Washington, DC: American Psychological Association.

Rozin, P., and A. E. Fallon. 1987. A perspective on disgust. *Psychology Review* 1:23–41.

Sallis, J. F., and K. Glanz. 2009. Physical activity and food environments: Solutions to the obesity epidemic. *Milbank Quarterly* 87(1):123–154.

Satter, E. 2000. *Child of mine: Feeding with love and good sense*. 3rd ed. Boulder, CO: Bull Publishing.

Savage, J. S., J. O. Fisher, and L. L. Birch. 2007. Parental influence on eating behavior: Conception to adolescence. *Journal of Law and Medical Ethics* 35(1):22–34.

Sclafani, A., and K. Ackroff. 2004. The relationship between food reward and satiation revisited. *Physiology and Behavior* 82(1):89–95.

Seale, J., A. Regmi, and J. Bernstein. 2003. *International evidence on food consumption patterns (Technical Bulletin No 1904)*. Washington, DC: U.S. Department of Agriculture, Economic Research Center.

Shepherd, R. 1999. Social determinants of food choice. *Proceedings of the Nutrition Society* 58(4):807–812.

Skinner, J. D., B. R. Carruth, B. Wendy, and P. J. Ziegler. 2002. Children's food preferences: A longitudinal analysis. *Journal of the American Dietetic Association* 102(11):1638–1647.

Small, D. M., and J. Prescott. 2005. Odor/taste integration and the perception of flavor. *Experimental Brain Research* 166(3–4):345–357.

Society for Nutrition Education. 1987. Recommendations for the Society for Nutrition Education on the academic preparation of nutrition education specialists. *Journal of Nutrition Education* 19(5):209–210.

Story, M., and S. French. 2004. Food Advertising and Marketing Directed at Children and Adolescents in the US. *International Journal of Behavioral Nutrition and Physical Activity* 1(1):3.

Stunkard, A. 1975. Satiety is a conditioned reflex. *Psychosomatic Medicine* 37(5):383–387.

Taras, H., M. Zive, P. R. Nader, C.C. Berrym, T. Hoy, and C. Boyd. 2000. Television advertising and classes of food products consumed in a pediatric population. *Journal of Advertising* 19:487–494.

Tepper, B. J. 1998. 6-*n*-Propylthiouracil: A genetic marker for taste, with implications for food preference and dietary habits. *American Journal of Human Genetics* 63(5):1271–1276.

———. 2008. Nutritional implications of genetic taste variation: The role of PROP sensitivity and other taste phenotypes. *Annual Review of Nutrition* 28:367–388.

Tepper, B. J., and R. J. Nurse. 1997. Fat perception is related to PROP taster status. *Physiology and Behavior* 61(6):949–954.

U.S. Department of Agriculture. 2000. Beliefs and attitudes of Americans towards their diet. In *Nutrition insight*. Washington, DC: Center for Nutrition Policy and Promotion, U.S. Department of Agriculture.

Ventura, A. K., and L. L. Birch. 2008. Does parenting affect children's eating and weight status? *International Journal of Behavioral Nutrition and Physical Activity* 5:15.

Wendel-Vos, W., M. Droomers, S. Kremers, J. Brug, and F. van Lenthe. 2007. Potential environmental determinants of physical activity in adults: A systematic review. *Obesity Reviews* 8(5):425–440.

An Overview of Nutrition Education: Facilitating Why and How to Take Action

OVERVIEW

This chapter introduces the reader to behavior-focused nutrition education and provides an overview of how behavioral science theory and nutrition education research can help increase nutrition education effectiveness.

CHAPTER OUTLINE

- Introduction
- Nutrition education
- Addressing the determinants of action and behavior change
- Addressing multiple influences on behavior
- Designing strategies for nutrition education
- A logic model approach for planning nutrition education
- Summary

LEARNING OBJECTIVES

At the end of the chapter, you will be able to:

- Explain what is meant by a behavior- or action-focused approach to nutrition education
- Appreciate the primary role of nutrition education in addressing the determinants of behavior
- Discuss how nutrition behavior theory and nutrition education research can provide a map for how to design effective nutrition education
- Critique the importance of theory in research and practice
- Describe the three components of nutrition education and the educational goal for each
- Describe a conceptual framework for theory-based nutrition education

■ INTRODUCTION

Alicia is a 19-year-old high school graduate who works in a busy dentist's office as an administrative assistant. She knows she should eat lots of fruits and vegetables, but at lunchtime she likes to eat food that is filling and can be picked up fast and eaten quickly. She would much rather eat a slice of apple pie than an apple.

Ray is in his mid-40s. His weight just crept up on him, a pound or two each year, and now he is about 40 pounds overweight. He would like to lose the weight, but it seems so hard.

If nutrition education is a combination of educational strategies and environmental supports to facilitate behaviors conducive to health, what can nutrition educators do to assist people like Alicia or Ray to eat more healthfully?

When health professionals first became interested in promoting health and facilitating change in health-related behavior, the emphasis was on providing information to patients and to the public. The assumption was that when individuals such as Alicia and Ray became well informed, they would take the necessary actions to avoid disease and improve their health, such as getting vaccinations, eating healthfully, attending health screenings, or stopping smoking. Consequently, much of health and nutrition education was knowledge-based. However, analyses of the results of health campaigns revealed that information alone was not sufficient to lead to the desired behavior. For most people, health is not an end in itself but a means to an end: the ability to do what they want to do in life to achieve the goals they have; for example, to do well in school or work, have a good relationship, or to enjoy sports or a vacation. Thus, taking actions related to health in the absence of symptoms is not a high priority for most. In the area of food, too, eating healthfully is not an end in itself for most people. Eating is about providing essential nourishment for life's many other activities and is a source of pleasure and enjoyment. And people's food choices are influenced by a myriad of factors. So, the question is, how can nutrition education programs best assist people to eat more healthfully? How can healthful eating become a source of pleasure and enjoyment? What factors contribute to making health behavior change programs more effective?

Elements Contributing to Nutrition Education Effectiveness

In a comprehensive review of nutrition education around the world between 1900 and 1970, Whitehead (1973) comes to some very broad conclusions about what made nutrition education effective: nutrition education was a factor in improving dietary practices when changing behavior was clearly specified as a goal, when appropriate educational methods were used, when individuals themselves were actively involved in problem solving, and when an integrated community approach was used. However, she notes that there was a need for better-designed studies to provide specific information on effective methods and techniques for nutrition education.

Increased interest in health promotion and chronic disease prevention in the 1970s led to the publication by the U.S. government of the first *Dietary Guidelines for Americans* in 1980, the Food Guide Pyramid in 1993 (now MyPyramid), and the first Healthy People policy document in 1990, all focusing on assisting the public to eat more healthfully to improve health and prevent chronic disease. Whereas prevention of nutrient deficiencies involved *adding* specific foods to the diet, health promotion and chronic disease or obesity prevention now requires *changes* in what is eaten and how much—a much more difficult task. Research in the area of diet and physical activity has been very active in the past two decades, partly because of government and public concerns about preventing chronic disease and obesity and improving health. Such research has generated findings that are very useful for nutrition education practice (Contento et al. 1995; Ammerman et al. 2002; Bowen & Beresford 2002; Baranowski et al. 2003; Pomerleau et al. 2005; Stables et al. 2005; Doak et al. 2006; Sharma 2006; Howerton et al. 2007; Lemmens et al. 2008; Shaya et al. 2008; Brown et al. 2009). These studies extend the earlier findings of Whitehead in a number of ways. They all agree that nutrition education is more likely to be effective when it includes the following:

- *A focus on behaviors/practices:* Nutrition education *focuses on specific individual actions and behaviors and community practices* that are of importance to the individuals themselves, to communi-

ties, or to the larger society. These behaviors may also serve larger goals of value to the individual or community.

- *Determinants of behavior:* Nutrition education *clearly identifies the factors influencing the behaviors* of the intended audience and makes modifying these influencing factors (determinants or potential mediators of the desired behavior change) the direct target of nutrition education interventions rather than merely providing general information.

- *Use of theory:* Nutrition education *uses theory and evidence* to design nutrition education.

- *Multiple levels and sufficient duration:* Nutrition education *attends to the multiple levels of determinants* of food choice and eating (and physical activity) behaviors and uses multiple channels to convey messages with significant intensity over a sufficient period of time.

- *Strategies:* Nutrition education *develops strategies to address the identified determinants* of behaviors or potential mediators of change and their environmental contexts at various levels of influence.

These elements of effectiveness are explored in the following sections. They also form the foundation of this book.

■ NUTRITION EDUCATION: A FOCUS ON BEHAVIORS, ACTIONS, AND PRACTICES

Nutrition education is more likely to be effective when the central focus of the program or activities is on addressing the specific food choice behaviors, nutrition-related actions, or community dietary practices that influence health and well-being rather than on simply disseminating food or nutrition information in a general manner. This behavior-focused approach to nutrition education is one that uses a set of educational strategies, accompanied by relevant environmental supports, to facilitate dietary behavior change or actions related to food and health. Dietary behaviors can include the following:

- Food choices or observable behaviors related to health, such as eating sufficient fruits and vegetables a day, following a lower-fat diet, consuming smaller portions of food, or even eating breakfast or healthy snacks

- Behaviors and practices related to food, such as food safety practices, food preparation or cooking, managing food-related resources, obtaining foods from farmers' markets, or vegetable gardening

- Behaviors related to other nutrition-related concerns, such as breastfeeding

- Specific physical activities, such as running, walking, bicycling, or playing baseball, because physical activity has been shown to be important for health and maintaining a healthy weight

Focusing on Specific Behaviors, Actions, or Practices Improves Effectiveness

A behavior-focused approach means that the outcomes expected are changes in behaviors, patterns of behavior/practices, or policies. The desired long-term outcomes are improvements in health or in quality of life for individuals or communities, or both. If an intervention seeks to reduce cardiovascular and cancer risk, it might focus on a pattern of behaviors that involves eating more fruits, vegetables, and whole grains and fewer foods high in saturated fat. If the intervention seeks to reduce excessive gain in weight, it can focus on these same behaviors along with the behaviors of controlling portions of high-energy-dense foods and increasing physical activity. If the intervention seeks to increase choice of local produce by low-income families, then a policy action or "behavior" results in Supplemental Nutrition Assistance Program electronic debit transfer (EBT) cards being accepted at farmers' markets.

The specific behaviors to be addressed are identified from the needs, perceptions, and desires of the intended audience, as well as from national nutrition and health goals and nutrition science–based research findings. Behaviors must of course be addressed and framed within their social context because behaviors both influence and are influenced by their social and environmental context.

Focusing on specific individual behaviors or patterns of behavior and community practices is especially important now that promoting health and reducing chronic disease and obesity have become major aims of nutrition education. As one research scientist said at the time the first *Dietary Guidelines* came out, "In the past, the message was, in essence, to eat more of everything. Now we are faced with the difficult problem of teaching the public to be more discriminating. Increasingly, the message will be to eat less" (Hegsted 1979). For those who are food insecure, a focus on specific patterns of behavior or practices can also contribute to improved health within the constraints they face.

Food and Nutrition-Related Behaviors Can Be Part of Broader Goals

For example, schools may institute gardens so as to increase children's fruit and vegetable intakes. But they could also help children learn where food comes from and serve science education goals. A school garden can also make the school grounds more attractive and make school children feel that the school cares. This may increase school attendance and hence academic achievement.

Critical Thinking Skills and Autonomy Are Still Important

A behavior- or action-focused approach does *not* mean that food and nutrition information is not important. Indeed, for many complex food and nutrition behaviors, a good deal of information may be needed, along with critical thinking skills. However, it does mean that the information provided by the intervention should be relevant to the behaviors and practices being targeted and should be designed to assist individuals to become willing and able to take action. Neither does it mean that nutrition education should be directed at manipulating people's behaviors to make them more healthful in the old behaviorist sense. Individuals change their behaviors only when they themselves see a need to do so and want to make a change. Nutrition education must both honor and foster such autonomy and self-responsibility through dialogue and debate (Buchanan 2004).

Popular author John C. Maxwell (2000) puts it this way: "People change when they hurt enough that they have to, learn enough that they want to, and receive enough that they are able to."

◼ ADDRESSING THE DETERMINANTS OF ACTION AND BEHAVIOR CHANGE

Nutritionists tend to think of nutrition knowledge and skills as the main (or even only) influence of importance to address in nutrition education.

Consequently, much of nutrition education has been knowledge-based. However, Chapter 2 demonstrates that there are many overlapping spheres of influence on or determinants of behavior. Thus, nutrition education must address these multiple determinants, as shown in **Figure 3-1**. Indeed, as shown in the figure, *knowledge and skills is only one category among many that influence behavior*. More specifically, human biology and experience with food and environmental factors exert their influence on food choice and dietary practices not only directly but also through people's interpretations of the world. These powerful psychological processes (perceptions, beliefs, values, and attitudes) are key influences on what people do. Nutrition education thus needs to be directed primarily at these powerful influences on behavior, along with supportive activities in the environment, such as ensuring that school lunches are healthy or that there are adequate playgrounds for children. Indeed, studies show that knowledge is clearly less important than these psychological processes (Shepherd & Towler 2007).

Need for Behavioral Sciences to Help

Because people's actions and behaviors are influenced by so many factors, we need help from our colleagues in the behavioral sciences, such as psychology, anthropology, economics, and communications, to help us understand and address these many influences. Indeed, research shows that nutrition education is more likely to be effective when it seeks to understand and address these numerous influences on behavior and behavior change. As has been noted, "it is a major paradigm shift to change the target of nutrition education from the goal of increasing knowledge to that of modifying factors that influence dietary behaviors" (Baranowski et al. 2003). The central mission of nutrition education, then, is to design activities that address the many influences on behavior that have personal relevance for a particular group.

Determinants and Mediators of Change

Influences on why people eat what they do are usually called *determinants of behavior*. In the context of nutrition education, this means *modifiable* determinants such as perceptions, attitudes, or feelings and even some environmental factors, as opposed to nonmodifiable ones such as socioeconomic status or educational level. Nutrition educators seek to understand not only the determinants of people's current eating and physical activity patterns but also determinants of why and how people make changes in these patterns. When these determinants of change are addressed in a nutrition education program, they are often called *potential mediators of behavior change* (Baranowski et al. 1997). The most effective way to assist people to make changes in their dietary practices is to identify the determinants of their current diets as well as the determinants that can potentially mediate behavior change.

To design and conduct nutrition education, therefore, we must identify the determinants of dietary behaviors and potential mediators of behavior change for a given group and prioritize them in order to develop strategies to address them (Baranowski et al. 2009).

Theory as a Guide for Nutrition Education

So, how shall nutrition educators go about designing these educational strategies and environmental support activities? Just knowing a list of the determinants of behavior or of potential mediators of behavior change does not necessarily help educators design more effective nutrition education strategies. Some factors may be more important than others in truly mediating behavior change for a given group or for a specific behavior. Given limited time and resources, we must choose the factors that are most relevant in mediating dietary change and tar-

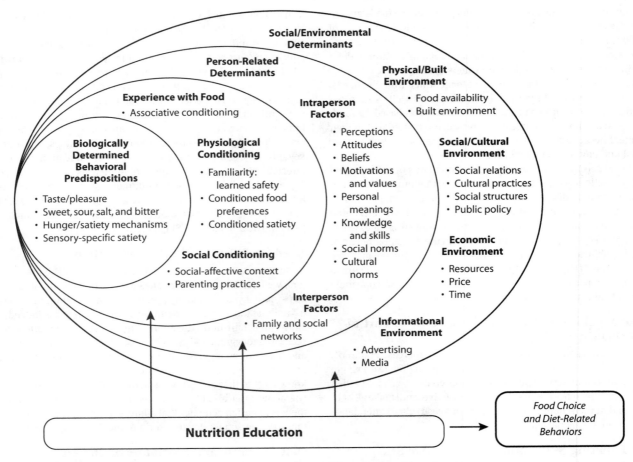

FIGURE 3-1 Factors influencing food choice and dietary behaviors and the role of nutrition education.

get them using appropriate educational strategies. How do we know which of the potential mediators are more important than others? Are these mediators related to each other? And if so, how do we know their relationships to each other?

This is where theory comes in: to act as a guide.

What Is Theory?

Just as a physical map is an abstract representation of some geographical space, so theory, in its simplest terms, is a *mental map* derived from evidence that helps us understand how some part of the world works. A comprehensive, and widely used, definition in the social sciences is that theory is a set of interrelated constructs (or concepts) that present a systematic view of phenomena (e.g., eating fruits and vegetables) by specifying relations among the constructs to *explain* and *predict* these phenomena (Kerlinger 1999). Theory in the area of behavioral nutrition and physical activity has also been described more simply as "a generalized and carefully interpreted, systematic summary of empirical evidence" (Brug, Oenema, & Ferreira 2005). That is, theory explains and/or predicts behavior.

Consequently, theory provides a map of how the many determinants of people's food choices or mediators of food- and nutrition-related behavior change (shown in Figure 3-1) are related to each other and to behavior. Behavioral nutrition and nutrition education research evidence then tells which of these determinants are more important than others for which behaviors and with which people. This kind of information

is very important so that we can better develop nutrition education programs that enable people to change their behavior if they choose to do so. (See **Box 3-1**.)

Theory Enhances Effectiveness

A founder of the field of social psychology, Kurt Lewin, said, "There is nothing so practical as a good theory" (Lewin 1935). Conducting nutrition education requires considerable resources in terms of time, money, and personnel, which are all usually in short supply. Thus, as nutrition educators we want to conduct nutrition education activities that make the most effective use of these resources. We can do that only if our nutrition education programs are based on evidence. If theory is the interpreted summary of evidence, presented in the form of a conceptual map, then we need theory to guide our work. If we do not use evidence-based theories, we must rely on guess-work or our own experience. These may be very effective, but also may not be—usually there is no evidence to know.

Theory Is Based on Evidence

Theories are developed when there is a need to find a solution to a problem or an explanation for some observation. In the case of nutrition education, the purpose of theory is to describe the nature and strength of the relationships of various hypothesized potential mediators (such as beliefs or barriers) to the behavior change or action. Theories can come from quantitative or interpretative investigations.

$\mathcal{B}ox$ 3-1   **Why Theory Is Important to Nutrition Educators: A Summary**

Theory is a conceptual model or a mental map representing how potential mediators influence behavior or behavior change. Mediators in real life are represented as constructs or variables in a theory. Theory is important to nutrition educators for the following reasons:

- Theory provides a mental map of *why* a behavior or behavior change occurs. It is not just a list of influences on behavior or behavior change. Such a map helps nutrition educators identify the specific set of mediators of behavior change that should be addressed in a nutrition education intervention.
- Theory specifies the *kinds of information* that need to be gathered before designing an intervention. It helps nutrition educators separate relevant from irrelevant mediators for a given group and behavior.
- Theory also provides nutrition educators guidance on exactly *how to design* the various intervention components and educational strategies to reach people more effectively.
- Theory provides guidance on exactly what to *evaluate* to measure the impact of the intervention, and how to design accurate measuring instruments.
- Theory is generated from research in nutrition education and related fields, using both qualitative and quantitative approaches.

Experimental Studies to Generate and Test Theory

Most behavioral science theories use experimental designs to examine the extent to which determinants or mediators explain and predict behaviors as hypothesized by theory; that is, to generate information on cause-and-effect relationships between determinants or potential mediators and behavior. These studies can involve quantitative research based on survey methods such as questionnaires or interviews, experiments, or randomized control trials, in which numerical data are analyzed quantitatively. Such methods can also be used to test theory and explore its generalizability to various populations.

Qualitative or Interpretative Studies to Generate Theory and Enhance Understanding

Qualitative studies can provide rich descriptions of food-related motivations and behaviors. In this formulation, theories are not developed for their predictive power but because they can be used to help provide a clearer understanding of people's life situations. Here, instead of reducing the information acquired from research into a small set of constructs and examining the quantitative relationships among them, in-depth interviews and other qualitative methods are used to generate a rich description of the ways people engage with food, incorporating their own meanings and understandings (Strauss & Corbin 1990). Themes that emerge are recorded, analyzed, and interpreted. Various procedures are used to ensure that findings are trustworthy.

Both Experimental and Interpretive Studies Are Important

Because both the experimental and interpretative approaches attempt to understand more clearly people's motivations and actions with respect to food and nutrition and are empirical in nature, both approaches are important to use, and they often converge. Thus, experimental and interpretive studies can both generate theories or abstract representations—conceptual models or mental maps—of some aspect of reality that can help nutrition educators better understand the world of the people with whom they work and better assist these people in attaining their own health and life goals. Reviews of nutrition education conclude that programs are more likely to be successful when they use appropriate theory and evidence to guide their choice of activities (Achterberg & Lytle 1995; Contento et al. 1995; Baranowski et al. 2003).

None of the research and the theories derived from them provides a complete explanation of food choice and dietary behavior change. Researchers can only infer the true reasons why people do what they do from what people say and what they do. Members of the public are not necessarily being untruthful about why they eat what they do; rather, people often do not know why they do what they do or how to go about making healthful changes. For example, individuals, particularly adolescents, insist that they are not influenced by others in their environment. Yet they all are. Knowing themselves is not easy! In addition, their reasons for what they do may change from time to time and differ by specific behavior.

Best Practices

Sometimes evidence accumulates from practice and can be generalized as "best practices" that can be useful to others.

All nutrition educators use theory. As nutrition educators, we all use theory and research or evidence to guide our work, whether we are aware of it or not. For example, there are hundreds of possible nutrition issues to discuss with consumers, students, or clients, and there are dozens of methods of doing so; the moment we choose a topic or a method, we are demonstrating that we have used a set of assumptions, or theory, to guide our choices and have drawn upon accumulated experience, or evidence. Indeed, it is impossible *not* to employ some kind of theory when making choices of what to cover and how.

Making Theory Explicit Is Important

It is helpful for us to make explicit the theory guiding our work, because we then have the opportunity to build in specific components based on the theory and to observe which components are useful and which are not. For example, will adding a module dealing with peer pressure, which theory suggests is important, enhance breastfeeding outcome compared with teaching only the basic information about the nutritional benefits of breastfeeding? Making a theory explicit also helps practitioners develop appropriate teaching activities (e.g., role playing of peer pressure situations and group suggestions of how to respond) and evaluation instruments (e.g., measurements of peer pressure as well as nutrition knowledge). The result is that we can draw conclusions from our work that will be helpful the next time around

Many Theories from the Behavioral Sciences Can Be Helpful

Nutrition education during the past two decades has increasingly drawn on theories from related fields to guide it, particularly psychosocial theories. The question often comes up, Why are there so many different theories used to study dietary behavior and design nutrition education? Why not just one? Most of the theories used in nutrition education originated in the behavioral sciences, food choice research, health education, or related fields. They were each developed to explain specific kinds of behavior that were of interest for different reasons:

- *Health behavior theories:* Psychologists interested in public health developed a few theories specifically to explain why people did or did not take some action that might prevent a negative health condition, such as participation in immunizations to prevent polio or screenings for HIV infection. These theories emphasize health beliefs.
- *Food choice theories:* Other researchers were interested in food choice. These researchers were not necessarily interested in health. They wanted to find out what people wanted in their foods—taste, cost, convenience, texture, and so forth. Health might or might not have been an important concern. These researchers produced theories of food choice (Conner & Armitage 2002).
- *Social behaviors:* Still other theories were originally developed to explain a variety of people's day-to-day behaviors, such as purchasing various goods, voting, participating in organizations, selecting a college to go to, and so forth. These theories sought to identify and understand both intrapersonal and interpersonal influences on behavior.

As nutrition educators, we recognize that eating behavior is complex, involving many settings and situations and influenced by many internal and external factors that often conflict with each other. We are interested in people's health beliefs with respect to food, nutrition, and physical activity. But we are also interested in why and how people make food choices in general. Because food is most often eaten in social contexts and may involve negotiations with others, we are keenly interested in theories of social interactions as well.

Thus, as nutrition educators we have to draw on all these theories to provide a more complete picture of why people eat what they do and how they change. No single behavioral theory, as an abstract representation of reality, may be able to capture all the factors influencing people's food- and activity-related behaviors. Different theories may be useful for different behaviors and different settings. We shall see, however, that there is some overlap among the various theories. Consequently, there has been a call for the use of multiple theories (Achterberg & Miller 2004) and more comprehensive theories (Triandis 1979; Kok et al. 1996; Fishbein 2000; Institute of Medicine 2002).

Components of Theory

Each of the influences on behavior is a determinant of behavior or a potential mediator of behavior change and hence can be represented as a construct in a theory. Some theories are more complex than are others, and some have been more thoroughly conceptualized and intensively studied than have others. Each theory uses unique terms to describe the factors influencing behavior or specific concepts that are important for the theory based on its origins. Often these terms are similar across theories; this is noted below where appropriate. Some of the themes generated from interpretive studies are also similar to constructs in standard health behavior change theories. Some clarifications are provided here.

Constructs and Variables

The influences on behavior that we have described so far as determinants of behavior or potential mediators of behavior change, such as beliefs, benefits, emotions, and attitudes, are the building blocks of theories.

- *Constructs:* When these determinants or mediators are systematically used in a particular theory they are called *constructs*, or

mentally constructed ideas about unobservable, intangible attributes (beliefs, attitudes) that are part of the theory. They exist in the mind as abstractions about some aspect of human experience. No one has observed "beliefs" about salt in the diet or "attitudes" toward breastfeeding. Yet, researchers can talk about them and measure them. For example, if a person believes that there are benefits to taking a specific health action, such as reducing salt intake reduces risk of hypertension, this belief can influence whether he adds salt to food. This belief about benefits becomes the "perceived benefits" construct in the health belief model.
- *Variables:* The term *variable* is often used synonymously with *construct*, but variables are really the operational definitions of constructs, specifying how a construct is to be measured for a specific situation. They are "variables" because they can vary in value. Thus, the perceived benefits of taking a specific action, such as the benefit of eating fruits and vegetables to reduce cancer risk, can be measured on a 1 to 5 scale. Individuals may judge the same specific benefit differently: some individuals may judge eating fruits and vegetables to reduce cancer risk as highly beneficial, giving it a score of 5, whereas others as only moderately so, giving it a score of 2 or 3.

These constructs are content-free in that the theory does not specify what the benefits are. Information about each construct must be obtained from any given audience or group through means such as in-depth interviews or quantitative surveys. For example, the benefits of eating fruits and vegetables for adults may be their role in prevention of chronic disease, but for adolescents the benefits may be clear skin and help in controlling weight.

Theory, Conceptual Model, and Theoretical Framework

The terms *model, conceptual model, theory,* and *theoretical framework* are often used to describe similar ideas:

- *Model* or *conceptual model* usually describes relationships between two or more constructs, focusing on *how* they relate. Sometimes a model is created by using constructs from several compatible theories, based on evidence.
- *Theory* is often used to describe a clearly stated set of relationships among core constructs, such as beliefs or emotions, to *explain* behavior or behavior change.
- *Theoretical framework* refers to a description of a set of concepts in relation to each other. It tends to be less formal than a theory.

However, these terms are similar to each other and overlapping, and definitions are not standardized. In this book, we use the terms as given by the researchers who developed and tested them. That is, if they refer to their mental map as a theory (e.g., the "theory of planned behavior"), we use the word *theory*; if they use the term *model* (e.g., the "health belief model"), we use the word *model*. The term *theory*, when used in a general sense in this book, refers to all these specific theories and models.

The *health belief model*, for example, provides a description or mental map of how various determinants of a health action or behavior are related to each other and to behavior. The *theory of planned behavior* attempts to explain a variety of behaviors not necessarily linked to health and provides mathematical relationships, based on research evidence, between the mediators of behavior and behavior itself.

Moderators

Sometimes determinants or mediators such as beliefs may be important for one group of people but not another. For example, in one study "overall health concern" was found to be an important determinant of food choice for husbands but not wives, whereas the opposite was true for the determinant "beliefs about convenience." In this case, gender was a moderator of the influence of the mediators "health concern" and "convenience" on the outcome, food choice.

Thus, *moderators* are factors that modify the influence of a determinant or potential mediator on the behavior. Examples of other possible moderators are ethnicity and educational level. That is, a nutrition education intervention may work in one ethnic group but not in another, or with those at some educational levels but not others.

Relationships Among Research, Theory, and Practice

Research has been defined as "careful or diligent search; investigation or experimentation aimed at the discovery and interpretation of facts; revision of accepted theories or practical application of such new or revised theories" (Merriam-Webster 2003). Research and theory are thus interrelated. Theory is a dynamic entity. Research generates theory; at the same time, theory is guided by, and tested through, research and practice. Stated more simply, theory is not divorced from practical experience but is in fact experience that has been systematically explored and reflected upon.

At the same time, theory can be tested, refined, and modified as it is applied in interventions in practice settings and its effectiveness is evaluated (Rothman 2004). Thus, theory, research, and practice all need each other.

An Overview of Theories of Dietary Behavior and Behavior Change

What can the theories generated from research tell about health and nutrition behaviors and behavior change that are useful for nutrition education? This section provides a general overview of relevant theory. Specific theories and their use in nutrition education are explored in greater detail in the following chapters.

The Knowledge-Attitude-Behavior Model

An approach commonly used in nutrition education, whether it is made explicit or not, is the knowledge-attitude-behavior (KAB) model. This model proposes that as people acquire knowledge in the nutrition and health areas, their attitudes change. Changes in attitude then lead to changes in behavior. Thus, the role of nutrition education is to provide a target audience with new information about nutrition or health, with the assumption that this information will lead to changes in attitudes, which in turn will result in improved dietary behavior or practices. The primary motivator is assumed to be accumulation of knowledge. This is shown in **Figure 3-2**. This would seem to be logical because knowledge at some level is essential for making healthful choices. The importance of information seems to be corroborated when millions can switch from eating "low-fat" diets to eating "low-carb" diets or the other way around in a matter of weeks, based on news reports that one is supposed to be better than the other for weight control. However, this phenomenon is really more about people's interest in the quick fix than about changed behaviors resulting from new scientific evidence or information. Witness the difficulty of getting people to eat more fruits and vegetables, despite health campaigns.

Different Kinds of Knowledge

Because humans are thinking beings, all their actions are related in some way to knowledge and understanding, often accompanied by feelings and emotions (Bandura 1986). However, there are many ways to conceptualize knowledge.

Instrumental or how-to knowledge: In most nutrition education programs, *knowledge* refers to understanding basic facts about food and nutrition, such as food groups or balanced diets; knowing the key features of MyPyramid; being able to read food labels; identifying food sources of nutrients; knowing how to store and prepare foods; shopping wisely; managing food budgets; and so forth. This kind of knowledge can be described as *instrumental* or *how-to knowledge*. It is essential for those already motivated to eat healthfully or who perceive some personal health risk. It may also be motivating for people who are highly disciplined or those who will eat according to accumulating scientific knowledge, who may be called cognitive or conscientious eaters. In this context, it should be noted that misinformation and misconceptions about food and nutrition can cause problems for those wishing to eat healthfully. Indeed, health literacy, an individual's ability to read, understand, and use health care information to make decisions and follow instructions for treatment, is very important for those with nutrition-related conditions who want to manage their conditions (Institute of Medicine 2004).

For most people, however, this kind of knowledge is not motivational. Such how-to knowledge is unlikely to lead to improved attitudes or behaviors in those who are not interested or motivated (Backett 1992; Moorman & Matulich 1993). Indeed, the scientific evidence for the link between the knowledge component of the KAB model and behavior is weak (Baranowski et al. 2003). In nutrition education intervention studies in which the "dissemination of information" or "teaching of skills" models were effective, the audiences were self-selected and already motivated (Contento et al. 1995).

Motivational or why-to knowledge: On the other hand, knowledge can be motivating and can lead to changes in attitudes and behaviors when it is about the consequences of the actions of individuals and communities. Thus, knowledge can be motivating when it consists of nutrition science–based evidence that eating certain foods, consuming nutrients, or eating according to certain patterns is related to specific health outcomes.

Such science-based information that has motivational power may be described as *why-to knowledge* because it provides reasons that nutrition educators can give to individuals about *why to* make a particular food choice or dietary change, such as why to eat more fruits and vegetables, why to eat more calcium-rich foods, or why to buy from local farmers. Such reasons are also called *outcome beliefs* because they are beliefs about the outcomes of a specific nutrition action such as eating fruits and vegetables. These outcome beliefs form the basis of the social psychological theories described later.

Social Psychological Theories of Health Behavior and Behavioral Change

Much of the work in the health behavior area is based on the pioneering thinking of Kurt Lewin, a leading social psychologist who emphasizes that the function of social psychology is to understand the relationships between an individual and the social environment (Lewin et al. 1944). He takes a phenomenological approach, which emphasizes that it is the world as it is perceived by the individual perceiver that most powerfully influences what the individual will do. He is thus interested in developing a psychological approach that explains both inner experiences and observable behavior from the person's own point of view. The environment or situation is also important. Lewin holds that "every psychological event depends upon the state of the person and at the same time on the environment, although their relative importance is different in different cases" (Lewin 1936). Recent nutrition education programs have used social psychological theories. See **Figure 3-3**.

The social psychological approach emphasizes the following:

- *The power of the situation:* People are creatures of their cultures and social contexts.
- *The power of the person:* At the same time, individuals construct their social world and have an impact on it. Facing the same situation, different people may react differently.
- *The power of cognition:* People's beliefs or cognitions about the world powerfully influence how they react to it. Social reality is something individuals subjectively construct. Their beliefs about themselves also matter.

When it comes to food, the social psychological approach is concerned with understanding how thoughts, feelings, and values affect food choices and dietary behaviors and with how the interactions with others and with the social environment can influence what and how much individuals eat (Conner & Armitage 2002; Rutter & Quine 2002). The purpose of understanding social psychological processes is not to manipulate individuals to make changes in their diets but rather to facilitate individuals' voluntary adoption of healthful behaviors by helping to increase awareness and reduce barriers to action, both personal and environmental.

The Importance of Motivation

The theories in this area emphasize motivation—which is based on expectations and values. (See **Box 3-2**.) They are called *expectancy-value theories.* The basic premise is that people all have internally determined goals. Motivation for behavior depends on the value individuals place on the goal and their expectations, or beliefs and estimates, that the given behavior will lead to this desired goal (Lewin et al. 1944). For example, some people may want to look attractive (the goal or value). If they expect that exercising (the action or behavior) will lead to the desired goal of looking attractive, then they will embark on the action. These beliefs are the *outcome beliefs* described earlier and are also called *outcome expectations.* Individuals also weigh the costs and

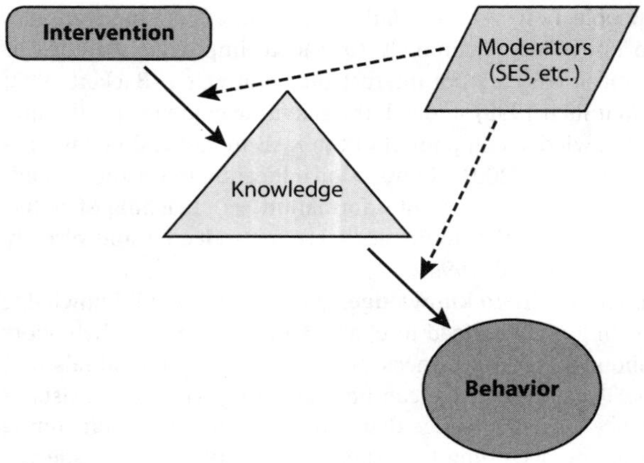

FIGURE 3-2 Knowledge-based programs: Knowledge as the mediator of behavior change.

Source: Adapted from Baranowski, T., T. O'Connor, and J. Baranowski. 2010. Initiating change in children's eating behaviors. In V. R. Preedy, R. R. Watston, and C. R. Martin (eds.). *International handbook of behavior, diet, and nutrition.* New York: Springer.

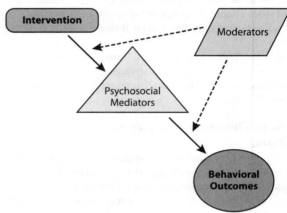

FIGURE 3-3 Theory-based programs: Psychosocial variables as the mediator of behavior change.

Source: Adapted from Baranowski, T., T. O'Connor, and J. Baranowski. 2010. Initiating change in children's eating behaviors. In V. R. Preedy, R. R. Watston, and C. R. Martin (eds.). *International handbook of behavior, diet, and nutrition.* New York: Springer.

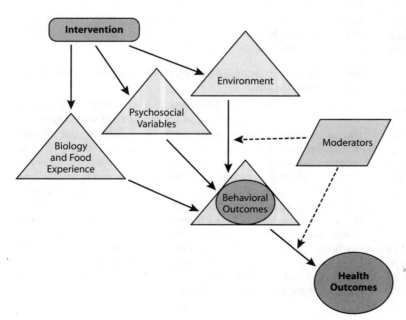

FIGURE 3-4 Social-ecological approach: Environmental theory-based psychosocial and biological variables as mediators of behavior change.

Source: Adapted from Baranowski, T., T. O'Connor, and J. Baranowski. 2010. Initiating change in children's eating behaviors. In V. R. Preedy, R. R. Watston, and C. R. Martin (eds.). *International handbook of behavior, diet, and nutrition.* New York: Springer.

Box 3-2 What Is Motivation?

Human motivation is very complex and research has generated many descriptions for it. In general, it is the internal condition that activates behavior and gives it direction; it energizes and directs goal-oriented behavior.

Some theories note that motivation ranges on a continuum from intrinsic to extrinsic. Motivation can come from experiencing intrinsic rewards inherent to a task or activity itself and satisfaction of basic needs. Motivation can come from beliefs about the self, others, and outcomes of the behavior. Extrinsic motivation comes from desire to meet expectations from outside of the person.

Expectancy-value theories, which are the foundation of social psychological theories, posit that we will engage in a behavior if we believe it will bring about outcomes that we desire or value. Outcomes can be internal or external.

motivation = beliefs about expected outcomes of behavior × the values we place on those outcomes

We want to maximize positive outcomes and minimize negative outcomes. These desired outcomes may serve immediate goals or larger intrinsic values that we possess.

---

benefits of the behavior (e.g., the inconvenience and exertion involved in exercising versus the improved muscle tone and decreased weight). The outcome of such cost-benefit analyses determines whether the individual takes action. In general, people are motivated to maximize the chances of desirable outcomes occurring and minimize the chances of undesirable outcomes occurring. That is, they ask the question, "What's in it for *me* (or for my family or my community)?" Only when they are convinced that there is something in it for them that is personally meaningful will they be motivated to act. Goals can be short term and immediate or may be more long term and global, involving values and ethics.

Beliefs About Outcome Expectations

Some important outcomes are as follows:

- *Health outcomes:* Health outcomes are beliefs that certain actions can enhance health outcomes or reduce risk of disease.
- *Social outcomes:* Social outcomes are expectations of what others will think when an individual performs the behavior.
- *Self-evaluative outcomes:* Self-evaluative outcomes, such as self-esteem or self-image, are also important for certain behaviors or situations.

Additional Factors

There are a few other important factors as well:

- *Self-efficacy:* Researchers who have studied a variety of social behaviors have found that in addition, individuals' estimates of whether they will be *able* to perform the behaviors are extremely important. This construct is called *self-efficacy* and is central to many theories.

- *Moderators:* Social psychological theory acknowledges that many factors that influence health behaviors, such as genetics, age, and gender, are not modifiable. Some of these factors may be moderators of the influences on behavior, as mentioned earlier. For example, men and women may perceive certain events differently, or certain health beliefs may differ by ethnicity or cultural context. These differences moderate the influence of beliefs on behavior.
- *Past experience:* Other factors that are not directly changeable by a nutrition education program, such as past experiences, life stage and life trajectories, personality, socioeconomic factors, place of residence, and social and cultural context, are not specifically part of these theories. However, expectancy-value theories propose that although early childhood experiences with food, past life experiences, life stage, place of residence, and cultural context cannot be changed, they do—if they are currently salient to the individual—influence behavior by influencing *current* preferences, beliefs, attitudes, values, expectations, motivations, sense of efficacy, and habits. These current beliefs, attitudes, and values can be captured by theory and research.
- *The importance of perceptions:* In general, social psychological theory proposes that although behavior certainly leads to objective consequences, the *interpretation* of these consequences by the individual has enormous influence on the person's intention to perform the behavior in the future (i.e., reinforce the behavior). Peer and family opinions are also important: these constitute the construct of *social norms*. Other social environmental and cultural forces also exist. However, social psychologist Triandis (1979) suggests that for any given individual, even such "external" factors as culture and social situations influence behavior because they are internalized by each individual. Thus, culture and social situations exist not only "out there" but also "in here," as subjective culture and subjective social situations that serve as mental maps that guide individuals' behavior by influencing their values, norms, roles, and so forth. All in all, then, a person's perception of the world appears to be a powerful influence on behavior. Indeed, often what people will or will not do is influenced as much by their *perception* of reality as by reality itself (Lewin et al. 1944; Bandura 1986).
- *Social psychological theory in outline:* In its simplest terms, then, research and theory suggest that for a particular dietary behavior to occur, we need to possess the following convictions about the particular behavior, such as eating more fruits and vegetables, referred to here as *X*. The first belief is this:
- I want to do *X* because it leads to the consequences I value. That is, we need to care about taking a particular action and feel that it is in our interest to do so. This statement is an expression of a *determinant* of behavior or a mediator of behavior change; it is the building block of several theories and is given the name *outcome expectations*.

The next belief is this:

- I can do *X*.

Once we are convinced that taking action has the desired consequences for us, once we *care*, once we are motivationally ready, we need to feel confident that we can carry out the action to obtain these benefits. This too is a construct that is common to most contemporary health behavior theories and is referred to as *self-efficacy*.

If both these convictions are strong, the likelihood is increased that the person will decide or intend to eat more fruits and vegetables. This is called a *behavioral intention* or *goal intention*:

● I will do *X*.

The role of other people also is important, leading to the following belief:

● Other people who are important to me think I should do *X*, and I value their opinion.

However, translating such intentions to action requires yet another step, the development of *implementation intentions* or an *action plan*:

● I will do *X* three times this coming week.

● *Food and nutrition knowledge and skills:* Translating intentions into actions also requires that we have the needed *food and nutrition knowledge and skills* to carry out the action. For example, we need to know how many servings of fruits and vegetables to eat, the need for eating a variety of colors, how to store fruits and vegetables so that they last longer, and how to prepare them in a way that tastes good to us.

● *Self-regulatory skills:* Maintaining the behavior over the long term requires a further step: the development of *self-direction skills*. Here, we set small achievable goals to achieve the outcomes we desire (such as "I will eat one extra serving of vegetables at lunchtime each day this week") and monitor our actions to evaluate how well we are fulfilling our action plans or goals. We then take corrective actions as necessary.

Behavior Change as a Process: Phases or Stages of Change

When nutrition education is examined closely, it seems nutrition educators frequently assume that diet-related change is a quick, one-step process. One day individuals are eating unhealthful diets, and the next day, after "nutrition education," they are model eaters. This assumption leads us to expect that people change quickly and thus expect that the typical four- to six-session program can change lifelong dietary habits. This is an unrealistic view of how we make changes in our lives, and it places unrealistic expectations on health promotion and nutrition education programs—and on ourselves.

When we carefully examine research in the health behavior and behavioral nutrition domains, it becomes evident that behavior change is a process. It may be a short one for some individuals or for some behaviors, and a long one for others. Although the process is continuous, with many factors interacting with each other, it can be described as occurring in two main phases: a motivational, pre-action or *thinking* phase, and an action or volitional or *doing* phase (Conner & Norman 1995; Schwarzer & Fuchs 1995; Norman, Abraham, & Conner 2000).

The Motivational, Pre-Action Phase

In the motivational, pre-action phase (or thinking phase), beliefs and attitudes or feelings are most important: beliefs such as whether individuals feel a sense of risk or threat regarding an issue; expectations about the outcomes of taking action, including perceived benefits and barriers; expectations of family and friends; and self-efficacy. These beliefs and attitudes can result in motivational readiness to take change, expressed in the form of a *behavioral intention*, or choice of a specific behavioral goal.

The Action Phase

In the action phase (or doing phase), individuals make *action plans* so that intentions can be translated into action. An action plan might be "I will add to my diet a fruit for a snack three days this coming week." In the early action phase, individuals may need to learn new food and nutrition information and new skills, such as learning about what constitutes a serving of fruits and vegetables, how to store and prepare them, how to read food labels, and how to handle family conflicts over food. However, behaviors need to be maintained for the long term, indeed for the rest of the individual's life, if individuals and communities are to see the benefits of these changes. For actions that are complex, as they are for dietary change, *maintenance* of the behaviors over the long term requires an additional set of skills involving a variety of self-management and self-regulation processes.

Other Phase or Stage Models

Other research suggests that the process can be divided into more specific phases or stages. Prochaska and DiClemente (1982) propose that change takes place through the stages of precontemplation, contemplation of change, the decision or preparation to change, action, and maintenance.

The diffusion of innovations framework (Rogers 1983) proposes that the process of change is initiated when individuals first become aware of the new idea or practice and gain some understanding of it. At the persuasion stage, individuals form a favorable or unfavorable attitude toward the practice. In the decision stage, individuals engage in activities, such as evaluating alternatives that lead to a choice to adopt or reject the new idea or practice. The individual may then go through a stage of trial adoption or implementation during which the innovation is tried out on a small scale before moving on to the final stage of full adoption or confirmation.

Understanding that dietary change occurs in phases or stages permits nutrition educators to better understand individuals' specific level of

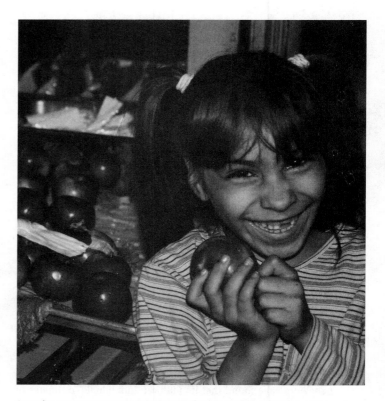

Providing opportunities to taste apples from local farms can help children to increase their fruit intake.

motivational readiness to take action and to tailor nutrition education to the individuals' stage in the change process. Stage models also proposes that individuals at different stages use different experiential and behavioral processes to make changes. Stage models are described in more detail in a later chapter.

Application to Diverse Population Groups

As described earlier, theories are abstract, symbolic representations of what is conceived to be reality based on evidence from research. As such, these theories can be used in nutrition education for a variety of population and cultural groups. For different population groups, the beliefs about desired outcomes may be different, based on cultural expectations, past life experiences, life stage (e.g., mothers of young children, postmenopausal women), or role in life (e.g., mothers, husbands, businesspeople). These beliefs must be carefully explored in formative research using these theories to understand the behavior from the perspective of the intended audience.

Researchers believe that when properly understood and applied, these theories can be used with many diverse cultural groups. Fishbein (2000) notes that each of the variables of the theory of planned behavior, for example, can be found in any culture, and that an integrative theory based on this theory has been used in HIV programs in more than 50 countries in both the developing and developed worlds. In the area of diet, the relative importance of the variables may differ for different groups (e.g., Liou & Contento 2001). For some groups, cultural beliefs regarding food may be more important than convenience is. For others, taste preferences are more important for motivating behavior change

than health considerations are. For others, the influence of family may override all other considerations.

■ ADDRESSING MULTIPLE INFLUENCES ON BEHAVIOR: A SOCIAL-ECOLOGICAL APPROACH

An important conclusion from recent research, which also supports the early conclusions of Whitehead (1973), is that nutrition education is more likely to be effective when it addresses the many levels of influences on behavior, ranging from food preferences and the sensory-affective responses to food to personal factors such as beliefs and attitudes and to the environmental context. (See **Figure 3-4** on page 50.)

For intentions or decisions to be translated into action and for the actions to be maintained for the long term, a supportive social and physical environment is required. At first, individuals may adopt the behavior only on a trial basis. Long-term maintenance of the behavior depends on whether they can fit it into their daily lives, whether there is social support for the behavior, and whether material conditions or social structures are in place or can be modified in some way to make it possible to carry out this new practice. Nutrition education programs thus seek to provide environmental support to individuals to enable them to act on their motivations and apply their skills.

As you can see in Figure 3-1, the role of nutrition education is to address the multiple and overlapping spheres of influence on food choices and dietary behaviors identified in Chapter 2. To do this, nutrition educators need to develop programs at several levels of intervention, shown in detail in **Figure 3-5**.

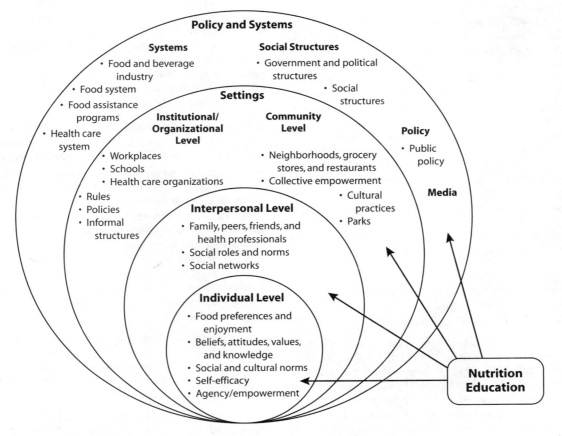

FIGURE 3-5 Social-ecological model: Levels of influence for nutrition education interventions.

- *Individual or intrapersonal level:* Focusing on the psychobiological core of experience with food, food preferences and enjoyment of food, beliefs, attitudes, values, knowledge, social and cultural norms, or life experience
- *Interpersonal level:* Focusing on family, friends, peers, interactions with health professionals, social roles, and social networks
- *Institutional/organizational level:* Focusing on rules, policies, and informal structures in workplaces, schools, or religious and social organizations to which individuals belong
- *Community level:* Focusing on social networks, norms, and community expectations, grocery stores, or restaurants
- *Social structure, policy, and systems level:* Focusing on policies and structure that regulate health actions

This approach is called the *social-ecological model* (McLeroy et al. 1988). The idea of directing interventions at various spheres of influence is now widely used in health promotion (Booth et al. 2001; Gregson et al. 2001; Wetter et al. 2001; Green & Kreuter 2004).

Sufficient Duration and Intensity of Intervention

Interventions with longer durations and more contact hours have resulted in more positive results. A notable illustration is the "Know Your Body" program, which was designed to reduce cardiovascular risk. This program involved 30 to 50 hours a year for three years and achieved improvements in serum cholesterol and blood pressure as well as diet (Walter 1989; Resnicow et al. 1992). The conceptually similar intervention, CATCH, involved 15 to 20 hours a year over three years (third through fifth grades) and resulted in behavior changes, though not in physiological parameters (Luepker et al. 1996). These behavioral changes were still in evidence in the eighth grade (Nader et al. 1999). Furthermore, many obesity prevention studies found that longer duration was important for effectiveness (Shaya et al. 2008).

A large-scale evaluation of health education programs in schools found that although large effect sizes could be achieved in program-specific knowledge in about 8 hours and general knowledge in about 20, only moderate effect sizes could be achieved in attitudes and behaviors even after 35 to 50 hours (Connell, Turner, & Mason 1985).

These studies suggest that nutrition education must be of sufficient duration and provide sufficient intensity to be effective. Yet many consumers often have short attention spans, and for many practical reasons nutrition education programs are of short duration. This presents a dilemma for nutrition educators. One way to resolve this dilemma is to use a coordinated and systematic approach delivered through multiple venues to provide nutrition education using many levels of intervention and through multiple channels so that, in total, sufficient duration and intensity are delivered to individuals and the public.

■ DESIGNING STRATEGIES FOR NUTRITION EDUCATION: A FRAMEWORK FOR LINKING BEHAVIORAL THEORY TO EDUCATION

The goal of nutrition education is to facilitate the adoption and maintenance of behaviors conducive to health and well-being. To do so effectively, we must shift the focus of nutrition education from simply increasing knowledge to addressing additional factors, both personal and environmental, that influence dietary behavior. As we have seen, these factors are determinants of behavior that can serve as potential mediators of behavior change. These determinants must be identified and prioritized so that educational strategies for addressing them can

be designed. Theories from behavioral nutrition and nutrition education research help us identify and prioritize these determinants because the determinants are constructs within these theories, and these theories are the mental maps we need to use.

Converting Spheres of Influence on Behavior to a Framework for Education

The way the information is presented in Figures 3-1 and 3-5 is not sufficient in itself to help nutrition educators design nutrition education activities. **Figure 3-6** converts the information into a diagram that shows exactly how nutrition education that is directed at the many influencing factors can make an impact on behavior and health outcomes. Chapter 2 describes how these influences on behaviors can be placed into three categories: biology and experience with food, person, and environment. Biology and experience with food and person-related determinants are often placed together because people's predispositions and experiences lead to sensory-affective responses that are individual and intrapersonal. These sets of determinants influence the enactment of food and nutrition-related behaviors, which then influence nutritional status and nutritional well-being and disease risk.

Figure 3-6 acknowledges that biological factors such as age, gender, and genetics and some external physical factors such as physical activity, concurrent infections, and other issues also have impacts on health and on behaviors that are not modifiable by nutrition education. At the same time, people's behaviors have effects on the kinds of food system in place, through consumer demand. For example, if individuals make food choices based primarily on taste, low cost, and convenience, then that is what the food system will provide. If people make choices based on quality or concern for the viability of local farms, then the food system will reflect those choices. People's food-related behaviors and practices also have impacts on society, such as on farmers and farm workers and on how food-related social structures and communities are organized. Figure 3-6 shows that behaviors are the focus of nutrition education and that addressing the influences on these behaviors or mediators of behavior change is the central mission of nutrition education.

A Conceptual Framework Linking Dietary Change and Nutrition Education: Facilitating Why and How to Take Action and Providing Environmental Support

For most people, change takes place gradually. Combining the information from Figure 3-6 with the notion of phases of change generates **Figure 3-7**. The research suggests that different processes are going on within individuals in these phases and hence nutrition education has different roles in each of these phases. To be effective, nutrition education must thus have a role in enhancing the *motivation* to act; facilitating *the ability or skills to act*; and promoting *environmental opportunities* to take the chosen action. Nutrition education can thus be conceptualized as consisting of three components with differing but complementary roles, all serving the educational or intervention goals of the program, as shown in Figure 3-7:

- *Motivational phase or component*, with a focus on why to take action
- *Action phase or component*, with a focus on how to take action
- *Environmental supports for action*, with an emphasis on changes in the environment

The conceptual framework that links the dietary change process to nutrition education as shown in Figure 3-7 is explored in greater detail in the following sections.

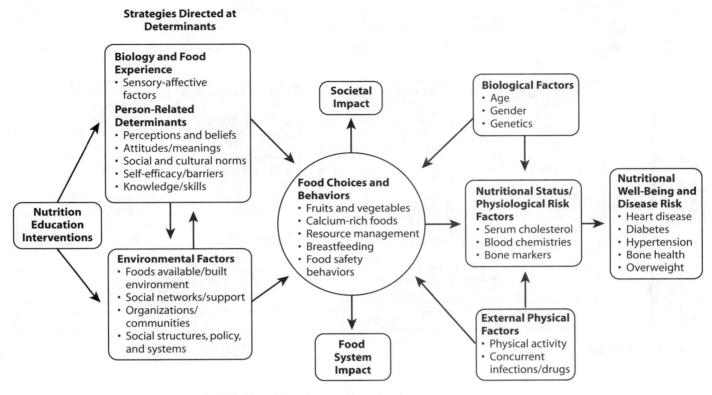

Strategies Directed at Determinants

Biology and Food Experience
- Sensory-affective factors

Person-Related Determinants
- Perceptions and beliefs
- Attitudes/meanings
- Social and cultural norms
- Self-efficacy/barriers
- Knowledge/skills

Nutrition Education Interventions

Environmental Factors
- Foods available/built environment
- Social networks/support
- Organizations/ communities
- Social structures, policy, and systems

Societal Impact

Food Choices and Behaviors
- Fruits and vegetables
- Calcium-rich foods
- Resource management
- Breastfeeding
- Food safety behaviors

Food System Impact

Biological Factors
- Age
- Gender
- Genetics

Nutritional Status/ Physiological Risk Factors
- Serum cholesterol
- Blood chemistries
- Bone markers

External Physical Factors
- Physical activity
- Concurrent infections/drugs

Nutritional Well-Being and Disease Risk
- Heart disease
- Diabetes
- Hypertension
- Bone health
- Overweight

FIGURE 3-6 Factors influencing nutritional well-being and the role of nutrition education.

The Motivational, Pre-Action Phase: A Focus on Why to Take Action

In the motivational, pre-action phase (thinking phase), beliefs and attitudes or feelings are most important.

- *Dietary change process:* As individuals begin to contemplate action, the behavior change process going on within the individual focuses on becoming motivated to consider action and deciding whether to take action. Many factors influencing motivational readiness to take action are important at this time and are listed in Figure 3-7. Theory and evidence from research suggest that the influencing factors, or potential mediators of behavior change, include awareness of risk or threat, beliefs about taking action, feelings about taking action, beliefs about self-efficacy or confidence in taking action, and beliefs about social environments. This phase may result in a decision-making phase in which individuals analyze the benefits versus the costs of taking action and clarify their values. When a decision is made, an intention is formed to take action.
- *Nutrition education program objective:* During this phase, the objective is to increase awareness, promote contemplation, enhance the motivation to act, and facilitate the intention to take action.
- *Focus of nutrition education strategies:* During the pre-action phase, the focus of the education program is on why to take action.

The Action Phase: A Focus on How to Take Action

In the action phase (doing phase), individuals make *action plans* so that intentions can be translated into action.

- *Dietary change process.* During the action phase, the behavior change process going on within the individual focuses on initiating action and maintaining it for the long term. Theory and evidence from research suggest that developing action plans is crucial for translating intentions into action. Food- and nutrition-related knowledge and cognitive, affective, and behavioral skills are also important, as are self-regulation skills or skills in setting goals and following through. These result in self-efficacy and a

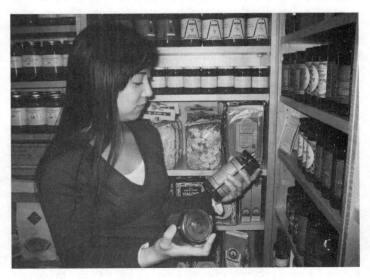

Food labels serve as a readily available source of how-to knowledge.

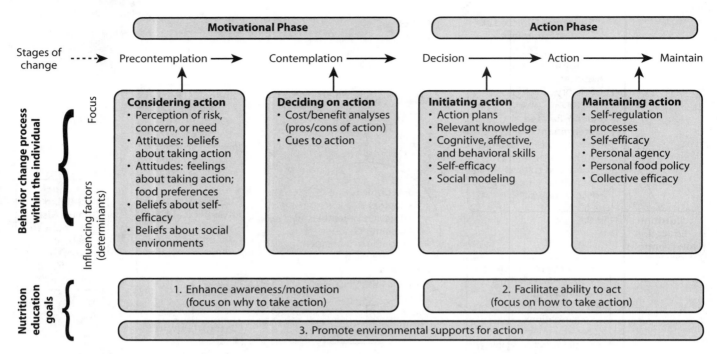

FIGURE 3-7 Conceptual framework for nutrition education.

sense of personal agency or ability to exert influence on one's behavior as well as one's environment that can lead to development of personal food policies and to acting with others to make changes in the community.

- *Nutrition education program objective:* During this phase, the objective is to facilitate the individual's ability to act.
- *Focus of nutrition education strategies:* During the action phase, the focus of the education program is on how to take action.

The Environmental Support Component

A supportive environment is important throughout the dietary change process. The nutrition education program objective is to educate decision makers, policy makers, and others who have power and authority to make changes in the environment about the importance of nutrition and health concerns and to work in collaboration with them to promote more supportive environments, including interpersonal social support, community activation, food and physical activity environments, and policy.

Putting It All Together

Nutrition educators can use the factors influencing the dietary change process just described and shown in Figure 3-7 to develop activities for individual nutrition education sessions or entire programs. It should be noted that for any given program or set of sessions or media materials, nutrition educators need to identify which of the nutrition education program objectives should predominate, based on the intended audience's state of readiness to change.

Why-To and How-To Knowledge: Motivation and Skills

Why-To Knowledge: Motivation

For an audience primarily in a pre-action phase, activities to increase awareness and enhance motivation should predominate. Why-to knowl-

edge is important here. It is often based on information from nutrition science studies about the health outcomes of taking action based on the relationship of nutrients or foods to health. Examples are the role of calcium in bone health or the role of antioxidants in reducing cancer risk. The stronger the evidence for health benefits, the more convincing is the case for taking action nutrition educators can make to their audience. The term *why-to knowledge* is a useful way to communicate to the lay public the kind of information that is motivational in nature and can serve as a potential mediator of change.

Why-to information also includes non-health-related information that is motivational and of personal importance, such as perceptions of convenience, taste, or cost; beliefs, attitudes, and feelings; values and personal meanings; social and cultural norms; and individual and ethnic identities. Why-to information may be particularly important for issues new to the audience. For familiar issues, nutrition educators need to think of exciting and fresh ways to enhance motivation.

How-To Knowledge: Skills

For those who are already motivated, how-to knowledge can be important. This includes information on basic facts about food and nutrition, such as knowing the key features of MyPyramid, knowing what is meant by balanced diets, being able to read food labels, identifying food sources of nutrients, shopping wisely, being able to practice safe food preparation methods, and so forth. Behavior change and self-regulation strategies should predominate.

In most audiences or groups, people are at different phases in the change process. Thus, nutrition education should generally begin with awareness and motivational activities. This should be followed by strategies to provide skills and information to assist individuals to take action. For all audiences, but particularly those ready to take action, environmental supports are important.

Applications of Why-To and How-To Knowledge

Low-Fat Lucy the Cow

Why-to and how-to approaches can be used in group settings such as shown in **Nutrition Education in Action 3-1**. This celebrity cow visited schools to provide motivation and skills to drink low-fat milk at school.

Sisters Together

Why-to information and how-to information can be used in brochures or website venues as well. An example is shown in **Nutrition Education in Action 3-2** about the Sisters Together campaign. The flyer begins with motivational, pre-action-phase nutrition education messages focusing on why-to information such as the positive outcomes or benefits to be expected from taking action. The flyer then focuses on perceived barriers to taking action and how to overcome them. It continues with action-phase nutrition education strategies, focusing on how-to information such as relevant food- and nutrition-related knowledge and skills, and concludes with the action-phase nutrition education strategy of goal setting.

The *Aha!* Moment in Behavior Change: Chaos Theory

You have probably experienced an *aha!* moment, when suddenly everything seems to come together and you can make the change you had wanted to make but could not seem to do for so long. Some researchers note that behavior change in individuals does not always follow paths as linear as the theories and models suggest. Through nutrition education efforts, individuals may become aware of their own motivations or their behaviors, but they do not immediately take action; when they do, they may not make the decision in the orderly sequence laid out previously and as described in various models. Researchers suggest that chaos theory from physics can make sense of these phenomena (Resnicow & Page 2008).

It is known, for example, that smokers on average make eight attempts to quit before they successfully do so. They experience an *aha!* moment. They cannot usually explain why they were successful this particular time. The theory constructs described earlier are still important and, on average, may work well. But for any given individual, the new information given about expected outcomes from taking action, the new feelings engendered, or the new skills provided may need to percolate in what may appear to be a chaotic fashion. From numerous occasions of nutrition education or individual counseling, after much rumination about the influences on their dietary or physical activity patterns and about what the individual wants out of life may come action. Because nutrition educators do not know when or why any given individual may choose to take action, we must use theory-based interventions to

---

NUTRITION EDUCATION IN ACTION 3-1

Celebrity Cow Promotes Low-Fat Milk to Elementary Schoolers

When studies revealed that children in New York City were eating too much saturated fat, the state health department and a university decided to do something about it: they launched a Low-Fat Milk Education Project. The problem was how to encourage children to make the switch from whole milk to low-fat milk, usually thought as being low in taste too. The solution was Low-Fat Lucy the Cow. Lucy became the celebrity "spokes-cow," played by a volunteer dressed in a black-and-white Holstein costume. Lucy put in live appearances in school assemblies. The message was "Choose low-fat milk in the school cafeteria and urge your parents to buy it at home." For two weeks prior to the assemblies, Lucy was promoted as a "mystery guest" via posters and announcements. On the day of her debut, students in the assemblies were primed for her appearance with a participatory game of Fat-BUSTERS, in which they were challenged to identify high- and low-fat foods from slides.

Lucy entered the school auditorium to the lively accompaniment of dance music. She carried two cartons of low-fat milk, which she displayed to the children as she danced down the aisle. Lucy then explained how changing to low-fat milk can help students keep their diets healthy and how, most of all, low-fat milk tastes great. In the auditorium after Lucy's presentation, the students were given low-fat milk, a low-fat cookie, and a pencil with Lucy's picture and the message "Drink Low-Fat Milk" in English and Spanish. This tasting helped to surmount a large obstacle to children switching milks: they do not like to try unfamiliar foods.

The children were then given handouts, refrigerator magnets to take home, and a simple puzzle. A week later, Lucy returned for a ceremony to select winners from students who had solved the puzzle. A second tasting took place, this one at school dismissal time, for both students and parents. Lucy also visited a parent association meeting about the same time.

Here you can see theory being used to design the program:

- Students were told that low-fat milk was good for their health and tasted great (outcome expectations).
- Children tasted low-fat milk to increase the liking for it (social-affective experience) and to create familiarity (food-related factor).
- Lucy the Cow was a celebrity (social norms and social modeling).
- School assembly setting indicated that the school was setting a social norm.
- Handouts, magnets, and puzzle (reinforcements) were used.
- A ceremony was held to select winners and give prizes (incentives and a reinforcement).
- Parental support (promoting a supportive environment) was encouraged.
- School support: the school now displayed low-fat milk prominently (promoting a supportive environment).

Did Lucy succeed? Before the project, 25% of the students who drank milk selected low-fat milk. That increased to 57%, whereas the control school students did not change.

Source: Wechsler, H., C. E. Basch, P. Zybert, and S. Shea. 1998. Promoting the selection of low-fat milk in elementary school cafeterias in an inner-city Latino community: Evaluation of an intervention. *American Journal of Public Health* 88:427–433.

NUTRITION EDUCATION IN ACTION 3-2

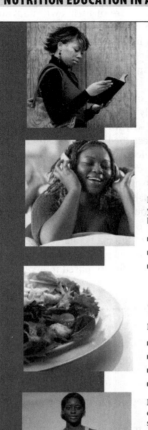

Celebrate the Beauty of Youth!

SISTERS together MOVE MORE EAT BETTER

Want to feel better, look better, and have more energy? Moving more and eating better is the best place to start.

Why Move More and Eat Better?

Being physically acti...
your health. But tha...
better. It can also he...

- Have more energ...
- Look good in hip...
- Tone your body...
  losing your curv...

Tips on M...

Physical activity...

- dancing
- rollerblading
- fast walking
- playing spor...

If you can, be...
can cheer each...
safer when yo...
you can walk...
you can work...

Think you do...
that you can...
and still ber...
activity is b...
small chang...

- Get off t...
  stop ear...
  the way...
- Park yo...
  and wa...

Celebrate the Beauty of Youth's WIN program provides women "why-to" and "how-to" information to improve their health and nutrition.

- Put physical activity on your to-do list for the day. For example, plan on exercising right after work, before you can get distracted by dinner or going out.

Look Good as You Get Fit

If you avoid physical activity because you do not want to ruin your hairstyle, try:

- a natural hairstyle
- a style that can be wrapped or pulled back
- a short haircut
- braids, twists, or locs

TIP: *Day-to-day activities can cause salt build-up in your hair. To remove salt, shampoo with a mild, pH-balanced product at least once a week.*

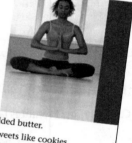
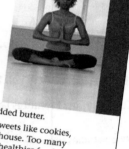

- Order a plain hamburger (without sauce or mayonnaise) or a grilled (not fried) chicken sandwich. Skip the fries and try a salad with fat-free or low-fat dressing instead.
- Go easy on mayonnaise, creamy sauces, and added butter.
- Do not keep a lot of sweets like cookies, candy, or soda in the house. Too many sweets can crowd out healthier foods.
- Rather than eliminate your favorite home-cooked foods, prepare them in slightly different ways: bake chicken instead of frying it; cook with extra herbs rather than extra butter; and reduce the amount of salt you use.

TIP: *Many food labels say "low-fat," "reduced fat," or "light." That does not always mean the food is low in calories. Sometimes fat-free or low-fat muffins or desserts have even more sugar than the full-fat versions. Remember, fat-free does not mean calorie-free, and calories do count!*

Many people think that bigger is better. We are so used to value-size servings that it is easy to eat more than our bodies need. Eating smaller portions will help you cut down on calories and fat (and might save you money too).

Even take-out and high-fat foods can be part of a balanced diet, as long as you do not eat them

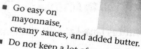

Tips on Eating Better

Eating right can be hard when you do not feel like cooking or there is a fast food place on every corner. Here are some simple things you can do to eat better:

- Start every day with breakfast. Try a low-fat, whole-grain breakfast bar; fat-free or low-fat yogurt; or whole-grain toast or bagel spread with a little peanut butter, jam, or low-fat cream cheese.
- Eat more fruits and vegetables, and choose whole grains like 100 percent whole-wheat bread, oatmeal, or brown rice instead of refined grains like white bread and white rice.
- Choose low-fat or fat-free milk instead of whole milk or a milkshake.

keep providing opportunities for individuals to contemplate and decide (Brug 2006).

The Cases of Alicia and Ray

Let us now examine the cases of Alicia and Ray. Alicia is not very concerned about her diet. She appears to be in a pre-action mode. Yet the nutrition science literature suggests that this is the time when eating a healthy diet could make a big difference in her health in the future. So, pre-action, motivational-phase nutrition education would likely be most appropriate for her, with an emphasis on why-to information and activities.

Ray, on the other hand, has thought about his situation. His problem seems to be related to how to translate interest and intention into action. For Ray, strengthening his beliefs about taking action and providing action-phase nutrition education may be appropriate.

The next few chapters describe theory and evidence from nutrition education and health behavior research that can help you determine the kinds of strategies that might work for Alicia and Ray.

■ A LOGIC MODEL APPROACH FOR PLANNING NUTRITION EDUCATION

Where and how, then, to begin? The task of nutrition education seems daunting, so nutrition educators need some systematic way to help them plan it effectively. Many planning models are used in different health-related programs, from the PRECEDE-PROCEED model for health promotion (Green & Kreuter 2004) to the Nutrition Care Process and Model of the American Dietetic Association (ADA 2008) to various health communication models (e.g., NCI Health Communications, CDCenergy) to social marketing models (Andreasen 1995). None of these is quite right for the purposes of this book—which is to assist nutrition educators to develop, deliver, and evaluate the kinds of educational interventions and programs that the vast majority conduct on an ongoing basis in their places of work.

A tool that is being used in many fields and that has been applied to nutrition education programs is helpful here: the *logic model*, which is a simplified but very logical model of how to plan a nutrition education program (Medeiros et al. 2005). It shows that in planning, nutrition educators need to think about the following:

- The resources that will go into a program (the *inputs*)
- The activities the program will undertake (the *outputs*)
- The changes or benefits that result (the *outcomes*)

In its simplest form, it thus consists of the components shown in **Figure 3-8**.

Based on the discussions so far, nutrition educators can use the logic model as follows. First, they must identify the specific behaviors,

patterns of behavior, or practices to address. Then, having considered what the resources are, they can design a set of activities that directly address the potential mediators of change for the specific behaviors or practices that they have identified.

Role of Theory in the Logic Model for Dietary Behavior Change

The logic model, however, does not—and is not designed to—tell us as nutrition educators *exactly how* to design the outputs component. That is, the model does not tell exactly how we should develop the educational activities and materials for which specific behaviors, directed at which multiple levels of influence, and on what basis they should be developed. This book is designed to fill this important gap. We incorporate this component into a logic model, as shown in **Figure 3-9**.

Nutrition educators first need to determine the behaviors or practices that will be the focus of the program, based on concerns or needs arising from nutrition science evidence, health policy, assessment of the intended audience, and other considerations. With the behavioral focus clearly delineated, we are ready to consider the inputs, outputs, and outcomes:

- *The inputs are what nutrition educators invest.* Inputs consist of the staff and volunteers of the program, time, materials, money, space, and partners and collaborators.
- *The outputs are what nutrition educators do.* Outputs consist of the activities that we are familiar with: conducting classes, facilitating groups, and developing materials, products, and other resources; working with families, community partners, and public policy makers; and working with media. But what we are less familiar with is the fact that these activities must be directed at the identified potential mediators of change that are suggested by theory. This means that these activities must be theory based, not just whatever is informative, fun, engaging, or familiar.

  How to design theory-based nutrition education intervention strategies, or outputs, is the major focus of this book. Developing motivation-phase, action-phase, and environmental support strategies is part of the outputs component of the logic model planning tool.
- *The outcomes are the results nutrition educators obtain from the theory-based strategies that they designed and implemented.* These outcomes become the basis of the evaluation. Although the ultimate desired outcomes are improved health, decreased disease risk, and other long-term benefits, such as community actions or revised policies to support the program's targeted core behaviors, many nutrition education programs are not intense enough or long enough to achieve such improvements. Therefore, they aim for changes in behaviors. They may even have to be satisfied with improvements in the mediating variables themselves, such as increased knowledge or more positive attitudes.

The Cooking with Kids Logic Model

How the logic model is used to plan nutrition education directed at several levels of influence is illustrated by the Cooking with Kids program, shown in **Figure 3-10**. The program consists of individual-level activities directed at students in the classroom; family-level activities; and institutional-levels activities designed to improve foods offered at school. The program is described in **Nutrition Education in Action 3-3**.

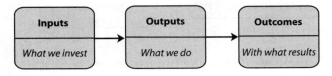

FIGURE 3-8 Components of the logic model.

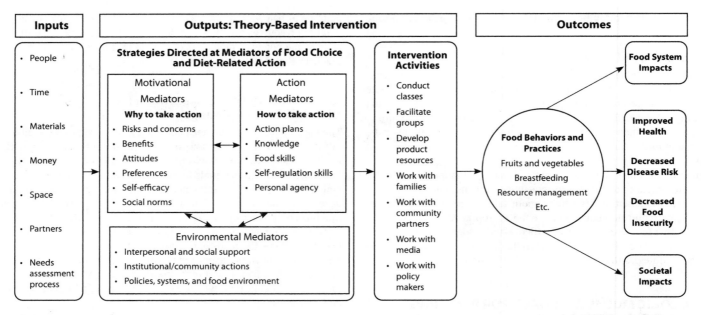

FIGURE 3-9 A logic model of theory-based nutrition education.

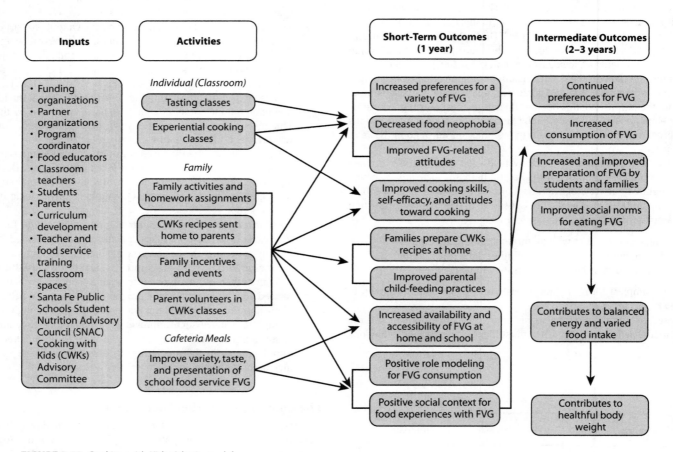

FIGURE 3-10 Cooking with Kids: A logic model.

Source: Walters, L., J. Stacey, and L. Cunningham-Sabo. 2005. *Learning comes alive through classroom cooking: Cooking with Kids.* Presented at the annual meeting of the Society for Nutrition Education. Orlando, FL. Used with the permission of Leslie Cunningham-Sabo.
(FVG = fruits, vegetables, and whole grains).

NUTRITION EDUCATION IN ACTION 3-3

Cooking with Kids

How the logic model is used to plan nutrition education directed at several levels of influence is illustrated by the Cooking with Kids program, shown in Figure 3-10. Cooking with Kids is a program designed to improve children's intakes of fruits, vegetables, and whole grains (the targeted behaviors) through several kinds of activities at various levels of intervention. These are shown in the logic model and described here:

- Individual-level intervention: Fruit- and vegetable-tasting activities for students in the classroom; cooking fresh, affordable foods from diverse cultures; nutrition information; foods in history; food journal activities; and take-home recipes
- Family-level activities: Volunteer participation; activities such as families getting together at the school during the evening and cooking and eating together; events; and incentives
- Institutional or environmental level: Improvements in the meals offered at school through collaboration with others, such as farm-to-table organizations; locally grown produce included in school meals; foods cooked in the classroom adapted and served in school meals

Evaluation

In a pilot evaluation, more than 80% of the students reported liking the foods cooked in the classroom, 75% chose the foods in the cafeteria, and 60% ate half or more of the lunch. About 50% of the parents reported that they used Cooking with Kids recipes at home, and 65% said their children now ate more fruits and vegetables at home.

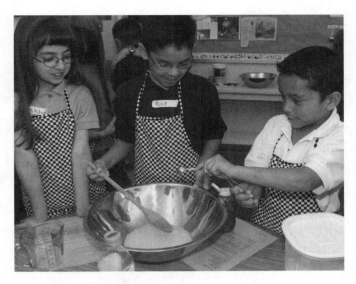

Cooking with Kids incorporates nutrition education into the classroom curriculum.

Sources: Walters, L., J. Stacey, and L. Cunningham-Sabo. 2005. *Learning comes alive through classroom cooking: Cooking with Kids.* Presented at the annual meeting of the Society for Nutrition Education. Orlando, FL; Walters, L., and J. Stacey. Cooking with Kids. http://www.cookingwithkids.net.

■ SUMMARY

This chapter shows that nutrition education is more likely to be effective if it includes the following key elements.

A Focus on Behaviors/Practices

Nutrition education needs to be carefully focused, usually on specific individual actions and behaviors or community practices that are of importance to individuals, to communities, or to the larger society. These behaviors may also serve larger goals of value to the individual or community. A focus on specific actions does not mean that nutrition educators use a behaviorist approach. It means they focus on actionable individual or community issues. Critical thinking is crucial.

Determinants of Behavior

Nutrition education needs to clearly identify the factors influencing the behaviors of the intended audience and makes modifying these influencing factors (determinants or potential mediators of the desired behavior change) the direct target of nutrition education interventions. Any knowledge that is provided needs to be relevant to the actions, practices, or issues targeted by the program rather than merely general information.

Theory

Nutrition education needs to *use theory and evidence* to design nutrition education. Theory, based on evidence, provides a mental map that tells us which determinants of behavior or mediators of change are more likely to result in changes in behavior by the intended audience.

Multiple Levels and Sufficient Duration

Nutrition education needs to attend to the multiple levels of influences on food choice and eating (and physical activity) behaviors. These include influences at the individual and interpersonal levels, at the community and organizational levels, and in the physical environment, social structures, systems, and policy. A coordinated and systematic approach of sufficient intensity and duration delivered through multiple venues is essential for nutrition education to have a significant impact.

Strategies

Nutrition education needs to design strategies that are based on theory to address the identified determinants of behavior or potential mediators of change and their environmental contexts at various levels of influence.

Nutrition educators should seek to use a combination of all these key elements to enhance their effectiveness.

Questions and Activities

1. Describe what is meant by "behavior-focused" nutrition education. Is it the same thing as a behaviorist approach? How or how not?

2. Describe four key elements that contribute to the effectiveness of nutrition education based on research.

3. Define *theory*. Give three reasons why theory is considered important in nutrition education.

4. What does the term *theory construct* mean? How is it related to the term *variable*?

5. Think back to a specific instance in which you gave a nutrition education session or discussed nutrition informally with others. Do you think you used theory? If so, describe the key features of your theory. If you did not use theory, explain what guided your session.

6. To what extent are you personally convinced that the use of theory and evidence will help you design more effective nutrition education? Why or why not?

7. In terms of behavior change, what does *motivation* mean? How can nutrition educators help individuals to become more motivated?

8. The knowledge-attitude-behavior (KAB) model of behavior change is quite commonly used. How effective has it been in nutrition education? Why?

9. Describe what is meant by expectancy-value theories. How might they differ from the KAB model?

10. Distinguish between why-to knowledge and how-to knowledge in the area of nutrition education.

11. Nutrition education has been described as consisting of two phases or components accompanied by environmental supports. What are the two phases and what is the primary focus of each phase?

12. Describe the key features of the logic model. If you have provided nutrition education before, no matter how small (e.g., one session) or large in scale, map it out according to the logic model. What are some of your reflections on the experience?

References

Achterberg, C., and L. Lytle. 1995. Changing the diet of America's children: What works and why. *Journal of Nutrition Education* 27(5):250–260.

Achterberg, C., and C. Miller. 2004. Is one theory better than another in nutrition education? A viewpoint: More is better. *Journal of Nutrition Education and Behavior* 36(1):40–42.

American Dietetic Association. 2008. Nutrition Care Process and Model Part I: The 2008 update. *Journal of the American Dietetic Association* 108:1113–1117.

Ammerman, A. S., C. H. Lindquist, K. N. Lohr, and J. Hersey. 2002. The efficacy of behavioral interventions to modify dietary fat and fruit and vegetable intake: A review of the evidence. *Preventive Medicine* 35(1):25–41.

Andreasen, A.R. 1995. *Marketing social change: Changing behavior to promote health, social development, and the environment*. Washington, DC: Jossey-Bass.

Backett, K. 1992. The construction of health knowledge in middle class families. *Health Education Research* 7:497–507.

Bandura, A. 1986. *Foundations of thought and action: A social cognitive theory*. Englewood Cliffs, NJ: Prentice Hall.

Baranowski, T., E. Cerin, and J. Baranowski. 2009. Steps in the design, development, and formative evaluation of obesity prevention–related behavior change. *International Journal of Behavioral Nutrition and Physical Activity* 6:6.

Baranowski, T., K. W. Cullen, T. Nicklas, D. Thompson, and J. Baranowski. 2003. Are current health behavioral change models helpful in guiding prevention of weight gain efforts? *Obesity Research* 11(Suppl):23S–43S.

Baranowski, T., L. S. Lin, D. W. Wetter, K. Resnicow, and M. D. Hearn. 1997. Theory as mediating variables: Why aren't community interventions working as desired? *Annals of Epidemiology* 7:589–595.

Booth, S. L., J. F. Sallis, C. Ritenbaugh, et al. 2001. Environmental and societal factors affect food choice and physical activity: Rationale, influences, and leverage points. *Nutrition Reviews* 59(3 Pt 2):S21–39; discussion S57–S65.

Bowen, D. J., and S. A. Beresford. 2002. Dietary interventions to prevent disease. *Annual Review of Public Health* 23:255–286.

Brown, T., and C. Summerbell. 2009. Systematic review of school-based interventions that focus on changing dietary intake and physical activity levels to prevent obesity: An update to the obesity guidance produced by the National Institute for Health and Clinical Excellence. *Obesity Reviews* 10(1):110–141.

Brug, J. 2006. Order is needed to promote linear or quantum changes in nutrition and physical activity behaviors: A reaction to 'A chaotic view of behavior change' by Resnicow and Vaughan. *International Journal of Behavioral Nutrition and Physical Activity* 3:29.

Brug, J., A. Oenema, and I. Ferreira. 2005. Theory, evidence and intervention mapping to improve behavior nutrition and physical activity interventions. *International Journal of Behavioral Nutrition and Physical Activity* 2(1):2.

Buchanan, D. 2004. Two models for defining the relationship between theory and practice in nutrition education: Is the scientific method meeting our needs? *Journal of Nutrition Education and Behavior* 36(3):146–154.

Connell D. B., R. R. Turner, and F. F. Mason. 1985. Summary of findings of the school health education evaluation: Health promotion effectiveness, implementation, and costs. *J School Health*. 55(8):316–321.

Conner, M., and C. J. Armitage. 2002. *The social psychology of food*. Buckingham, UK: Open University Press.

Conner, M., and P. Norman. 1995. *Predicting health behavior*. Buckingham, UK: Open University Press.

Contento, I., G. I. Balch, Y. L. Bronner, et al. 1995. The effectiveness of nutrition education and implications for nutrition education policy, programs, and research: A review of research. *Journal of Nutrition Education* 27(6):279–418.

Doak, C. M., T. L. Visscher, C. M. Renders, and J. C. Seidell. 2006. The prevention of overweight and obesity in children and adolescents: A review of interventions and programmes. *Obesity Reviews* 7(1):111–136.

Fishbein, M. 2000. The role of theory in HIV prevention. *AIDS Care* 12(3):273–278.

Green, L.W., and M.W. Kreuter. 2004. *Health promotion planning: An educational and ecological approach*. 4th ed. New York: McGraw-Hill Humanities/Social Sciences/Languages.

Gregson, J., S. B. Foerster, R. Orr, et al. 2001. System, environmental, and policy changes: Using the social-ecological model as a framework for evaluating nutrition education and social marketing programs with low-income audiences. *Journal of Nutrition Education* 33(Suppl 1):S4–S15.

Hegsted, M. 1979. Interview quoted in: Anders, H. J. Nutrition and health. *Chemical and Engineering News*, March 26:27.

Howerton, M. W., B. S. Bell, K. W. Dodd, D. Berrigan, R. Stolzenberg-Solomon, and L. Nebeling. 2007. School-based nutrition programs produced a moderate increase in fruit and vegetable consumption: Meta and pooling analyses from 7 studies. *Journal of Nutrition Education and Behavior* 39(4):186–196.

Institute of Medicine. 2002. *Speaking of health: Assessing health communication strategies for diverse populations*. Washington, DC: National Academy Press.

———. 2004. *Health literacy: A prescription to end confusion*. Washington, DC: National Academy Press.

Kerlinger, F. N., and H. B. Lee. 1999. *Foundations of behavioral research*. New York: Cengage Learning.

Kok, G., H. Schaalma, H. De Vries, G. Parcel, and T. Paulussen. 1996. Social psychology and health. *European Review of Social Psychology* 7:241–282.

Lemmens, V. E., A. Oenema, K. I. Klepp, H. B. Henriksen, and J. Brug. 2008. A systematic review of the evidence regarding efficacy of obesity prevention interventions among adults. *Obesity Reviews* 9(5):446–455.

Lewin, K. T. 1935. *A dynamic theory of personality*. New York: McGraw-Hill.

Lewin, K. T. 1936. *Principles of topological psychology*. New York: McGraw-Hill.

Lewin, K. T., T. Dembo, L. Festinger, and P. S. Sears. 1944. Level of aspiration. In *Personality and the behavior disorders*, edited by J. M. Hundt. New York: Roland Press.

Liou, D., and I. R. Contento. 2001. Usefulness of psychosocial theory variables in explaining fat-related dietary behavior in Chinese Americans: Association with degree of acculturation. *Journal of Nutrition Education* 33(6):322–331.

Luepker, R. V. et al. 1996. Outcomes of a field trial to improve children's dietary patterns and physical activity. The Child and Adolescent Trial for Cardiovascular Health. CATCH Collaborative Group. *Journal of the American Medical Association* 275(10):768–776.

Maxwell, J. C. 2000. *Failing forward: Turning mistakes into stepping stones for success*. Nashville, TN: Thomas Nelson Publishers.

McLeroy, K. R., D. Bibeau, A. Steckler, and K. Glanz. 1988. An ecological perspective on health promotion programs. *Health Education Quarterly* 15:351–377.

Medeiros, L. C., S. N. Butkus, H. Chipman, R. H. Cox, L. Jones, and D. Little. 2005. A logic model framework for community nutrition education. *Journal of Nutrition Education and Behavior* 37(4):197–202.

Merriam-Webster. 2003. *Merriam-Webster's collegiate dictionary*. 11th ed. Springfield, MA: Merriam-Webster.

Moorman, C., and E. Matulich. 1993. A model of consumers' preventive health behaviors: The role of health motivation and health ability. *Journal of Consumer Research* 20:208–228.

Nader, P. R., E. J. Stone, L. A. Lytle, et al. 1999. Three-year maintenance of improved diet and physical activity: The CATCH cohort. Child and Adolescent Trial for Cardiovascular Health. *Archives of Pediatric and Adolescent Medicine* 153(7):695–704.

Norman, P., C. Abraham, and M. Conner. 2000. *Understanding and changing health behavior: From health beliefs to self-regulation*. Amsterdam: Harwood Academic Publishers.

Pomerleau, J., K. Lock, C. Knai, and M. McKee. 2005. Interventions designed to increase adult fruit and vegetable intake can be effective: A systematic review of the literature. *Journal of Nutrition* 135(10):2486–2495.

Prochaska, J. O., and C. C. DiClemente. 1982. Transtheoretical therapy: Toward a more integrative model of change. *Psychotherapy: Theory, Research, Practice* 19:276–288.

Resnicow, K., Cohen, L., Reinhardt, J., et al. 1992. A three-year evaluation of the Know Your Body program in inner-city schoolchildren. *Health Education Quarterly* 19:463–480.

Resnicow, K., and S. E. Page. 2008. Embracing chaos and complexity: A quantum change for public health. *American Journal of Public Health* 98(8):1382–1389.

Rogers, E. M. 1983. *Diffusion of innovations*. New York: Free Press.

Rothman, A. J. 2004. "Is there nothing more practical than a good theory?" Why innovations and advances in health behavior change will arise if interventions are used to test and refine theory. *International Journal of Behavioral Nutrition and Physical Activity* 1(1):11.

Rutter, D. R., and L. Quine. 2002. *Changing health behaviour: Intervention and research with social cognition models*. Buckingham, UK: Open University Press.

Schwarzer, R., and R. Fuchs. 1995. Self-efficacy and health behaviors. In *Predicting health behavior*, edited by M. Conner and P. Norman. Buckingham, UK: Open University Press.

Sharma, M. 2006. International school-based interventions for preventing obesity in children. *Obesity Reviews* 8:155–167.

Shaya, F. T., D. Flores, C. M. Gbarayor, and J. Wang. 2008. School-based obesity interventions: A literature review. *Journal of School Health* 78(4):189–196.

Shepherd, R., and G. Towler. 2007. Nutrition knowledge, attitudes and fat intake: Application of the theory of reasoned action. *Journal of Human Nutrition and Dietetics* 20(3):159–169.

Stables, G. J., E. M. Young, M. W. Howerton, et al. 2005. Small school-based effectiveness trials increase vegetable and fruit consumption among youth. *Journal of the American Dietetic Association* 105(2):252–256.

Strauss, A. L., and J. Corbin. 1990. *Basics of qualitative research: Grounded theory procedures and research*. Newbury Park, CA: Sage Publications.

Triandis, H. C. 1979. Values, attitudes, and interpersonal behavior. In *Nebraska symposium on motivation*, edited by H. E. How. Lincoln: University of Nebraska Press.

Walter, H. J. 1989. Primary prevention of chronic disease among children: The school-based "Know Your Body" intervention trials. *Health Education Quarterly* 16:201–214.

Wetter, A. C., J. P. Goldberg, A. C. King, et al. 2001. How and why do individuals make food and physical activity choices? *Nutrition Reviews* 59(3 Pt 2):S11–20; discussion S57–S65.

Whitehead, F. 1973. Nutrition education research. *World Review of Nutrition and Dietetics* 17:91–149.

CHAPTER 4

Foundation in Theory and Research: Increasing Awareness and Enhancing Motivation

OVERVIEW   This chapter describes key theories and research that help readers understand the important role of motivation in food choice and nutrition-related behavior change. It also describes how each theory can be translated into effective nutrition communication and education. It focuses on motivation to act and the key role of beliefs, feelings, and attitudes in providing *why-to* nutrition education.

CHAPTER OUTLINE
- Increasing awareness and enhancing motivation
- The health belief model
- The precaution adoption process model
- Theory of planned behavior
- Self-determination theory
- Translating behavioral theories into educational strategies for why to take action
- Summary

LEARNING OBJECTIVES   At the end of the chapter, you will be able to:
- Describe key theories that help nutrition educators understand motivation for health and nutrition behaviors, in particular the health belief model and the theory of planned behavior
- Describe how these theories have been used in research to investigate determinants of food choice and nutrition-related behaviors
- Discuss how theories and research have been used in nutrition education programs to increase awareness and enhance motivation
- Demonstrate understanding that the major task of nutrition education is to use theory to identify and design strategies to address potential mediators of change
- Identify implications for designing nutrition education to increase interest, enhance motivation, promote active contemplation, and facilitate formation of intentions to take action

■ INCREASING AWARENESS AND ENHANCING MOTIVATION: WHY TO TAKE ACTION

People's food choices and eating patterns develop over a lifetime and are embedded in many aspects of their lives. Many people may not be entirely satisfied with how they are eating, but their patterns generally work for them, given their life circumstances and the trade-offs they need to make. Given the many competing desires and priorities in people's lives, health is not always uppermost. The first crucial step in making specific changes is for individuals to become aware of a need to change and to see what's in it for them to do so. When aware, interested, and motivated, people are more ready for information and skills that assist them to take action.

Research suggests that the adoption and maintenance of health behaviors are a process involving two main phases: a decision-making or deliberative phase, and an action or implementation phase (Schwarzer 1992; Abraham & Sheeran 2000). This means that nutrition education programs should consist of both a motivational pre-action phase or component and a postdecision action and maintenance component. It is recognized, of course, that humans are thinking, feeling, and acting wholes, so motivation or willingness to take action and the ability to act are closely related, each enhancing the other. It may be that for many individuals, problems with getting started and maintaining action rather than motivation or forming intentions prevent them from engaging in recommended healthful behaviors. Nevertheless, thinking about the behavior change process as two phases or components helps with the conceptualization and design of nutrition education programs.

Why take action? This chapter focuses on the first phase or component. It examines what nutrition behavior research and theory have found about how individuals become aware, interested, and motivated. Armed with that knowledge, nutrition educators can design programs to assist individuals move from not even considering action to thinking about it.

Cultural and social psychological beliefs are important here. People's beliefs, values, feelings, attitudes, and perceptions of social and cultural norms influence their health behaviors. These cognitive-motivational factors come from cultural, social, family, or personal sources. Prior life experiences, life stage, personality, family structure, and sociodemographic and historic factors also influence individuals' behavior. These, of course, are not modifiable by educational means. However, these factors affect *current* beliefs, attitudes, or self-identities that influence behavior, and these *can* be addressed by nutrition education.

Cultural Context

Consideration of cultural context is important in planning nutrition education. All humans are cultural creatures. People experience culture from the moment they are born; for example, in some cultures girl babies get pink clothes and boy babies, blue. Culture is concerned with shared knowledge and shared meanings, where *meanings* implies some complexity of belief or knowledge and a connection of values or feelings with beliefs (D'Andrade 1984). Cultural knowledge and values develop over time for the group or society in ways that help to promote its survival (LeVine 1984). Food, which is essential to survival, is not surprisingly very much part of culture. Culture defines what people should or should not eat and prescribes how to prepare food; where, when, and with whom it should be eaten; who does the shopping and cooking; and whose opinions are most important in the choice of family meals (Rozin 1982; Sanjur 1982; Kittler & Sucher 2001).

Differences in cultural values about health in general can also influence dietary practices. For example, some cultures, such as mainstream American culture, emphasize personal responsibility or self-help in promoting individual health or preventing illness, whereas others may believe that chance or fate is more important. Although mainstream culture may emphasize personal choice in matters of food and eating, others emphasize the role of family in decisions related to food and health. Some view health from a biomedical viewpoint; others, experiential or psychosocial (Chesla et al. 2000). Some of these differing cultural norms are shown in **Table 4-1**.

Interactions of Culture and Social Psychological Factors

Children acquire their culture's beliefs and values both directly and indirectly (Spiro 1984). Direct influence occurs when the child is told explicitly about "facts," norms, values, and so forth about the culture (e.g., "We don't eat pork"). Indirect acquisition occurs through observing what other people do (norms), whether in interpersonal settings or

TABLE 4-1	**Comparison of Some Common Cultural Values Relevant to Dietary Behavior**
Mainstream American Culture	**Other Cultural Groups**
Health and illness are located in the person.	Health and illness are long-term, fluid, and continuous expressions of relationships between an individual and others.
Illness is caused by natural etiological agents such as genes, viruses, bacteria, and stress.	Illness is caused by quasi-natural agents such as weather or various states of one's blood (e.g., thin, weak, or bad), or by violations of religious or moral expectations, emotions such as envy or jealousy, or punishment for misconduct.
Personal responsibility for health; importance of sense of control.	Chance, fate, and God influence health, illness, and healing.
Nutritional health is the result of deficiencies and imbalances in food components and nutrients in food.	Health is the result of the balance of forces in the body, such as hot–cold; imbalances cause illness, and health can be restored by balancing of hot and cold foods.
Self-help.	Societal or community obligation to assist.
Emphasis is on individualism/privacy.	Welfare of the group, interpersonal harmony are important.
Time is highly important.	Personal interactions are highly important.
Future orientation.	Past or present orientation; tradition is important.
Interactions emphasize directness and openness.	Interactions emphasize indirectness, importance of "face."
Informality and egalitarianism.	Status, formal relationships are important.

through media such as television, and making inferences from norms and cultural artifacts about the values of the culture. For example, if families within a culture spend a lot of time preparing healthful food (norms) and enjoying it, or if their kitchens are equipped for making healthful foods (artifacts), children growing up in that culture are likely also to value healthful food. Anthropologists suggest that this outcome is likely in part because there is a tendency for the descriptive understanding of one's culture—how things are—to become fused with a normative understanding—how things should be. LeVine (1984) comments, "The fusion of what is and ought to be in a single vision . . . gives distinctive cultural ideologies their singular psychological power, their intimate linkages with individual emotion and motivation" (p. 78).

Given these definitions and observations, culture can be seen as connected intimately with the intra- and interpersonal cognitive-motivational factors in food choice that are discussed later in this chapter. That is, the beliefs, attitudes, and values to be discussed are the same ones under discussion here; culture may be considered their primary source. The relation of culture to the food and physiological factors discussed in earlier chapters has been explored by Rozin (1982), who describes how mild social pressure may maintain the consumption of initially unpalatable foods until preference becomes internalized by liking for the taste, as with chili, or by other factors, such as addiction to coffee.

Social pressure of this kind tends to be consistent with the beliefs, values, and practices of the culture or subculture (e.g., adolescents, ethnic groups). However, cultural and social influences are distinguishable to some degree through the concept of internalization. Culture involves beliefs and values that are internalized or believed in widely among members of the group; as children acquire these beliefs and values, they become acculturated. Deutsch and Gerard (1955) distinguish two kinds of social influence: with *normative* social influence, people conform to others' wishes to gain social acceptance. Conformity to the family's wishes is of some importance earlier in life; later, the key reference group consists of peers. With *informational* social influence, people learn about reality from what others say and do. This learning, then, also influences people's values, attitudes, and actions.

Culture "Out There" and "In Here"

Researchers point out that culture "out there" is interpreted by the family and passed down to their children as family cultural traditions (Triandis 1979; Ventura & Birch 2008). Children in turn filter these family cultural traditions through their own personal experience with food to develop their own interpretations of their culture (Rozin 1982). Likewise, traditional cultures of immigrants and subcultures are interpreted by communities and families to varying degrees. Individuals filter these family and community interpretations of traditional culture through their own experiences with food and mainstream culture to create their own personal or family interpretations of their traditions and cultures. These interpretations result in different degrees of acculturation to mainstream culture, which need to be considered in nutrition education (Satia et al. 2002).

For example, some cultures believe that foods have "hot" and "cold" (or yin and yang) qualities and must be eaten to balance hot and cold body conditions to maintain health. However, individuals within a culture differ in the strengths of their beliefs about this interpretation of health and consequently on the extent to which these beliefs influence their health behaviors. Knowledge about the strength of these beliefs for a given audience can be useful in planning nutrition education (Liou & Contento 2004). Likewise, fate in some cultures is an important determinant of health behaviors. Again, members of the culture may

differ considerably in the strength of this belief. For other subcultures—where religiosity, racial pride, sense of time, and sense of community are important—individual differences exist and individual cognitive-motivational factors remain very important (Kreuter et al. 2003). In the case of breastfeeding, although cultural and family expectations are very important, individuals *still* differ in their opinions about these expectations (Bentley, Dee, & Jensen 2003).

All these considerations help nutrition educators recognize that individuals *internalize* the beliefs, norms, and values of their culture, and it is these personal interpretations that are powerful in people's lives (Triandis 1977). Some of these internalized cultural beliefs, norms, and values can be considered to be determinants of behavior and can be included as constructs in the theories and models described in this chapter, which can then be addressed in nutrition education research and activities directed at individual change.

Acculturation and Social Psychological Determinants to Study Food-Related Behaviors

Degree of acculturation may modify the social psychological mediators of diet-related behavior. Thus, a study of Chinese Americans examining health beliefs used the lens of culture and found that the social psychological mediators derived from theory were useful for all study participants, but were more predictive of behavior among those who were more acculturated (Liou & Contento 2004). A study of Latino adolescents found that gender and acculturation significantly modified the social psychological theory-based predictors of behavioral intention to eat a healthful diet (Diaz et al. 2009). Other cultural values may need to be more specifically addressed in nutrition education.

Understanding Motivations for Health Behavior Change

Centuries ago, the Greeks described both *logos* (reason) and *pathos* (emotion) as important in the human experience and key bases for ac-

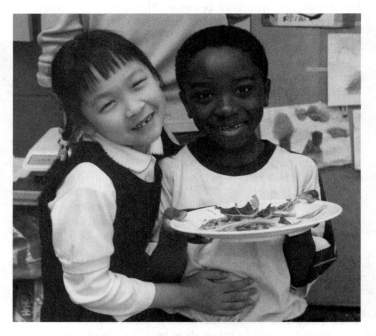

Attitude-change theories can help develop nutrition education activities to motivate students in group settings.

Theory in nutrition education provides a conceptual map, derived from evidence, to help us understand how the various influences on food- and nutrition-related behavior change are related to each other and to the behavior itself. These influences or potential mediators of change in the real world are thus "constructs" in the conceptual maps or theories.

mediators of behavior change = constructs in theories

Some theories were developed to explain behaviors undertaken for health reasons (e.g., health belief model). Other theories are needed to understand food choices and dietary behaviors undertaken for a variety of reasons in addition to health (e.g., theory of planned behavior). Still other theories are needed to understand how individuals can translate attitudes and intention into long-term dietary change (e.g., self-regulation models, social cognitive theory).

tion. Social psychological theories address both aspects of human motivation. Some theories were developed because researchers were studying health-related behaviors specifically, whereas others were investigating other social behaviors (such as consumer behaviors, including food choice) not necessarily related to health. Thus, the health belief model was developed specifically to understand and predict health behaviors. Its main constructs—perceived threat, perceived benefits, and perceived barriers (described in greater detail later in this chapter)—have proved to be very important and are widely used in interventions. However, the model does not help nutrition educators understand food choices and dietary behaviors that are undertaken for a variety of reasons other than health. For such understanding, other related social psychological theories prove very helpful.

These social psychological theories focus on beliefs, attitudes, and motivations and are very useful for designing nutrition education activities to increase interest and assist people to acquire the motivation to move from nonaction to the intention to take action on food- and nutrition-related issues. They are useful for group settings as well as mass media health communication campaigns. (See **Box 4-1**.)

Why Focusing on Motivation Is Important

Research shows that those who develop strong and stable intentions are more likely to be motivated to take action on their intentions. Most people have intentions for many health-related behaviors, but the intentions are not always very strong—as seems to be the case for Alicia and Ray, who you met in Chapter 3. People want to eat more healthfully, be more active, or get more sleep. But, for any given action, there also are many beliefs and emotions that can compete with the intention to eat more healthfully (cake is tasty but fattening; walking is healthy but takes time and effort). Thus, it is not always easy for people to develop strong and stable motivations or intentions.

Acting on these weak health intentions is made even more difficult in the face of strong environmental forces to act otherwise, from television advertising or the conveniently located less-than-healthful foods

at work to family members who have other needs and tastes. Thus, a motivational component in nutrition education is important for a wide range of people:

1. Those who are not aware of the importance of specific food-related actions that they could take to protect their health
2. Those who are aware but are uncommitted to taking action
3. Those with weak intentions, whom nutrition educators can stimulate to reexamine their intentions and assist to develop stronger intentions
4. Those who were taking action but have not maintained their motivation to do so.

The theories described in this chapter can help us as nutrition educators understand how to help our audiences reflect on their decisions and develop strong intentions for targeted behaviors or actions.

■ THE HEALTH BELIEF MODEL

In simplest terms, the health belief model states that people's beliefs influence their health-related actions or behaviors. The health belief model is a framework for understanding individuals' psychological readiness or intention to take a given health action. It was one of the earliest conceptual models to address health behavior specifically and is the most well-known theory in the field of public health. It is used widely around the world.

The model was developed in the 1950s by social psychologists working in the Lewin tradition, who were interested in using social science to solve practical public health problems (Becker 1974; Rosenstock 1974). They were committed to building theories for long-term use and not merely to solving practical health problems one at a time. The model is intuitively appealing, easy for nonpsychologists to understand and apply, and inexpensive to implement. Its commonsense constructs (beliefs) are clearly stated, manageable in number, and easily measured in a variety of ways, from interviews to surveys. The model focuses health professionals' attention on modifiable factors influencing behavior. (See **Box 4-2**.)

The health belief model proposes that readiness to take action is based on the following beliefs or convictions:

- I am susceptible to this health risk or problem.
- The threat to my health is serious.
- I perceive that the benefits of the recommended action outweigh the barriers or costs.
- I am confident that I can carry out the action successfully.
- Cues to action are present to remind me to take action.

Constructs of the Model

The model proposes that people's likelihood of taking a specific health-related action is primarily motivated by the following perceptions, considerations, or beliefs:

- *Perceived severity:* The construct of perceived severity refers to our beliefs about the seriousness of contracting an illness or other health-related condition. It may include an evaluation of the personal medical consequences (such as pain, disability, or death) or social consequences (impact on work, family life, and so forth) of the health condition.
- *Perceived susceptibility:* Perceived susceptibility is our belief about the possibility or likelihood of *personally* contracting this illness or health-related condition.
- *Perceived threat or risk* is the combination of perceived severity and personal susceptibility. These perceptions together result in our psychological state of readiness to take action.
- *Perceived benefits:* Perceived benefits are our opinions of whether a particular action or behavior is useful or effective in reducing the risk or threat of getting the condition. The behaviors may be eating fruits and vegetables to reduce cancer risk or safe food handling practices to reduce foodborne illness.
- *Perceived barriers:* Perceived barriers are our perceptions of the difficulties of performing the behavior, which can be psychological as well as physical. These may include perceptions of the cost and inconvenience of eating fruits and vegetables or the perception that some fruits and vegetables may not be agreeable. The barriers or obstacles may also be environmental, such as perceptions of the lack of availability and accessibility of healthful foods or options for physical activity. We tend to weigh costs of action against the benefits of action before taking action, even if we are not always conscious of doing so. Changing these beliefs through nutrition education, such as by increasing the perceived benefits and decreasing perceived barriers, should increase the likelihood of our taking a given health action.
- *Self-efficacy:* The health belief model was originally developed to explain simple health behaviors such as vaccinations or screenings, and hence did not include the influence of other people in the environment or the role of perceived skill or ability to perform the behavior (called self-efficacy). The role of self-efficacy has now been added to the model to explain long-term behaviors such as dietary behaviors. Self-efficacy is the confidence we have that we can perform the behavior (such as selecting, storing, or preparing fruits and vegetables).
- *Cues to action:* External events, such as the illness of a friend or family member or news stories on a scientific study about the issue, or internal events, such as personal symptoms and pains, are cues that remind us to act. These cues may influence our perceived threat for the condition and increase the likelihood that we will take action.

The model also postulates that demographic variables such as age, sex, and ethnicity indirectly influence behavior through their impact on perceived threat or perceived benefits and barriers. Likewise, sociopsychological variables such as personality, socioeconomic status, and peer and reference group pressure also influence behavior indirectly through their impact on perceived threat or perceived benefits and barriers.

Overcoming Optimistic Bias

Based on this model, then, making people aware of threat or risk is an important task of nutrition education. Indeed, studies have found that many people are falsely optimistic about their diets (Shim, Variyam, & Blaylock 2000). Many think that their diets are appropriately low in fat when in fact their diets are high in fat (Glanz, Brug, & van Assema 1997). Nutrition educators can use risk appraisals and self-assessments to elucidate personal risk information. Such personalized feedback counters people's tendency to be optimistically biased and encourages them to make changes in their dietary behaviors based on their true risk. A review of studies found that knowing personal risk may indeed spur lifestyle changes (McClure 2002).

A summary of the model is shown in **Figure 4-1**. An example of how this theory was used in developing educational materials for those with HIV/AIDS (Hoffman et al. 2005) is described in **Nutrition Education in Action 4-1**.

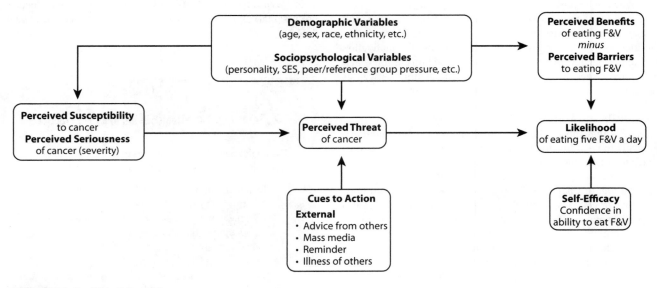

FIGURE 4-1 Health belief model.

(F&V = fruits and vegetables)

NUTRITION EDUCATION IN ACTION 4-1

Use of the Health Belief Model in the Development of Food Safety Materials for People with HIV/AIDS

Theory Construct/Determinant or Mediator of Behavior	Application to Food Safety Materials
Perceived susceptibility	Provided statistics and stated that people living with HIV/AIDS are more at risk for foodborne illness
Perceived severity	Stated that a foodborne illness can result in long-term health problems and even death
Perceived benefits	Provided positive, action-oriented effects of properly preparing and eating food safely; gave information on how to act, what to do
Perceived barriers	Gave enough information on food preparation and pathogens to correct misinformation; gave information to assist in properly preparing; gave reassurance
Cues to action	Gave explanations for issues brought up in discussion groups, for example, why some foods are risky, how to reduce risk for some foods by reheating, and substitutes for risky foods
Self-efficacy	Provided positive, action-oriented food selection and handling tips designed to reduce anxiety, and guidance in performing food safety actions to prevent foodborne illness

Source: Modified from Hoffman, E. W., V. Bergmann, J. Armstrong Schultz, P. Kendall, L. C. Medeiros, and V. N. Hillers. 2005. Application of a five-step message development model for food safety education materials targeting people with HIV/AIDS. *Journal of the American Dietetic Association* 105:1597–1604. Used with permission of the American Dietetic Association.

Evidence from Research and Intervention Studies

Because the health belief model is concerned with beliefs and concerns that can be changed through the means of communication or education, the model has been used as a framework to guide a variety of health behavior and nutrition education investigations.

Research Studies Using the Model

In a comprehensive review of 29 prospective and retrospective health belief model–related investigations undertaken during the decade following the publication of the health belief model in 1974, Janz and Becker (1984) found that the beliefs that were the most powerful determinants in predicting health behavior across all studies were as follows: perceived barriers to taking action (significant in 91% of studies), perceived benefits of taking action (81%), perceived susceptibility to the condition (71%), and perceived seriousness of the condition (59%).

- One study found that the health belief model was a moderately good predictor of fat intake, accounting for about 30% of the variance in behavior between groups (Shafer, Keith, & Schafer 1995). This model included the construct of self-efficacy, with items stated in terms of difficulty or perceived barriers: "Even though I know that my way of eating is not good for me, I just can't seem to change my habits." In another study of individuals' likelihood to reduce their fat intake to reduce heart disease risk, *perceived barriers* also emerged as most important, followed by self-efficacy (Liou & Contento 2001).
- In a study with older adults, the *perceived threat* of foodborne illness was important, but safe food handling behaviors were most strongly influenced by the cues to action from news stories or labels on food packages (Hanson & Benedict 2002).
- A study found that for wives the costs of, or barriers to, a healthy diet in terms of expense, time, unpleasantness, and confusion about recommendations had a significant effect on fat intake,

whereas for their husbands, perceived threat of disease and self-efficacy had a significant effect (Shafer et al. 1995).

These studies show that although most health belief model constructs are important mediators of dietary behavior, their relative importance differed by study, most likely reflecting the specific behavior in question and the nature of the particular groups of people in the different studies. The specific beliefs may also differ by cultural heritage. For example, one study found that barriers to eating healthfully among African Americans included the social and cultural symbolism of certain foods along with taste and expense (James 2004).

These studies show that a sense of threat or perceived risk of disease (e.g., heart disease) *and* perceived benefits of taking action are important. Benefits in this context are effective responses or actions individuals can take to reduce the threat or avoid the danger—actions such as eating a healthier, low-fat diet or eating organic foods. Hence the term *response efficacy* is also used. An understanding of barriers to action and a feeling of *self-efficacy* in overcoming barriers are also paramount.

Intervention Studies Using the Model

Numerous intervention programs based on the health belief model have been developed and implemented in the public health arena, including dietary change. Indeed, the constructs of *benefits* and *barriers* are widely used in interventions. You shall see later that they are similar to constructs in other theories, such as the pros and cons of change in the transtheoretical model, and beliefs about outcomes (or *outcome expectations*) in the theory of planned behavior and social cognitive theory. What the health belief model adds is the construct of perceived risk, which is regarded as the motivational factor that initiates the psychological readiness to take action. How the main constructs of the health belief model can be converted into practical activities is shown in **Table 4-2**. A few example intervention studies are described next.

TABLE 4-2	Health Belief Model: Major Concepts and Implications for Nutrition Education Interventions	
Construct of Theory/Mediator of Behavior Change	**Definition**	**Applications to Practice**
Perceived severity	Beliefs about the seriousness of the consequences of a health condition	Provide messages about the serious personal impacts (medical and social) of conditions such as heart disease or diabetes.
Perceived susceptibility	Chances of experiencing a risk or getting a condition	Provide messages or activities to personalize risk for individuals based on family history or behavior through self-assessment tools.
Perceived benefits	Beliefs that a given action is effective in reducing risk	Provide messages about benefits of engaging in a behavior to reduce risk based on scientific evidence on the efficacy of the behavior to reduce risk and other benefits, such as taste or convenience.
Perceived barriers	Beliefs about the psychological or tangible costs or obstacles to taking the action	Identify and reduce perception of barriers to engaging in the action. For example, fruits and vegetables can be inexpensive if eaten in season and can be filling. Correct misconceptions.
Self-efficacy	Confidence in one's ability to carry out the action	Messages that provide guidance on how to make behavior or action easy to do.
Cues to action	Strategies to activate readiness to take the action	Provide reminders about the behavior: posters, community billboards, and media campaigns.

Group Interventions

Older Adults: One study focused on increasing consumption of whole-grain foods by older adults (Ellis et al. 2005). The program was delivered in congregate meal sites and consisted of five sessions that addressed variables or constructs of the health belief model as follows:

- *Perceived susceptibility and severity:* Emphasizing the health conditions that occur frequently in older people that are associated with low intake of whole grains
- *Perceived benefits:* Describing the potential benefits in terms of decreasing the risk of certain health conditions
- *Perceived barriers:* Providing information on how to overcome barriers; taste testing many different whole-grain foods to overcome the barrier of taste
- *Self-efficacy:* Demonstrating and reinforcing during the sessions various ways to include whole-grain foods, teaching label reading skills, and correcting misinformation about the labeling of whole grains
- *Cues to action:* Recipes, tip sheets, and other handouts to provide continuing cues to action at home

The program resulted in increased frequency of eating whole-grain foods. The participants' knowledge improved (although it was high to begin with), and they believed more strongly than before that whole-grain foods would reduce risk of disease.

University Employees: Likewise, an eight-session program with university employees that focused on perceived risk for cardiovascular disease and cancer, perceived benefits to taking action, and perceived barriers resulted in significant behavioral change in terms of reduced intakes of calories, fat as a percentage of calories, saturated fat, and cholesterol (Abood, Black, & Feral 2003). Intakes of fruits and vegetables also increased but did not reach significance.

Social Marketing Campaigns: Two social marketing campaigns based on the health belief model are described here: one, called Project LEAN (Low-Fat Eating for Americans Now), was a national campaign designed to promote low-fat eating and emphasized the perception of risk. The other, called Pick a Better Snack, was designed to increase fruit and vegetable consumption among low-income groups in Iowa and emphasized the positive message of how to reduce barriers. Adding group education enhanced the effectiveness of the media campaign. These two campaigns are described in **Nutrition Education in Action 4-2** and **Nutrition Education in Action 4-3**.

Take-Home Message about Health Belief Model

- When people experience a personal threat about a health condition they will likely take action, but only if the benefits of taking action outweigh the barriers, actual and psychological. Having the ability to take action also is crucial.
- You will find this theory especially useful for designing nutrition education activities to enhance awareness and motivation to take action to reduce risk of a health-related condition.

■ THE PRECAUTION ADOPTION PROCESS MODEL

In its simplest terms, the precaution adoption process model (PAPM) describes how people come to the decision to adopt a new precautionary behavior through a series of stages from unawareness, through decision making, to action and maintenance.

The goal of PAPM is to explain how individuals come to the decision to take action about a risk and how they translate that decision into action (Weinstein 1988; Weinstein & Sandman, 1992). The model proposes that behavior change proceeds through a series of stages, starting with individuals being unaware of a health- or food-related risk (e.g.,

NUTRITION EDUCATION IN ACTION **4-2**

The Project LEAN (Low-Fat Eating for Americans Now) Campaign

This national social marketing campaign was designed to promote low-fat eating: Project LEAN (Samuels 1993). The program consisted of several components to heighten public awareness about the risk of diets high in dietary fat, especially saturated fat:

- Media campaign
- Participation of chefs and food journalists in demonstrations to show health professionals how to help the public appreciate the taste of low-fat foods
- Community programs and private voluntary organization activities to reinforce the message

Theoretical Framework

Dietary fat was chosen because of its health risks and because surveys showed it was a concern of the public. A series of 10 focus group interviews revealed that knowledge of sources of fat was high. However, convenience, habit, and taste were major obstacles. It was decided that the media component would consist of a national public service advertising campaign based on the health belief model and sponsored by the Advertising Council.

Motivational Messages

Given that lack of motivation was considered the major obstacle to eating lower-fat foods, the campaign consisted of two components: motivational messages to enhance the sense of perceived risk (why to change) and a toll-free hotline (1-800-EATLEAN) that people could call to receive a booklet that provided information on effective actions individuals could take to reduce the risk, including recipes (how to change). The 15- and 30-second television spots used a Hitchcock-like, humorous approach to emphasize the impact of fat in the diet. The public service print advertisements are shown here.

Evaluation

The messages were broadcast through various channels, including television, radio, newspapers, and media events. It was estimated that the public service advertising component reached 50% of the viewing audience, and the print publicity more than 35 million readers. The hotline received more than 300,000 calls, and numerous local campaigns were implemented.

Source: Samuels, S. E. 1993. Project LEAN: Lessons learned from a national social marketing campaign. *Public Health Reports* 108:45–53.

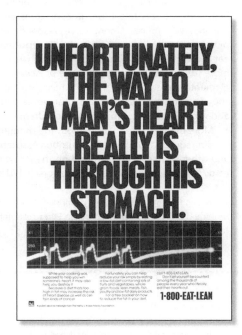

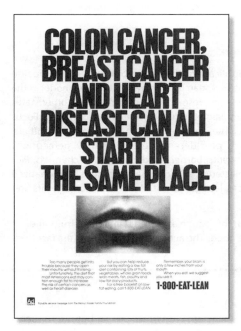

Public service advertisements for Project LEAN.

NUTRITION EDUCATION IN ACTION 4-3

The Pick a Better Snack™ Campaign

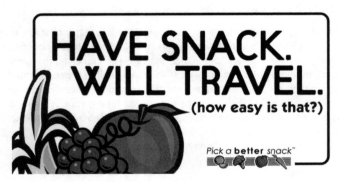

The *Pick a* **better** *snack* campaign was developed by the partners in the Iowa Nutrition Network to increase fruit and vegetable consumption among children in Iowa by promoting a switch from high-fat, low-nutrient snacks to nutrient-dense, low- or no-fat fruits and vegetables. Intended audiences were low-income parents, providers of early childhood education, and schools, as well as children themselves. The campaign included monthly classroom lessons that featured the fruits and vegetables most available or seasonal that month, as well as simple graphics with colorful fruits and vegetables that were used on recipe cards, posters, grocery-store signage, bookmarks, brochures, and billboards.

Theoretical Framework

In terms of theory application, the *Pick a* **better** *snack* campaign originated from formative research, with the health belief model as the foundation. Social marketing research and materials from other states were reviewed, and campaign themes were selected for testing. Focus groups were then held. They included groups of low-income mothers, fathers, and child-care providers to determine their perceptions about motivations, benefits, barriers, and information channels. *Pick a* **better** *snack* was selected as a key message because it emphasized a simple action that can lead to increased consumption of fruits and vegetables.

- *Perceived benefits:* The focus was on the benefit that fruits and vegetables "taste good." The audience already knew the fact that

fruits and vegetables are also good for your health. In the school component, students tasted different fruits and vegetables in monthly classes to increase familiarity with and enjoyment of the sensory-affective aspects of these foods.
- *Perceived barriers:* Messages through the mass media focused on making eating fruits and vegetables easy to do. Recipes were provided where appropriate.

Examples of messages are as follows:

- Bananas: Peel. Eat. (how easy is that?)
- Tomatoes: Slice. Eat. (how easy is that?)
- Apples: Wash. Bite. (how easy is that?)

Evaluation

Two communities were selected for implementation of intense media efforts in early 2003 to determine which strategies would best reach the targeted low-income audience. Media buys were secured for billboards, bus signs, radio, and local shopper newspapers. Surveys were conducted in Food Stamp offices ($n = 600$) and with customers in the front of grocery stores in low-income neighborhoods ($n = 500$). Surveys indicated that the most effective implementation channels were billboards, schools, television, grocery stores, and Women, Infants, and Children (WIC) offices. Among survey respondents, 51% recalled hearing or seeing the campaign messages, 25% reported they were starting to eat more fruits and vegetables, and 36% were thinking about eating more fruits and vegetables because of *Pick a* **better** *snack*. Surveys of elementary age students ($n = 1455$) receiving the classroom component showed a statistically significant improvement in attitudes toward fruit and vegetable snacks among these children.

More detailed information about the program, its partners, and its funding sources (Supplemental Nutrition Assistance Program Education and other sources) can be found on the *Pick a* **better** *snack* website, http://www.idph.state.ia.us/pickabettersnack/default.asp.

Source: Logo and graphics used with permission of Iowa Department of Public Health and Iowa Department of Education, Bureau of Nutrition Programs and Transportation.

---

osteoporosis, heart disease), and then becoming aware but unengaged and believing that the risk may apply to other people but not to themselves. Here, they have an *optimistic bias*. Individuals who reach the decision-making stage are engaged with the issue and are considering their response, such as whether to take calcium supplements or whether to reduce their saturated fat intake as a precaution. They can choose to take action or not to act. If they decide to act, they then initiate the behavior. The model is shown in **Figure 4-2**.

The model is especially useful in helping nutrition educators understand that those not currently taking action on an issue that health

professionals think is important are not all the same. Some are not taking action because they have not heard about the threat or issue. Media messages are important here in helping people become aware of a threat and the precautions they can take. However, there also is a group that is aware but unengaged, believing the precaution does not apply to them personally. An optimistic bias is in operation. For this group, engagement in the action may require targeted communications about risk or some personal experience that makes the issue salient or relevant to them. There are still others who may feel that they just do not have the confidence (self-efficacy) or skills to engage in the behav-

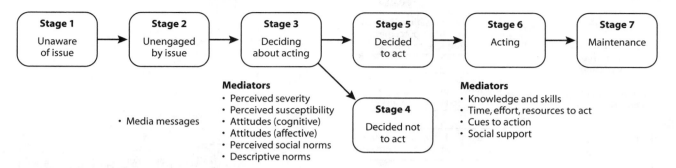

FIGURE 4-2 Stages of the precaution adoption process model.

ior, so there is no point trying. Finally, among those who are not taking action are those who have thought about the issue but have rejected taking action. They may be quite well informed, or they have tried the behavior many times before (e.g., dieting) and have given up. This is a difficult group to reach.

At the point of deciding whether to take action, the many mediators from the health belief model and theory or planned behavior are important in facilitating a decision: perceived susceptibility and threat in terms of the health or food issue; perceived benefits to taking action; attitudes, including worry and fear; perceived social norms; and the behaviors and recommendations of others (descriptive norms).

Once the decision has been made, taking action then requires time, effort, resources, detailed how-to knowledge and skills, social support, and cues to action. Nutrition education has an important role here.

THEORY OF PLANNED BEHAVIOR

In its simplest terms, the theory of planned behavior states that people's behaviors are determined by their intentions, which in turn are influenced by attitudes, social norms, and perception of control over the behavior.

The theory of planned behavior (Ajzen 1991; Fishbein & Ajzen 1975), with its emphasis on attitudes, was developed to try to understand a number of social behaviors such as participation in community organizations or attendance at college or church. It has been found to be very useful for understanding food choice and voluntary health and dietary behaviors. Like other social psychological theories based on expectancy-value considerations, the theory assumes that people make decisions in a reasonable manner. Despite its name, the theory does not imply that behaviors are necessarily rational, planned, or appropriate from an objective point of view—only that they make sense to the person. For example, eating a large piece of chocolate cake to feel good is rational from the cake eater's point of view, whatever the nutritional merits of the act.

Understanding underlying reasons for action. The theory of planned behavior permits nutrition educators to discern these underlying reasons for action and understand a given group's own reasons that motivate the behavior. The theory does not specify what these beliefs are, only which categories of beliefs or which constructs to explore. It is thus a content-free model that can be used with a variety of health behaviors and groups. The actual beliefs must be obtained from the groups themselves, using open-ended elicitation interviews or other means.

Neither does the theory imply that people consciously and systematically go through all the processes described here every time they act. Obviously, many health-related behaviors have become automatic or habitual, such as smoking or eating cereal at breakfast. However, the theory does suggest that the attitudes and beliefs underlying these behaviors can be brought to awareness and hence changed. It is thus important for nutrition educators to understand the nature of attitudes and beliefs, how they are formed, and how they might be changed.

A summary of the model is shown in **Figure 4-3**, and how the main constructs of the theory can be used in nutrition education practice are described in **Table 4-3**.

Behavior

The theory of planned behavior calls for the behaviors to be stated specifically: the more specifically the behavior is stated, the more predictive the theory is of the behavior. Questions regarding very specific behaviors are "How many times do you eat fruit as part of your noon

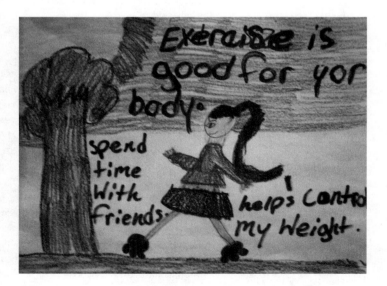

The theory of planned behavior allows us to understand what motivates us to exercise.

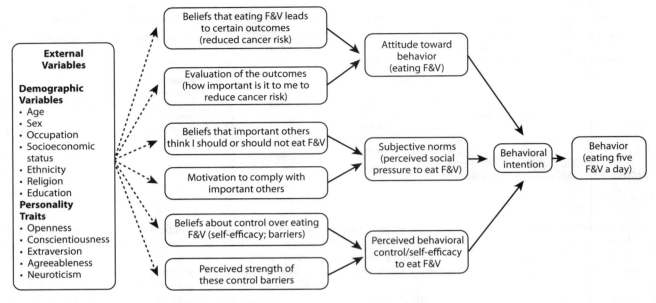

FIGURE 4-3 Theory of planned behavior: Example of behavior of eating fruits and vegetables.

(F&V = fruits and vegetables)

TABLE 4-3	Theory of Planned Behavior and Extensions: Major Concepts and Implications for Nutrition Education Interventions	
Construct of Theory/Potential Mediator of Behavior Change	**Definition**	**Applications to Practice**
Behavioral intentions	Perceived likelihood of taking a given action	Lead group through decision-making activities to assess personal positive and negative expectations (pros and cons) of change and commitment to try the new behavior.
Attitudes	Favorable or unfavorable judgments about a given behavior	Messages and images can show healthful behavior in positive light.
Outcome expectations (basis of cognitive attitudes)	Beliefs about the outcomes of performing the behavior	*Enhance positive expectations:* Provide messages or use strategies in groups to enhance people's expectations about taste, health benefits, and convenience of eating F&V, including through tasting, preparing, or cooking them. *Decrease negative expectations:* F&V can be inexpensive if eaten in season and can be filling; correct misconceptions.
Affective attitudes (experiential attitudes)	Emotional response to the idea of performing the behavior	Provide opportunities to experience and enjoy healthful food through food tastings or food preparation and cooking experiences accompanied by eating the food prepared with others. Explore anticipated regret if action is not taken.
Subjective norms (injunctive norms)	Beliefs that people who are important to the group either approve or disapprove of them performing a behavior	For adolescents, show that eating F&V is cool; use peer or valued models to encourage eating F&V.
Descriptive norms	Beliefs about other people's *attitudes* or *behaviors* in regard to the behavior	In groups, collect or give data showing that many teens do eat F&V and/or value health; correct misconceptions.
Perceived behavioral control	Perceptions of how much control people have over the behavior, whether there are environmental barriers to action	Provide messages that eating F&V can be easy and convenient (e.g., for bananas: "Peel, eat; how easy is that?"). Provide information on how to prepare F&V to carry to school or work.

Note: F&V = fruits and vegetables.

day meal each month?" (Conner & Norman 1995) and "How often do you eat vegetables each week?" However, many studies state behaviors more generally, reflecting practical considerations, such as "eating a low-fat diet" or "eating a healthy diet." In the area of diet or physical activity, frequency questionnaires or behavioral checklists are often used to measure behaviors. In cross-sectional studies, behaviors and the determinants of the behaviors (described later in this chapter) are measured at the same time, whereas in prospective studies determinants are measured first, followed by the behavior some time later, such as the next day, or two or four weeks later, as specified.

Behavioral Intention

The theory of planned behavior proposes that we are more likely to engage in a behavior, such as eating low-fat foods or engaging in physical activity, if we intend to do so. That is, when we make plans to do something, we are more likely to do it than if we do not. This most immediate mediator of behavior change is called *behavioral intention* (BI). This state of mind can be stated simply as "I intend to eat more fruits and vegetables" or "I intend to eat fewer high-fat snacks in the next month" (on a scale from "definitely do not" to "definitely do"). Sometimes intentions are stated in terms of how likely a person is to engage in an *expected action*, such as "How likely are you to eat organic foods in the next week?" (Sparks, Shepherd, & Frewer 1995). It has been suggested that *desires* ("I would like to eat fruit as part of my midday meals") may be either a precursor to behavioral intention or another way to state behavioral intention.

Research evidence has found that reported intentions are reliably and moderately correlated with a range of health actions (Armitage & Conner 2001) and hence are a key mediator of behavior or indicator of level of commitment or motivation. Individuals are certainly not likely to engage in a behavior if they do *not* intend to do so. Intention is in turn determined by attitudes, social norms, and a sense of control over the behavior.

Attitudes

Attitudes are favorable or unfavorable judgments about a given behavior, such as "Eating fruits and vegetables would be good/bad, enjoyable/unenjoyable," often rated on a 5- or 7-point scale.

Attitudes have both a *cognitive/evaluative component*, also called *instrumental attitudes*, such as how good or bad for health it would be to lose weight, and an *affective component*, also called *experiential attitudes*, such as how good or bad a person would feel about him- or herself losing weight. Both components influence intentions (Trafimow & Sheeran 1998; Ajzen 2001).

Cognitive/Evaluative Component (or Instrumental Attitudes)

Attitudes are strongly influenced by our beliefs about the outcomes or consequences of our actions and how important these consequences are.

Beliefs About Expected Outcomes or Consequences of Behavior

We do what fulfills a value that has meaning for us. These values can be quite immediate or more enduring, quite personal or all-pervasive and global. The immediate, or instrumental, values are beliefs and expectations that a behavior (such as eating fruits and vegetables) will lead to certain outcomes and are usually called *outcome beliefs* or *outcome expectations* (OEs). Examples are "Eating fruits and veg-

etables will increase how much energy I have"; or "will reduce my risk of cancer" and "if I eat this food, I will feel comforted or it will relieve my depression." These beliefs are really *reasons* why to engage in the behavior.

Expected outcomes or reasons for a given action or behavior are of two general kinds: health outcomes based on scientific evidence, and personally meaningful outcomes including social and self-evaluative outcomes:

- *Health outcomes* are based on the scientific evidence on diet and health or diet and disease relationships, such as between eating calcium-rich foods and bone health, breastfeeding and the health of the infant, antioxidants in food and cancer, and so forth. For example, those who believed that there was a connection between diet and cancer risk decreased their intake of fat over a three-year period (Kristal et al. 2000).
- *Personally meaningful outcomes* might be taste, convenience, preparation/cooking needs, cost, good value for money, contribution to personal appearance, having more energy, and so forth. Expected outcomes can be positive (e.g., good taste) or negative (e.g., high cost), as well as cognitive (e.g., "Eating fruits and vegetables will decrease my risk of cancer") and affective (e.g., "Eating fruits and vegetables will make me feel good about myself").
- *Larger, global end goals* might include such values as family cohesion, empowerment of communities, support of local farmers, or conservation of resources (discussed later).

Value of Outcomes to Individuals

Our judgments about how desirable (for example, from "not desirable" to "very desirable") the outcomes of a behavior are also influence whether we take action.

Motivation

$$\text{motivation} = \text{beliefs about expectations} \times \text{values}$$

Motivation to initiate a behavior thus depends on our beliefs about both the *expected outcomes* and the *value* to us personally of future outcomes from the behavior. Future events cannot serve as determinants of behavior in the present. However, their representations in our minds in the present can have powerful causal impacts on present action. That is, we want to maximize positive outcomes such as health, taste, or not wasting food and minimize negative outcomes of engaging in food or nutrition behavior, such as cost or inconvenience.

Attitudes and Their Underlying Beliefs

Attitudes toward a behavior can be considered our summaries of our decision-making processes about the behavior. We come to judge whether we are positively or negatively inclined toward a given behavior, such as eating at fast food restaurants or breastfeeding, based on *underlying beliefs* about the outcomes of the behavior and how much we value these outcomes. It has been found that attitudes and their underlying beliefs are often quite interchangeable in studies: they often yield the same predictive power (Schwarzer 1992). Thus, beliefs about expected outcomes of behavior are major mediators of behavioral intention (through attitude formation) and hence are motivators of behavior.

In designing nutrition education interventions, nutrition educators can then design activities to address directly people's specific expectations about the outcome of the behavior, such as taste, cost, or convenience. These are often abbreviated OE for *outcome expectations*.

Affective Component: Emotions and Enjoyment of Food (or Experiential Attitudes)

Although the cognitive component of attitudes based on beliefs about outcomes of a behavior is a major motivator of behavioral intention, the affective component of attitudes, reflecting people's feelings or emotions about performing the behavior, is also a powerful—some would say more powerful—motivator of dietary behaviors (Salovey & Birnbaum 1989). People's emotions and feelings reflect their more enduring values and "hot buttons." Affective beliefs or feelings are more likely to be derived from direct experience, such as physiological reactions to food (e.g., taste, smell, sight, or fillingness of food) and familiarity through frequent exposure. *Emotions* have been described as a state of arousal involving both conscious thought and physiological or visceral changes. The result of this internal process of emotion is a feeling toward a food, behavior, object, or situation.

Food Preferences and Enjoyment

Sensory-affective responses to food powerfully influence food choice and dietary behavior (Rozin & Fallon 1981). Consumers consistently rate taste preferences or liking as a leading motivator of their dietary choices. It was also demonstrated in a study using the theory of planned behavior to study the choice of low-salt breads (Tuorila-Ollikainen, Lahteenmaki, & Salovaara 1986). The theory predicted 38% of buying intentions and 21% of actual selections. However, the individuals were also given a taste test and asked to rate breads in terms of "liking." When this rating of liking was included in the theory, the values were improved to 52% and 32%, respectively. In fact, liking was by itself the best predictor of the behavior.

Anticipated Positive Feelings

Feelings and emotions about involvement in a behavior also contribute to attitudes. For example, our attitudes toward losing weight may be motivated not only by our belief that it will make us healthier or look better (the cognitive aspect of attitudes) but also that it will make us feel good about ourselves because we are able to take control of our lives. Helping children enjoy eating more vegetables may make parents feel good about themselves.

Anticipated Regret

Anticipated regret or worry about the consequences of acting or failing to act also has been shown to be a mediator of preventive health behavior. A study showed that anticipated regret influenced the intention to eat junk foods (Richard, van der Pligt, & de Vries 1996). Another example might be our anticipated regret or worry that regularly eating foods high in saturated fat may increase our risk of getting heart disease later.

Relationship Between the Cognitive/Thinking and Affective/Feeling Components

The cognitive and affective components of attitudes are inextricably linked to each other. Studies have found that when beliefs and feelings are consistent with each other, both are equally good at predicting attitudes and behavior. However, when they are not consistent, feelings are primary (Ajzen 2001). For example, one study found that positive affective reactions to fast food, convenience, and self-serving thoughts overrode cognitive analyses of the longer-term health risks associated with frequent fast food consumption (Dunn et al. 2008).

Individuals may differ in their tendency to base their attitudes on beliefs or feelings. In studies on social issues, the attitudes of those identified as "thinkers" were better predicted by their beliefs than by their feelings, whereas the reverse was true for individuals identified as "feelers" (Ajzen 2001). In a parallel fashion, attitudes toward some foods or issues (e.g., specific foods such as chocolate) may be based largely on feelings, whereas attitudes toward others (e.g., eating foods produced through gene biotechnology) may be based largely on reasoning and the evaluation of scientific information.

Strong and Stable Attitudes

Studies have shown that strong attitudes toward foods are more predictive of behavioral intentions than are weak attitudes (Sparks, Hedderley, & Shepherd 1992). Information that is personally relevant to people leads to the formation of stronger attitudes. Stronger attitudes are less susceptible to change. Stable attitudes are also more predictive of dietary behaviors. For example, stable attitudes were predictive of eating a low-fat diet three months later (Conner et al. 2000) and of eating a healthier diet six years later (Conner, Norman, & Bell 2002). More stable attitudes are also more resistant to persuasion.

The downside of these findings is that nutrition education is less likely to change strong and stable attitudes toward less nutritious foods or diets. The upside is that once people form strong and stable attitudes toward more healthful food practices—through nutrition education, for example—these are likely to last and to be predictive of behavior.

Conflicting Attitudes: Ambivalence

The coexistence of both positive and negative beliefs about outcomes of behavior may cause ambivalence (Armitage & Conner 2000b; Ajzen 2001). This is especially true for food choices and dietary behaviors. For example, individuals may believe that eating fruits and vegetables is desirable because doing so reduces the risk of cancer, but fruits and vegetables may also be expensive and inconvenient to carry around or eat. Animal products may taste good, but individuals may have concerns about animal welfare issues.

Ambivalence may also result from a conflict between the cognitive component (chocolate cakes are fattening) and the affective component of attitudes (I love the taste of chocolate). The relative strengths of these thoughts and feelings influence whether a person takes action. For example, greater ambivalence about eating meat, vegetarianism, or vegan diets resulted in weaker associations between attitudes and intentions (Povey, Wellens, & Conner 2001). The same was found for ambivalence about eating chocolate (Sparks et al. 2001). Ambivalent attitudes are weak and are more susceptible to persuasive communication.

Subjective Norms (Perceived Social Pressure)

Subjective norms, or perceived social pressure, are our beliefs that most people who are important to us either approve or disapprove of us performing a behavior (e.g., "People who care about me think that I should/should not breastfeed"). These also are called *injunctive norms* (other people's injunctions).

Subjective or injunctive norms are in turn determined by the following:

- *Normative beliefs:* The strength of our beliefs that specific important people approve or disapprove of the behavior ("My close friends/parents think that I should/should not eat meat").
- *Motivation to comply:* The strength of our desire to comply with these people's opinions ("How much do you want to do what your friends think you should do?"). This strength may range from "not at all" to "very much." Because individuals' motivations may be related to the approval of a range of specific others, the variety of

people (e.g., peers, family) whose approval is important for the particular behavior (e.g., eating fruits and vegetables or drinking soda) and the particular population (e.g., teenagers) must be assessed to design effective nutrition education.

Descriptive Norms

It has been shown that *descriptive norms* can be as important as injunctive ones in motivating health behaviors (Sheeran, Norman, & Orbell 1999). Descriptive norms include beliefs about other people's *attitudes* toward the behavior in question (group attitude), such as attitudes of individuals' personal or social network toward drinking soda, and perceptions of other people's *behavior* (group behavior), such as how many in an individual's social circle drink soda. This construct captures the strong impact of social or cultural attitudes and practices.

Are Attitudes or Subjective Norms More Important?

Individuals differ on the relative weight they place on attitudes and on the opinions of others. These relative weights also differ across behaviors. For example, subjective norms may be more important in cultures that are more collectivist in nature, whereas attitudes may be more important in individualistic cultures (Ajzen 2001). Some food behaviors (such as eating low-fat foods) may be more influenced by attitudes, whereas others (such as breastfeeding) are more influenced by social norms. (See **Box 4-3**.)

Perceived Behavioral Control

We also act in accordance with our perceptions of how much control we have over the behavior, or *perceived behavioral control* (PBC). This theory construct also includes the notion of whether we can overcome barriers or can perform the behavior. For example, healthier foods may not be easily available in the local grocery store, or people may not know how to cook. Perceived behavioral control influences both intention and behavior, probably because *perception* of control is likely to increase our effort to successfully carry out an intention and because perception of control may reflect *actual* control (refer to Figure 4-2).

Perceived Behavioral Control and Self-Efficacy

Perceived behavioral control is similar to the self-efficacy construct of social cognitive theory (Armitage & Conner 1999, 2001). Self-efficacy is generally defined in terms of *personal competence or confidence* in being able to carry out a given behavior ("I am confident that I could successfully eat five fruits and vegetables a day if I wanted to") whereas perceived behavioral control includes the notion of *perceived difficulties*, including personal resources and external barriers. Many researchers, however, consider the terms to be interchangeable (Ajzen 1991, 1998; Bandura 2000; Fishbein 2000), with some using the term *self-efficacy* (Fishbein 2000) in models and others, its complement, *barriers* (Lien, Lytle, & Komro 2002; Kassem et al. 2003). Examples are "I am confident that I can eat fruit at work even if it is not readily available" and "I can avoid eating attractive, high-fat foods, even at a party."

Extensions of the Theory of Planned Behavior

Research has led to investigations of possible extensions of the theory of planned behavior by incorporating mediators of behavior that reflect on the self, such as moral norms and self-identity. In the area of food and nutrition, these mediators have been found to make some additional independent contribution to the prediction of behavior.

Box 4-3   Theory of Planned Behavior in Practice

The theory of planned behavior proposes that individuals are likely to take a specific action if they *intend* to take that action. Intention to take action is based on the following beliefs and feelings:

- I believe that taking this action will lead to outcomes I desire.
- I perceive that the positive outcomes of taking this action outweigh the negative outcomes.
- I have positive feelings about taking this action, and taking action will make me feel good about myself.
- People important to me think that I should take this action and their opinions are important to me.
- I am confident that I can carry out the action, despite difficulties.

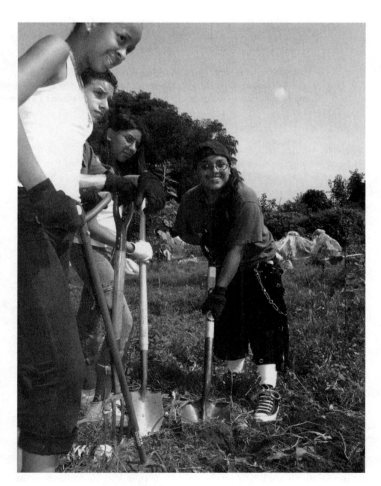

Participating in a community urban farming project improves youths' attitudes toward food and nutrition.

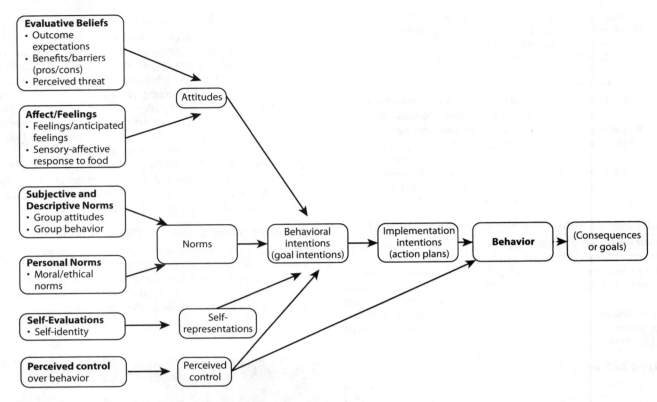

FIGURE 4-4 Extended theory of planned behavior.

Source: Based on Abraham, C., and P. Sheeran. 2000. Understanding and changing health behaviour: From health beliefs to self-regulation. In *Understanding and changing health behaviour from health beliefs to self-regulation*, edited by P. Norman, C. Abraham, and M. Conner. Amsterdam: Hardwood Academic Publishers.

Figure 4-4 summarizes the many constructs of the extended theory of planned behavior and how they are related to and predict behavioral intentions and behavior.

Personal Normative Beliefs: Perceived Moral or Ethical Obligation

A number of researchers have found that *personal normative beliefs* are important (Armitage & Conner 2000b). An example might be "I feel I should breastfeed my baby." Studies have shown that *moral and ethical considerations* make some contribution to prediction of behavior, such as parents giving milk to their children ("I feel it is my moral obligation to feed my child milk/healthful foods") (Raats, Shepherd, & Sparks 1995). A review has found that moral norms are important in bridging the intention–behavior gap (Godin, Conner, & Sheeran 2005). A related concept is perceived personal responsibility, such as "I feel that I have a responsibility to buy organic foods to improve the health of the natural environment," which was found to be related to behavior (Bissonette & Contento 2001).

Self-Identity

Related to the focus on personal norms are other thoughts we have about ourselves, including self-concept or self-identity, which refers to the relatively enduring characteristics people ascribe to themselves (Sparks 2000). These *self-referent factors* have been shown to contribute some to the prediction of behavior: "I think of myself as someone who is

concerned about environmental issues" or "green issues" or "a health-conscious consumer" (Sparks et al. 1992; Sparks et al. 1995; Bissonette & Contento 2001; Robinson & Smith 2002). Individuals' identities in food choice tend to be both stable and dynamic over time and were shaped by life experiences (Bisogni et al. 2002).

Ideal-self versus actual-self discrepancies, resulting in disappointment, sadness, or depression, and *ought-to-be self versus actual-self discrepancies*, resulting in fear and anxiety, have been studied in other domains (Abraham & Sheeran 2000). In nutrition, surveys of consumers often reveal these kinds of considerations when individuals think about their diets. For example, one survey found that people's predominant emotions about their diets were guilt, worry, helplessness, anger, and fear: "I feel like a bad mom. I know that my kids should have better things to eat" (IFIC Foundation 1999). These considerations are especially strong relative to weight issues.

From "I Wish" to "I Will": Implementation Intentions (Action Plans)

Personal experience suggests, and research confirms, that behavioral intentions are not sufficient to initiate difficult behaviors such as dietary change. Our intentions or wishes are more likely to be carried out if they are first translated into *implementation intentions*, specifying exactly when, where, and how we will undertake the particular behavior (Armitage 2006; Garcia & Mann 2003). These are called *action plans* in other theories. The general behavioral intention may be to eat five fruits and vegetables a day. However, to make that a reality, we need to make more specific plans, such as "I will have a midmorning snack of fruit and add one vegetable to my lunch each day this week."

Note, however, that setting an implementation intention for a healthy behavior (e.g., eating more fruit for a snack) by itself does not necessarily drive out a habit that might be counter to this intention (e.g., eating fatty snacks and sweets) (Verplanken & Faes 1999).

Habits, Routines, and Behaviors Without Conscious Planning

Many behaviors appear to occur without much thought. We do not seem to consciously and systemically go through a decision-making process based on beliefs, peer pressure, or sense of control every time we make a choice. We develop routines or habits that seem to be automatic responses to situations and are often the driving force in behavior. Indeed, for many behaviors, past behavior has been shown to be a good predictor of future behavior (Triandis 1977; Ajzen & Madden 1986; Conner et al. 2000; Ajzen 2001; Nilsen, Bourne, & Verplanken 2008). This is especially true of frequently performed behaviors, such as eating behavior (Kumanyika et al. 2000).

Motivations and Cues

Research suggests that when we repeatedly perform a behavior in a particular situation, both the overall motivation, such as our liking for cereal in the morning, and the instructions for its implementation—preparing the cereal—may become integrated in our thinking about the situation. Thus, both the motivation and the cues are automatically triggered in memory when we are faced with the same situation (e.g., eating cereal in the morning) (Fazio 1990).

Time and Circumstances

We may use reasoned processes under certain circumstances, and habitual or automatic processes in others (Fazio 1990). For example, we may use deliberate processes when the behaviors are perceived to have serious personal consequences, such as choosing whether to breast-feed a baby. However, when consequences are perceived not to be very serious, as is the case of many everyday food choices, automatic processes occur. The time available to make a decision may also be a factor. When there is very little time to make a decision, such as may occur in supermarket purchases, spontaneous processes may be more important than reasoning processes are. For example, roughly 65% of supermarket decisions are made in the store and, of those that are unplanned, 67% are due to retail displays and other manufacturing factors (Abratt & Goodey 1990). Marketing practices, such as the ambiance in restaurants or how food is described on menus, also can influence individuals without their being conscious of it (Wansink 2006; Cohen 2008).

Habit Versus Intention

Intention and habit may be competing with each other. However, studies show that although past behavior is predictive of eating a low-fat diet, stable intentions can also be powerful, if not more so, in mediating future behavior (Conner et al. 2000; Conner & Abraham 2001). Thus, targeting both intentions and perceived control over the behavior is likely to influence future behavior *despite* past behavior. Nutrition education can assist individuals to make specific plans or make personal policy decisions about their habitual patterns to make them more healthful, such as to eat whole-grain cereals for breakfast each morning rather than high-sugar cereals. There is evidence that current habit strength can significantly predict healthful eating, such as of fruit (Brug et al. 2006).

Evidence for the Theory from Research and Intervention Studies

Research on Food Choice and Dietary Behaviors

The theory of planned behavior has been studied extensively and rigorously in the social psychology field and used widely to understand health issues, including food choice and dietary and physical activity behaviors (Godin & Kok 1996). The effectiveness of the theory may depend on how specifically the behavior is defined as well as on the nature of the group being studied.

A few specific studies are described here to indicate the range of behaviors and groups with whom the theories have been used. As noted earlier, the theory is content-free: it does not specify what the specific beliefs are, only which constructs to explore, because the actual beliefs differ by group and by behavior. (See **Box 4-4**.) Here are a few studies as examples.

Box 4-4   **Understanding Jason and His Friends Using the Theory of Planned Behavior**

Jason is a 25-year-old salesperson in a clothing store. To determine the reasons, insights, or feelings that would motivate Jason and individuals like him to think seriously about why to take action now about eating more fruits and vegetables, you would have to conduct some interviews. From these, the reasons or outcome expectations, attitudes or feelings, and larger values or hot buttons in the following list might emerge. Modify and add to the following list those that you think would be powerful for Jason and his friends:

- *Attitudes:* Their attitude toward eating fruits and vegetables is positive, but weakly so.
- *Outcome expectations:* There are competing beliefs or outcome expectations about eating fruits and vegetables: these foods are known to be healthful, but they don't taste as good as other foods, they are not convenient to eat during the day, and they are expensive.
- *Social norms:* Jason and youth like him are busy, vibrant young people who do things together—eating fruits and vegetables is not one of them! It is just not part of their mind-set.
- *Values or hot buttons:* They feel they are now adults, able to make their own choices. Eating fruits and vegetables seems like what "good children" do. They are no longer children.
- *Self-identity:* They do not see themselves as "health-conscious eaters." They know people like that and don't want to be like them.

Nutrition education for this group thus needs to address all these determinants that are potential mediators of behavior change, helping Jason and his friends to see "what's in it for me" to eat fruits and vegetables.

Studies with Adolescents

Studies with adolescents have examined a variety of behaviors:

- *In a study of "eating a healthful diet"* (defined in terms of calories, fat, and fruit and vegetable consumption), results showed that the constructs of the theory of planned behavior together predicted 42% of intention and 17% of behavior (Backman et al. 2002). *All three constructs* of the theory of planned behavior were good predictors. The underlying outcome beliefs that were most important were as follows: like the taste of healthful foods, feel good about self, tolerate giving up liked foods, and lose or maintain a healthy weight.
- *For soft drink consumption*, which is a very specifically defined behavior, the predictions by the constructs of the theory of planned behavior were high: 64% for intention and 34% for behavior (i.e., soda consumption) (Kassem et al. 2003). The strongest predictors of soda consumption were *attitude* and the subjects' underlying outcome beliefs (feel healthy, become hyper, gain weight, quench thirst), followed by *perceived behavioral control* (availability at home and school, money) and *subjective norms*.
- *One study examined the role of an expanded theory* of planned behavior on buying or eating local and organic foods by adolescents (Bissonette & Contento 2001). It found that behavior was best predicted by *behavioral intention*, *beliefs about outcomes*, and *perceived social influences*. Also significant were *perceived responsibility* for buying and eating organic foods and *self-identity* for buying and eating local food.

Studies with Adults

Numerous studies have also been conducted with adults both with the general population and those at risk of chronic disease:

- *In an adult population*, the importance of eating vegetables, health benefits, convenience, and the taste of vegetables (*outcome expectations*) were highly associated with eating vegetables in a variety of situations in one study (Satia et al. 2002).
- *In a longitudinal study* of young adults, all psychosocial factors assessed among young adults appeared predictive of one or more eating behaviors reported eight years later (Kvaavik et al. 2005).
- *For those at risk of diabetes*, the theory of planned behavior was found to be useful in explaining the diet and physical activity intentions (Blue 2007).
- *In a study of self-care behavior* in persons with type 2 diabetes, it was found that participants reported high *perceived behavioral control* in relation to medication taking, but low perceived control in relation to exercise and dietary behaviors (Gatt & Sammut 2008).
- *Cultural beliefs*. Theory constructs can incorporate cultural beliefs (Blanchard et al. 2009). One study found that barriers included the *outcome beliefs* that to eat healthfully meant giving up part of their cultural heritage and trying to conform to the dominant culture. Friends and relatives (*social norms*) were also not supportive of dietary changes (James 2004).

Table 4-3 shows how the constructs of the theory can be applied to nutrition education practice.

An example of how the constructs of the theory of planned behavior were used to explain milk consumption in a sample of pregnant women enrolled in, or eligible for, the Women, Infants and Children program is shown in **Nutrition Education in Action 4-4** (Park & Ureda 1999). Nutrition educators can use their understanding of these beliefs or motivations as the basis for designing nutrition education programs that are relevant to such women.

Intervention Studies

Using the theory of planned behavior to develop interventions involves two stages. In the first stage, nutrition educators can use the theory to identify which of the constructs or mediators of behavior are relevant for the target group and thus should be addressed. They obtain such information by extensive open-ended interviews or focus groups, or both, to gain insight into the factors important to the group with respect to food or physical activity. In the second stage, nutrition educators design the message content based on these relevant beliefs. If the model is used in a strict way, with all the variables, then both of these stages can be quite labor intensive and time-consuming. However, numerous interventions have used the key elements of the theories with some success, focusing on outcome beliefs, social norms, and self-efficacy.

Group-Based Interventions

- *A review of two studies with preschoolers* directed at increasing fruit and vegetable intakes found that the potential mediators of change were preference for fruit (expected outcomes), parental facilitation of vegetables, and family rules for eating and availability at home of vegetables (behavioral control) (Tak, Te Velde, & Brug 2008).
- *A middle school intervention* designed to improve behaviors related to obesity prevention found that students significantly decreased the frequency of sweetened beverages, packaged snacks, and eating at a fast food restaurant. They also decreased their screen time. Their outcome beliefs and overall self-efficacy, but not their attitudes, became more positive (Contento et al. 2007).
- *A school-based weight gain prevention* intervention for adolescents based on the theory of planned behavior and accompanied by environmental supports positively influenced several measures of body composition among both girls and boys (Singh et al. 2007).
- *A gardening program* that was effective in improving youth fruit and vegetable consumption found that perceived behavioral control was predictive of behavior in girls (Lautenschlager & Smith 2007).

Media-Based Interventions

Mass media campaigns often have drawn on expectancy-value theories to develop messages that are motivating. Such messages are in essence "arguments" or reasons for the behavior, providing information on expected outcomes, including perceived benefits. Here are several examples:

- *The 5 A Day fruits and vegetables national program* in the United States also used outcome beliefs (or reasons for taking action) for its main message: eating five servings of fruits and vegetables daily can improve health. National monitoring data showed a modest increase in consumption (Potter, Finnegan, & Guinard 2000).
- *A media campaign called "1% or Less"* encouraged people to switch from higher-fat milk to milk with 1% or less fat (Booth-Butterfield & Reger 2004). The campaign targeted behavioral beliefs and found significant effects on intention, attitudes, and behavioral beliefs; these were related to changes in self-reported milk use.

NUTRITION EDUCATION IN ACTION 4-4

Using the Theory of Planned Behavior to Understand Milk Consumption Among Pregnant Women Enrolled in the Women, Infants and Children (WIC) Program

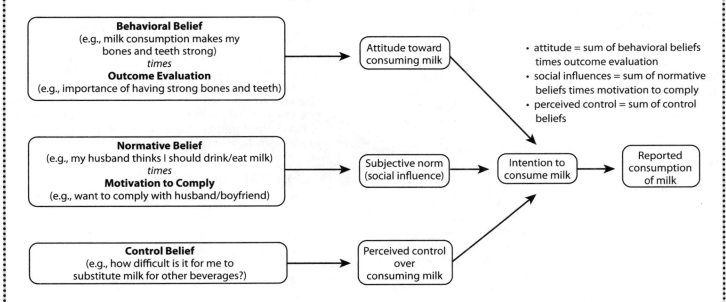

Target Audience and Behavior

- *Audience:* Pregnant women enrolled in, or eligible for, the WIC program
- *Behavior:* Consumption of milk and of milk used in cooking or added to cereal, quantified as the number of cups per day

Theory Constructs/Mediators

- *Behavioral intention:* "How likely is it that you will drink at least 2 cups of milk a day (including milk from milk-containing foods) for the next month?" and "How often do you plan to drink/eat milk for the next month?"
- *Outcome expectations:* Fifteen belief items, such as taste, provides my baby with necessary nutrients, makes me fat, quenches my thirst, makes me feel great, good for my skin and hair.
- *Normative beliefs:* Six items, such as my best friend, mother/parents, sister/brother, or nurse/WIC staff/nutritionist think I should drink milk.

- *Beliefs about control:* Twelve items such as able to buy/get whenever I want, difficult to drink milk.

Results

The following beliefs were among the most predictive of milk consumption:

- *Behavioral beliefs:* Taste, provides my baby with necessary nutrients, quenches my thirst, makes me feel sick/upsets my stomach, makes my bones and teeth strong, causes constipation
- *Social influence:* None significant
- *Control beliefs:* Able to buy/get whenever I want, able to drink 2 cups per day, able to keep milk fresh, kept at home for me

Source: Park, K., and J. R. Ureda. 1999. Specific motivations of milk consumption among pregnant women enrolled in or eligible for WIC. *Journal of Nutrition Education* 31(2):76–86. Diagram used with permission of the Society for Nutrition Education.

- A *brief telephone-delivered message* followed up by three mailings compared beliefs regarding individuals' personal responsibility and social responsibility to eat five fruits and vegetables (Williams-Piehota et al. 2004). Both types of messages increased intake substantially, with the social message slightly more effective over a longer term.

Other Potential Mediators of Food Choice and Dietary Behavior Change

Global Values and Hot Buttons

Values are an important basis for action. The social psychological theories described so far posit that individuals are motivated to take action if the action will lead to outcomes or goals they value (Lewin et al. 1944). These goals about certain immediate ends, such as taste, seeming cool, losing weight, or being liked by one's friends are called *outcome expectations*, as noted. Other goals are more global and are called *terminal* or *end-state values*. These are often set by a person's culture or subculture and are relatively enduring.

Global Values of Rokeach

A widely used set of end-state values is that of Rokeach (1973): an exciting life, a world of beauty, inner harmony, a sense of accomplishment, social recognition, national security, a comfortable life, pleasure, a world at peace, equality, family security, freedom, happiness, mature love or sexuality, salvation, self-respect, true friendship, and wisdom. He does not include health as a value because he believes that health was important for everyone and thus did not differ among people. However, health has been incorporated in the list of values by others.

Global Values of Kahle

Marketers often use Kahle's list of values (Kahle 1984; Andreasen 1995): self-respect, sense of accomplishment, self-fulfillment, fun and enjoyment in life, security, being well respected, a warm relationship with others, and excitement. Other lists include additional values such as novelty, independence, or sense of belonging.

Other Basic Values

The needs for competence, autonomy, and sense of being related to others are seen as basic values, common to all cultures, in self-determination theory (Deci & Ryan 2000).

Other values may also be important, such as family cohesion, empowerment of communities, support of local farmers, social justice, or conservation of resources. For example, a study with adults found that individuals who cleaned their plates felt they did not want to waste food because it was linked to a larger value of not wasting resources (Pelican et al. 2005). Values may also differ by age group, so values for children, teens, and adults may differ.

Notice that these values are based on people's emotions or deepest feelings about themselves or the world around them. Consequently, they are sometimes referred to as people's *hot buttons* in the mass media literature.

Personal Meanings Given to Food

Out of our values and specific past experiences may emerge very personal meanings we attach to the foods we eat. Foods may be eaten because they are comfort foods that remind us of positive childhood experiences or because we want to use them to manage feelings. For example, a study with teenagers found that although they knew that eating sweets might be unhealthy, bad for their teeth, or fattening, it was also a way to deal with frustration, stress, or anger (Spruijt-Metz 1995). Eating junk food or skipping lunch was a way to assert their independence and personal will and to challenge (parental) authority and test boundaries. Nutrition educators must explore and consider these personal meanings of food when they plan nutrition education programs.

Take-Home Message about Theory of Planned Behavior

- People are likely to take action if they expect the action will lead to outcomes they desire, thus improving their attitudes; if other people they value think it is a good idea; and if they feel they have some control over taking action. Developing specific implementation plans can help them translate intention to action.
- You will find this theory especially useful for designing nutrition education activities and mass media programs to increase awareness of issues and enhance motivation for action. The theory is also useful for designing strategies to help people set specific plans to implement their intention to take action.

■ SELF-DETERMINATION THEORY

In its simplest terms, self-determination theory proposes that individuals have innate psychological needs for autonomy, competence, and relatedness, which, when satisfied, enhance their autonomous motivation and well-being. The enhancement of growth and well-being requires the satisfaction of these basic needs and supportive social conditions.

Self-determination theory (SDT) is a general theory of human motivation, which begins with the assumption that people are active organisms, with innate tendencies toward psychological growth and development, who strive to master ongoing challenges and to integrate their experiences into a coherent sense of self. The theory focuses on the degree to which human behaviors are volitional or self-determined—that is, the degree to which people are able to reflect on and engage in actions with a full sense of choice (Deci & Ryan 1985, 2000, 2008; Ryan & Deci 2000). For example, self-determined individuals choose to behave in a manner that reflects their autonomy. Their behavior is not to achieve an external reward or escape aversive stimuli in the environment.

Components of the Theory

This natural human tendency toward growth and development requires ongoing (1) satisfaction of basic psychological needs and (2) supports from the social environment to function effectively.

Basic Psychological Needs

Basic psychological needs are a natural aspect of human beings that apply to all people, regardless of gender, group, or culture. These are innate, universal, and essential for health and well-being. To the extent that the needs are satisfied people will function effectively and develop in a healthy way, but to the extent that they are thwarted, people will not function optimally or in a healthy way. According to Deci and Ryan, three psychological needs motivate the self to initiate behavior and specify "nutriments" that are essential for psychological health and well-being of an individual: the need for competence, need for autonomy, and the need for relatedness to others (Deci & Ryan 2000, 2008).

- *Need for competence:* The need for competence refers to the need to experience ourselves as capable and competent in controlling the environment and being able to reliably predict outcomes.
- *Need for autonomy* (or self-determination): The need for autonomy refers to our need to actively participate in determining our own behavior. It includes the need to experience our actions as result of autonomous choice without external interference.
- *Need for relatedness:* The need for relatedness refers to our need to care for and be related to others. It includes the need to experience authentic relatedness from others and to experience satisfaction in participation and involvement with the social world.

Different Types of Motivation: Autonomous and Controlled

The degree to which individuals are self-determined depends on the degree to which these needs are met and how individuals handle pressures from the environment. Different *types* of motivations have been described based on the degree to which motivations are autonomous or controlled.

Autonomous motivation is when individuals initiate an activity or behavior for its own sake because it is interesting and satisfying in itself, as opposed to doing an activity to obtain an external goal. The individuals experience a full sense of choice and fully endorse the activity. Intrinsic motivation is a prototype of this experience. People engage in behaviors because of passion, pleasure, and interest. Autonomous motivation is not the same as independence, which means to function alone and not rely on others. Independent action can be undertaken autonomously and yet include engagement with and relying on others because it is satisfying. In contrast, people may be independent because they feel pressured to be independent or because they do not like being engaged with or dependent on others. In both cases, the motivation is not autonomous.

Controlled motivation is when individuals engage in activities in response to external pressure or to achieve an external goal. These pressures and goals are extrinsic motivators, which can often undermine intrinsic motivation because they are experienced as controlling.

Amotivation is when individuals have no motivation or intention to engage in a particular action or behavior. This may result from not valuing the behavior or outcome, not believing that the behavior will lead to desired outcomes, or not feeling competent to engage in the behavior.

Continuum of Motivations

Internalization and integration refers to the process by which individuals internalize and actively attempt to transform externally driven motivations (extrinsic motives) and feeling controlled into personally endorsed values and thus assimilate and integrate ways to regulate behaviors that were originally external. Based on the degree of autonomy and control, motivations can be aligned along a continuum ranging from being highly controlled by external motivators to autonomous motivation based on intrinsic motives (Ryan & Deci 2000, Deci & Ryan 2008):

- *External regulation:* On one end of the continuum is external regulation, which refers to doing something for the sole purpose of achieving a reward, avoiding a punishment, or living up to external expectations.
- *Introjected regulation:* Introjected regulation refers to partial internalization of extrinsic motives. However, these motivations are still somewhat alien to the person, who feels controlled by them.

Individuals feel guilt, shame, and self-criticism when they fail and pride and self-aggrandizement after success.
- *Identified regulation:* Next on the continuum is identified regulation. Individuals accept the importance of the behavior for themselves and accept it as their own. They identify with the value of the activity and willingly accept responsibility for the behavior. They engage in the behavior with a greater sense of autonomy and thus do not feel pressured or controlled by external factors to do the behavior.
- *Integrated regulation:* Further along the spectrum is integrated regulation, when individuals have identified with the values and meanings of the activity or behavior to the extent that it becomes fully internalized and autonomous (Deci & Ryan 2008). The behavior is personally relevant and meaningful. This is the means through which externally motivated behaviors become truly autonomous or self-determined.
- *Intrinsic motivation:* At the far end of the spectrum is intrinsic motivation, where individuals engage in the behavior because it is interesting and satisfying. They experience positive feelings from the behavior itself.

External and introjected ways of regulating behavior are clearly controlled by external motivators and may be described as forms of *controlled motivation*. Identified, integrated, and intrinsic modes of regulating behavior are forms of *autonomous motivation*. Use of integrated regulation bears some resemblance to intrinsic motivation because both are accompanied by a sense of volition and choice. However, the integrated mode of regulation is based on the person, though having fully integrated the value of the behavior, still wanting to achieve some other outcome whereas intrinsic motivation is based on interest in the behavior itself.

Energy and Vitality

Deci and Ryan (2008) define vitality as energy available to the self either directly or indirectly from basic psychological needs. This energy allows individuals to act autonomously. Deci and Ryan point out that many theorists have posited that self-regulation depletes energy, but SDT researchers have proposed and demonstrated that only controlled regulation depletes energy. Autonomous regulation can actually be vitalizing (e.g., Moller, Deci, & Ryan 2006).

Facilitating Internalization and Integration

Both autonomous motivation and well-internalized forms of extrinsic motivation are associated with more positive human experience, performance, and health consequences. Extrinsic motivation is more likely to become intrinsic when individuals feel competent (able to perform a behavior), have a sense of autonomy (where they have choice and control), and experience relatedness or connection to others.

Support for Autonomy

Studies show that self-determined behavior is enhanced by (1) providing individuals with a meaningful rationale so that they understand why the specific behavior or activity is important, (2) acknowledging the individuals' feelings and perceptions about the behavior so that they feel understood, and (3) supporting their experience of choice and minimizing the use of pressure to do the behavior while at the same time pointing out discrepancies between individuals' behaviors and their stated desires.

Research and Interventions Using Self-Determination Theory

Some studies have been conducted with self-determination theory in the health domain:

- *A study with urban adolescents* found that perceived autonomy and competence in physical education were interrelated and functioned as a whole for enhancing leisure-time physical activity intentions and behaviors (Shen, McCaughtry, & Martin 2008).
- *Another study with school children* found that extrinsic goals (pressure to lose weight) negatively predicted whereas intrinsic goals positively predicted self-determined motivation to be active, which in turn positively predicted quality of life and exercise behavior (Gillison, Standage, & Skevington 2006).
- *A test of SDT in school physical education* (PE) found that need satisfaction predicted intrinsic motivation, which in turn linked to adaptive PE-related outcomes. In contrast, need satisfaction negatively predicted amotivation, which in turn was positively predictive of feelings of unhappiness (Standage, Duda, & Ntoumanis 2005).
- *An obesity-prevention curriculum for middle school youth* called Choice, Control, and Change, which is designed to enhance autonomous motivation focused on dietary behaviors that youth had control over (such as sweet drinks and packaged snacks). The intervention provided a meaningful rationale for healthy behaviors through inquiry-based science activities, and guided goal setting where youth selected which goals to work on, promoting autonomy. Results showed that youth improved their food choices and increased their sense of competence and autonomy (Contento et al. 2007).
- *Diabetes patients* who perceived that they received autonomy support from their health care providers showed increased autonomous motivation, competence, and improved blood glucose levels (Williams, Freedman, & Deci 1998).
- *Providing choice to patients with eating disorders* during the first few weeks of inpatient treatment reduced the drop-out rates (Vandereycken & Vansteenkiste 2009).

Take-Home Message about Self-Determination Theory

- All people have an innate tendency toward growth and development. Maintenance of this tendency requires ongoing satisfaction of basic needs for competence, autonomy, and relatedness to others and a supportive social environment.
- Nutrition education needs to focus on supporting autonomous motivation by providing a meaningful rationale for behavior, acknowledging participants' feelings so that they feel understood, and supporting their experience of choice.

■ TRANSLATING BEHAVIORAL THEORIES INTO EDUCATIONAL STRATEGIES FOR WHY TO TAKE ACTION

Translating theory into practical strategies is a crucial process for the effectiveness of the nutrition education intervention. This section lists the mediators of behavior change derived from theory along with potential practical, theory-based educational strategies that nutrition educators might use to address them. You would only select those strategies that operationalize the theory-based potential mediators of change that are a part of the intervention model you have chosen. The process of linking mediators of behavior change with educational practice is the central focus of this book and is described more fully in Part II.

Translating the Health Belief Model into Educational Strategies

The health belief model emphasizes the importance of enhancing awareness of perceived susceptibility and severity (together they constitute perceived threat or risk) of a condition by assessment of individual behaviors or community practices so as to have a clear understanding of the situation. It also emphasizes the role of perceived benefits and barriers in whether individuals will actually take action on their sense of threat. The following strategies are useful for operationalizing mediators from the theory.

Awareness of Risk, Concern, or Need

Nutrition educators can design interventions to increase the salience of specific issues of concern or perceived risk related to personal health, community practices, or the sustainability of food system practices. People need enough knowledge of potential concern to warrant action but not so much as to paralyze them from action. They need accurate perceptions and understandings of their own behaviors or community practices in relation to the risk or concern. Effective strategies and specific activities for this mediator might involve the following:

- *Increasing the salience of issues and problems:* Nutrition educators can use trigger films, striking national or local statistics, pictures and charts, personal stories, and other strategies to make salient issues of concern, such as the increase in obesity rates, how much of school lunches are thrown away, the portion sizes of food products, the prevalence of bone loss or metabolic syndrome in adolescents, or the rate of loss of farm land.
- *Providing self-assessment compared to recommendations:* Individuals can complete checklists, food frequency questionnaires, or 24-hour food intake recalls and compare intakes to a standard, such as MyPyramid servings, to give themselves an accurate picture of their intake. They can also complete checklists to see how "green" their food shopping practices are (e.g., where the food comes from, degree of packaging). Such personalized feedback helps counteract optimistic bias and encourages individuals to consider changes in their dietary behaviors based on their true risk.
- *Making a community assessment of practices:* Information about community food practices could provide a true picture of the extent of risk or severity of an issue. Nutrition educators can use existing data or surveys, formal and informal.

Fear-Based Communications

The use of fear-based communications in health promotion activities to increase perceived risk has been the subject of some debate and discussion. Fear and threat are conceptually distinct: *fear* is defined as a negative emotion accompanied by a high level of arousal, whereas *threat* is a cognition. They are, however, intricately related, such that the higher the threat, the greater the fear experienced.

Reviews of studies have found that, overall, fear appeals have a moderate effect on changing attitudes, intentions, and behavior (Leventhal 1973; Witte & Allen 2000). It may also be that some individuals are more likely than others to respond to appeals based on threat. Strong fear appeals produce high levels of perceived seriousness and susceptibility and are more persuasive than low or weak fear appeals—the stronger the fear aroused by a fear appeal, the more persuasive it is. However, fear appeals result in two competing responses that interfere with each other: an adaptive response to deal with the risk or danger, or a maladaptive response of denial or defensiveness.

Effective Use of Fear

Fear appeals are effective only if people also feel that they can do something to protect themselves. Thus, fear appeal messages can be effective in bringing about behavior change when they do the following: (1) depict a significant and relevant threat, but only when the messages also (2) clearly specify that there are effective strategies in which people can engage to reduce the threat or fear, and that (3) these strategies appear easy to accomplish. Nutrition educators need to provide specific instructions on exactly when, where, and how to take action.

For example, a campaign providing cancer risk information should be accompanied by information on actions people can take to reduce the risk, such as eating more fruits and vegetables, increasing physical activity, and getting regular checkups with physicians. It is important for nutrition educators to consider the social contexts of individuals and explore these with the intended audience in formative research (Salovey, Schneider, & Apanovitch 1999).

Perceived Benefits and Barriers

Explore Benefits and Barriers

In group settings, nutrition educators can help participants understand the benefits of taking action. For breastfeeding, these might include health of the baby, convenience, mother–child bonding, and so forth. Also nutrition educators must identify barriers, such as pain of first breastfeeding, embarrassment in public situations, or wishes of others in the family. These can be identified through presentations or group discussion. These theory constructs can also be explored through the media, such as the campaign to eat five fruits and vegetables a day.

Gains and Losses

How messages are framed in terms of gains and losses may be important. For example, there is some evidence that health communications about the need for people to get checkups (e.g., mammograms) are more persuasive if they are framed in terms of guarding against health losses (breast cancer), but that to get people to adopt preventive actions, communications are more effective if they are framed in terms of health benefits or gains.

Case Study Using the Health Belief Model

Alicia has learned that her mother had a heart attack. This is a cue to action. She decides to attend a nutrition education session—which happens to be based on the health belief model. The session outline is shown in **Case Study 4-1**.

Translating the Theory of Planned Behavior into Educational Strategies

The theory of planned behavior emphasizes the importance of attitudes (which are based on beliefs), social norms, and perceived control over being able to take action. These factors influence people's decision making and intention to take action. If the individuals choose to take action, making specific implementation intentions or action plans can help translate intentions into action. The following strategies are useful for operationalizing mediators from the theory.

Analyze Behaviors and Practices

Use of the theory in nutrition education begins by identifying the food or health issue and behaviors or practices that will be the focus of the nutrition education program. Individuals and groups need to be clear about their own behaviors and community practices in relation to a given issue. Nutrition educators can obtain this information using existing literature or data or can obtain the information from the groups with interviews, behavioral checklists, 24-hour dietary or physical activity recalls, and so forth. These should be specific, such as eating vegetables, breastfeeding, snacks, beverages, breakfast, shopping at a farmers' market, walking, playing basketball, and so forth.

Understand Behavioral Intention

Nutrition educators can use survey instruments, interviews with key individuals, focus groups, or group discussion to estimate the degree to which the members of the audience are ready to take action. Following this, they investigate and address the determinants of intention to engage in the behaviors or practices, as described in the following subsections.

Attitudes and Beliefs About Taking Action

A major task in enhancing motivation is to design activities that focus on beliefs about the potential desirable outcomes of behaviors, such as the benefits of eating healthful foods or sustainable or "green" food choices. Such beliefs are powerful motivators of behavior through their impact on attitudes, intentions, and formation of goals.

Identify Relevant Beliefs and Attitudes

The first step is to identify which *beliefs* and *attitudes* are relevant to the recommended nutrition- or food-related behavior in the given group through a thorough needs analysis. Nutrition educators can identify these beliefs and attitudes by surveys, focus groups, interviews, or other methods. This is a crucial step and is similar to market research in the social marketing process.

Select Potential Mediators of Change for the Group

The nutrition educator can then select a series of key beliefs determining intentions as intervention targets. The relative importance of different beliefs, or reasons for action, will differ depending on the behavior and the group or audience. For example, in the case of eating fruits and vegetables, being cool may be important for teenagers, improving the health of the baby may be important for pregnant women, reducing cancer risk may be important for men, and ease of preparation may be important for women. In focus groups before the 5 A Day campaign was launched, the benefits of feeling better, health, and weight control were determined to be most salient to consumers. Despite scientific evidence, the stated benefit that eating fruits and vegetables would "cut my risk of getting cancer in half" was not considered credible or relevant to their eating choices (pollution and genetics were more important) (Loughrey et al. 1997), affirming the importance of identifying motivating beliefs and attitudes from the target audience before designing an educational program.

Design Messages: The Elaboration Likelihood Model (ELM)

Nutrition educators then convert these beliefs about valued outcomes to be achieved from the recommended behavior (such as breastfeeding or eating fruits and vegetables) into messages for the mass media or into educational activities for groups. The elaboration likelihood model

CASE STUDY 4-1

The Case of Alicia: Nutrition Education Using the Health Belief Model

Alicia, you recall, is a 19-year-old high school graduate who works as a receptionist in a busy dentist's office. She grabs a quick lunch each day—something filling. She doesn't cook much and so tends to snack and eat fast food. Her mother recently had a heart attack and was hospitalized. Alicia was alarmed. Until now she had not thought much about her health or her diet. In her view, medical conditions were caused by biology, mostly, or luck. Now she wants to learn more about the condition and whether and how she might prevent such an attack in herself. This is a "cue to action" in the health belief model. The staff in the office told her about educational sessions offered by the nearby community clinic.

One session was called "Eat Right for Your Heart." Alicia decides to attend. Here is a sample of what the session might be like. Note that it focuses on specific behaviors—eating snacks and fast foods.

"Eat Right for Your Heart"

Potential Mediator of Change	Nutrition Education Activities
Perceived susceptibility	Self-assessment: As they come in, participants are asked to write down everything they ate and drank in the past 24 hours. Then, they are to circle the foods that are high in fat.
Perceived severity	The instructor shows the group some examples of popular fast foods and snacks. Then, she asks a volunteer to come up and measure out, with estimates provided by the group, how many teaspoons of fat (from a container of solid cooking fat) they think is in each snack. *Alicia and the others are shocked at the amount of fat in the food items.*
	The instructor then conducts a demonstration using a plastic tube to represent a blood vessel. She pours some "blood" through—it moves quickly through the tube. Then, she places some of the solid fat in the tube, and the blood now trickles through. She discusses this as illustrating the impact of a dietary pattern with large amounts of snacks and fast foods that are high in saturated fat. *Alicia and the others are moved by the visual demonstration and their perceived risk of disease is heightened.*
Perceived benefits of taking action	The instructor provides the evidence showing that eating a healthy diet low in saturated fat and high in whole grains and fruits and vegetables can reduce risk of chronic disease. *Alicia is now very concerned about her diet and thinks she will do something about it.*
Perceived barriers	The group reviews their dietary recalls and discusses barriers to reducing the number of unhealthy snacks they eat.
Overcoming barriers	The group brainstorms ways to reduce the number of unhealthy snacks and fast food items they eat and substitute with healthier snacks, such as fruits and vegetables or whole-grain snacks and healthier options at fast food restaurants.
State likelihood of taking action	The instructor asks group members to write down one action they will take to reduce their consumption of unhealthy snacks and fast foods and replace them with healthier ones. *Alicia is pleased that there are some actions she can take to protect her heart. She decides that she will take fresh fruit or bagged baby carrots to work each day. She thinks that she will also commit to a second behavior: she will select a healthier option at least once a week when she goes to fast food restaurants.*

(ELM) proposes that individuals will process messages through either a central route or a peripheral route (Petty & Cacioppo 1986):

- *Central or mindful route:* The effectiveness or persuasiveness of nutrition educators' messages about the perceived benefits or desirability of the outcomes of the recommended behavior (breastfeeding, parents feeding their children healthy foods), whether delivered through group educational activities, mass media messages, or brochures and newsletters, depends on many factors, chief among them being whether the messages are constructed in such a way as to induce individuals to *think*

about the messages or *elaborate* on them. In this "central processing" of the message, individuals understand and evaluate the benefits or other outcomes of behavior in light of their own established beliefs and attitudes. Beliefs and attitudes changed by this route are well thought out and become integrated into individuals' belief or attitude structure, such as "It is desirable for me to eat more locally grown foods because it will support local farmers."

Individuals are more likely to think about the message if they judge it to be personally relevant and there are few barriers to in-depth processing of the message; that is, when the message is easy to understand, people have time to think about it, and there are not many distractions.

- *Peripheral or mindless route:* When the health message is difficult to process or does not seem relevant, individuals tend to judge the message by more superficial aspects, such as the attractiveness or credibility of the source or the associations of the food with other desirable attributes, such as a picture of a slender, attractive woman. This is the "peripheral," or "mindless," route to changes in beliefs and attitudes.

Attitudes and Feelings

One important way to increase motivation to eat healthful food is to provide opportunities for individuals to experience and enjoy healthful food, for example, through food tastings or food preparation and cooking experiences in groups accompanied by eating the prepared food together. These food experiences need to be long term to have full impact. Repeated experiences and familiarity are more likely to lead to positive sensory-affective responses to new foods. Indeed, an intervention study found that after 16 weeks eating lower-fat foods, individuals' reported desires to eat low-fat foods increased and their desires to eat high-fat foods decreased (Grieve & Vander Weg 2003).

When appropriate, groups can explore their feelings about food, understand these feelings, and seek ways to enjoy substituting less healthful with more healthful foods. In addition, because people's feelings and emotions are closely related to their deeply held values, emotion-based messaging has been proposed as a way to build on people's values and hot buttons, such as about being a good parent (McCarthy & Tuttelman 2005).

Anticipating positive feelings and anticipated regret is important. Nutrition educators can help the group members explore how they would feel about themselves for taking the recommended action—would they feel good about themselves? Would they anticipate regret if they did not take action?

Misconceptions

Misconceptions should also be identified through formal or informal assessment and addressed at this time. Very often individuals do not initiate behaviors because of erroneous beliefs about expected outcomes, such as the belief that whole grains and beans are difficult to digest. The 5 A Day campaign found that many of those surveyed believed people needed only one or two fruit and vegetable servings a day. Consequently, the need for five a day became a central message.

Social Norms and Social Expectations

Nutrition educators can make groups with whom they work aware of the influence of social norms on their behaviors through group activities identifying what important others think that they should be doing (e.g., perceptions of the spouse's or partner's approval or disapproval of breastfeeding). In addition, educators can use materials, films, posters, and statistics to indicate how individuals similar to the group are engaging in the healthful behaviors, such as other WIC women breastfeeding, teenagers drinking water, and so forth (descriptive norms).

Personal Norms, Moral Norms, or Internal Standards

Nutrition educators can explore the group's personal norms or internal standards and sense of responsibility through various values clarification activities. Individuals can reflect on and evaluate the importance of health in their lives and make choices about the values they wish to place on health. Moral issues can also be explored.

Beliefs About Self-Efficacy and Control: Barriers and Difficulties

Beliefs about self-efficacy or control over the behavior are important in the motivational phase of decision making about diet as well as in the postdecisional phase when individuals are attempting to carry out the behavior. In the motivational phase, self-efficacy can be seen as the mirror image of perceived barriers or difficulty in taking action. It involves recognition of the need for skills to take action. In group settings, nutrition educators can elicit perceptions of the barriers to taking action from group members, and then share and discuss ways to reduce those barriers. In mass media approaches and materials, difficulties can be addressed in the messages themselves. For example, a statewide program placed a series of messages on billboards about eating fruits and vegetables. These included pictures of bananas with the message "Peel, eat; how easy is that!" and tomatoes with the message "Slice, eat; how easy is that!" (http://www.idph.state.ia.us/pickabettersnack/default.asp).

Beliefs About the Self

Many other related beliefs are also potential mediators of behavior change, such as perceived responsibility or moral obligation and personal meanings given to food and eating. Nutrition educators should identify and address these needs in the nutrition education activities where they are relevant and salient for a given audience. Such beliefs can be identified for a given group in a personal setting or through surveys, or information may be found in the published literature.

The educational strategies used also depend on the channel and on the behavior. Active methods of self-exploration and understanding are likely to be most effective. One strategy might be facilitated group dialogue (Norris 2003) (see Chapter 17). This is similar to motivational interviewing for individuals (Rollnick, Miller, & Butler 2007). Films, discussions, or debates of the pros and cons of the behavior may be useful here. Self-presentations such as self-identity or social identity can be explored. Ideal-self versus actual-self discrepancies and ought-to-be self versus actual-self discrepancies can be explored through activities that bring to awareness these discrepancies, and strategies can be provided for handling them.

Habits or Routines

Many behaviors appear to occur without much thought. As we have seen, this results from the frequent pairing of foods and the situations in which they are consumed. Such habits or routines are also important motivators of behavior. Nutrition education can be directed at bringing such attitude–situation cues to awareness so that individuals can choose to change behaviors if they wish. Nutrition education activities can be designed to bring the less positive habits or routines (e.g., being a couch potato) to consciousness so that they can be considered and replaced by more positive habits or routines. Because these may require more effort (e.g., exercising regularly), nutrition educators can design tip sheets, checklists, or activities to assist individuals to develop these new routines.

Decision Making and Resolving Ambivalences

Nutrition educators can help the group explore the benefits and costs of taking action as well as not taking action. This can be done verbally as a group or through an activity where individuals write out the pros and cons. In addition, educators can help group participants explore their own values by providing the group with a series of value statements

CASE STUDY 4-2

The Case of Maria: Nutrition Education Using the Theory of Planned Behavior

Maria is a 23-year-old who works in a construction company office. She eats lunch each day from a mobile vendor who sells hotdogs, hamburgers, and sandwiches and drinks a soda pop or two each day for a quick pick-me-up. She has a 4-year-old daughter who goes to a Head Start program. She and her husband are divorced. She knows that she and her daughter should eat more fruit each day, but they both like sweets and soda, which are cheap and convenient. Pamphlets at Head Start encourage parents to provide healthy snacks and drinks for children at home. She wants to be a good mother and she is becoming concerned about her daughter's teeth; her daughter also is getting a little chubby. She sees that there will be a session for moms offered at the site titled "Give your child the smile of a lifetime—healthy snacking." Notice that it is on a specific behavior.

Here is a sample of what the session might be like:

"Give Your Child the Smile of a Lifetime—Healthy Snacking"

Potential Mediator of Change	Nutrition Education Activity
Beliefs about outcomes of current behavior	The participants are asked to write down everything their child ate and drank in the past 24 hours (Head Start provides menus for foods/drinks offered there). Then, they are to circle the drinks high in sugar and snacks high in sugar and fat.
Beliefs about outcomes of current behavior	The instructor brings out a variety of popular sugared drinks. Then, she asks a volunteer to come up and measure out, with estimates provided by the group, how many teaspoons of sugar (from a container of sugar) they think is in each drink.
	Maria and the other parents are shocked at the amount of sugar in drinks and the number of calories. She always thought that liquids had no calories.
	The instructor then shows the group a chicken bone that she has let sit in a glass of soda pop for several days. The bone is rubbery and soft compared to a bone placed in water. She points out that the same can happen to teeth, particularly when children take a sweetened drink to bed with them in a bottle.
	Maria and the other parents are again surprised that sweetened carbonated drinks could have such an effect.
	The instructor then shows participants various packaged snacks. She asks them to read the label to find out how much sugar is in each. Again, she has volunteers measure out the amount of sugar in each.
	Maria takes note of the calories in the cookies and packaged snacks she and her daughter often eat.
Beliefs about positive outcomes of potential behavior (potential motivators or mediators of change)	The instructor provides the evidence showing that drinking water and milk instead of sugared drinks and eating low-fat dairy products in the context of a healthy diet including whole grains and fruits and vegetables can help children develop strong bones and maintain a healthy weight. She shows pictures of strong bones and children with beautiful teeth and smiles, and being active and full of energy.
	Maria likes the pictures she sees and her attitude becomes more positive.
Social norms	The instructor shows a film clip showing similar moms offering their children healthy snacks and talking about their experiences.
Perceived control over behavior, including barriers or difficulties	The group reviews the dietary recalls for their children. They discuss the difficulties in getting children to drink milk and water rather than sweetened drinks and to eat healthy snacks.
Overcoming barriers	The group discusses the authoritative parenting style, where the parent offers healthful drinks such as 100% juice, milk, and water and lets the child choose, or the parent provides several healthy snacks and lets the child choose which to eat. The group brainstorms different kinds of good (and tasty) substitutes for unhealthy snacks.
Behavioral intention/ implementation intentions	The instructor asks group members to write down at least one action they will take during the coming week to make their child's diet healthier. She asks them to be very specific.
	Maria feels motivated to take action. She decides that she will offer a couple of healthful snacks when her daughter comes home after Head Start each day instead of the usual less healthy ones. She decides on a second action: she will not stock soda pop in the house so that she and her daughter will only drink it occasionally. She believes her implementation plan is feasible.

to which they can respond. This is to seek to elicit their ambivalences, and then assure them that this is normal.

At the end of these activities, individuals can come to closure and write out their intention with respect to the issue or behavior that is the focus of the program.

Case Study Using the Theory of Planned Behavior

Maria is a 23-year-old mother of a preschool child. She has not been interested much in health for herself but wants to make sure that her child eats well. She decides to attend a nutrition education session—which happens to be based on the theory of planned behavior. The session outline is shown in **Case Study 4-2**.

Translating Self-Determination Theory into Educational Strategies

The focus of nutrition education using self-determination theory is to facilitate internalization of motivation and autonomous enactment of behaviors. Nutrition educators can do this by providing conditions that are supportive of the basic needs for competence, autonomy, and relatedness. The processes are very similar to motivational interviewing for individuals (Rollnick et al. 2007) and facilitated dialogue (Norris 2003) described in Chapter 17.

Autonomy support involves the following:

- Eliciting the understandings and feelings of the participants through reflective listening.
- Providing individuals with a meaningful rationale for taking action.
- Providing structure for explorations.
- Helping individuals explore and resolve their ambivalences, assuring them that ambivalences are normal; expressing empathy. At the same time, point out discrepancies between their current behavior and what they say they would like to do.
- Minimizing control or pressure; roll with the resistance.
- Emphasizing choice, and providing a menu of effective options, including the option of not making a change.

■ SUMMARY

A major task in the thinking phase or component of nutrition education is to increase awareness and enhance motivation, promote active contemplation, and facilitate formation of intentions to take action. Several theories are useful here and research evidence provides support for use of the theories in nutrition education and physical activity programs.

Taken together, theory and research suggest that it is effective for nutrition educators to design activities that focus on helping people understand personal and community risks and the benefits of specified healthful food choices and diet- and physical activity–related behaviors;

helping participants identify potential barriers to carrying out the behaviors; and exploring ways to overcome barriers.

The Health Belief Model

The health belief model proposes that when people experience a personal threat about a health condition they will likely take action, but only if the benefits of taking action outweigh the barriers, actual and psychological. Having the ability to take action is also crucial. The health belief model is especially useful for adults who are at risk for health conditions or who are beginning to think about their health. It may be less useful for children, for whom health is not a motivator.

The Precaution Adoption Process Model

The precaution adoption process model proposes that the decision as to whether to take precautionary action in response to a risk depends on individuals' stage of awareness, which can range from unaware, to awareness without engagement, to being undecided, to active decision making. Nutrition education strategies need to differ for these different groups, who all appear to be in a pre-action phase. Mediators from other theories are helpful in explaining the active decision-making process as well as providing strategies for those initiating and maintaining the chosen precautionary action. Thus, nutrition education interventions should be tailored to the stages of decision making.

The Theory of Planned Behavior

The theory of planned behavior is useful to enhance motivation for healthful eating and active living. It states that people are likely to take action if they expect the action will lead to outcomes they desire, thus improving their attitudes; if other people they value think it is good idea; and if they feel they have some control over taking action. Developing specific implementation plans can help them translate intention to action. Both group nutrition education and media communications are useful strategies to deliver effective messages in this phase of nutrition education. Affect or feelings are particularly important in the case of food and eating. Thus, individuals should be provided with opportunity to taste and experience healthful foods and explore and understand their emotions with respect to food or being physically active. Media messages should be personally relevant to the intended audience, memorable, and easy to understand and process. Nutrition educators can help individuals set specific plans to implement their intention to take action.

Self-Determination Theory

Self-determination theory suggests that supporting individuals' basic needs for competence, autonomy, and relatedness to others can enhance autonomous motivation.

By addressing all these mediators of behavior change, nutrition education interventions can enhance motivation to act, activate decision making, and assist people to consider intentions to act.

Questions and Activities

1. The first step in making diet-related behavior changes is considered to be becoming motivated. What does it mean to be motivated? What is the main educational goal of nutrition education in this first step? How can nutrition educators best achieve this goal?

2. Describe briefly what you think are the essential features of each of the following theories in terms of how they explain health motivations:
   a. The health belief model
   b. The theory of planned behavior
   c. Self-determination theory

3. Describe in your own words the following theory constructs. How are the terms related to motivation?
   a. Outcome expectations
   b. Perceived severity
   c. Perceived susceptibility
   d. Perceived benefits
   e. Perceived barriers
   f. Attitudes
   g. Behavioral intentions
   h. Subjective norms
   i. Self-efficacy
   j. Self-identity
   k. Perceived behavioral control

4. Several of the constructs listed in Question 3 are similar in concept but have different names because of the different origins of the theories. Which are they?

5. Think of a health-related behavior you have been trying to change:
   a. Write a list of the reasons you would like to make this change and also a list of the difficulties you are having trying to make the change. You can use the following space to write your answers.
   b. Can you match up *each* of the reasons and difficulties that you listed with at least *one construct* of one of the theories described?

Reasons and Difficulties You Stated	Name of Theoretical Construct	Justification for Assignment

   c. In what ways do the theories help you understand your food choices and eating behaviors better?

6. If you were asked to design media messages for a group of young people like Jason, who you met in Box 4-4, what do you think would be one key message you would want to get across?

7. Describe five key strategies that nutrition educators can use to enhance motivation for healthy eating and active living.

References

Abood, D. A., D. R. Black, and D. Feral. 2003. Nutrition education worksite intervention for university staff: Application of the health belief model. *Journal of Nutrition Education and Behavior* 35(5):260–267.

Abraham, C., and P. Sheeran. 2000. Understanding and changing health behaviour: From health beliefs to self-regulation. In *Understanding and changing health behaviour from health beliefs to self-regulation*, edited by P. Norman, C. Abraham, and M. Conner. Amsterdam: Harwood Academic Publishers.

Abratt, R., and S. D. Goodey. 1990. Unplanned buying and in-store stimuli in supermarkets. *Managerial Decisions and Economics* 11:111–121.

Ajzen, I. 1991. The theory of planned behavior. *Organizational Behavior and Human Decision Processes* 50:179–211.

———. 1998. Models of human social behaviour and their application to health psychology. *Psychology and Health* 13:735–739.

———. 2001. Nature and operation of attitudes. *Annual Review of Psychology* 52:27–58.

Ajzen, I., and T. J. Madden. 1986. Prediction of goal-directed behavior: Attitudes, intentions and perceived behavioral control. *Journal of Experimental Social Psychology* 22:453–474.

Andreasen, A. R. 1995. *Marketing social change: Changing behavior to promote health, social development, and the environment.* Washington, DC: Jossey-Bass.

Armitage, C. J. 2006. Evidence that implementation intentions promote transitions between the stages of change. *Journal of Consulting Clinical Psychology* 74(1):141–151.

Armitage, C. J., and M. Conner. 1999. Predictive validity of the theory of planned behaviour: The role of questionnaire format and social desirability. *Journal of Community and Applied Social Psychology* 9:261–272.

———. 2000a. Attitudinal ambivalence: A test of three key hypotheses. *Personality and Social Psychology Bulletin* 26(11):1421–1432.

———. 2000b. Social cognition models and health behavior: A structured review. *Psychology and Health* 15:173–189.

———. 2001. Efficacy of the Theory of Planned Behaviour: A meta-analytic review. *British Journal of Social Psychology* 40(Pt 4):471–499.

Backman, D. R., E. H. Haddad, J. W. Lee, P. K. Johnston, and G. E. Hodgkin. 2002. Psychosocial predictors of healthful dietary behavior in adolescents. *Journal of Nutrition Education and Behavior* 34(4):184–192.

Bandura, A. 2000. Health promotion from the perspective of social cognitive theory. In *Understanding and changing health behavior: From health beliefs to self-regulation*, edited by P. Norman, C. Abraham, and M. Conner. Amsterdam: Harwood Academic Publishers.

Becker, M. H. 1974. The health belief model and personal health behavior. *Health Education Monographs* 2(4):324–473.

Bentley, M. E., D. L. Dee, and J. L. Jensen. 2003. Breastfeeding among low income, African-American women: Power, beliefs and decision making. *Journal of Nutrition* 133(1):305S–309S.

Bisogni, C. A., M. Connors, C. M. Devine, and J. Sobal. 2002. Who we are and how we eat: A qualitative study of identities in food choice. *Journal of Nutrition Education and Behavior* 34(3):128–139.

Bissonette, M. M., and I. R. Contento. 2001. Adolescents' perspectives and food choice behaviors in relation to the environmental impacts of food production practices. *Journal of Nutrition Education* 33:72–82.

Blanchard, C. M., J. Kupperman, P. B. Sparling, et al. 2009. Do ethnicity and gender matter when using the theory of planned behavior to understand fruit and vegetable consumption? *Appetite* 52(1):15–20.

Blue, C. L. 2007. Does the theory of planned behavior identify diabetes-related cognitions for intention to be physically active and eat a healthy diet? *Public Health Nursing* 24(2):141–150.

Booth-Butterfield, S., and B. Reger. 2004. The message changes belief and the rest is theory: The "1% or less" milk campaign and reasoned action. *Preventive Medicine* 39(3):581–588.

Brug, J., E. de Vet, J. de Nooijer, and B. Verplanken. 2006. Predicting fruit consumption: Cognitions, intention, and habits. *Journal of Nutrition Education and Behavior* 38(2):73–81.

Chesla, C. A., M. M. Skaff, R. J. Bartz, J. T. Mullan, and L. Fisher. 2000. Differences in personal models among Latinos and European Americans: Implications for clinical care. *Diabetes Care* 23(12):1780–1785.

Cohen, D. A. 2008. Obesity and the built environment: Changes in environmental cues cause energy imbalances. *International Journal of Obesity* 32:S137–S142.

Conner, M., and C. Abraham. 2001. Conscientiousness and the theory of planned behavior: Towards a more complete model of the antecedents of intentions and behavior. *Personality and Social Psychology Bulletin* 27:1547–1561.

Conner, M., and P. Norman. 1995. *Predicting health behavior*. Buckingham, UK: Open University Press.

Conner, M., P. Norman, and R. Bell. 2002. The theory of planned behavior and healthy eating. *Health Psychology* 21(2):194–201.

Conner, M., P. Sheeran, P. Norman, and C. J. Armitage. 2000. Temporal stability as a moderator of relationships in the Theory of Planned Behaviour. *British Journal of Social Psychology* 39(Pt 4):469–493.

Contento, I. R., P. A. Koch, H. Lee, W. Sauberli, and A. Calabrese-Barton. 2007. Enhancing personal agency and competence in eating and moving: Formative evaluation of a middle school curriculum—Choice, Control, and Change. *Journal of Nutrition Education and Behavior* 39(5 Suppl):S179–S186.

D'Andrade, R.G. 1984. Cultural meaning systems. In *Culture theory: Essays on mind, self, and emotion*, edited by R. A. Shweder and R. A. LeVine. Cambridge, UK: Cambridge University Press.

Deci, E. L., and R. M. Ryan. 1985. *Intrinsic motivation and self-determination in human behavior*. New York: Plenum.

———. 2000. The "what" and "why" of goal pursuits: Human needs and the self-determination of behavior. *Psychological Inquiry* 11(4):227–268.

———. 2008. Facilitating optimal motivation and psychological well-being across life's domains. *Canadian Psychology* 49:14–23.

Deutsch, M., and H. B. Gerard. 1955. A study of normative and informational social influences upon individual judgement. *Journal of Abnormal Psychology* 51(3):629–636.

Diaz, H., H. H. Marshak, S. Montgomery, B. Rea, and D. Backman. 2009. Acculturation and gender: Influence on healthy dietary outcomes for Latino adolescents. *Journal of Nutrition Education and Behavior* 41(5):319–326.

Dunn, K. I., P. B. Mohr, C. J. Wilson, and G. A. Wittert. 2008. Beliefs about fast food in Australia: A qualitative analysis. *Appetite* 51(2):331–334.

Ellis, J., M. A. Johnson, J. G. Fischer, and J. L. Hargrove. 2005. Nutrition and health education intervention for whole grain foods in the Georgia older Americans nutrition programs. *Journal of Nutrition for the Elderly* 24(3):67–83.

Fazio, R. H. 1990. Multiple processes by which attitudes guide behavior: The MODE model as an integrative framework. In *Advances in Experimental Social Psychology*, edited by M. P. Zana. San Diego: Academic Press.

Fishbein, M. 2000. The role of theory in HIV prevention. *AIDS Care* 12(3):273–278.

Fishbein, M., and I. Ajzen. 1975. *Belief, attitude, intention and behavior: An introduction to theory and research*. Reading, MA: Addison-Wesley.

Garcia, K., and T. Mann. 2003. From "I Wish" to "I Will": Social-cognitive predictors of behavioral intentions. *Journal of Health Psychology* 8(3):347–360.

Gatt, S., and R. Sammut. 2008. An exploratory study of predictors of self-care behaviour in persons with type 2 diabetes. *International Journal of Nursing Studies* 45(10):1525–1533.

Gillison, F. B., M. Standage, and S. M. Skevington. 2006. Relationships among adolescents' weight perceptions, exercise goals, exercise motivation, quality of life and leisure-time exercise behaviour: A self-determination theory approach. *Health Education Research* 21(6):836–847.

Glanz, K., J. Brug, and P. van Assema. 1997. Are awareness of dietary fat intake and actual fat consumption associated?—a Dutch-American comparison. *European Journal of Clinical Nutrition* 51(8):542–547.

Godin, G., M. Conner, and P Sheeran. 2005. Bridging the intention-behavior "gap": The role of moral norm. *British Journal of Social Psychology* 44(Pt 4):497–512.

Godin, G., and G. Kok. 1996. The theory of planned behavior: A review of its applications to health-related behaviors. *American Journal of Health Promotion* 11(2):87–98.

Grieve, F. G., and M. W. Vander Weg. 2003. Desire to eat high- and low-fat foods following a low-fat dietary intervention. *Journal of Nutrition Education and Behavior* 35(2):98–102.

Hanson, J. A., and J. A. Benedict. 2002. Use of the Health Belief Model to examine older adults' food-handling behaviors. *Journal of Nutrition Education and Behavior* 34(Suppl 1):S25–S30.

Hoffman, E. W., V. Bergmann, J. A. Shultz, P. Kendall, L. C. Medeiros, and V. N. Hillers. 2005. Application of a five-step message development model for food safety education materials targeting people with HIV/AIDS. *Journal of the American Dietetic Association* 105(10):1597–1604.

IFIC Foundation. 1999. Are you listening? What consumers tell us about dietary recommendations. *Food insight: Current topics in food safety and nutrition.* Sept./Oct.:1–6.

James, D. C. 2004. Factors influencing food choices, dietary intake, and nutrition-related attitudes among African Americans: Application of a culturally sensitive model. *Ethnicity and Health* 9(4):349–367.

Janz, N. K., and M. H. Becker. 1984. The Health Belief Model: A decade later. *Health Education Quarterly* 11(1):1–47.

Kahle, L. R. 1984. The values of Americans: Implications for consumer adaptation. In *Personal values and consumer psychology*, edited by R. E. Pitts Jr. and A. G. Woodside. Lexington, MA: Lexington Books.

Kassem, N. O., J. W. Lee, N. N. Modeste, and P. K. Johnston. 2003. Understanding soft drink consumption among female adolescents using the Theory of Planned Behavior. *Health Education Research* 18(3):278–291.

Kittler, P. G., and K. P. Sucher. 2001. *Food and culture*. 3rd ed. Belmont, CA: Wadsworth/Thomson Learning.

Kreuter, M. W., S. N. Lukwago, R. D. Bucholtz, E. M. Clark, and V. Sanders-Thompson. 2003. Achieving cultural appropriateness in health promotion programs: Targeted and tailored approaches. *Health Education and Behavior* 30(2):133–146.

Kristal, A. R., K. Glanz, B. C. Tilley, and S. Li. 2000. Mediating factors in dietary change: Understanding the impact of a worksite nutrition intervention. *Health Education and Behavior* 27(1):112–125.

Kumanyika, S. K., L. Van Horn, D. Bowen, et al. 2000. Maintenance of dietary behavior change. *Health Psychology* 19(1 Suppl):42–56.

Kvaavik, E., N. Lien, G. S. Tell, and K. I. Klepp. 2005. Psychosocial predictors of eating habits among adults in their mid-30s: The Oslo Youth Study follow-up 1991–1999. *International Journal of Behavioral Nutrition and Physical Activity* 2:9.

Lautenschlager, L., and C. Smith. 2007. Understanding gardening and dietary habits among youth garden program participants using the Theory of Planned Behavior. *Appetite* 49(1):122–130.

Leventhal, H. 1973. Changing attitudes and habits to reduce risk factors in chronic disease. *American Journal of Cardiology* 31(5):571–580.

LeVine, R. A. 1984. Properties of culture: An ethnographic view. In *Culture theory: Essays on mind, self, and emotion*, edited by R. A. Shweder and R. A. LeVine. Cambridge, UK: Cambridge University Press.

Lewin, K., T. Dembo, L. Festinger, and P. S. Sears. 1944. Level of aspiration. In *Personality and the behavior disorders*, edited by J. M. Hundt. New York: Roland Press.

Lien, N., L. A. Lytle, and K. A. Komro. 2002. Applying theory of planned behavior to fruit and vegetable consumption of young adolescents. *American Journal of Health Promotion* 16(4):189–197.

Liou, D., and I. R. Contento. 2001. Usefulness of psychosocial theory variables in explaining fat-related dietary behavior in Chinese Americans: Association with degree of acculturation. *Journal of Nutrition Education* 33(6):322–331.

————. 2004. Health beliefs related to heart disease prevention among Chinese Americans. *Journal of Family and Consumer Sciences* 96:21–22.

Loughrey, K. A., G. I. Balch, C. Lefebvre, et al. 1997. Bringing 5 A Day consumers into focus: Qualitative use of consumer research to guide strategic decision making. *Journal of Nutrition Education* (29):172–177.

McCarthy, P., and J. Tuttelman. 2005. Touching hearts to impact lives: Harnessing the power of emotion to change behaviors. *Journal of Nutrition Education and Behavior* 37(Suppl 1):S19.

McClure, J. B. 2002. Are biomarkers useful treatment aids for promoting health behavior change? An empirical review. *American Journal of Preventive Medicine* 22(3):200–207.

Moller, A. C., E. L. Deci, and R. M. Ryan. 2006. Choice and ego-depletion: The moderating role of autonomy. *Perspectives of Social Psychology Bulletin* 32(8):1024–1036.

Nilsen, P., M. Bourne, and B. Verplanken. 2008. Accounting for the role of habit in behavioural strategies for injury prevention. *International Journal of Injury Control and Safety Promotion* 15(1):33–40.

Norris, J. 2003. *From telling to teaching.* North Myrtle Beach, SC: Learning by Dialogue.

Park, K., and J. R. Ureda. 1999. Specific motivations of milk consumption among pregnant women enrolled in or eligible for WIC. *Journal of Nutrition Education* 31(2):76–86.

Pelican, S., F. Vanden Heede, B. Holmes, et al. 2005. The power of others to shape our identity: Body image, physical abilities, and body weight. *Family and Consumer Sciences Research Journal* 34(1):57–80.

Petty, R. E., and T. Cacioppo. 1986. *Communication and persuasion: Central and peripheral routes to attitude change.* New York: Springer-Verlag.

Potter, J. D., J. R. Finnegan, and J. X. Guinard. 2000. *5 A Day for Better Health program evaluation report.* Bethesda, MD: National Institutes of Health, National Cancer Institute.

Povey, R., B. Wellens, and M. Conner. 2001. Attitudes towards following meat, vegetarian and vegan diets: An examination of the role of ambivalence. *Appetite* 37(1):15–26.

Raats, M. M., R. Shepherd, and P. Sparks. 1995. Including moral dimensions of choice within the structure of the theory of planned behavior. *Journal of Applied Social Psychology* 25:484–494.

Richard, R., J. van der Pligt, and N. K. de Vries. 1996. Anticipated affect and behavioral choice. *Basic and Applied Social Psychology* 18:111–129.

Robinson, R., and C. Smith. 2002. Psychosocial and demographic variables associated with consumer intention to purchase sustainably produced foods as defined by the Midwest Food Alliance. *Journal of Nutrition Education and Behavior* 34(6):316–325.

Rokeach, M. 1973. *The nature of human values.* New York: Free Press.

Rollnick, S., W. R. Miller, and C. C. Butler. 2007. *Motivational interviewing in health care: Helping patients change behavior.* New York: Guilford Publications.

Rosenstock, I. M. 1974. Historical origins of the health belief model. *Health Education Monographs* 2:1–8.

Rozin, P. 1982. Human food selection: The interaction of biology, culture, and individual experience. In *The psychobiology of human food selection*, edited by L. M. Barker. Westport, CT: Avi Publishing.

Rozin, P., and A. E. Fallon. 1981. The acquisition of likes and dislikes for foods. In *Criteria of food acceptance: How man chooses what he eats*, edited by J. Solms and R. L. Hall. Zurich: Foster Lang.

Ryan, R. M., and E. L. Deci. 2000. Self-determination theory and the facilitation of intrinsic motivation, social development, and well-being. *American Psychologist* 55(1):68–78.

Salovey, P., and D. Birnbaum. 1989. Influence of mood on health-relevant cognitions. *Journal of Personality and Social Psychology* 57(3):539–551.

Salovey, P., T. R. Schneider, and A. M. Apanovitch. 1999. Persuasion for the purpose of cancer risk reduction: A discussion. *Journal of the National Cancer Institute Monographs* (25):119–122.

Sanjur, D. 1982. *Social and cultural perspectives in nutrition.* Englewood Cliffs, NJ: Prentice Hall

Satia, J. A., A. R. Kristal, R. E. Patterson, M. L. Neuhouser, and E. Trudeau. 2002. Psychosocial factors and dietary habits associated with vegetable consumption. *Nutrition* 18(3):247–254.

Schwarzer, R. 1992. Self-efficacy in the adoption of maintenance of health behaviors: Theoretical approaches and a new model. In *Self-efficacy: Thought control of action*, edited by R. Schwarzer. Washington, DC: Hemisphere.

Shafer, R. B., P. M. Keith, and E. Schafer. 1995. Predicting fat in diets of marital partners using the Health Belief Model. *Journal of Behavioral Medicine* 18:419–433.

Sheeran, P., P. Norman, and S. Orbell. 1999. Evidence that intentions based on attitudes better predict behaviour than intentions based on subjective norms. *European Journal of Social Psychology* 29:403–406.

Shen, B., N. McCaughtry, and J. Martin. 2008. The influence of domain specificity on motivation in physical education. *Research Quarterly in Exercise and Sport* 79(3):333–343.

Shim, Y., J. N. Variyam, and J. Blaylock. 2000. Many Americans falsely optimistic about their diets. *Food Review* 23(1):44–50.

Singh, A. S., A. Paw, M. J. Chin, J. Brug, and W. van Mechelen. 2007. Short-term effects of school-based weight gain prevention among adolescents. *Archives of Pediatric and Adolescent Medicine* 161(6):565–571.

Sparks, P. M. 2000. Subjective expected utility-based attitude-behavior models: The utility of self-identity. In *Attitudes, behavior, and social context: The role of norms and group membership*, edited by D. J. Terry and M. A. Hoggs. London: Lawrence Erlbaum.

Sparks, P., M. Conner, R. James, R. Shepherd, and R. Povey. 2001. Ambivalence about health-related behaviours: An exploration in the domain of food choice. *British Journal of Social Psychology* 6(Pt 1):53–68.

Sparks, P., P. Hedderley, and R. Shepherd. 1992. An investigation into the relationship between perceived control, attitude variability, and the consumption of two common foods. *European Journal of Social Psychology* 22:55–71.

Sparks, P., R. Shepherd, and L. J. Frewer. 1995. Assessing and structuring attitudes toward the use of gene technology in food production: The role of perceived ethical obligation. *Basic and Applied Social Psychology* 163:267–285.

Spiro, M. E. 1984. Some reflections on cultural determinism and relativism with special reference to emotion and reason. In *Culture theory: Essays on mind, self, and emotion*, edited by R. A. Shweder and R. A. LeVine. Cambridge, UK: Cambridge University Press.

Spruijt-Metz, D. 1995. Personal incentives as determinants of adolescent health behavior: The meaning of behavior. *Health Education Research* 10(3):355–364.

Standage, M., J. L. Duda, and N. Ntoumanis. 2005. A test of self-determination theory in school physical education. *British Journal of Educational Psychology* 75(Pt 3):411–433.

Tak, N. I., S. J. Te Velde, and J. Brug. 2008. Are positive changes in potential determinants associated with increased fruit and vegetable intakes among primary schoolchildren? Results of two intervention studies in the Netherlands: The Schoolgruiten Project and the Pro Children Study. *International Journal of Behavioral Nutrition and Physical Activity* 5:21.

Trafimow, D., and P. Sheeran. 1998. Some tests of the distinction between cognitive and affective beliefs. *Journal of Experimental Social Psychology* 34:378–397.

Triandis, H. C. 1977. *Interpersonal behavior.* Monterey, CA: Brooks/Cole.

————. 1979. Values, attitudes, and interpersonal behavior. In *Nebraska symposium on motivation*, edited by H. E. How. Lincoln: University of Nebraska Press.

Tuorila-Ollikainen, H., L. Lahteenmaki, and H. Salovaara. 1986. Attitudes, norms, intentions and hedonic responses in the selection of low salt bread in a longitudinal choice experiment. *Appetite* 7(2):127–139.

Vandereycken, W., and M. Vansteenkiste. 2009. Let eating disorder patients decide: Providing choice may reduce early drop-out from inpatient treatment. *European Eating Disorder Reviews* 17(3):177–183.

Ventura, A. K., and L. L. Birch. 2008. Does parenting affect children's eating and weight status? *International Journal of Behavioral Nutrition and Physical Activity* 5:15.

Verplanken, B., and S. Faes. 1999. Good intentions, bad habits, and effects of forming implementation intentions on healthy eating. *European Journal of Social Psychology* 29:591–604.

Wansink, B. 2006. *Mindless eating: Why we eat more than we think.* New York: Bantam Dell.

Weinstein, N. D. 1988. The precaution adoption process. *Health Psychology* 7:355–386.

Weinstein, N. D., and P. M. Sandman. 1992. A model of the precaution adoption process: Evidence from home radon testing. *Health Psychology* 11:170–180.

Williams, G. C., Z. R. Freedman, and E. L. Deci. 1998. Supporting autonomy to motivate patients with diabetes for glucose control. *Diabetes Care* 21(10):1644–1651.

Williams-Piehota, P., A. Cox, S. N. Silvera, et al. 2004. Casting health messages in terms of responsibility for dietary change: Increasing fruit and vegetable consumption. *Journal of Nutrition Education and Behavior* 36(3):114–120.

Witte, K., and M. Allen. 2000. A meta-analysis of fear appeals: Implications for effective public health campaigns. *Health Education and Behavior* 27(5):591–615.

CHAPTER 5

Foundation in Theory and Research: Facilitating the Ability to Take Action

OVERVIEW

This chapter describes key theories and research that can help readers understand the behavior change process within individuals. It also describes how each theory is translated into nutrition education practice. It focuses on the key role of self-regulation processes and knowledge and skills in enhancing the ability to act and applications to nutrition education.

CHAPTER OUTLINE

- Introduction
- Understanding the mediators of action and procedures for behavior change
- Social cognitive theory
- Self-regulation/self-efficacy models
- Grounded theory approach
- Transtheoretical model and the stages of change construct
- Translating behavioral theories into educational strategies to facilitate the ability to take action
- Summary

LEARNING OBJECTIVES

At the end of the chapter, you will be able to:

- Describe key theories of health behavior change, including social cognitive theory, self-regulation models such as the health action process model, and stage models such as the transtheoretical
- State key concepts in these theories and their application to practice
- Demonstrate understanding of how theory and research have been used in interventions to assist people take action and maintain change
- Describe implications for nutrition education strategies to facilitate initiating and maintaining action or behavior change

■ INTRODUCTION: FACILITATING THE ABILITY TO TAKE ACTION

Numerous factors influence our food choices and eating patterns on a daily basis, as we have seen. To take action or change dietary and physical activity patterns, we have to be convinced of the desirability, effectiveness, and feasibility of the action. Once convinced, we may state an intention to carry out the behavior. But stating an intention to take action does not by itself lead to action. We still need a way to translate intentions into action.

Bridging the Intention–Action Gap

There are many people, including nutrition educators at times, for whom problems with getting started and maintaining action rather than their beliefs and attitudes prevent them from engaging in behaviors that they themselves have concluded are important to them (Gollwitzer 1999;

Gollwitzer & Oettingen 2000). How can we as nutrition educators help individuals bridge the intention–behavior gap? How do we help individuals move from motivation to action, from intention to reality, from thinking to doing?

The major way to bridge the intention–behavior gap is to make the desired action easier to understand and do. Nutrition educators can do that in two major ways: we can build individuals' abilities and skills to act on their motivations, and we can make the environment more supportive of the behavior. Facilitating the ability to take action is the topic of this chapter. Making the environment more supportive is the subject of the next.

UNDERSTANDING THE MEDIATORS OF ACTION AND PROCEDURES FOR BEHAVIOR CHANGE

What can research and theory tell us that is useful in assisting individuals and groups to translate their intentions or goals into action?

Research and theory suggest that just as beliefs and affect or feelings predominate in the pre-action, motivational, or thinking phase, so food- and nutrition-specific knowledge and skills and self-regulatory processes predominate in the action and maintenance, or doing, phase of the behavior change process. The most useful theories or models for this phase of nutrition education are social cognitive theory; self-regulation or self-influence models (Bagozzi 1992; Gollwitzer 1999), such as the health action process approach (Schwarzer & Fuchs 1995; Sniehotta, Scholz, & Schwarzer 2005); and the transtheoretical or stages of change model (Prochaska & DiClemente 1984). These models identify factors that explain motivation for health behaviors, as do the theories described in the last chapter. However, in addition, these theories provide guidance on ways to facilitate people's ability to take action and make changes in their behavior.

Again, the question might be: why are there several theories instead of just one? And again the reason is that they were developed under different circumstances to understand different behaviors but can be applied to nutrition education. There is remarkable agreement among them, however, about the importance of the self-regulation process (or skills in self-direction) for taking and maintaining action. A few key theories that have been found useful to nutrition education are described here.

SOCIAL COGNITIVE THEORY

In its simplest terms, social cognitive theory proposes that behavior is the result of personal, behavioral, and environmental factors that influence each other in a dynamic and reciprocal fashion. Environments shape behaviors, but individuals also have the capacity to exert influence over the environment as well as their own behaviors through self-reflection and self-regulatory processes.

Social cognitive theory, as proposed and developed by Bandura (1977, 1986, 1989, 1997, 2000, 2004) to analyze and understand human thought, motivation, and action in general, has become the most widely used theory for designing nutrition education and health promotion programs. In addition to providing a unified and comprehensive framework for understanding the determinants of *behaviors*, it describes potential mediators and procedures for *behavioral change* that can be used to design strategies to assist people to take action.

Social cognitive theory proposes that personal, behavioral, and environmental factors work in a dynamic and reciprocal fashion to influence health behavior. *Personal factors* involve people's thoughts and feelings. *Behavioral factors* include their food-, nutrition-, and health-related knowledge and skills, together called *behavioral capability* and their skills in regulating and taking charge of their own behaviors, called *self-regulation skills*. *Environmental factors* include those factors external to individuals, such as the physical and social environments.

Constructs of the Theory

The constructs of the theory and their relationships to each other and to behavior are shown in **Figure 5-1**. **Table 5-1** provides a summary of the constructs of the theory and how they can be used in the design of nutrition education.

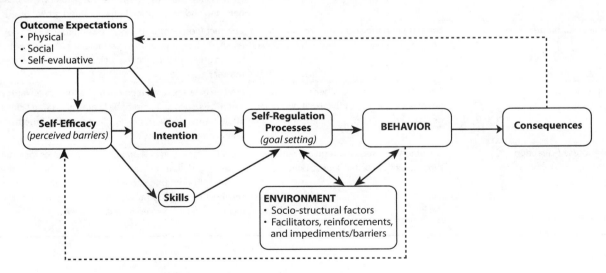

FIGURE 5-1 Social cognitive theory.

Source: Based on Bandura, A. 2000. Health promotion from the perspective of social cognitive theory. In *Understanding and changing health behavior: From health beliefs to self-regulation*, edited by P. Norman, C. Abraham, and M. Conner. Amsterdam: Harwood Academic Publishers.

TABLE 5-1 **Social Cognitive Theory: Major Concepts and Applications to Nutrition Education Interventions**

Theory Construct/Potential Mediator of Behavior Change	Definition	Applications to Practice
Outcome expectations (physical or material)	Beliefs about the likelihood and the value of physical outcomes or consequences that can be expected from a behavior	Provide activities to enhance awareness of negative outcomes such as risk of disease (perceived threat) or enhance the importance of positive outcomes (perceived benefits) of taking action such as messages about effect of F&V on cancer risk reduction.
Outcome expectations (social)	Beliefs about the likelihood and the value of social outcomes or consequences that can be expected from a behavior	Supply messages about social norms and activities on how to handle them (e.g., make eating F&V cool for teens).
Outcome expectations (self-evaluative)	Beliefs about the likelihood and the value of self-evaluative outcomes or consequences that can be expected from a behavior	Emphasize self-satisfaction and self-worth from behavior (e.g., "By eating F&V, I am being good to myself").
Barriers or impediments	Including the perceptions of *personal* barriers or challenges to taking action (which are integral to self-efficacy assessments) and actual *environmental* barriers (which reside in socio-structural factors)	Help individuals identify the *perceived barriers* that impede their ability to take health actions and provide strategies, knowledge, and skills to make the actions easy to understand and do. For *environmental barriers*, assist group to develop collective efficacy to take collective action; work with policy makers and decision-makers to create supportive environments.
Self-efficacy	Beliefs about personal ability to perform the given behavior that brings the desired outcomes.	Assist individuals to achieve success by making changes in small steps. Create modeling and mastery experiences about food and nutrition (e.g., cooking, gardening, advocacy). Provide feedback and encouragement. Assist individuals to interpret physiological responses to the new food or behavior correctly.
Behavioral capability	The food- and nutrition-related knowledge and cognitive, affective, and behavioral skills needed to enact the behavior	Provide necessary knowledge and cognitive skills for taking action through presentations, handouts, demonstrations, videos, and other channels, as well as discussions and debates to develop critical thinking skills. Also provide affective skills, such as handling stressful situations, and behavioral skills such as food purchasing and storage, cooking skills, safe food handling and preparation behaviors, and growing vegetables.
Observational learning/modeling	Learning to perform a behavior through peer modeling	Conduct food demonstrations relating to the behavior being enacted, such as making a low-fat recipe. Provide opportunities for the group to practice the recipe, with guidance, to enhance mastery.
Reinforcement	Responses to individuals' behavior that increases or decreases the likelihood of its occurrence	Provide external reinforcement in the form of rewards or incentives, such as T-shirts, key chains, and raffle tickets, for goal attainment. Provide opportunities to develop internal or self-reinforcement for own accomplishments.
Self-regulation/self-direction	The ability to direct and regulate behavior through skills of self-influence	Provide instruction and practice opportunities for individuals to develop skills in self-regulation of behavior: assessing their values, self-monitoring, goal setting, self-rewards, and problem solving. Emotion coping and stress-management skills are also included and ways to enlist social support.

Personal Factors

Social cognitive theory posits that our behavior is influenced by a host of thoughts or beliefs about ourselves. We demonstrate forethought and are thus capable of intentional or purposive action. Future events cannot serve as determinants of current behavior, but their cognitive representations in the present through our symbolic capability can have a strong motivating impact on current behavior. We are self-reflective and able to evaluate our actions, and we can exercise influence over our behavior. Among the many person-related factors, two major constructs that are important in motivating behavior are outcome expectations and self-efficacy.

Outcome Expectations/Beliefs About Outcomes

Social cognitive theory posits that much of our behavior is regulated by our beliefs about anticipated outcomes from engaging in a behavior or pattern of behavior and the degree to which we value these outcomes. As such, outcome expectations are similar to beliefs about outcomes of behavior in the theory of planned behavior and to perceived benefits of behavior in the health belief model. *Outcome expectancies* are the values people place on these outcomes and are also called *incentives* by Bandura (1986).

Social cognitive theory states that we will choose to perform an action that maximizes the anticipated positive outcomes and minimizes the anticipated negative outcomes. Outcome expectations can take three forms:

- *Physical outcomes:* Physical outcomes are the physical and health effects that accompany the behavior. According to Bandura (2000, 2004), in the health domain, negative physical outcomes include perceived risk of disease from not engaging in healthy behaviors, similar to the perceived threat construct of the health belief model. Positive outcomes are similar to the perceived benefits construct, including pleasant sensory experiences, such as from the pleasant taste of fruits.
- *Social outcomes:* Social outcomes are the social consequences of the behavior. Behaviors that fulfill social norms bring positive reactions, such as soda drinking among teenagers, whereas those that violate social norms bring social censure, such as breastfeeding in public in cultures where this is not the norm.
- *Self-evaluative outcomes:* Self-evaluative outcomes are the positive and negative reactions we have to our own behaviors. We engage in behaviors that bring satisfaction and a sense of self-worth; for example, "By eating fruits and vegetables I am being good to myself." We avoid behaviors that lead to dissatisfaction, such as "I avoid eating junk foods because if I eat them, I am not doing the right thing for myself." Bandura (2000) believes that self-satisfaction for personal accomplishments is one of the more powerful regulators of behavior, often more important than tangible rewards. Examples are success in breastfeeding or in being able to walk an hour a day.

With each form, anticipated positive outcomes serve as incentives, and negative outcomes serve as disincentives (Bandura 2000, 2004). Refer to Figure 5-1.

Self-Efficacy

Self-efficacy is considered to be the major motivator of action and mediator of behavior change. Although beliefs about health outcomes or risks of behavior are a precondition for change, self-efficacy is needed to overcome impediments or barriers to adopting and maintaining healthy behaviors (Bandura 1989, 2000). Self-efficacy is the confidence we have that we can carry out the intended behavior successfully or overcome barriers to engaging in the behavior. Self-efficacy involves both the skills and the confidence that we can effectively and consistently use these skills. Extensive research indicates that the higher the level of perceived self-efficacy, the more effort we will expend and the longer we will persist in a new learned behavior, especially in the face of difficulties. See **Box 5-1** for strategies to enhance self-efficacy in individuals.

Self-efficacy has been shown through research to be especially important in the initiation, modification, and maintenance of complex behaviors such as healthful eating and physical activity. Self-efficacy tends to be domain specific. Examples in the health area might be an individual's confidence that he or she can eat a healthful diet, run 3 miles a day, change his or her eating pattern/shopping practices to be more supportive of sustainable food systems, or organize his or her work situation to be able to breast-feed even when it is difficult to do so. Thus, the concept of self-efficacy has been incorporated into the more recent versions of other theories such as the health belief model, theory of planned behavior, and the transtheoretical model as applied to the area of diet and health.

Taking Charge of Our Lives: Personal Agency

Social cognitive theory extends the notion of self-efficacy further to the notion of personal agency—a strong sense of our ability to *exercise in-*

$\mathcal{B}ox$ 5-1   Methods for Enhancing Self-Efficacy

Beliefs in personal efficacy can be strengthened through four main sources of influence:

1. *Personal mastery experiences:* Enabling individuals to master the behavior by setting and achieving increasingly challenging action goals. Practice is thus the most effective way of creating a strong sense of personal efficacy.
2. *Social modeling:* Showing that others similar to themselves can succeed. This includes detailed demonstrations of the steps involved.
3. *Social persuasion:* Providing encouragement that they can do it. Such encouragement can overcome self-doubts. Included here are also efforts to structure the situation so that individuals can succeed and to help them measure success against their own improvement.
4. *Modification of emotional or physical responses to the behavior:* People rely partly on information from their physiological states to judge their own abilities. Self-efficacy can thus be strengthened by assisting individuals in modifying their emotional or physical responses to the behavior where these are stressful or caused by misinterpretations of the experience. Fear can be relabeled as excitement and (mis)perceptions can be corrected.

Source: Adapted from Bandura, A. 1997. *Self-efficacy: The exercise of control.* New York: WH Freeman.

fluence over our own behaviors and over external events that affect our lives to produce a desired effect. These judgments of personal agency have far-reaching influences on thought patterns, emotional reactions, and behavior. Unless we believe that we can achieve desired outcomes through our own actions, we have little incentive to take action. According to Bandura (1989, 2000), such a sense of personal agency is not just confidence in knowledge and skills to carry out a given action but is also the ability to regulate motivations, thought processes, feelings, and behavioral patterns or to change environmental conditions, depending on what is needed in the context of the particular domain of action.

Social cognitive theory thus views individuals as agents who are able to take charge of their lives. Bandura (1989) points out that a robust sense of personal agency and the ability to recover quickly from difficulties and setbacks help people succeed in their endeavors. For example, James Joyce's book *The Dubliners* was rejected by 22 publishers and a manuscript by E. E. Cummings was rejected 12 times, but each author kept sending them in for consideration. They are now both considered major writers.

Collective Efficacy
Social cognitive theory has extended the notion of self-efficacy to collective efficacy, which emphasizes the human capacity for collective action. Collective efficacy is the ability for individuals to work in a group to bring about changes in environments, including social structures and policy, to benefit the entire group (Bandura 1997). This construct is described in detail in Chapter 6.

Impediments or Barriers
Some barriers are *personal*, including our judgments of our self-efficacy—or lack thereof—to surmount obstacles (such as lack of confidence to cook healthful foods) (see Figure 5-1). According to Bandura (2004), assessing barriers is part of self-efficacy assessments because they allow us to judge whether we will be able to carry out a behavior even under difficult circumstances, such as cooking a low-fat meal even when we are busy or tired from a day at work. Some impediments are *external* or reside in the environment, such as lack of availability or accessibility of healthful foods or venues for physical activity and lack of health resources.

Goals and Goal Intentions
Goals can refer to valued end states (or values) that serve an orienting function for the long term, such as being healthy, enjoying a high quality of life, living an ethical life, and so forth. These are extremely important because they represent internal standards or values we develop from a variety of sources, against which we can judge our current behaviors. However, sometimes they may be too broad to guide specific actions.

Goals also can refer to proximal or immediate goals that contribute to our long-term goals. Such goals are similar to the behavioral intention construct of the theory of planned behavior. In the context of a behavior change process, this represents a commitment to take action. When our outcome expectations are positive (perceived benefits) and self-efficacy is high, we are motivated to form proximal goals and develop action plans to carry them out. This process is part of the self-regulation or self-direction process described later in this chapter.

Reinforcements
Reinforcements are the responses to a person's behavior that increase or decrease the likelihood of occurrence of that behavior. This term is used to describe positive reinforcements or rewards, which can be external or internal. External reinforcement is providing an action or item that is known to have reinforcement value for the individual or group, such as gold stars for children completing a task in school, or T-shirts or other rewards for completing a health program or a task such as goal setting. Internal reinforcement is individuals' own perceptions that the behavior had some value for them.

Relapse Prevention
Relapse prevention focuses on strategies to maintain the new behaviors. These strategies include cognitive restructuring, which involves substituting alternative thoughts and behaviors for less healthful eating behaviors; controlling the environment by removing or avoiding cues to less healthful eating (such as avoiding going into the ice cream store) and adding cues for more healthful eating (such as leaving washed fruit out on the counter at home); and setting new goals.

Behavioral Factors
According to social cognitive theory, behavioral factors are equally important. These include food-related *knowledge and skills* needed to engage in the behavior, such as eating low-fat foods, when desired. In addition, initiation and maintenance of the behavior for the long term requires *self-regulation skills*, including individuals' ability to exercise influence and control over their own behavior.

Behavioral Capabilities: Nutrition Knowledge and Skills/Health Literacy
Behavioral capabilities are the food- and nutrition-related knowledge and skills that individuals need to carry out the behavior or practice the behavioral goals that they have selected. Here knowledge is of the instrumental or how-to kind:

- *Factual knowledge:* Factual knowledge includes food and nutrition information and how to use it, such as information about nutrients and food sources, MyPyramid, the *Dietary Guidelines*, or the *Physical Activity Guidelines*. The information must be specific to the behavior that has been chosen if it is to be helpful to the individuals attempting to carry out the behavior.
- *Procedural knowledge:* Procedural knowledge is the knowledge about *how* to do something, or decision rules for solving given cognitive tasks. Included are relatively simple skills, such as how to read food labels, and more complex critical thinking skills, such as evaluating the advantages and disadvantages of breast-feeding. It would also include information on how exactly to breast-feed. Through the acquisition of such knowledge, people develop *knowledge structures*, or schemas—personal conceptual frameworks, if you will—for given areas of information.
- *Behavioral skills.* Additional mechanisms are needed to get from knowledge structures to skilled action. Learning by doing (or "enactive learning") is the translating vehicle, according to Bandura (1986). This means people need to develop *behavioral skills* through performing the behaviors and practicing them, such as preparing healthful snacks, cooking low-fat recipes, practicing safe food handling behaviors, or breastfeeding. Nutrition educators can facilitate the acquisition of such skills by first demonstrating the skills and then providing the opportunity for individuals to practice them. This is sometimes referred to as *modeling and guided practice*. With continued practice these skills can become easy to do and routinized and hence can be performed without much additional thought.

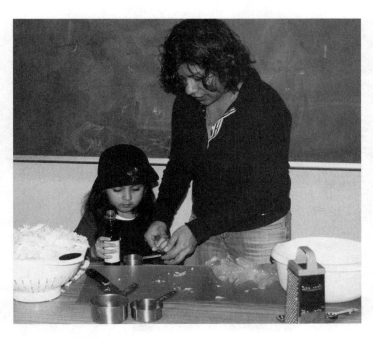

One mom helps her daughter cook at a WIC center.

- *Health literacy:* Health literacy is an individual's ability to read, understand, and use health care information to make decisions and follow instructions for treatment. This is very important for those with nutrition-related health conditions who want to manage their conditions (Institute of Medicine 2004; Osborne 2005). It is especially important for nutrition educators to use appropriate literacy level, plain language, and graphics with low-literacy audiences to ensure understanding. Such communication issues are discussed in detail in Chapters 16 and 17.

Self-Regulation and Goal-Setting Processes

Motivation alone is not sufficient to initiate health-promoting personal change. Self-regulation, or our ability to direct and influence our own behavior, is also required. This is not achieved through willpower but by learning skills for self-influence. Self-regulation or self-direction of behavior involves the following components: we must first observe the behavior we seek to change (e.g., we observe that we eat only two servings of fruits and vegetables each day). This provides the information we need for setting realistic goals. We then set specific behavioral change or action goals and learn the food and nutrition skills needed to achieve them. We monitor our own progress toward achieving these action goals and reward ourselves when we meet them. This reward may be the satisfaction of doing the right thing for our health. This process is called *goal setting* (Bandura 1986; Cullen, Baranowski, & Smith 2001; Shilts, Horowitz, & Townsend 2004a, 2004b, 2009).

Why goal-setting is important. Goal setting is important because setting action goals or action plans increases our motivation to act by building our perceptions of our self-efficacy and mastery, creating self-satisfaction and a sense of fulfillment from having achieved the goals, and cultivating intrinsic interest through active involvement in the process. Goal setting is similar to implementation or action plans in other self-regulation theories. These theories point out that such planning ahead means that we have decided on the behavior ahead of

time and will not need to make a new decision in each new situation, thus reducing stress and effort (Gollwitzer 1999).

In the self-regulation process, when we do not attain our action goals, we engage in problem solving and decision making to find more effective ways to attain the goals we set or set new ones that are more attainable. Evidence shows that those who are successful at self-directed change are highly skilled at enlisting these self-regulatory skills to work for them. Maintenance of personal change requires not only a set of behavioral and self-regulation/ self-direction skills but a resilient sense of efficacy. If we are not convinced of our sense of personal efficacy, we may abandon the skills we have been taught when we experience difficult situations or do not get quick results.

In general, social cognitive theory places great importance on mastery experiences for individuals. There is a difference between self-efficacy and actual skills, and individuals must have the opportunity to learn and practice the behavioral skills to achieve their goals.

Environmental Factors

Social cognitive theory distinguishes between *situation*, which is people's perception or cognitive representation of the environment, and *environment*, which relates to the objective factors affecting their behavior that are external to them.

Influences of the Environment on Behavior

Numerous environmental factors influence behavior, as we saw in Chapter 2 (Bandura 1997). Many physical and sociostructural environments have an impact on us whether we like it or not. Examples in the area of food-related behaviors are the physical availability of specific healthy foods at school and at the workplace or in the local corner store, and the social environment, such as whether family or friends eat fruits and vegetables.

People's Influences on the Environment

At the same time, we can control how we react to environments, act within them, or work to change them. For example, we might influence what the family purchases or advocate for policies within workplaces or schools to improve nutrition at the site. We might advocate for legislators to enact policies to improve the built environment such as more supermarkets in food deserts or more walkable streets. We also can create environments, for example, by organizing a nutrition committee to make changes in a school or at a worksite. We are constantly interacting with our environments, choosing how to interpret and react to them, negotiating with them, or changing them, so that we influence our environments even as our environments influence us. Nutrition education thus seeks to work with policymakers to create environments that are supportive.

Observational Learning from the Environment

The environment is also the source for *modeling* of behaviors. Trial-and-error learning from experiences—that is, feedback from the consequences of our own behavior—is one source of learning. However, we also learn by observing the behavior of others and the consequences that follow from their behavior. Such observational learning is a very important construct in social cognitive theory. For example, children, who are trying to figure out the world, learn from observing their parents. Teenagers learn from observing the food-related behaviors of their peers, valued adults, and relevant celebrities and public figures. Nutrition educators can use modeling as a strategy by pointing to positive role models or by teaching people food-related skills, such as through cooking demonstrations.

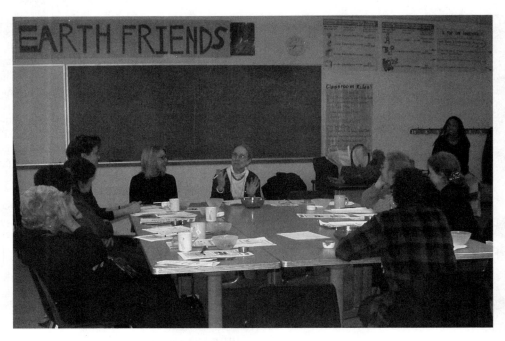

Learning to set action plans for healthy living.

Human Agency Perspective on Social Cognitive Theory

Social cognitive theory gives special emphasis to individuals' ability to think and plan ahead, to be reflective about their own abilities and actions, and to be reflective about the meaning and purposes of their life pursuits. This ability to exercise influence over their lives or to take control Bandura describes as human agency (Bandura 1989, 2001). As we have seen, there is personal agency but also collective agency, where people work together with others to bring about goals they all desire. Nutrition education can be designed to enhance both personal and collective agency.

Relationship to Biological Variables

In the area of food choice and dietary behaviors, biological variables are also important, as we saw in Chapter 2. Food choice may be influenced by biology, just as foods eaten have an impact on physiological systems or biology. Clearly, physiological processes such as hunger and satiety are crucial in influencing the quantity of foods individuals eat. People's biologically and genetically determined taste propensities also influence their choice of different kinds of foods (Keller et al. 2002; Mennella, Pepino, & Reed 2005). Some researchers have therefore suggested that in the food and health areas biology should be added as another set of influences in reciprocal determinism (Thoresen 1984; Bandura 1986, 1997; Baranowski et al. 2003) to yield interacting influences of person, behavior, biology, and environment.

Evidence from Research and Intervention Studies

Research Studies Using the Theory

A few research studies illustrate how social cognitive theory has been used to study dietary behaviors:

- *Children:* One study examined the three social cognitive theory components for their usefulness in predicting fruit and vegetable consumption in elementary school children (Reynolds et al. 1999). It is summarized in **Nutrition Education in Action 5-1**. As you can see from the information in the feature, the study found that availability and motivation each had a significant direct effect on consumption, but knowledge did not. Motivation had a significant relationship to knowledge.
- *Adults:* A study in adults examined the relationships of the constructs of social environment, reinforcement, modeling, knowledge, and outcome expectations to the consumption of four beverages: whole milk, low-fat/skim milk, regular soda, and diet soda (Lewis, Sims, & Shannon 1989). They found that the factors influencing consumption varied by forms of the beverage and by the two age groups they studied, students and adults. Clearly, then, both the behavior and the intended audience are important considerations when the theory is applied.
- *Questionnaires:* Theory can also be used as the basis of questions in open-ended interviews or in questionnaires. **Table 5-2** gives an example of how social cognitive theory was used to construct questions to determine the influences on fruit and vegetable consumption by low-income black American adolescents (Molaison et al. 2005).

Intervention Studies Using the Theory

Numerous intervention studies in the domain of food and diet have been conducted using social cognitive theory, although the full model is not usually used in all studies. A few studies are described here to illustrate the theory.

Studies with Children

- *The Child and Adolescent Trial for Cardiovascular Health (CATCH)* program was a large randomized controlled trial with third- to fifth-graders designed to reduce risk for cardiovascular disease (Luepker et al. 1996). The educational activities were based on

NUTRITION EDUCATION IN ACTION 5-1

Using Social Cognitive Theory to Understand Fruit and Vegetable Consumption by Elementary School Children

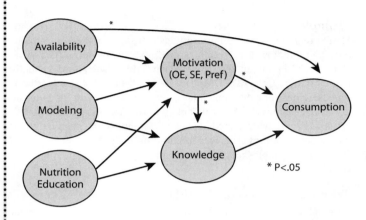

Using social cognitive theory to understand fruit and vegetable consumption in elementary school children.

This study used social cognitive theory to examine factors that would explain why third-grade children did or did not eat fruits and vegetables. The constructs of the theory, how they were measured, and the results of the study are summarized here.

Behavior: 24-hour recalls, analyzed for fruits and vegetables.

Environmental component: The environmental component was measured by three constructs:

- Availability of fruits and vegetables at home, measured by parents' response about the presence of 31 items in the home

- Social modeling, measured as the sum of the number of people that the child indicated he or she saw eating fruits and vegetables (e.g., friends their age, teacher)
- Nutrition education, measured as the number of sources that the children said taught them about fruits and vegetables from a choice of six persons (e.g., teachers, parent) and four sources (e.g., poster, TV)

Person-related component: This component consisted of two constructs: motivation and knowledge.

- *Motivation* was measured as a composite, latent construct made up of three constructs put together:
  - Outcome expectancies (OE), measured with items such as "eating fruits and vegetables will make me smarter"
  - Self-efficacy (SE), measured with items such as "I can drink a glass of my favorite juice with my dinner"
  - Preference (Pref), measured as liking for 20 items
- *Knowledge* was measured with 10 true or false and multiple-choice questions related to fruits and vegetables.

Results: Results are shown in the accompanying diagram, which depicts the relationship between theory constructs in environmental and personal components and the behavior—consumption of fruits and vegetables. You can see that availability and motivation each had a significant direct effect on consumption, but knowledge did not. Motivation had a significant relationship to knowledge.

Source: Reynolds, K. D., A. W. Hinton, R. Shewchuk, et al. 1999. A social cognitive model of fruit and vegetable consumption in elementary school children. *Journal of Nutrition Education* 31(1): 23–30. Figure used with permission of the Society for Nutrition Education.

---

social cognitive theory constructs and emphasized the behaviors of reduction in fat intake and increase in physical activity.

The program resulted in a significant reduction in fat intake and increased physical activity compared with controls. It also resulted in changes in food choices; social reinforcement by parents, friends, and teachers; and in self-efficacy for diet and physical activity (Edmundson et al. 1996; Hoelscher et al. 2004).

- *Planet Health* is an obesity prevention program for middle school students that focuses on decreasing television viewing, decreasing consumption of high-fat foods, increasing fruit and vegetable intake, and increasing moderate and vigorous physical activity (Gortmaker et al. 1999). In an evaluation study, it was taught through four subject areas and included increased physical education time. Results showed there was a reduced prevalence of obesity and increase in fruit and vegetable intake in girls, and decreased leisure screen time in both boys and girls.

- *Choice, Control, and Change* is an obesity prevention program (also for middle school students) that focuses on fostering personal agency by using an inquiry-based science education to address outcome expectations or why to take action, and goal-setting and self-regulation skills for how to take action. An evaluation found that students in intervention schools compared to the controls reported consumption of significantly fewer sweetened drinks and packaged snacks, smaller sizes of fast food, increased intentional walking, and decreased leisure screen time, although it found no increases in their intakes of vegetables and water (Contento et al. 2007; Sauberli et al. 2008). See Nutrition Education in Action 12-2 in Chapter 12 for further details.
- *EatFit*, an intervention with middle school students, was directed at both dietary and physical activity behaviors (Horowitz, Shilts, & Townsend 2004). It was found that adding a guided goal-setting component to the intervention improved students'

TABLE 5-2	Using Social Cognitive Theory to Guide Questions About Influences on Fruit and Vegetable Consumption in a Sample of Low-Income Black American Adolescents	
Open-Ended Questions		**SCT Construct**
Home		
If you looked in the refrigerator or the kitchen cabinet of your home right now, what kinds of fruits (vegetables) would you find?		Environmental
Do you ever eat fruits (vegetables) away from home? What are some other places that you eat fruit (vegetables)?		Environmental
Behavior		
Do you help prepare the meals and snacks in your home?		Behavior
Personal beliefs		
What do you think would happen if you don't eat fruit (vegetables)?		Outcome expectancies
What would make you want to eat more fruit (vegetables)?		Outcome expectancies
If you wanted to eat more fruit or vegetables, would you be able to? Why or why not? How would you get them?		Self-efficacy
Family and friends		
Do you think your friends (family members) would help you eat more fruits and vegetables?		Social support
What would you do if no one is eating fruits (vegetables), but you would like to eat fruit (vegetables)?		Social expectations
What are some reasons you and your friends eat fruit (vegetables)?		Social expectations

Source: Molaison, E. F., C. L. Connell, J. E. Stuff, M. K. Yadrick, and M. Bogle. 2005. Influences on fruit and vegetable consumption by low-income black American adolescents. *Journal of Nutrition Education and Behavior* 37(5): 246–251. Used with permission of the Society for Nutrition Education.

dietary behavior, physical activity behavior, and physical activity self-efficacy compared with the same intervention without goal setting (Shilts et al. 2009). See **Nutrition Education in Action 5-2**.

Studies with Adults

- *ALIVE* was a randomized control using e-mail to reach employees with a 16-week program involving individually tailored, small-step goals; a personal homepage with tips; educational materials; and tracking and simulation tools, similar to the program described in Nutrition Education in Action 5-4. Results showed increases in moderate and vigorous physical activity and walking and in fruit and vegetable intake, and decreases in saturated fat intake (Sternfeld et al. 2009).

- *A community-based diabetes education program* resulted in positive impacts on knowledge, health beliefs, and the self-reported behaviors of using herbs in place of salt, cooking with olive or canola oil, and using artificial sweeteners in baking. Participants increased their self-efficacy in changing their diet and preparing healthful meals (Chapman-Novakofski & Karduck 2005).

Examples from Practice

Many programs in community settings focus on outcome expectations plus skill building. An example is the "Just Say Yes to Fruits and Vegetables" (JSY) program, discussed in **Nutrition Education in Action 5-3**. Another is the *Little by Little* CD-ROM discussed in **Nutrition Education in Action 5-4**. The usefulness of a one-time interactive experience with the latter program was examined for low-income women. The CD-ROM included a self-assessment with immediate feedback to make the need for change individually relevant. This was followed by suggestions on how to add fruits and vegetables to the diet and finally goal setting and individual commitment.

Take-Home Message about Social Cognitive Theory

- Social cognitive theory states that individuals' personal agency and their environments interact dynamically, resulting in personal and social change. In addition to being convinced that taking a given behavior will be effective in leading to the outcomes they desire, people must also believe that they can carry out the behavior even in the face of difficulties and setbacks. Therefore, self-efficacy is a major mediator of change, and behavioral and self-regulation/self-direction skills development is the major procedure for change. The environment both influences and is influenced by people's behaviors.

- This theory is especially useful in designing nutrition education that proposes to address both motivation and skills, and both the individual and the environment.

■ SELF-REGULATION/SELF-EFFICACY MODELS

Many other researchers have found from research that our ability to regulate, exercise control, or generally take charge of our behaviors is a key process in initiating and maintaining health behavior change. Self-efficacy becomes very important in this process (Bagozzi 1992; Gollwitzer 1999; Gollwitzer & Oettingen 2000; Rothman 2000). The processes described are similar to those in social cognitive theory. However, these models note that becoming motivated to initiate a behavior requires a different mind-set and different tasks from maintaining a behavior once we have started taking action. In the motivation phase, a deliberative—or thinking—mind-set predominates, and in the action phase an implementation—or doing—mind-set predominates (Abraham, Sheeran, & Johnson 1998; Gollwitzer & Oettingen 2000). Self-efficacy is important in both phases, with motivational self-efficacy in the first, and coping self-efficacy in the second phase.

Health Action Process Approach Model

This section describes the health action process approach model because it is a simple model and includes a time dimension (Schwarzer & Fuchs 1995; Schwarzer & Renner 2000; Sniehotta et al. 2005; Ziegelmann & Lippke 2007). It is shown in **Figure 5-2**. The model proposes two phases—a pre-action phase and an action phase—and focuses on the important

NUTRITION EDUCATION IN ACTION 5-2

EatFit: A Goal-Oriented Intervention that Challenges Adolescents to Improve Their Eating and Fitness Choices

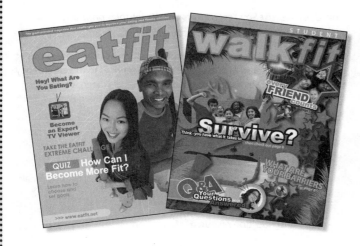

Surveys show that the diets of youth do not meet those recommended by the Dietary Guidelines, and neither do youth engage in recommended amounts of physical activity. This program was designed to improve the dietary and physical activity behaviors of middle school students. It consisted of a classroom for the teacher or leader, a workbook for each student, a Web-based interactive program in which students received personalized assessment based on a 24-hour diet record that they had completed, personalized dietary feedback, goal setting, and a contract. The program was based on social cognitive theory:

Outcome expectancies: Motivators identified from focus groups were as follows: improved appearance, increased energy, and increased independence. These were used in the lessons.

Self-efficacy: Students were provided opportunity to practice skills (recipe preparation and tasting, physical activities), receive encouragement, and develop social support among the group.

Self-regulation:

- Self-monitoring of their own diets and physical activity patterns
- Setting goals
- Monitoring their progress toward the goals
- Problem-solving activities to overcome perceived barriers (e.g., how to select fast foods that support their goals)
- Rewards or positive reinforcements for attaining goals

   Details of how the food choice determinants or theory constructs were operationalized in the program are shown in the following table.

Source: Horowitz, M., M. K. Shilts, and M. S. Townsend. 2004. EatFit: A goal-oriented intervention that challenges adolescents to improve their eating and fitness choices. *Journal of Nutrition Education and Behavior* 36:43–44. Used with permission of the Society for Nutrition Education.

Examples of Use of Social Cognitive Theory in EatFit

Theory Construct/ Strategy	Theory-Based Activities
Self-efficacy/skills mastery	Students increase their self-efficacy in choosing foods that meet their selected dietary goals. They learn how to read food labels and practice those skills by answering questions on dozens of foods that are specific to their goals.
Modeling	Students interview a parent or guardian about their goal-setting experiences.
Barriers counseling	During the parent interview, students ask about barriers/hurdles encountered during parent's goal progress and the resolution of those hurdles.
Self-monitoring	Students complete self-assessments of current dietary and fitness practices.
Goal setting	Students set physical activity goals using results from the self-assessments.
Contracting	Students complete contracts for their dietary and fitness goals. This contract specifies the goal and the motivation for attainment and has space for signatures from student, a friend, and a parent.
Cue management	A teacher-led discussion asks "What are some negative cues that may prevent you from reaching your fitness goal?"
Social support	To strengthen social support networks, students are placed into groups based on chosen goals.
Reinforcement	Students receive raffle tickets for goal attainment.
Cognitive restructuring	By restructuring the way students think about breakfast, options open up for their morning meal such as leftover pizza or a microwaveable burrito, thus making breakfast easier to obtain.
Relapse prevention	The student workbook includes a section devoted to helping students maintain, set, and achieve new goals after the completion of the intervention.
Environment/ reciprocal determinism	Homework assignments focus on the role of the environment on behavior change. For example, students identify five locations where they could exercise after school, the hours of operation, and cost. Students find one food from an on-campus source that meets their dietary goals.

NUTRITION EDUCATION IN ACTION 5-3

Just Say Yes to Fruits and Vegetables

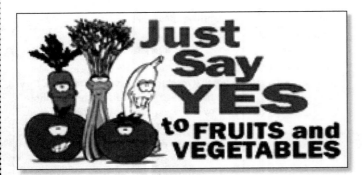

The Just Say Yes to Fruits and Vegetables (JSY) project, in partnership with organizations that serve the food insecure, is dedicated to improving the health and nutritional status of Supplemental Nutrition Assistance Program (SNAP) populations in the state of New York. The project accomplishes this by providing comprehensive nutrition education programs for SNAP populations in a variety of community settings.

About JSY: Nutrition Education Sessions

- Does your organization work with SNAP eligibles, recipients, or applicants?
- Is your organization interested in offering free nutrition education programs to your clients?
- Do your clients want to know what to do with some of the produce you give them?
- Do your clients need help with preparing healthy meals on a budget?

If you said "Yes" to these questions, then the Just Say Yes to Fruits and Vegetables project would love to visit your site!

How does the Just Say Yes to Fruits and Vegetables program work with food pantries and other communities?

Nutritionists from this program provide nutrition education sessions at local food pantries and agencies that provide services to the emergency feeding network. Sessions emphasize the use of frozen, canned, and dried products as well as fresh in-season fruits and vegetables. Each session offers the following:

- Easy, low-cost recipes
- A taste sample of a recipe made with the featured fruit or vegetable
- Tips and ideas for planning and preparing delicious, healthy meals
- Information on stretching food dollars
- Food safety information
- Food and nutrition resource information

What is the purpose of a nutrition education session?

Nutritionists from the JSY program provide nutrition education sessions at a variety of sites across the state of New York. The purpose of this program is to

- Empower low-income New Yorkers to make healthier food choices
- Convey the message that consumption of fruits and vegetables may reduce the risk of chronic diseases (such as heart disease, diabetes, and cancer)
- Enhance nutrition knowledge and skills in purchasing and preparing the best-quality fruits and vegetables
- Improve food safety skills

Source: New York State Department of Health. 2005. Just Say Yes to Fruits and Vegetables. http://www.jsyfruitveggies.org. Logo used with permission.

---

role of self-efficacy at various points in the dietary change process, as shown in the figure.

Motivational Phase

The focus in the motivational phase is on beliefs and affect or feelings, and a deliberative mind-set prevails. In this model, the motivational phase involves the relationships among potential mediators of behavior change, as shown in Figure 5-2. Individuals' intention to adopt a valued health behavior (such as eating a low-fat, high-fiber diet) depends on three sets of beliefs:

- *Risk perceptions:* The belief that we are at risk for disease (e.g., heart disease).
- *Outcome expectancies:* The belief that a change in behavior would reduce the health threat ("If I eat healthful foods, I will reduce my risk for heart disease").

- *Perceived self-efficacy:* The belief that we are sufficiently capable of exercising control over a difficult behavior, such as "I am capable of controlling my diet to make it healthful in spite of temptations to eat sweets." This can be called *motivational self-efficacy.*

Planning

Strategic planning has been found to greatly enhance the translation of intentions into action (Ziegelmann & Lippke 2007; Scholz et al. 2008). Here people begin to make plans to carry out the behavior and developing confidence in being able to make plans becomes important.

Action Phase

In the action phase, the mind-set is one of implementation (or doing), and the focus is on self-regulatory processes (Gollwitzer & Oettingen 2000).

NUTRITION EDUCATION IN ACTION 5-4

The *Little by Little* CD-ROM: Eat Better for a Better You

People find it hard to change dietary behavior. So, asking them to eat four and a half cups of fruits and vegetables per day may be overwhelming, and many may be afraid to undertake any change at all if they believe it will be too difficult. The *Little by Little* CD-ROM program encourages small dietary changes to move people in the right direction toward a better diet. It is brief and easy and takes only about 12 to 15 minutes.

Program

The program has three components:

- *Self-assessment and feedback:* Participants complete a 10-item survey on their usual intake of fruits and vegetables and get immediate feedback on their intake so as to make the need for change personally meaningful.
- *Modules on suggestions for specific situations:* Individuals click on only those modules that are relevant to them. The program is thus very flexible. For example, those who think that time is the issue can go to the Time section. Those who eat out a lot can find hints on getting more fruits and vegetables when eating out. If money is an issue, they can go to that section. If they pack lunches for themselves or their children, the program offers ideas. The whole point is giving people something easy that they can do to improve their diets.
- *Goal setting and individual commitment:* To facilitate goal setting, the program suggests several goals to work toward, guided by options that the participant had chosen throughout the

program, and the participant is asked to choose one or two of them.

Evaluation

The program was evaluated though a randomized trial in which one group used the interactive CD-ROM program, a second group used the CD-ROM program and also received reminder phone calls, and a third (control) group received a stress management CD-ROM. The study participants were low-income African American and white women, mean age 50.1 years (SD 7.22, range 39–65).

Results

Two months after the one-time experience with the CD-ROMs, both intervention groups reported significantly higher intakes of fruits and vegetables than the control group did. The *Little by Little* group with reminder calls increased daily intake by 1.32 fruits/vegetables, an 86% greater increase than the control group ($P = .016$). The *Little by Little* group without reminder calls increased daily intake by 1.20 fruits/vegetables, a 69% greater increase than the control group ($P = .052$). Significantly greater movement in stage of readiness for change also occurred in the *Little by Little* groups compared with the control group.

Source: Block, G., P. Wakimoto, D. Metz, et al. 2004, July. A randomized trial of the *Little by Little* CD-ROM: Demonstrated effectiveness in increasing fruit and vegetable intake in a low-income population. *Preventing Chronic Disease* [online serial] 1(3). http://www.cdc.gov/pcd/issues/2004/jul/04_0016.htm.

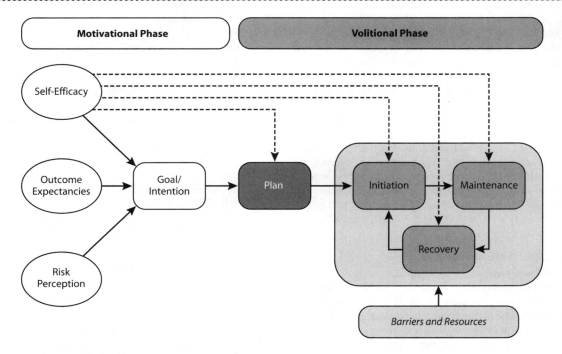

FIGURE 5-2 The health action process approach.

Source: R. Schwarzer, Freie Universitat Berlin, Germany. Used with permission.

Box 5-2 **Action Plans/Goal Setting: Why They Help Individuals Translate Intentions into Action**

Action plans (or implementation intentions) are highly effective in bridging the intention to behavior gap for many reasons:

- Stating a clear action plan means committing to an action, resulting in a sense of control, of determination, and also obligation to realize the action or behavior.
- The decision is made ahead of time so that when the situation arises the individual does not have to think and make a new decision each time. Such *planning ahead* means the behavior will require less mental effort each time.
- Because the action plan is made in advance, it is also on the person's mind.
- Developing action plans increases an individual's intrinsic interest through active involvement in the process.
- Action plans increase motivation through anticipation of self-satisfaction in achieving the goals

The action initiation subphase is a planning phase in which we first convert intentions (e.g., eating four and a half cups of fruits and vegetables a day) into *action plans* or *implementation intentions, specifying when, where, and how we will take action* ("I will add orange juice at breakfast each day next week; I will have a fruit for a snack three days this coming week"). Making very specific action plans has been shown to be effective in assisting individuals to initiate action (Gollwitzer 1999; Armitage 2004; de Nooijer et al. 2006). See **Box 5-2** for more details about why planning ahead helps people translate intentions into action.

The action maintenance subphase is a behavioral maintenance phase in which we develop the ability to influence and take charge of our own actions or behavior through our own efforts. See **Box 5-3** for details. A major challenge for us at this stage—indeed, an ongoing challenge in maintaining healthful practices—is setting priorities between conflicting goals or desires. We may want to eat more healthfully, but we also have work-related aspirations that do not leave much mental and physical time for planning and eating healthfully. At this time, the chosen behavioral goal, such as to eat healthful lunches at work, needs to be protected from being interrupted or given up prematurely because of competing intentions, such as the desire to be a productive worker and hence to work through lunch. Higher-order thinking or metacognitive activity is needed for us to stick with our chosen behavior and ignore the distracting action imperatives.

Self-Regulation and Self-Efficacy

Self-regulatory skill development thus relies on conscious control and attention. It also relies on strategies for coping with our emotions, such as the ability to ignore feelings of worry or of disappointment in not meeting the set goals. These skills are important because many desirable food- and nutrition-related practices require effort, for example, learning to cook so as to gain control over what ingredients are in the food eaten. Nutrition educators should note that implementing a new, more health-

ful behavior, such as adding fruit to the diet, does not automatically reduce less healthful habits such as eating high-fat, high-sugar snacks (Verplanken & Faes 1999).

Coping Self-Efficacy

Optimistic beliefs about our ability to deal with barriers, although a major hindrance in getting us motivated, may be helpful here because a new behavior may turn out to be much more difficult to adhere to than we had anticipated. These beliefs are sometimes referred to as *coping self-efficacy*. An example is "I can stick with a healthful diet even if I have to try several times until it works" or "even if I need a long time to develop the necessary routines" (Schwarzer & Renner 2000). The aim here is for the new behavior to become habitual and routine.

Just as initiation of a behavior is based on our *anticipation* of the satisfaction we can obtain from a behavior, so maintenance of the new behavior is based on our experience of the satisfaction of the *actual outcomes* we obtain from the new behavior (Rothman 2000).

Recovery

Individuals may not be able to maintain their goal behaviors at all times. Recovery self-efficacy—the conviction that they are able to get back on track after being derailed from the goal or after they experience setbacks—now becomes important. High recovery self-efficacy enables individuals to get back on track.

Evidence for the Model from Research Studies

Several studies have examined the importance of these variables in relation to diet and physical activity (Taylor, Bagozzi, & Gaither 2005; Ziegelmann, Lippke, & Schwarzer 2006; Schwarzer et al. 2007; Lippke, Ziegelmann et al. 2009):

- A study of four health behaviors, including dietary behavior and physical activity, found that self-efficacy and planning were the immediate predictors of behavior, while risk perception was an early phase factor (Schwarzer et al. 2007).
- For physical activity behavior, planning was found to be useful only if individuals held sufficiently high self-efficacy (Lippke, Wiedemann et al. 2009).
- In a study of fruit and vegetable intake, outcome expectations predicted progression from pre-intention to intention, whereas social support predicted progression to the action phase. Low levels of planning were associated with relapse to the pre-action phase. Self-efficacy emerged as a universal predictor of phase transitions (Wiedemann et al. 2009).

■ GROUNDED THEORY APPROACH: PERSONAL FOOD POLICIES

Some studies using a grounded theory approach or interpretative approach to studying dietary behavior have found that individuals develop personal food policies or systems to manage, over the long term, the numerous and conflicting values they hold about their food choices (Connors et al. 2001; Bisogni et al. 2005; Contento et al. 2006).

For example, some people balance criteria for food choice:

- One study found that individuals can choose one value and use it predominantly, such as choosing the least expensive option, the one that tastes the best, or the healthiest, regardless of other criteria (Connors et al. 2001). Or they can prioritize by various

---

$\mathscr{B}$ox 5-3   Meeting the Challenge of Maintaining Healthful Behaviors

Maintaining chosen behaviors over the long term requires "self-regulatory skills" by which individuals develop the ability to influence and take charge of their own actions through their own efforts. Some of the strategies that are helpful are listed here.

Maintaining Goals

- *Prioritizing competing goals:* Individuals all have competing goals at any one time. To maintain their chosen behavioral goal, they need to protect it from being interrupted or given up prematurely as a result of competing intentions. They can also seek ways of satisfying both their health goal and other goals at the same time.
- *Mindful eating: protecting action goals from distractions:* Individuals can become busy and distracted by the presence of friends or colleagues or of nonhealthful foods, and, without thinking, they fail to follow their action plan. Sticking with their plan is not about being rigid or about denial. It is about being mindful about their eating and thinking about whether this is what they really want to be doing. In the current environment, eating healthfully and being physically active require conscious attention.
- *Focusing on the big picture in the achievement of action goals:* Individuals can remember that if they eat foods they had not planned to on one occasion, they can always compensate for it on another occasion so that overall they achieve their goal.
- *Linking action goals to their self-identity:* Sometimes it can help for individuals to remember that they now have a new identity—for example, as individuals who want to take care of themselves, or as active people.
- *Correctly attributing their successes and failures:* This allows individuals to claim successes and feel good about them and recognize that failures may be caused by circumstances beyond their control.

Developing Routines and Habits

- Sticking with action plans can make the chosen behavior become more routine; new habits are developed.

Countering

- Individuals can substitute alternative thoughts and behaviors for less healthful eating behaviors.

Coping Self-Efficacy

- Optimistic beliefs about their ability to deal with barriers—the conviction that they can carry out their intentions even under difficult circumstances—can be very helpful at this stage.

Creating Personal Environments to Achieve Goals

- *Stimulus control:* Individuals can restructure their personal environment to make it more supportive by removing cues to less healthful eating and adding cues for more healthful eating.
- *Seeking social support:* Individuals can seek the help of those around them.

Enjoying Healthful Food: Coming to Like What One Eats

- Eating healthfully becomes enjoyable as healthful foods become familiar and when individuals learn the skills to make them tasty.

Developing Personal Policies: Expressing Agency

- Individuals can develop personal food policies or systems to manage, over the long term, the numerous and conflicting values they hold about their food choices. For example, they may have a policy that they will always have breakfast before leaving the house, even if it is modest.

---

values or criteria, such as using cost as the criterion for home meals, but relaxing this criterion when guests are coming for dinner; using health as the main criterion, but building in occasions (e.g., eating out) when health will be relaxed in favor of taste; or accommodating the needs of others rather than their personal values to manage social relationships, such as when invited out to dinner.

- A study with adolescents obtained similar kinds of personal policies: they balanced "unhealthy foods" with "healthy foods" within a meal, between meals (less-healthy lunches with peers and healthful dinners at home), and between weekdays and weekends (Contento et al. 2006).

Following are examples of people's personal policies for managing healthy eating over the long term:

- Managing healthy eating for a sample of adults meant being concerned about balance, low fat, weight control, whether foods

were natural, disease management, or disease prevention (Falk et al. 2001). Strategies to ensure healthful eating were avoidance or limitation of foods that were less healthful, substitution with others, and using appropriate food preparation methods.

- For those experiencing food insecurity, personal food policies were chosen to cope with the lack of sufficient quantity of wholesome, nutritious food. Here the personal food policies included substituting less expensive foods for more expensive (e.g., dried beans instead of canned beans, or canned fruits instead of fresh), reducing or omitting unaffordable ingredients, looking for foods from atypical sources such as food pantries, and putting children's food needs first (Hoisington, Shultz, & Butkus 2002).

- People who are diagnosed with type 2 diabetes as adults need long-term maintenance of behavior change. People with diabetes are required to adopt and maintain a number of dietary patterns and self-care behaviors to achieve and sustain control of their blood sugar. They use many of the strategies described

---

NUTRITION EDUCATION IN ACTION 5-5

Food Selection and Eating Patterns Among People with Type 2 Diabetes

People with type 2 diabetes are required to adopt and maintain for the long termmany dietary and self-care behaviors to achieve and sustain control of their blood sugar. This study used semistructured, in-depth interviews to explore the beliefs and perspectives of those with type 2 diabetes about dietary requirements, food selection and eating patterns as well as their attitudes about self-management practices. These interviews were analyzed for themes, which are captured in the accompanying diagram.

Prior history with food selection and weight control efforts are linked to current challenges involving avoiding favorite foods and choosing more healthful alternatives, managing weight, dining out, and exercising restraint in terms of portions. Their prior knowledge was helpful in using strategies to manage their diets.

The mediators that facilitated or impeded their food selection behaviors and eating patterns were as follows:

- Level of social support, particularly support of spouse.
- Degree of self-efficacy or confidence that they would be able to stay with their eating plans even in difficult situations, such as when eating with coworkers who were eating fast foods they liked or resisting rich baked goods at family gatherings.
- Time management, which was a problem because they always had to plan ahead of time what they were going to eat and stick with a schedule. They had to time their insulin or oral medication to food intake.

In general, they developed specific practices, routines, or personal policies to support their self-management efforts.

Source: Savoca, M., and C. Miller. 2001. Food selection and eating patterns: Themes found among people with type 2 diabetes mellitus. *Journal of Nutrition Education* 33:224–233. Figure used with permission of the Society for Nutrition Education.

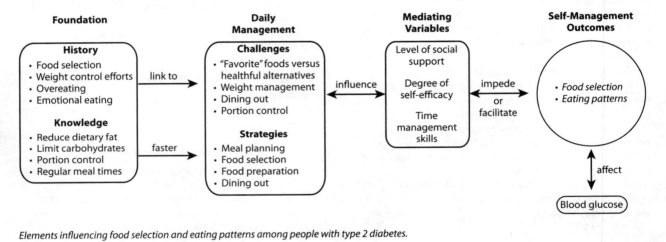

Elements influencing food selection and eating patterns among people with type 2 diabetes.

---

previously: making action plans and protecting their action plans from competing goals, being mindful about their eating so that they are not distracted by alternative intentions, and making personal food policies. A study that examined diabetics' beliefs and perceptions about their diets and how to manage them is described in **Nutrition Education in Action 5-5**.

■ **TRANSTHEORETICAL MODEL AND THE STAGES OF CHANGE CONSTRUCT**

In its simplest terms, the transtheoretical model (TMM) proposes that self-change in behavior is a process that occurs through five stages and that individuals use a variety of psychological and behavioral processes in making changes.

The transtheoretical model has become one of the most widely used models in the study of health behavior change (Prochaska & DiClemente 1984; Prochaska & Velicer 1997; Wright, Velicer, & Prochaska 2009). It originated from an analysis of 18 systems of psychotherapy that identified common processes that individuals use to make changes in their own behavior (Prochaska & DiClemente 1984), hence the name *transtheoretical*. During this analysis, Prochaska and DiClemente found that behavior change seemed to occur through a series of stages. The model has now been applied to a range of health behaviors, including safer sex practices, mammography screening, weight control, and diet and physical activity behaviors.

The transtheoretical model proposes that self-change in behavior is a process that occurs through five stages. It also proposes that there are 2 mediators of change (decisional balance based on pros and cons of change, and self-efficacy) and 10 processes of change. The transtheoretical model is a model of behavior *change*, not a model predicting behavior. It is shown in **Figure 5-3**.

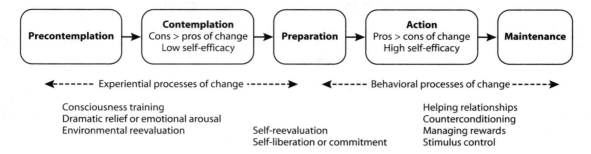

FIGURE 5-3 Transtheoretical model.

The Stages of Change Construct

The transtheoretical model proposes that health behavior change is a gradual, continuous, and dynamic process that can be seen as occurring through a series of stages based on people's readiness to change. Knowledge of the stage or readiness of individuals and groups can be used to inform intervention design. Many studies use the stages of change construct without using the transtheoretical model's "processes of change," making the underlying theory a stages of change model. In some studies, the stages are collapsed into pre-action and action/maintenance stages, resulting in a stage structure similar to some of the theories described earlier.

The stages as are follows:

1. *Precontemplation (PC):* Precontemplation is the time during which individuals are not aware of, or not interested in, a behavior or practice that might enhance their health. Also included in this category are those who have tried and failed to make the behavior change, perhaps many times, and no longer want to think about it.
2. *Contemplation (C):* Contemplation is the stage in which individuals are considering making a change sometime in the near future, usually defined as within the next six months. They are more aware of the pros of changing but are especially aware of the costs of changing. They struggle between thinking about the positive outcomes of the behavior and the amount of time, energy, and other resources that will be needed to change. This can cause enormous ambivalence, resulting in "chronic contemplation" or procrastination (Prochaska, DiClemente, & Norcross 1992). Individuals at this stage need motivational activities rather than action-oriented, behavioral change strategies.
3. *Preparation (P):* Preparation is the stage in which individuals intend to make a change in the immediate future, usually defined as one month, and may have already taken some steps in that direction. Individuals in this stage are ready for action-oriented strategies that will help them initiate action.
4. *Action (A):* Action is the stage in which individuals have started to engage in the new behavior or practice (often defined as within the previous six months). They may adopt the practice (e.g., eat less fat) on a small scale at first or try out alternative practices, such as eating less meat rather than using low-fat milk in place of whole milk, to find one at which they can be successful and that fits into their usual routine. Action-oriented strategies are particularly helpful here.
5. *Maintenance (M):* Maintenance refers to the period in which people have performed the new behavior or practice for long enough (usually defined as longer than six months) to be comfortable with incorporating it as part of their way of life (e.g., they now routinely buy and use nonfat milk or eat five fruits and

vegetables a day). Individuals may need to continue to exert effort to maintain the behavior and avoid relapse.

For addictive behaviors, a sixth stage, *termination*, is included, during which individuals no longer succumb to any temptation and feel total self-efficacy. For dietary behaviors, this stage may not be practical or applicable because everyone has to eat; hence, a more realistic goal is a lifetime of maintenance.

Different Stages for Different Behaviors

Nutrition educators should note that individuals can be, and usually are, at different stages of change for different diet-related behaviors. For example, individuals wanting to "eat more healthfully" may be at the action stage in terms of adding fruits and vegetables to their diets but still contemplating cutting down on high-fat, high-sugar food products. Or people may have started making changes in diet but not physical activity (Boudreaux et al. 2003). There are also considerable spontaneous changes in stages among people over time, both forward and backward (Kristal et al. 2000; De Nooijer et al. 2005).

Nutrition Education for Different Stages

A major contribution of the stages of change construct is a reminder that most nutrition education programs are "action centered," assuming a certain degree of readiness to take action on the part of program participants. They thus fail to address the needs of those who are not yet emotionally prepared to act.

Changes in stage are not always linear. The transtheoretical model acknowledges that change is more like a spiral than a straight line, with a great deal of back and forth movement and recycling between the stages. Research studies are also finding that in the area of diet, the stages are often not clearly delineated.

Mediators of Change

The theory proposes two mediators of change: the pros and cons of change and self-efficacy.

Decisional Balance: The Pros and Cons of Change

Decisional balance, or the weighing of the pros and cons of change, is an important construct in the transtheoretical model. Pros are people's beliefs about the anticipated benefits of changing, and cons are the costs of changing. Decisional balance is based on a model of decision making that proposes that behavior change emerges when the pros, or anticipated benefits, outweigh the cons, or costs, of the change. The pros and cons of change are similar to the perceived benefits and barriers constructs of the health belief model and the outcome expectations construct of the theory of planned behavior and social cognitive theory.

Examples of pros of change are "Eating healthy food is helpful in preventing cancer" and "Eating healthful food will improve the way I look." Examples of cons of change include "I would find it hard to give up some of my favorite foods to follow a healthier diet" and "It is too expensive to eat organic foods."

In the pre-action stages, the cons of change have been found to be higher than the pros. In the action stages, the pros of change are higher than the cons (Steptoe et al. 1996; Prochaska & Velicer 1997). The crossover point in the diet and physical activity areas is generally between the contemplation and the preparation and action stages. Thus, it can be concluded that only when perceived benefits outweigh perceived barriers will contemplators move into preparation and action. Some studies indicate that the pros of change have to increase twice as much as the cons must decrease for action to be initiated. This suggests that considerable emphasis may need to be placed on raising the benefits of change to overcome the barriers to change.

Self-Efficacy

The self-efficacy construct was integrated into the stages of change model from social cognitive theory. It is the confidence that people have that they can carry out the behavior across different challenging situations and not relapse to their previous, less healthy behavior. Self-efficacy tends to decrease between the precontemplation stage and contemplation stage, probably because in the precontemplation stage individuals have an optimistic bias about what they can do, and it is during the contemplation stage that they first realize how difficult the new behavior may be. Self-efficacy then steadily increases through the action and maintenance stages (Sporny & Contento 1995; Steptoe et al. 1996; Campbell et al. 1998; Ma et al. 2002).

Temptation is a construct that reflects the urge to engage in a less healthful behavior in difficult situations, such as individuals might experience at a party laden with high-fat, high-sugar foods when they are watching their weight. Temptation is low in precontemplation, as would be expected; people only perceive temptation as a problem if they have become concerned about eating high-fat, high-sugar foods and are trying to avoid them. Temptation is especially strong during the contemplation and preparation stages and declines substantially in the maintenance stage.

The Processes of Change

The processes of change are overt and convert strategies that individuals use to move themselves through the stages of change. Each of the change processes is a category of similar activities and experiences that facilitate individuals' progress through the stages. Ten processes have been proposed. These include *experiential* or *cognitive processes* that focus on thoughts, feelings, and experiences and *behavioral processes* that focus on behaviors and reinforcement. The transtheoretical model proposes that behavior change is facilitated if interventions focus on change processes that are matched to the stage of change of individuals.

The processes associated with change are as follows:

Experiential Processes

- *Consciousness-raising:* When we increase our awareness about the causes, consequences, and cures for a health issue and seek new information about healthy behaviors. For example, "I seek out magazine articles to learn more about how eating fruits and vegetables can affect health."
- *Dramatic relief or emotional arousal:* When we experience and express the negative emotions or feelings (fear, anxiety, worry, sense of threat) about our problems, followed by reduced emotion if appropriate action is seen as possible. For example, "Warnings

about how diet can contribute to the risk of developing heart disease make me anxious."
- *Self-reevaluation:* When we reassess our beliefs, knowledge, feelings, or self-image about a particular unhealthy food-related behavior or practice in relation to ourselves (e.g., an image of self as a junk food eater). For example, "I think about how I would be a healthier person if I ate more fruits and vegetables."
- *Environmental reevaluation:* When we examine our positive and negative beliefs and feelings about the impact of our personal diet-related behaviors on others. This could also include evaluation of ourselves as a role model to others, positive or negative. For example, "I realize that I may be able to keep local farmers in business if I join a community-supported agriculture farm" or "I realize that I would be a role model to my children if I ate more fruits and vegetables daily."
- *Self-liberation or commitment:* When we believe that we can change and make a conscious choice and firm commitment to make the change. For example, "I am committed to eating more fruits and vegetables each day."

Behavioral Processes

- *Helping relationships:* When we enlist the trust, caring, and acceptance in our relationships with others to help us change (such as making pacts with coworkers not to eat donuts for snacks).
- *Counterconditioning:* When we learn to replace less healthful behaviors with more healthful ones, such as eating fruit instead of high-fat, high-sugar desserts.
- *Managing rewards:* When we reevaluate the way in which we use food as a reward or punishment. Evidence suggests that self-changers use rewards more than punishment to manage their behaviors.
- *Stimulus or environmental control:* When we remove cues or triggers for undesirable behavior (e.g., avoiding walking past a bakery that makes our favorite pastries) and add cues or prompts for more healthful alternatives, such as putting on the office calendar a reminder to walk during lunch hour.
- *Social liberation:* When we become aware of environmental factors that influence our dietary patterns and use the external environment to help us get started or to stay with a change. For example, if individuals are trying to eat more vegetables, they will choose a restaurant that offers salads and vegetable entrées for lunch. This process also involves the notion of advocacy, for example, to increase the availability of more healthful foods in schools and communities.

Processes of Change at Different Stages

Studies have provided evidence that individuals use these processes in self-change to different extents as they move through the stages (Prochaska & Velicer 1997). In the area of diet, it has been found that experiential and behavioral processes often increase together through the stages (Greene et al. 1999; Rosen 2000).

Precontemplation

The transtheoretical model proposes, and research evidence confirms, that when people are in the precontemplation stage, they use all of these processes significantly less than in all the other stages.

Contemplation

In the contemplation stage, people become open to consciousness-raising strategies, such as observations, self-assessments, and other strategies to raise awareness about their behavior. For example, they may conduct self-assessments of their fruit and vegetable intakes per day and look for information about the benefits of fruits and vegetables for health or disease risk.

During contemplation, people are also open to emotionally arousing experiences, such as stories about the impact of diabetes on given individuals, which can lead to dramatic relief as they make changes (e.g., based on information about the efficacy of fruits and vegetables for reducing disease risk). As individuals become more conscious of themselves and the nature of their food-related issues, they are more likely to reevaluate themselves, their values, and their problems both cognitively and affectively. They also evaluate the effects of their behaviors on those around them and on the physical environment. Movement through the contemplation stage involves increased use of the cognitive, affective, and evaluative processes of change.

Action

People begin to take action when they believe that they have the autonomy to make changes through a self-liberation process, and then make a firm commitment to change. As they take action, they call on skills in counterconditioning (substituting more healthful foods for those less healthful) as well as environmental or stimulus control such as making sure not to keep large supplies of energy-dense foods in the house to help them maintain their weight.

Maintenance

Successful maintenance of change involves the use of behavioral processes to prevent relapse to less healthy patterns of behavior. Here nutrition education can assist individuals to acquire and practice these skills. Social support can be important, as well as rewards given by others or by individuals themselves. Most important to maintenance is the sense people have that they are becoming who they want to be.

Research and Intervention Examples

A number of studies show support for the stages of change construct in the area of diet. For example, those individuals in the action and maintenance stages have lower intakes of fat and higher intakes of fiber and of fruits and vegetables compared with those in the pre-action stages (Brug et al. 1994; Glanz et al. 1994; Sporny & Contento 1995; Steptoe et al. 1996; Glanz et al. 1998). In studies, the stage of change is useful as a predictor of health behavior change, as a way to stratify people so as to match interventions to individuals on the basis of their readiness to change, and as an intermediate outcome measure to indicate progress toward health behavior change.

Mediators and Stages

The motivating forces for movement through the stages (or mediators of change), according to the transtheoretical model, are the balance of pros and cons of change (perceived benefits and barriers) and self-efficacy.

Numerous cross-sectional studies have examined the relationship between these variables and stages of change in the area of diet and physical activity. Psychosocial constructs from the other theories are often also included (Sporny & Contento 1995; Brug, Glanz, & Kok 1997; Campbell et al. 1998; Campbell, Reynolds, et al. 1999; De Nooijer et al. 2005; Kavookjian et al. 2005; Henry et al. 2006; Buchanan & Coulson 2007; Wright et al. 2009). Taken together, these and other studies suggest that although there is considerable moving back and forth among stages, perceived benefits or pros are especially important in the early stages, where they serve a motivational role, and must become greater than cons if change is to take place. Self-efficacy has been found to influence movement through the stages (O'Hea et al. 2004; Henry et al. 2006).

Stage-Matched Interventions Tailored to Individuals

One of the main implications of the stages of change model is that nutrition educators should use different kinds of nutrition education activities with individuals at different stages of psychological readiness to change (Velicer & Prochaska 1999). Here the stages of change construct is used to design interventions that are specifically tailored to *individuals* at different stages of change (Prochaska et al. 1993). Tailoring differs from targeting in that *targeted* interventions are directed at groups or populations with similar characteristics, whereas *tailored* interventions are directed at individuals within target populations. Here individuals complete a questionnaire by phone, paper, or computer to assess their pros and cons, self-efficacy, and stages of change and are then provided with individualized feedback reports based on their responses. They are next provided with information (e.g., through newsletters, email, or the Internet) on the processes of change that they can use, appropriate to their stage.

In the area of diet, tailored interventions have been conducted in a variety of settings, such as primary care settings (Campbell et al. 1994; Salmela et al. 2009), health departments (Jacobs et al. 2004), worksites (Campbell et al. 2002; Brug, Oenema, & Campbell 2003; De Bourdeaudhuij et al. 2007), after-school programs with youth (Di Noia, Contento, & Prochaska 2008), and families (De Bourdeaudhuij et al. 2002). Other channels have also been used, such as the Web (Oenema, Tan, & Brug 2005; Park et al. 2008) and multimedia programs (tailored soap opera and interactive infomercials) (Campbell, Honess-Morreale, et al. 1999). These studies suggest that tailoring the intervention to a given individual's stage of psychological readiness to take action can enhance the effectiveness of nutrition education.

Stage-Matched Interventions with Groups

In a group or population-wide setting, nutrition educators cannot provide interventions that are specific to each individual's stage of readiness to change. However, assuming that there will be people at all stages of change in a group, educators can sequence activities in a stepwise fashion:

1. Promotional activities to promote awareness and enhance motivation, targeting those in the pre-action stages
2. Action and skills training, targeting those in the action stage
3. Social support and maintenance of behavior
4. Environmental supports

Such strategies, if effective, should accelerate movement from pre-action stages into the action and maintenance stages. Consequently, intervention outcomes can be measured in two ways: change in the targeted behavior, such as reduction in fat intake or increase in fruit and vegetable intake, or progression to a later stage of change (Glanz et al. 1998; Kristal et al. 2000; Prochaska 2007). Use of stage-matched group activities in studies with diet have indeed found that those in pre-action stages at baseline were much more likely to move into action and maintenance stages than controls were. Changes in stage were associated with decreases in fat intake and increases in fiber, fruit, and vegetable intake, for example (Glanz et al. 1998; Kristal et al. 2000).

Interventions have also been conducted in which the activities have been specifically based on the 10 processes of change delineated by the transtheoretical model. A few are described here:

- *Study with college students:* One study with college students was delivered in a group setting (Finckenor & Byrd-Bredbenner 2000). The first half of the sessions focused on the processes of consciousness raising and emotional arousal. The later sessions focused on self-evaluation and social liberation, which included some skill building.

- *Study with adolescents:* A computer-based program for urban youth in after-school community programs resulted in improved intakes of fruits and vegetables (Di Noia, Contento, & Prochaska 2008). The intervention activities are described in **Nutrition Education in Action 5-6**.
- *Clinic-based program:* In another study, the transtheoretical model processes of change were used in a clinic-based program that focused on a healthy lifestyle approach to weight management that also included exercise. It was successful in promoting changes in exercise and dietary behaviors, weight loss, increased cardiorespiratory fitness, and improved lipid profiles (Riebe et al. 2003).

Take-Home Message about the Transtheoretical Model

- The transtheoretical model emphasizes that individuals are at different stages in terms of their readiness to engage in a health- or food-related behavior and that, consequently, nutrition education interventions must be designed to meet the needs of individuals at each stage of change. The majority of people is not ready for action in terms of healthy behaviors and will not be well served by traditional action-oriented programs.

- To enhance effectiveness, nutrition education interventions can address the mediators of change—pros and cons of change and self-efficacy—and base activities on the 10 processes of change, matched to the individual's or group's stage of change.

■ TRANSLATING BEHAVIORAL THEORIES INTO EDUCATIONAL STRATEGIES TO FACILITATE THE ABILITY TO TAKE ACTION

Nutrition educators need to translate information about potential mediators of the targeted behavior changes into appropriate practical theory-based and educational strategies to ensure the effectiveness of nutrition education interventions.

Translating Social Cognitive Theory into Educational Strategies

Translating theory into practical strategies is crucial for the effectiveness of the nutrition education. Social cognitive theory emphasizes that taking a health-related action requires that people become aware of health

---

NUTRITION EDUCATION IN ACTION 5-6

Computer-Based Program to Increase Consumption of Fruits and Vegetables in Teens Using the Transtheoretical Model

This program was designed to increase fruit and vegetable consumption among economically disadvantaged urban youth attending after-school programs in community sites. It consisted of four 30-minute sessions of CD-ROM-mediated intervention content that was based on the four constructs of the transtheoretical model: stages of change, decisional balance of perceived pros and cons of change, self-efficacy, and processes of change.

Program

In Session 1, all users completed an introductory session, which provided information on health benefits of fruit and vegetable consumption. Youth also completed a staging questionnaire. Sessions 2–4 differed depending on the youth's stage of change:

Precontemplation: Activities designed to enhance awareness of lower-than-recommended intakes and promote acceptance of need for dietary change. These included the following:

- *Consciousness raising:* Interactive dietary assessment with personalized feedback on their intakes
- *Dramatic relief:* Personal testimonial about losing a loved one and discussion of lifestyle habits associated with increased cancer risk
- *Environmental reevaluation:* Vignette of boy increasing his intake of fruits and vegetables and impact on family and friends

Contemplation/Preparation:

- *Self-evaluation:* Guided imagery to understand health consequences of not eating enough fruits and vegetables
- *Self-liberation:* Selecting a daily goal and developing action plan for reaching goal

Action/Maintenance:

- *Reinforcement management:* Multimedia presentation of ways of rewarding oneself and being rewarded by others for eating fruits and vegetables
- *Helping relationships:* "Buddy contract" with someone else to maintain consumption
- *Counterconditioning:* Interactive activity to identify problem behaviors and multimedia presentation of healthy replacement behaviors to try instead
- *Stimulus control:* Assessment of home, school, and neighborhood environments that encourage unhealthy eating and discussion of how to handle

Evaluation

The program was evaluated using a pretest, post-test quasi-experimental design in which adolescents in youth service agencies were assigned to the computer intervention condition or the control condition. Measures were self-reported fruit and vegetable consumption and stages, pros, cons, and self-efficacy.

Results

Youths who completed the computer program increased their pro scores and fruit and vegetable consumption compared to control youths. In addition, more of them progressed to later stages of readiness to take action and maintained recommended intake levels.

Source: Di Noia, J., I. R. Contento, and J. O. Prochaska. 2008. Computer-mediated intervention tailored on transtheoretical model stages and processes of change increases fruit and vegetable consumption among urban African-American adolescents. *American Journal of Health Promotion* 22:336–341.

risks, believe in the benefits of taking action, and set goals to make changes. They then need relevant food- and nutrition-related knowledge to accomplish goals as well as self-regulation skills to exercise control over their health-related behaviors (Bandura 1989, 2004). Self-efficacy is key. Changes in the environment to support these changes are also important; individuals and groups can advocate for these changes and

develop collective efficacy. Nutrition education strategies for addressing these mediators are described here.

Some of these strategies are used in the case study of Ray. You remember him from earlier chapters. He decides to attend a nutrition education session. A hypothetical lesson plan for his session is shown in **Case Study 5-1.**

CASE STUDY 5-1

The Case of Ray: Nutrition Education Using Social Cognitive Theory

Ray, you recall, is in his mid-40s. His weight just crept up on him, a pound or two each year, and now he is about 40 pounds overweight. His job is as a salesman in a large appliance store, where he is mostly on the phone or stands around and is not very active. He buys packaged snacks from the vending machine and nibbles when he is bored or anxious. He goes to a nearby fast food restaurant for lunch with a couple of coworkers most days. When he goes home he wants to just sit and watch TV and drink a

few beers. His wife is interested in eating more healthfully, but he likes a hearty meal and always a dessert.

His doctor tells him that he is at risk of diabetes and that his "bad" serum cholesterol is on the high side. The physician tells Ray that the clinic offers nutrition education sessions and he might benefit from attending. Ray sees one session titled "Small size it!" and decides to attend. Here is a sample of what the session might be like:

"Small Size It!"

Potential Mediator of Change	Nutrition Education Activities
Perceived physical outcomes (self-assessment of risk)	Self-assessment: The participants are asked to write down everything they ate and drank in the past 24 hours. Then, they are to circle the sweetened beverages, snacks, and fast food they consumed.
Perceived physical outcomes (health risk)	The instructor uses a slide presentation to tell the participants about the scientific evidence about the impact of excess weight on health.
Perceived physical outcomes (health risk)	Instructor shows the group bottles (empty) of different sizes of a popular drink. Then, she asks a volunteer to come up and measure out, with estimates provided by the group, how many teaspoons of sugar they think is in each size of bottle. She then converts teaspoons of sugar to calories. She provides them with a worksheet where they check which size of beverage they usually drink and how often. They then calculate how many calories a year that would be for each bottle size. She also explained that whenever people consume about 3,500 calories in the diet beyond need, their bodies deposit the extra calories as a pound of fat.
	Ray and the others are surprised at the number of calories in drinks. He did not think liquids had calories. He asks if beer also has calories and learns that it does indeed. At about 300 calories a day in beverages he is consuming, that would be about 10,000 calories a year. That would translate to nearly 3 pounds a year. He now understood how his extra weight crept up.
Perceived physical outcomes (health risk)	The instructor then shows participants a slide presentation that depicts the number of calories in some key fast food items. For example, a medium cheeseburger had 650 calories, a large french fries had 500 calories, and a medium milkshake had 500 calories.
	Ray and the others are shocked by the presentation, and their perceived risk of disease is heightened.
Perceived benefits of taking action	The instructor provides the evidence showing that choosing healthier options and smaller sizes can help them control their weight.
Impediments or perceived barriers to taking action	Group members review their dietary recalls and discuss barriers to making changes.
Overcoming barriers	The group brainstorms ways to select healthier options.
Goal setting/action plan	The instructor asks group members to write down one action they will take in the coming week to reduce the size of their portions.
	Ray is now very concerned about his diet and energized /motivated do something about it. He chooses two actions he will take: he will switch from a cheeseburger to a grilled chicken sandwich for lunch; and he will have only one beer at home and make that a near beer with very few calories (all he really wants is the bubbly bitter taste). He intends to come back to a session next week to learn about reading food labels and plans on setting additional goals for actions he could take.

Outcome Expectations: Awareness of Risk or Benefits of Diet and Physical Activity Practices

Interventions can be designed to increase the relevance of specific issues of concern or perceived risk related to personal health, community practices, or the sustainability of food system practices. Benefits of current practices can also be explored. Effective strategies and specific activities for this mediator might involve the following:

- *Increasing the relevance of risks or concerns:* Trigger films, striking national or local statistics, pictures and charts, personal stories, and other strategies can be used to make salient issues of concern, such as the increase in obesity rates, the portion sizes of food products, or the prevalence of metabolic syndrome in adolescents.
- *Providing self-assessment compared to recommendations:* Individuals can complete checklists, food frequency questionnaires, or 24-hour food intake recalls and compare intakes to a standard, such as MyPyramid servings, to give themselves an accurate picture of their intake.
- *Making a community assessment of practices:* Information about community food practices could provide a true picture of the extent of risk of a condition. Existing data or surveys, formal and informal, can be used.
- *Physical outcomes:* In group settings, nutrition educators can help participants understand the pleasurable and aversive outcomes of taking action. For breastfeeding, these might include health of the baby, convenience, mother–child bonding, and so forth. Also, they can identify costs or barriers, such as pain of first breastfeeding. These can be identified through presentations, videos, or group discussion.
- *Social outcomes:* Behavior is partly regulated by the social approval and disapproval of others. In the case of breastfeeding, this might include embarrassment in public situations or wishes of others in the family.
- *Self-evaluative outcomes:* Self-evaluative outcomes are the positive and negative outcomes people expect of their own behaviors. In the case of breastfeeding, this might include the satisfaction mothers get from feeling they are being good mothers.

Behavioral Capability: Food- and Nutrition-Related Knowledge and Cognitive Skills

Knowledge

After individuals become motivated to take a nutrition-related action, they need specific knowledge and skills to act on their decision. For example, individuals need to know how to select foods for optimal health from the 50,000-item supermarket; evaluate the nutrition information that bombards them from magazines, newspapers, advertising, and friends; and interpret personal medical information provided by their physicians. Food and nutrition education must therefore provide information and opportunity to develop the cognitive skills that enhance people's power to act on their desire to change.

Now is the time to provide how-to information (factual knowledge) about foods, nutrients, dietary guidelines, label reading, or MyPyramid and ways to apply this information in people's daily eating plans (procedural knowledge). If a low-fat diet is the focus of the program, important knowledge is the fact that chicken eaten with skin has 3 times the calories as chicken without skin and is 5 to 10 times as caloric (because of fat) if it also is battered and deep fried. Lectures, handouts, tip sheets, newsletters, flyers, and Web-based programs are all suitable here, depending on the behavior or practice and the channel chosen (e.g., mass media or in person).

Critical Thinking Skills

Food and nutrition issues are often complex. The nutrition research findings are sometimes contradictory. Individuals need the ability to evaluate evidence and understand reasoned arguments for different options, such as whether to reduce dietary fat or carbohydrate to lose weight. They need critical thinking skills to evaluate controversial issues or to understand complex issues related to health and food policies. Nutrition education activities such as written or oral critiques, debates, and trigger films for discussion can be useful here.

Self-Efficacy and Building Behavioral Skills in Foods and Nutrition

Self-efficacy may increase with increased levels of skills, but self-efficacy is not the same thing as physical skills such as food preparation or safe food handling. Self-efficacy involves both skills and the confidence that individuals can consistently use them even in the face of impediments or barriers. To develop food- and nutrition-related behavioral skills, nutrition educators should model the behavior, such as through food demonstrations accompanied by clear instructions. However, individuals learn best and their self-efficacy is enhanced if educators also provide them with opportunities to practice the behavior. Verbal encouragement by the nutrition educator can overcome self-doubts. This process is often called guided mastery experience. If active living is included in the program, nutrition educators can provide information on how to exercise safely. Social cognitive theory emphasizes that it requires actual experience to develop physical skills, such as cooking, safe food preparation practices, and other food-related skills. Refer to Box 5-1 for details.

Goal Setting

Behavior change requires not only behavioral skills but also the ability of individuals to exercise self-influence or self-direction over their own behavior. This ability does not involve willpower so much as a set of self-regulation skills or skills for directing our behaviors, including goal setting (Bandura 1986; Cullen et al. 2001; Shilts, Horowitz, & Townsend 2004a). Nutrition education interventions need to teach individuals the skills of goal setting and provide opportunities to practice them, with guidance. Goal setting is a process involving the following steps (Shilts et al. 2004b, 2009):

- *Performing self-assessment or observation:* The purpose is to identify ways in which individuals' current actions or behaviors contribute to the issue or problem they are concerned about.
- *Setting action goals:* Individuals then need to set action goals to address their concern or problem, for example, to eat more fruits and vegetables.
- *Contracting:* Commitment to the action goal is strengthened by believing in the value of the behavior, perceiving that the goal is attainable, and making binding pledges, often called *contracts*. Such pledges have motivational impact because there are consequences or costs to not following through on an agreement. These consequences may be personal, such as self-reproof, or social, if the commitments were made in public or involve others, where the costs may include embarrassment or social disapproval.
- *Acquiring relevant knowledge and skills:* Information and skills to attain the goal are needed next.

- *Monitoring of progress toward the goal:* The focus should be on positive accomplishments rather than failures.
- *Attaining goals:* Attaining a goal can result in a sense of self-efficacy, self-satisfaction, and accomplishment that sustains effort or leads to the setting of increasingly more difficult behavior change goals.
- *Using problem-solving and decision-making strategies:* These strategies are mobilized if the goal is not achieved. The goal can be modified, or a new, more achievable one can be set.

The use of contracting was specifically studied in a pilot program with low-income women (Heneman et al. 2005). It was shown to increase the effectiveness of nutrition education: women significantly increased their fruit intake. In terms of their stages of change, they moved toward acceptance of vegetable consumption. The "Contract for Change" that was used in the study is shown in **Figure 5-4**.

Self-Regulation Skills and Personal Food Policies for Maintaining Change

Nutrition education activities designed to assist individuals to maintain their chosen action should focus on teaching individuals the strategies that are shown in Box 5-2 and Box 5-3.

Translating the Transtheoretical Model into Educational Strategies

The construct of stages of change, along with the mediators of pros and cons of change, can be used to tailor nutrition education to individuals through a variety of media as described earlier. The 10 processes of change are also useful in nutrition education. Nutrition Education in Action 5-6 presents an example of how the constructs were used to tailor nutrition education to increase fruit and vegetable intake in youth. **Table 5-3** describes in detail how transtheoretical model constructs are translated into educational strategies.

■ SUMMARY

Once convinced of the desirability, effectiveness, and feasibility of an action, individuals may state an intention to take action. However, to help individuals convert their intentions to action, nutrition educators can build individuals' abilities and skills to act on their motivations. This chapter focuses on facilitating the ability to take action. Several theories are useful here.

Social Cognitive Theory

Social cognitive theory states that in addition to being convinced that taking a given behavior will be effective in leading to the outcome individuals desire, they must also believe that they can carry out the behavior even in the face of difficulties and setbacks. The environment both influences and is influenced by people's behaviors. Therefore, self-efficacy and skills are the major facilitators of change. Individuals need skills in self-regulation, which consist of setting goals for themselves and monitoring their progress toward their goals. They need the knowledge and cognitive, affective, and behavioral skills that will enable them to achieve their goals. These skills help contribute to a sense of personal agency where they can take charge of their lives. Individuals also need

---

The aim of this is to help you make and keep healthy eating habits.

1. Goals: List two ways you can eat more fruits and vegetables.

1) _____

2) _____

2. Setting a goal: Choose one goal from the above two lines and make it into something you can do.

Action goal: _____

What will you do differently? _____

_____

How often?_____

How much?_____

Where?_____

With whom?_____

3. Make a plan: List two reasons why this change may be hard.

1) _____

2) _____

What will you do to beat these problems?

1) _____

2) _____

Let's Try to Make This Change!

FIGURE 5-4 Example of a contract for setting goals.

Source: Heneman, K., A. Block-Joy, S. Zidenberg-Cherr, et al. 2005. A "contract for change" increases produce consumption in low-income women: A pilot study. *Journal of the American Dietetic Association* 105(11):1793–1796.

	TABLE 5-3	**Transtheoretical Model: Application to Nutrition Education Interventions**	

Stage of Readiness to Change	Important Processes for Moving to Next Stage	Nutrition Education Intervention Strategies
Precontemplation	Increased awareness, sense of risk, understanding, and recognition of emotional adjustments needed for change	Provide personalized information on own eating pattern (e.g., fruit and vegetable intake) through self-assessment and feedback (e.g., group 24-hour recall); personalize risk; and help individuals understand and express emotions about the need for change. Media: trigger films, personal testimonies, and media campaigns to address feelings and personalized risks.
Contemplation	Recognition of ambivalence but increased appreciation for benefits of behavior, and confidence in one's ability to enact the recommended behavior	Messages or strategies in groups to enhance people's pros/benefits of change (e.g., taste, health benefits, convenience); discuss barriers to change; assist individuals to recognize own ambivalence; and provide positive feedback about individuals' current abilities and assets.
Preparation	Making a commitment to change; resolving ambivalence	Have individuals state goal intention (e.g., to eat more fruits and vegetables); develop specific action plans; and start taking small steps toward goal; reinforce attempts to change.
Action	Building skills and seeking social support	Teach food- and nutrition-specific knowledge and skills needed for behavior change; goal setting and self-monitoring skills; provide encouragement and support; and encourage seeking of social support network.
Maintenance	Self-management and relapse prevention skills creating social and environmental support	Teach new ways of thinking about behavior, restructuring environment, and rewarding themselves; anticipate and plan for potential difficult situations; create buddy systems; problem-solve if they lapse; and strengthen skills to advocate for environments that support healthful food practices.

a supportive environment and collective efficacy to work to change the environment.

Other Self-Regulation Models

Other models such as the health action process model emphasize that the ability to regulate, exercise control, or generally take charge of behaviors is a key process in initiating and maintaining health behavior change. Self-efficacy is very important in this process and planning is an important strategy.

Transtheoretical Model

The transtheoretical model emphasizes that individuals are at different stages in terms of their readiness to engage in a health- or food-related behavior and that consequently, nutrition education interventions must be designed to meet the needs of individuals at each stage of change. The mediators of change are the pros and cons of change and self-efficacy. To enhance effectiveness, nutrition education interventions can base activities on the 10 processes of change, matched to the individual's or group's stage of change.

Main Focus for Nutrition Education

Nutrition educators' main focus is to assist individuals to develop nutrition-related skills, skills in self-regulation of their behaviors, including goal setting and planning, and developing personal food policies to cope with their life situations and maintain the changes they have sought.

Questions and Activities

1. Social cognitive theory is widely used in nutrition education and health promotion. Why do you think this is so—what specific features of the theory make it so useful?

2. Describe in your own words the following theory constructs. How are the terms related to people's ability to take action or to change their behaviors? Be specific.
   a. Outcome expectations
   b. Self-efficacy
   c. Modeling
   d. Behavioral capability
   e. Environment
   f. Pros and cons of change

3. Describe what is meant by the "processes of change" in the transtheoretical model.

4. Compare social cognitive theory, the transtheoretical model, and the health action process approach in terms of (a) what motivates behavior, (b) what facilitates the ability to change one's behavior, and (c) how change occurs. In what ways are the constructs similar or different in the three theories?

5. What strategies can be used to increase self-efficacy in individuals?

6. Why is goal setting (or stating action plans) so important? What does it accomplish? What are some key steps?

7. Interview one person who successfully took action on a diet- or activity-related behavior change he or she wished to make and one who was not successful. Ask them what they think contributed to their success or lack of success.
   a. How would you now describe the factors involved in the failures and successes using the language of social cognitive theory constructs described in this chapter?

Reasons Given for Being Successful/Not Successful	Name of Construct of Theory	Justification for Assignment

   b. Can you now explain why one was successful whereas the other was not?
   c. For the person who was not successful, what five tips can you give him or her to help that individual be more successful in the future?

8. Maintaining the health-related changes people make is not easy. Describe five tips you would provide in a nutrition education session on the issue.

References

Abraham, C., P. Sheeran, and M. Johnson. 1998. From health beliefs to self-regulation: Theoretical advances in the psychology of action control. *Psychology and Health* 13:569–591.

Armitage, C. J. 2004. Evidence that implementation intentions reduce dietary fat intake: A randomized trial. *Health Psychology* 23(3):319–323.

Bagozzi, R. P. 1992. The self-regulation of attitudes, intentions, and behavior. *Social Science Quarterly* 55:178–204.

Bandura, A. 1977. *Social learning theory*. Englewood Cliffs, NJ: Prentice Hall.

——. 1986. *Foundations of thought and action: A social cognitive theory*. Englewood Cliffs, NJ: Prentice Hall.

——. 1989. Human agency in social cognitive theory. *American Psychologist* 44:1175–1184.

——. 1997. *Self efficacy: The exercise of control*. New York: WH Freeman.

——. 2000. Health promotion from the perspective of social cognitive theory. In *Understanding and changing health behavior: From health beliefs to self-regulation*, edited by P. Norman, C. Abraham, and M. Conner. Amsterdam: Harwood Academic Publishers.

——. 2001. Social cognitive theory: An agentic perspective. *Annual Review of Psychology* 51:1–26.

——. 2004. Health promotion by social cognitive means. *Health Education and Behavior* 31(2):143–164.

Baranowski, T., J. Baranowski, K. W. Cullen, et al. 2003. Squire's Quest! Dietary outcome evaluation of a multimedia game. *American Journal of Preventive Medicine* 24(1):52–61.

Bisogni, C. A., M. Jastran, L. Shen, and C. M. Devine. 2005. A biographical study of food choice capacity: Standards, circumstances, and food management skills. *Journal of Nutrition Education and Behavior* 37(6):284–291.

Boudreaux, E. D., K. B. Wood, D. Mehan, I. Scarinci, C. L. Taylor, and P. J. Brantley. 2003. Congruence of readiness to change, self-efficacy, and decisional balance for physical activity and dietary fat reduction. *American Journal of Health Promotion* 17(5):329–336.

Brug, J., K. Glanz, and G. Kok. 1997. The relationship between self-efficacy, attitudes, intake compared to others, consumption, and stages of change related to fruit and vegetables. *American Journal of Health Promotion* 12(1):25–30.

Brug, J., A. Oenema, and M. Campbell. 2003. Past, present, and future of computer-tailored nutrition education. *American Journal of Clinical Nutrition* 77(4 Suppl):1028S–1034S.

Brug, J., P. van Assema, G. Kok, T. Lenderink, and K. Glanz. 1994. Self-rated dietary fat intake: Associations with objectively assessed intake, psychosocial factors and intention to change. *Journal of Nutrition Education* 26:218–223.

Buchanan, H., and N. S. Coulson. 2007. Consumption of carbonated drinks in adolescents: A transtheoretical analysis. *Child Care and Health Development* 33(4):441–447.

Campbell, M. K., B. M. DeVellis, V. J. Strecher, A. S. Ammerman, R. F. DeVellis, and R. S. Sandler. 1994. Improving dietary behavior: The effectiveness of tailored messages in primary care settings. *American Journal of Public Health* 84(5):783–787.

Campbell, M. K., L. Honess-Morreale, D. Farrell, E. Carbone, and M. Brasure. 1999. A tailored multimedia nutrition education pilot program for low-income women receiving food assistance. *Health Education Research* 14(2):257–267.

Campbell, M. K., K. D. Reynolds, S. Havas, et al. 1999. Stages of change for increasing fruit and vegetable consumption among adults and young adults participating in the national 5-A-Day for Better Health community studies. *Health Education and Behavior* 26(4):513–534.

Campbell, M. K., M. Symons, W. Demark-Wahnefried, et al. 1998. Stages of change and psychosocial correlates of fruit and vegetable consumption among rural African-American church members. *American Journal of Health Promotion* 12(3):185–191.

Campbell, M. K., I. Tessaro, B. DeVellis, et al. 2002. Effects of a tailored health promotion program for female blue-collar workers: health works for women. *Preventive Medicine* 34(3):313–323.

Chapman-Novakofski, K., and J. Karduck. 2005. Improvement in knowledge, social cognitive theory variables, and movement through stages of change after a community-based diabetes education program. *Journal of the American Dietetic Association* 105(10):1613–1616.

Connors, M., C. A. Bisogni, J. Sobal, and C. M. Devine. 2001. Managing values in personal food systems. *Appetite* 36(3):189–200.

Contento, I. R., P. A. Koch, A. Calabrese-Barton, H. Lee, and W. Sauberli. 2007. Enhancing personal agency and competence in eating and moving: Formative evaluation of a middle school curriculum—*Choice, Control, and Change*. *Journal of Nutrition Education and Behavior* 39:S179–S186.

Contento, I. R., S. S. Williams, J. L. Michela, and A. B. Franklin. 2006. Understanding the food choice process of adolescents in the context of family and friends. *Journal of Adolescent Health* 38(5):575–582.

Cullen, K. W., T. Baranowski, and S. P. Smith. 2001. Using goal setting as a strategy for dietary behavior change. *Journal of the American Dietetic Association* 101(5):562–566.

De Bourdeaudhuij, I., J. Brug, C. Vandelanotte, and P. Van Oost. 2002. Differences in impact between a family- versus an individual-based tailored intervention to reduce fat intake. *Health Education Research* 17(4):435–449.

De Bourdeaudhuij, I., V. Stevens, C. Vandelanotte, and J. Brug. 2007. Evaluation of an interactive computer-tailored nutrition intervention in a real-life setting. *Annals of Behavorial Medicine* 33(1):39–48.

De Nooijer, J., E. de Vet, J. Brug, and N. K. de Vries. 2006. Do implementation intentions help to turn good intentions into higher fruit intakes? *Journal of Nutrition Education and Behavior* 38(1):25–29.

De Nooijer, J., P. Van Assema, E. De Vet, and J. Brug. 2005. How stable are stages of change for nutrition behaviors in the Netherlands? *Health Promotion International* 20(1):27–32.

Di Noia, J., I. R. Contento, and J. O. Prochaska. 2008. Computer-mediated intervention tailored on transtheoretical model stages and processes of change increases fruit and vegetable consumption among urban African-American adolescents. *American Journal of Health Promotion* 22(5):336–341.

Edmundson, E., G. S. Parcel, H. A. Feldman, et al. 1996. The effects of the Child and Adolescent Trial for Cardiovascular Health upon psychosocial determinants of diet and physical activity behavior. *Preventive Medicine* 25(4):442–454.

Falk, L. W., J. Sobal, C. A. Bisogni, M. Connors, and C. M. Devine. 2001. Managing healthy eating: Definitions, classifications, and strategies. *Health Education and Behavior* 28(4):425–439.

Finckenor, M., and C. Byrd-Bredbenner. 2000. Nutrition intervention group program based on preaction-stage-oriented change processes of the Transtheoretical Model promotes long-term reduction in dietary fat intake. *Journal of the American Dietetic Association* 100(3):335–342.

Glanz, K., A. R. Kristal, B. C. Tilley, and K. Hirst. 1998. Psychosocial correlates of healthful diets among male auto workers. *Cancer Epidemiology, Biomarkers, and Prevention* 7(2):119–126.

Glanz, K., R. E. Patterson, A. R. Kristal, et al. 1994. Stages of change in adopting healthy diets: Fat, fiber, and correlates of nutrient intake. *Health Education Quarterly* 21(4):499–519.

Gollwitzer, P. M. 1999. Implementation intentions—strong effects of simple plans. *American Psychologist* 54:493–503.

Gollwitzer, P. M., and G. Oettingen. 2000. The emergence and implementation of health goals. In *Understanding and changing health behaviour from health beliefs to self-regulation*, edited by P. Norman, C. Abraham, and M. Conner. Amsterdam: Harwood Academic Publishers.

Gortmaker, S. L., K. Peterson, J. Wiecha, et al. 1999. Reducing obesity via a school-based interdisciplinary intervention among youth: Planet Health. *Archives of Pediatric and Adolescent Medicine* 153(4):409–418.

Greene, G. W., S. R. Rossi, J. S. Rossi, W. F. Velicer, J. L. Fava, and J. O. Prochaska. 1999. Dietary applications of the stages of change model. *Journal of the American Dietetic Association* 99(6):673–678.

Heneman, K., A. Block-Joy, S. Zidenberg-Cherr, et al. 2005. A "contract for change" increases produce consumption in low-income women: A pilot study. *Journal of the American Dietetic Association* 105(11):1793–1796.

Henry, H., K. Reimer, C. Smith, and M. Reicks. 2006. Associations of decisional balance, processes of change, and self-efficacy with stages of change for increased fruit and vegetable intake among low-income, African-American mothers. *Journal of the American Dietetic Association* 106(6):841–849.

Hoelscher, D. M., H. A. Feldman, C. C. Johnson, et al. 2004. School-based health education programs can be maintained over time: Results from the CATCH Institutionalization study. *Preventive Medicine* 38(5):594–606.

Hoisington, A., J. A. Shultz, and S. Butkus. 2002. Coping strategies and nutrition education needs among food pantry users. *Journal of Nutrition Education and Behavior* 34(6):226–233.

Horowitz, M., M. K. Shilts, and M. S. Townsend. 2004. EatFit: A goal-oriented intervention that challenges adolescents to improve their eating and fitness choices. *Journal of Nutrition Education and Behavior* 36(1):43–44.

Institute of Medicine. 2004. *Health literacy: A prescription to end confusion*. Washington, DC: National Academy Press.

Jacobs, A. D., A. S. Ammerman, S. T. Ennett, et al. 2004. Effects of a tailored follow-up intervention on health behaviors, beliefs, and attitudes. *Journal of Women's Health* 13(5):557–568.

Kavookjian, J., B. A. Berger, D. M. Grimley, W. A. Villaume, H. M. Anderson, and K. N. Barker. 2005. Patient decision making: Strategies for diabetes diet adherence intervention. *Research Social Administration and Pharmacy* 1(3):389–407.

Keller, K. L., A. Pietrobelli, S. Must, and M. S. Faith. 2002. Genetics of eating and its relation to obesity. *Current Atherosclerosis Reports* 4(3):176–182.

Kristal, A. R., K. Glanz, B. C. Tilley, and S. Li. 2000. Mediating factors in dietary change: Understanding the impact of a worksite nutrition intervention. *Health Education and Behavior* 27(1):112–125.

Lewis, C. J., L. S. Sims, and B. Shannon. 1989. Examination of specific nutrition/health behaviors using a social cognitive model. *Journal of the American Dietetic Association* 89(2):194–202.

Lippke, S., A. U. Wiedemann, J. P. Ziegelmann, T. Reuter, and R. Schwarzer. 2009. Self-efficacy moderates the mediation of intentions into behavior via plans. *American Journal of Health Behavior* 33(5):521–529.

Lippke, S., J. P. Ziegelmann, R. Schwarzer, and W. F. Velicer. 2009. Validity of stage assessment in the adoption and maintenance of physical activity and fruit and vegetable consumption. *Health Psychology* 28(2):183–193.

Luepker, R. V., C. L. Perry, S. M. McKinlay, et al. 1996. Outcomes of a field trial to improve children's dietary patterns and physical activity. The Child and Adolescent Trial for Cardiovascular Health. CATCH Collaborative Group. *Journal of the American Medical Association* 275(10):768–776.

Ma, J., N. M. Betts, T. Horacek, C. Georgiou, A. White, and S. Nitzke. 2002. The importance of decisional balance and self-efficacy in relation to stages of change for fruit and vegetable intakes by young adults. *American Journal of Health Promotion* 16(3):157–166.

Mennella, J. A., M. Y. Pepino, and D. R. Reed. 2005. Genetic and environmental determinants of bitter perception and sweet preferences. *Pediatrics* 115(2):e216–e222.

Molaison, E. F., C. L. Connell, J. E. Stuff, M. K. Yadrick, and M. Bogle. 2005. Influences on fruit and vegetable consumption by low-income black American adolescents. *Journal of Nutrition Education and Behavior* 37(5):246–251.

Oenema, A., F. Tan, and J. Brug. 2005. Short-term efficacy of a Web-based computer-tailored nutrition intervention: Main effects and mediators. *Annals of Behavioral Medicine* 29(1):54–63.

O'Hea, E. L., E. D. Boudreaux, S. K. Jeffries, C. L. Carmack Taylor, I. C. Scarinci, and P. J. Brantley. 2004. Stage of change movement across three health behaviors: The role of self-efficacy. *American Journal of Health Promotion* 19(2):94–102.

Osborne, H. 2005. *Health literacy from a to z: Practical ways to communicate your health message.* Sudbury, MA: Jones and Bartlett.

Park, A., S. Nitzke, K. Kritsch, et al. 2008. Internet-based interventions have potential to affect short-term mediators and indicators of dietary behavior of young adults. *Journal of Nutrition Education and Behavior* 40(5):288–297.

Prochaska, J. M. 2007. The transtheoretical model applied to the community and the workplace. *Journal of Health Psychology* 12(1):198–200.

Prochaska, J. O., and C. C. DiClemente. 1984. *The transtheoretical approach: Crossing the traditional boundaries of therapy.* Homewood, IL: Dow Jones-Irwin.

Prochaska, J. O., C. C. DiClemente, and J. C. Norcross. 1992. In search of how people change. Applications to addictive behaviors. *American Psychologist* 47(9):1102–1114.

Prochaska, J. O., C. C. DiClemente, W. F. Velicer, and J. S. Rossi. 1993. Standardized, individualized, interactive, and personalized self-help programs for smoking cessation. *Health Psychology* 12(5):399–405.

Prochaska, J. O., and W. F. Velicer. 1997. The transtheoretical model of health behavior change. *American Journal of Health Promotion* 12(1):38–48.

Reynolds, K. D., A. W. Hinton, R. Shewchuk, et al. 1999. A social cognitive model of fruit and vegetable consumption in elementary school children. *Journal of Nutrition Education* 31(1):23–30.

Riebe, D., G. W. Greene, L. Ruggiero, et al. 2003. Evaluation of a healthy-lifestyle approach to weight management. *Preventive Medicine* 36(1):45–54.

Rosen, C. S. 2000. Is the sequencing of change processes by stage consistent across health problems? A meta-analysis. *Health Psychology* 19:593–604.

Rothman, A. J. 2000. Toward a theory-based analysis of behavioral maintenance. *Health Psychology* 19(1 Suppl):64–69.

Salmela, S., M. Poskiparta, K. Kasila, K. Vahasarja, and M. Vanhala. 2009. Transtheoretical model-based dietary interventions in primary care: A review of the evidence in diabetes. *Health Education Research* 24(2):237–252.

Sauberli, W., H. Lee, I. R. Contento, P. Koch, and A. Calabrese-Barton. 2008. Enhancing personal agency and competence in eating and moving: An outcome evaluation of choice, control, and change (C3), an inquiry-based middle school science curriculum to reduce obesity. *Journal of Nutrition Education and Behavior* 40, 4(Suppl):536.

Scholz, U., B. Schuz, J. P. Ziegelmann, S. Lippke, and R. Schwarzer. 2008. Beyond behavioural intentions: Planning mediates between intentions and physical activity. *British Journal of Health Psychology* 13(Pt 3):479–494.

Schwarzer, R., and R. Fuchs. 1995. Self-efficacy and health behaviors. In *Predicting health behavior*, edited by M. Conner and P. Norman. Buckingham, UK: Open University Press.

Schwarzer, R., and B. Renner. 2000. Social-cognitive predictors of health behavior: Action self-efficacy and coping self-efficacy. *Health Psychology* 19(5):487–495.

Schwarzer, R., B. Schuz, J. P. Ziegelmann, S. Lippke, A. Luszczynska, and U. Scholz. 2007. Adoption and maintenance of four health behaviors: Theory-guided longitudinal studies on dental flossing, seat belt use, dietary behavior, and physical activity. *Annals of Behavioral Medicine* 33(2):156–166.

Shilts, M. K., M. Horowitz, and M. S. Townsend. 2004a. Goal setting as a strategy for dietary and physical activity behavior change: A review of the literature. *American Journal of Health Promotion* 19(2):81–93.

———. 2004b. An innovative approach to goal setting for adolescents: Guided goal setting. *Journal of Nutrition Education and Behavior* 36(3):155.

———. 2009. Guided goal setting: Effectiveness in a dietary and physical activity intervention with low-income adolescents. *International Journal of Adolescent Medicine and Health* 21(1):111–122.

Sniehotta, F. F., U. R. Scholz, and R. Schwarzer. 2005. Bridging the intention–behaviour gap: Planning, self-efficacy, and action control in the adoption and maintenance of physical exercise. *Psychology and Health* 20:143–160.

Sporny, L. A., and I. R. Contento. 1995. Stages of change in dietary fat reduction: Social psychological correlates. *Journal of Nutrition Education* 27:191–199.

Steptoe, A., S. Wijetunge, S. Doherty, and J. Wardle. 1996. Stages of change for dietary fat reduction: Associations with food intake, decisional balance, and motives for food choice. *Health Education Journal* 55:108–122.

Sternfeld, B., C. Block, C. P. Quesenberry Jr., et al. 2009. Improving diet and physical activity with ALIVE: A worksite randomized trial. *American Journal of Preventive Medicine* 36(6):475–483.

Taylor, S. D., R. P. Bagozzi, and C. A. Gaither. 2005. Decision making and effort in the self-regulation of hypertension: Testing two competing theories. *British Journal of Health Psychology* 10(Pt 4):505–530.

Thoresen, C. E. 1984. Strategies for health enhancement overview. In *Behavioral health: A handbook of health enhancement and disease prevention*, edited by J. D. Matarazzo, S. M. Weiss, J. A. Herd, and N. E. Miller. New York: Wiley.

Velicer, W. F., and J. O. Prochaska. 1999. An expert system intervention for smoking cessation. *Patient Education and Counseling* 36(2):119–129.

Verplanken, B., and S. Faes. 1999. Good intentions, bad habits, and effects of forming implementation intentions on healthy eating. *European Journal of Social Psychology* 29:591–604.

Wiedemann, A. U., S. Lippke, T. Reuter, B. Schuz, J. P. Ziegelmann, and R. Schwarzer. 2009. Prediction of stage transitions in fruit and vegetable intake. *Health Education Research* 24(4):596–607.

Wright, J. A., W. F. Velicer, and J. O. Prochaska. 2009. Testing the predictive power of the transtheoretical model of behavior change applied to dietary fat intake. *Health Education Research* 24(2):224–236.

Ziegelmann, J. P., and S. Lippke. 2007. Planning and strategy use in health behavior change: A life span view. *International Journal of Behavioral Medicine* 14(1):30–39.

Ziegelmann, J. P., S. Lippke, and R. Schwarzer. 2006. Adoption and maintenance of physical activity: Planning interventions in young, middle-aged, and older adults. *Psychology and Health* 21:145–163.

CHAPTER 6

Foundation in Theory and Research: Promoting Environmental Supports for Action

OVERVIEW

This chapter describes key issues and approaches for addressing environmental determinants or mediators of healthful food and nutrition actions. The focus of this chapter is on providing environmental and policy supports to increase opportunities for individuals to take healthful action.

CHAPTER OUTLINE

- Introduction
- Interpersonal environment
- Organizational-level environmental change
- Community-level activities
- Policy and systems change activities
- Strategies to improve environmental and policy supports for action or behavior change
- Summary

LEARNING OBJECTIVES

At the end of the chapter, you will be able to:

- Identify approaches to address environmental determinants of healthful food and nutrition actions
- Describe interventions that have addressed interpersonal, organizational, and community influences on behavior to make them more supportive of healthful eating and active living
- Recognize the importance of collaborations and partnerships for promoting environmental and policy supports for action
- Define the concepts of social networks, social support, collaboration, partnership, empowerment, and collective efficacy and describe how they have been used in nutrition education
- Describe how nutrition education can address several levels of influence to support people's willingness and ability to take action

■ INTRODUCTION: MAKING HEALTHFUL CHOICES THE EASY ONES

The nation is concerned about the high rates of obesity and chronic disease and has increasingly recognized that the environment has a hand in this situation. There has been considerable interest in addressing this environment. From the surgeon general to public health officials to food companies, all say that they are interested in being part of the solution rather than part of the problem. Research has been extremely active in this area (Glanz et al. 2005; Matson-Koffman et al. 2005; Story et al. 2008; Jordan 2008; American Academy of Pediatrics Committee on Environmental Health 2009; Sallis, Orleans, & Buchner 2009).

However, high-calorie foods are everywhere, convenient and cheap, escalators and elevators are ubiquitous, and attractive and safe parks are not readily available. All of this makes it difficult to eat healthfully and be physically active. Often individuals are willing and able to take action and have the intention to do so but find that taking action is very much influenced by environmental factors—by whether the desired foods are available at a price they can afford or accessible when they need them, by what other members of their families do, by policies at their schools or places of work, and by the structure of their communities. Thus, helping individuals bridge the intention–behavior gap requires that nutrition educators seek ways to make the healthful actions the easy ones. This chapter focuses on environmental determinants that facilitate or hinder individuals from being able to act on a condition or issue of concern to them. It examines approaches and recent studies that suggest strategies for promoting environments that are supportive of action.

What Does the Term *Environment* Mean?

The terms *environment* and *ecology* can have different meanings.

Environment

This book uses the term *environment* to refer to factors that are *external* to the individual. For example, a social norm is a perception that influences behavior but is not classified as an environmental determinant of behavior because it is our *perception* of the environment and is not external to us. Social networks and social support, on the other hand, are external to us, so are considered potential environmental mediators of behavior. Culturally based institutional practices and social structures such as family meals or community holiday practices are also considered part of the environment.

Environmental interventions are those that involve strategies for changing the physical surrounding, social climate, information environment, organizational systems, or policy to provide support for healthy eating and active living.

Ecology

The term *ecology* is derived from the biology literature, where it refers to the relationship between organisms and their natural environments. In this book, the term *ecological* refers to issues within the field of food and nutrition related to the natural environment. Ecological concerns are thus concerns about the impact of food production, marketing, and consumption practices on the natural environment, and hence the ability of the food system to produce wholesome food in a way that remains sustainable. Examples are issues related to the availability and accessibility of foods produced using sustainable practices or to the vibrancy of local farms.

In the health promotion field, the contexts in which people live are often also called *ecologies*. Thus, *social ecological models* refers to approaches that address several social ecologies or levels of influence on behavior at once. The term is used in that sense here. These levels are labeled intrapersonal factors, interpersonal processes and primary groups, institutional factors, community factors, and public policy and legislation (McLeroy et al. 1988; Green & Kreuter 2004). In the social ecological model, activities and initiatives are designed to change institutions, communities, policy, and legislation to foster individual and community health. Such social ecological approaches to intervention thus address both environmental and personal determinants of behaviors or mediators of change.

Policy

Policy activities are part of environmental supports for action. *Policy* usually refers to a deliberate plan of action to guide decisions and achieve rational outcomes. Policies can be seen as the arrangement of political, management, and financial mechanisms to reach specified goals—a set of rules and understandings that govern behavior and practice. *Public policy* usually refers to a course of action taken by governmental entities with respect to a particular issue or set of issues—a set of agreements about how government will address societal needs and spend public funds.

How Might the Environment Influence Individuals?

The physical availability and accessibility of healthful foods and the means to be physically active are of course paramount. The fact that healthful foods are present, though, does not mean that people will eat them. How does the environment affect individuals' behaviors? It has been proposed that the environment affects people through conscious and unconscious processes (Kremers, de Bruijn, Visscher et al. 2006).

- *Conscious processes* result in impacts on behavior through psychosocial cognitions. For example, the lack of healthful foods in a neighborhood may reduce our sense of self-efficacy, and high prices for such foods may result in a negative attitude toward healthful foods. Changes in these cognitions can become mediators of change in intentions and behavior.
- *Unconscious processes* operate through a "mindless" or automatic route in which behaviors are automatically elicited by the environment through environment–behavior links (Wansink 2006). This route exists because our cognitive capacity is limited and automatic processes free our conscious capacity from having to consider, make choices, and deal with every aspect of our lives all the time. We automatically and unconsciously engage in actions in response to environmental cues. For example, whenever there is an advertising break in a television program, we may head for the refrigerator for a snack. In addition, marketing practices and environmental cues often are arranged so as to unconsciously influence our choices. For example, many purchases in supermarkets are unplanned and, of those, about two thirds are influenced by visual displays and other marketing devices (Abratt & Goodey 1990). Restaurant ambiance and how the food is described also can influence the amount people spend on food and drink (Wansink 2006; Cohen 2008). Thus, even with motivation, knowledge, and skills, people often still face difficulties in taking action because of automatic responses to the environment and environmental obstacles. Consequently, the environment must be addressed if nutrition education is to be effective.

Addressing Environmental Determinants: A Social Ecological Approach

Dietary behaviors are complex and the influences on them are many, as we saw in Chapter 2. Nutrition education is more likely to be effective if it focuses on specific actions, practices, or issues, identifies the determinants of those actions, uses theory to design strategies to address them, and attends to the multiple levels of influences on these behaviors or issues by using multiple channels to assist people to eat more healthfully and be more active.

Different theories and approaches are relevant for these different levels of intervention, as shown in **Figure 6-1**.

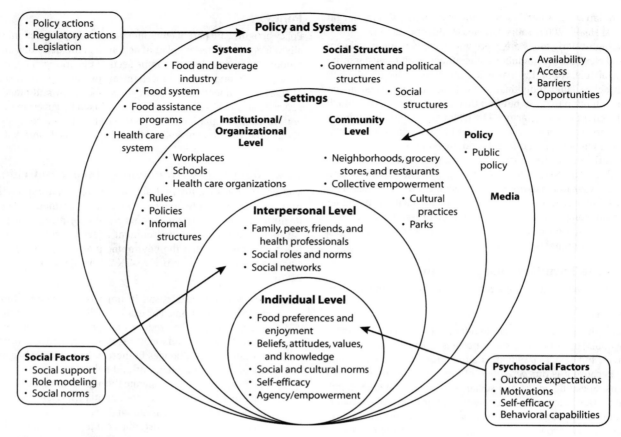

FIGURE 6-1   Social ecological model: Approaches at different levels of action.

Individual Level

The social psychological theories discussed in detail so far are very important for interventions directed at individuals. Nutrition education based on these theories focuses on beliefs or outcome expectations and motivations for why to take action and food and nutrition-related skills for how to take action as well as self-efficacy and self-regulation skills for how to take charge and direct our behaviors.

Interpersonal Level

Approaches at this level focus on understanding people's social networks and helping to provide social support for healthy living. Strategies might include creating support groups for the program participants, working with peer educators, and developing a family component to support school- and worksite-based programs.

Organizational and Community Settings

The role of nutrition educators here is to educate decision makers in these settings about the importance of issues that are the focus of our programs and to develop collaborations with them to bring about access, availability, and opportunities in the relevant food and activity environments. These may include food service directors in schools and workplaces or leaders in the community.

Policy, Systems, and Social Structures

Creating supportive environments often requires that nutrition educators educate new audiences about the importance of actions or issues of concern and work in collaborations and partnerships with them so as to bring about supportive action. These may include those who have decision-making power and authority in other fields that affect the lives of program participants, such as school and workplace administrators, community leaders, policy makers, legislators, and regulators. Studies show that activities directed at both the individual and the environment are important because the barriers to healthful living are both personal and environmental.

This chapter explores each of these levels of influence in greater detail.

■ INTERPERSONAL ENVIRONMENT: FAMILY, PEERS, AND SOCIAL SUPPORT

Individuals live within a network of social relationships. These networks involve family, peers, coworkers, and those in various organizations to which individuals belong. These social relationships greatly influence individuals' food choices and dietary behaviors. Thus, strategies to promote supportive environments usually address these social relationships.

Homes

Americans eat about two thirds of their calories from foods prepared in the home. Among the factors associated with healthful dietary behaviors, the most important are foods present in the home (household food availability), whether foods are easily accessible to family members, the frequency of family meals, and parents' own intakes and parenting practices when it comes to children (Cullen et al. 2003; Fulkerson et al. 2008; Burgess-Champoux et al. 2009).

Social Environmental Influences in the Home

Family practices are important influences on health. Although youth frequently eat outside the home, they still eat many of their meals with the family, particularly when they are younger. Surveys show that about three quarters of those ages 12 to 14 still eat five meals a week with their families, declining to about 60% for those ages 15 to 16, and about 40% for those ages 17 to 19 (Council of Economic Advisers 2000). Modeling of healthful eating and activity behaviors by parents and siblings and authoritative parenting style (where parents set limits but also are nurturing) can be very important, particularly with younger children (Ventura & Birch 2008). A large population-based study with diverse adolescents found that parenting style (authoritarian and neglectful) and parental modeling practices were complexly related to body mass index and differed for sons and daughters (Berge et al. 2009). A study found that the resemblance between food choices of teens and their parents was 76% to 87%, depending on the food, whereas between teens and their peers it was 19% (Feuenekes et al. 1998).

Decision-making patterns within families also are important. It has been proposed that family food and eating practices can be thought of as consisting of a family food decision-making system (FFDS). For any given food event, goals need to be decided and may involve negotiating limits and trade-offs among competing food and eating goals; choosing among alternatives as to where to acquire food; how it should be prepared and presented; and implementing the chosen alternatives. Out of these experiences, family food routines and policies emerge (Gillespie & Gillespie 2007; Gillespie & Johnson-Askew 2009). A study found that adolescents negotiate with their families as to what to eat and balance the less healthful foods they eat with their peers with healthier meals at home (Contento et al. 2006). Thus, family eating patterns are very important and can be addressed by nutrition education, which can assist families to become more aware of their food decisions and develop strategies for effective decision-making.

Family Involvement in School Programs

Many interventions in schools have focused on *family involvement* as a way to enhance home support for health. However, nutrition educators often find that parents are busy and cannot attend regular classes designed for them. Likewise, newsletters sent home have not been found to be effective. Hence, the strategies described in the following paragraphs have been found to be more effective. In each of these examples, the parents were considered a new audience for which a separate set of educational goals and objectives, educational strategies, and evaluation measures had to be designed.

- *Student–parent activities at home with third graders.* In a large study with third graders, school and school-plus-family interventions were compared (Edmundson et al. 1996). Packets containing games and activities that required parental or adult involvement to complete were sent home to families each week for five weeks.

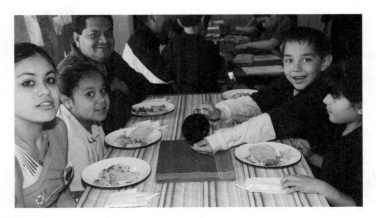

Parents and their children enjoy a meal they cooked together at their school's "Family Night."

Rewards were given for completed lessons that were returned. There were also two family fun nights. Results showed that there was a greater improvement in dietary intentions and usual food choices for lower-fat and lower-sodium foods for those who had the additional family interventions.

- *Behavioral coupons with teens.* The family component of a different study, this time with middle school students, consisted of three newsletters and a set of 10 behavioral coupons with simple messages such as "Serve a fruit or vegetable with dinner tonight" (Lytle et al. 2004). About 30% of parents completed at least one set of behavioral coupons.
- *Family fun nights.* A more intense family component was Family Fun Nights, in which families actually came together over a meal for a food-and-game experience (Harrington et al. 2005). Each of the seven sessions offered a game, new recipe choices, intervention messages to parents, a children's fun page that reinforced program themes, optional conversation topics, and menu suggestions.

Social Networks and Social Support

It has been shown that social relationships influence health status, probably both through direct effects and through their ability to buffer the negative effects of life stressors on health (Gottlieb 1985; Berkman & Glass 2000). In particular, emotional support is related to good health and to reduced all-cause mortality.

Social Networks

Social networks refers to the web of social relationships that surround individuals. In the area of diet, food choices and eating patterns are directly influenced by social networks. The resemblances of food choices within the family are significantly greater than between family members and their friends. On the other hand, family members and others who live together may not all like or want to eat the same foods. Thus, there is a need to negotiate with the family or others about what to buy or eat (Furst et al. 1996; Feuenekes et al. 1998; Contento et al. 2006). Relationships with peers and those with whom people work also have an impact on individuals' day-to-day choices. Researchers characterize social networks as follows (Israel & Rounds 1987):

- *Structure:* The size and number of members in the network
- *Density:* The extent to which members know and interact with each other

- *Proximity:* The degree to which individuals in the network are similar to each other or located in close proximity
- *Interaction:* The frequency of contact, the variety of functions that the network serves (complexity), and how close members are emotionally (intensity)
- *Reciprocity:* The extent to which individuals help each other with resources and support

Some individuals are within very extensive social networks of family and friends who are in frequent contact with each other, whereas others have few friends and family with whom they interact.

Social Support

Social support refers to the support that individuals in social networks provide each other in various areas:

- *Emotional support:* Involves empathy, trust, caring, and esteem. This may be found in expressions such as "he listens to me when I talk to him about things," "some people look down on you: well, she doesn't," "she is someone I trust and I know she will keep what I tell her confidential."
- *Instrumental support:* Involves money or other tangible resources and help, such as with babysitting or shopping. This is reflected in "she helped me by talking with the owners and convincing them to wait a while for the rent money."
- *Informational support:* Involves advice and information useful in solving problems. This might include "he offered suggestions about what I could do."
- *Appraisal support:* Involves constructive feedback and self-evaluation. This is reflected in statements such as "he seems to have faith in me."

Again, individuals differ in the degree to which they receive social support for their eating and physical activity patterns.

Nutrition education interventions can seek to strengthen existing social networks to make them more supportive of health (such as involving the family in the intervention), provide structured social support groups, or initiate new social networks in which individuals participating in the intervention can help each other (such as regular meetings of participants, walking groups, or buddy systems). Social support is incorporated into many health interventions and indeed was identified in a review of nutrition education as one of the elements that contributed to effectiveness (Ammerman et al. 2002). Weight loss interventions (e.g., Weight Watchers) routinely incorporate social support groups. Interventions in schools and workplaces have also incorporated social support in various forms. A few illustrations are provided here.

Social Support in Workplaces

In worksite interventions, social support has been operationalized as peer support at the worksite and involvement of family. The interventions have attempted to make these existing social networks more supportive of health. Most of the interventions have used group education classes along with other strategies. When intervention components were compared in one study, it was found that interactive strategies such as group education classes and contests were more effective in terms of nutritional outcomes (e.g., eating more fruits and vegetables) than were one-time activities such as kickoffs or more passive efforts such as use of printed materials (Patterson et al. 1997).

Workplace-Plus-Family Support

In a study in which a family component was included (the Treatwell 5 A Day study), results show that total fruit and vegetable intake in-creased by 19% in the worksite-plus-family group, 7% in the worksite intervention-only group, and 0% in the control group, suggesting that including a family component can be an effective strategy (Sorensen et al. 1999). This study also measured coworker support for healthful eating, asking questions such as how often coworkers "encourage you to eat vegetables," "complement your attempts to eat a healthy diet," or "bring fruit to work for you to try." Coworker support increased significantly in both intervention conditions compared with the control condition. Taken together, these studies suggest that incorporating social support into nutrition education interventions is an important strategy to increase effectiveness.

Peer Educators as Social Support

Peer educators have served an important role in nutrition education in several settings. In schools, the use of peers has been found to be very accepted and popular among the peer leaders themselves, their classmates, and teachers (Story et al. 2002). Their role is not only to teach sessions and serve as models, but also to provide social support to classmates.

The Expanded Food and Nutrition Education Program of the U.S. Department of Agriculture (USDA) serves several hundred thousand low-income youth and families each year and is based on the use of paraprofessionals and peers, many of whom are indigenous to the target population. These peer educators work with small groups, often in their homes, thus providing modeling and social support as well. Results show that this approach is effective in improving eating patterns (U.S. Department of Agriculture 2003). Use of peer counselors also increased breastfeeding duration, as did support at home (Kistin, Abramson, & Dublin 1994; Sciacca et al. 1995). Peer educators were also effective among older adults (Ness, Elliot, & Wilbur 1992).

Support Groups

Often nutrition educators have the opportunity to provide individuals with social support by the creation of a new support group as part of the intervention. Many of the facilitated discussion groups in the Women, Infants and Children (WIC) program and other programs serve this function. Weight management groups that meet over a long period can also provide support to members.

The social support approach is especially useful for those who have been diagnosed with type 2 diabetes. Controlling blood sugar and preventing complications are unending challenges and require changes in diet for a lifetime. Consequently, the impact of receiving a diagnosis can be devastating. Nutrition educators can provide group members an opportunity to process their feelings with others like them through a series of structured activities. Nutrition educators can also help individuals develop action plans, and group members can meet to share challenges and successes. Such groups can provide emotional support, involving empathy and caring; informational support in the form of advice and information useful in solving problems; and appraisal support in terms of accurate feedback. They do not usually provide instrumental support.

■ ORGANIZATIONAL-LEVEL ENVIRONMENTAL CHANGE

To make the food environment in organizations more supportive of healthful action, nutrition educators can work in collaboration with those who have power and authority to make healthful foods more available and accessible in the given setting, such as in schools and workplaces.

School Settings

The school food environment can have a large impact on the quality of children's food choices and intakes because they eat a large proportion of their daily calories at school. For example, foods eaten at school constitute 35% to 40% of students' daily calorie intake, through eating foods obtained from the school meals program, à la carte offerings, vending machines, and school stores. Participation in the National School Lunch Program (NSLP) declines with age, with about two thirds of elementary school children participating, down to about half in middle school, and then to one third in high school. Foods available in venues that are alternatives to the NSLP, called *competitive foods*, tend to be higher in fat and sugar and less nutritious. For example, the availability of vending machines and snack bars lowers the level of participation in the NSLP, and at the same time, these venues tend to stock high-fat, high-sugar items such as snack chips, candy, and soda and are low in fruits and vegetables. Because it has been shown that the availability and accessibility of fruits and vegetables increases consumption of such foods (Hearn et al. 1998), it is not surprising that when students move from an elementary school, where only the NSLP is available, to a middle school with à la carte and snack bar meals, their intakes of fruit, vegetables, and milk decrease and their consumption of sweetened beverages and high-fat, high-sugar foods increases (Cullen & Zakeri 2004).

Many nutrition education interventions with school-aged youth have worked with school staff to increase the availability and accessibility of targeted foods in the school meals program, such as lower-fat foods, fruits, and vegetables (French & Stables 2003; French & Wechsler 2004). The interventions share many features, so only a few are described here to illustrate. For all of them, the outcomes were improved intake of the targeted foods or nutrients by students.

Fruit and Vegetable Interventions

Numerous interventions have focused on increasing fruit and vegetable intake. For example, two studies based on social cognitive theory and conducted with fourth and fifth graders involved not only a classroom component but also a number of changes in the school environment: improved variety and attractiveness of the fruits and vegetables served at lunch, availability of an extra fruit item at lunch when a dessert was served, and point-of-purchase signs in the cafeteria (Perry et al. 1998; Reynolds et al. 2000). Results showed that the interventions increased the intake of fruits and vegetables combined.

Fresh Fruit and Vegetable Program (USDA)

Eligible schools that apply can be funded by the USDA to receive baskets of fresh fruits and vegetables each day for each classroom. Surveys at the end of the academic year showed that high school students in intervention schools compared to those in schools not receiving the program were more likely to report eating more fruit and to be drinking 100% fruit juice. There was no change in vegetable intake (Davis et al. 2009).

ProChildren Study

In a group-randomized trial among 10- and 11-year-old children from schools in Norway, the Netherlands, and Spain, it was found that adjusted fruit and vegetable intake reported by the children from intervention schools was 20% higher than fruit and vegetable intake reported by children from control schools, particularly in the schools that more fully implemented the program (Te Velde et al. 2008).

Interventions Directed at Several Dietary Behaviors

Other interventions have addressed several dietary behaviors at once.

The Child and Adolescent Trial for Cardiovascular Health (CATCH)

CATCH was a large randomized study with third to fifth graders based on social cognitive theory and designed to lessen cardiovascular disease risk factors by focusing on decreasing fat intake, increasing intake of higher-fiber foods, and increasing physical activity (Luepker et al. 1996). It consisted of a classroom education component, physical education intervention, food service cafeteria intervention, and a parent/home component.

The food service intervention (the environmental component) focused on decreasing total fat, saturated fat, and sodium in the school meals through training of staff in the areas of menu planning, food purchasing, food preparation methods, and program promotion (e.g., posters, taste tests, table tests). The food service intervention successfully reduced the fat, sodium, and calories and increased the content of fiber and vitamins A and C in meals (Osganian et al. 1996). The success was due to methods that were used to change the staff's food preparation behaviors, a finding that has made this intervention a model for school cafeteria interventions (Hoelscher et al. 2003). The intervention was able to achieve a significant reduction in fat intake in the children and an increase in targeted mediators of behavior: behavior-relevant knowledge, behavioral intention, food choices, and perceived support from teachers and parents (Edmundson et al. 1996; Lytle et al. 1996).

Cookshop

An intervention study with children in kindergarten to the sixth grade, called Cookshop, was designed to increase preferences for and consumption of minimally processed whole grains and fresh vegetables; it combined cooking these foods in the classroom with multiple exposures to these same foods in the same recipes in the cafeteria (Liquori et al. 1998). Using fresh vegetables meant that children were actively involved in the food preparation process, such as cutting and chopping. Nutrition educators worked with school food service directors to provide training to the staff to also cook these same recipes from scratch. The study compared cooking as an educational strategy with an active hands-on educational strategy that did not involve food, but both groups received the environmental cafeteria component. All students took parent newsletters home. Monthly newsletters were available to all parents to pick up, with shopping tips and low-cost recipes.

The intervention was based on social cognitive theory and emphasized that eating a plant-based diet was not only important for personal health but also encouraged a more resource-conserving and sustainable food system. The results showed that actual cooking experiences and eating with peers in the classroom resulted in increased consumption of targeted foods as measured by plate waste observations in the lunchroom. Control classes, receiving the environmental intervention only, did not increase their intake of these foods, suggesting that increased awareness and motivation through education are needed along with environmental opportunities for action.

Dutch Obesity Intervention in Teenagers (Do-iT) Program

This was a multicomponent health promotion intervention for Dutch adolescents directed at influencing body composition and aerobic fitness by influencing the following behaviors: reduced consumption of sweetened beverages and high-calorie sacks, decreased sedentary behaviors, and increased physical activity (Singh et al. 2007). School cafeterias were asked to serve healthier products, restrict access to vending machines, serve smaller portions, and use labels on foods signifying better not (red label), sometimes (yellow label), and DO-iT (green label) foods. Schools increased time devoted to physical activity. Results showed a positive impact on weight but not on fitness and also on sweetened beverages but not other targeted behaviors. It also had an impact on some of the mediators (Singh et al. 2006; Singh et al. 2007).

Environmental-Change-Only Interventions

Several studies have focused on changes in the food environment only.

Elementary Grades

One study designed to increase fruits and vegetables intake among first- and third-grade students used as its intervention strategy increasing the availability and attractiveness of fruits and vegetables and having the school food service and staff daily encourage students to eat them. The intervention included special events, such as kickoffs, samplings, challenge weeks, a theater production, and a final meal (Perry et al. 2004). Students in the intervention schools significantly increased their total fruit intake. Researchers concluded that although this intervention was partly successful, multicomponent interventions are more powerful than cafeteria programs alone.

Studies that focused on increasing the availability or offerings of lower-fat entrées in the school lunch, with and without promotional activities, were able to moderately increase consumption of lower-fat entrées, but researchers concluded that including promotional activities was more effective (Whitaker et al. 1994).

Middle School Students

An environmental intervention in middle schools was directed at increasing physical activity and providing and marketing low-fat food items in all school food sources, including à la carte sources, school stores, and bag lunches (Sallis et al. 2003). It was successful in increasing physical activity in boys, but was not able to reduce fat intake of students at the schools, partly because of barriers to full implementation of the program.

Summary

These findings suggest that interventions involving the cafeteria and competitive foods are difficult to implement and, even when implemented, are more likely to be successful in improving student intakes of targeted foods if they are accompanied by promotional or educational activities and classroom curriculum that draw attention to the importance and availability of healthier options.

Farm to School Programs

Farm to School programs connect schools with local farms (Center for Food and Justice 2010). Schools buy and feature foods such as fruits, vegetables, eggs, honey, meat, and beans on their menus or offer farm-fresh salad bars as part of the National School Lunch Program. These programs also provide students experiential learning opportunities through farm visits, classroom visits by farmers, cooking demonstrations, school gardens, and recycling and composting programs. Through these programs, farmers have access to a new market and participate in a program designed to educate children about local food and agriculture. Such programs require the participation of a wide variety of people and organizations, and nutrition educators can have a key role. Other participants include parents, school principals, school board members, school food service staff, and students. In the United States, legislation now makes some funds available for such projects.

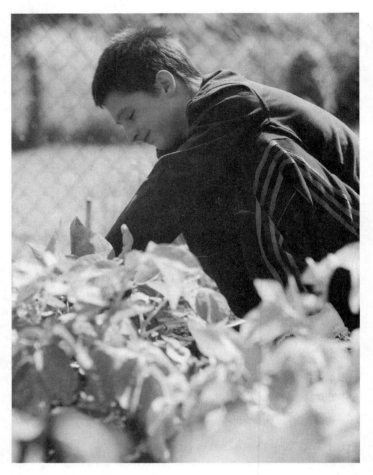

Community gardens, where youths can grow fresh produce, support healthy behaviors.

Food Pricing and Promotions in Schools

To educate decision makers about the importance of healthful food in their organizations, nutrition educators have to convince them that making the food environment more healthful is feasible financially. To do so, several nutrition education interventions have explored the role of changing pricing structure and promotions on sales of targeted foods in high schools and workplaces as a way to create an enabling environment.

Short-Term Study

One short-term study of three weeks found that when prices on fresh fruit, carrots, and salad were reduced 50%, sales of fruit went up 400% and carrots 200%. Salad sales did not change (French et al. 1997). Contextual factors were important—where the items were placed in the cafeteria area and how the items were presented (e.g., whether the baby carrots were prepackaged with an accompanying low-fat dip or were unlabeled in plastic cups with plastic wrap).

Longer-Term Study

A longer-term study of one school year found that increasing prices slightly on three popular high-fat foods as a way to subsidize lower prices on more healthful foods resulted in stable food service revenues and more nutritious foods being sold (Hannan et al. 2002). Another one-year study with both high schools and workplaces found that lower prices were effective in promoting choices of targeted food items in vending machines and that signage had a smaller but significant independent effect on sales (French et al. 2001). By providing such information to school administrators or school food service mangers, nutrition educators can help them in their decisions.

Promotional Activities

A study in high schools focused on implementing a large number of school-wide promotional activities rather than pricing. It found that over a two-year period, the number of promotions was associated with the increase in percentage of sales of lower-fat foods in à la carte areas of school cafeterias (Fulkerson et al. 2004). These results suggest that intense promotion can be an effective strategy in both elementary and secondary schools.

Awards to Health Promoting Schools

Some communities have initiated awards to recognize schools that make efforts to improve the food environment. One example is the Healthy Eating Champions Award for Elementary Schools program that recognizes and rewards schools for their outstanding commitment to the promotion of nutrition, for nutrition education, and for making healthy foods and beverages available (He et al. 2009). It was found that schools that participated had increased student awareness about healthy eating, more student involvement in healthy eating initiatives, and the creation of opportunities for goal setting and spirit boosting.

Workplaces

A majority of adults are employed in workplaces of some sort. Hence, what is available in and around such places can have an impact on food choices. A number of health promotion interventions in workplaces have attempted to make changes in the food environment by increasing the number of healthful low-fat and high-fiber foods and fruits and vegetables available in the employee cafeteria and other sources of food at work, such as vending machines (e.g., Sorensen et al. 1990; Sorensen et al. 1996). Nutrition and health professionals work with worksite decision makers to develop a variety of activities for the worksite. Along with other educational, promotional, organizational, and policy activities, these interventions have had a positive impact on eating patterns (Sorensen et al. 1999; Engbers et al. 2005). Here are a couple of examples.

Treatwell Program

An example of a worksite program to increase fruit and vegetable consumption that addressed multiple levels of influence is summarized in **Nutrition Education in Action 6-1**. The Treatwell program randomly assigned 22 worksites into three groups: minimal intervention controls, worksite intervention, and worksite-plus-family (Sorensen et al. 1998; Sorensen et al. 1999). The worksites were community health centers with racially and ethnically diverse employees, providing services to low-income community residents. The behavioral goal of the program and hence the expected outcome of the intervention was that the employees in these worksites would increase their consumption of fruits and vegetables. Nutrition Education in Action 6-1 lists the theoretical models that were used. The study also tested whether the intervention had an impact on the potential mediators of behavior change. These are shown in the table, along with how the changes were measured. (The results were

described earlier in this chapter in the section titled "Social Support in Workplaces.")

Local Foods at Workplaces

Increasing the purchase of locally grown produce through worksite sales was the objective of another intervention (Ross et al. 2000). Here, workers were given the opportunity to order local produce, which was then delivered to the worksite. This environmental change was accompanied by promotional materials about the farms that grew the produce and an opportunity to sample the produce. The delivery was very public so that friends' ordering and satisfaction could be observed to provide a social normative influence. Results showed that workers who ordered local foods at the worksite were motivated to purchase locally grown produce outside the worksite as well.

■ COMMUNITY-LEVEL ACTIVITIES

A *community* refers to both a physical locality where a group of people live and to a group of people who share common interests. Nutrition educators work in almost every community, so community projects abound.

Community Capacity Building

Community capacity may be described as the characteristics of communities that affect their ability to identify, mobilize, and address social and public health problems (Goodman et al. 1999). It is similar to the idea of social capital, where the structure of social relationships facilitates coordination and cooperation for mutual benefit. Nutrition educators can participate in the process by working in coalition with others to enhance collective efficacy and empowerment to increase community capacity.

Collective Efficacy

Collective efficacy is the belief of groups and community members that they have the capacity to take collective action to create change in their environment. Bandura (2001) notes that because human functioning is rooted in social systems, personal agency operates within a broad network of social structures that individuals, in turn, also help to create. Thus, personal agency and social structures operate interdependently. According to Bandura (2001), personal agency is not about self-centered individualism; rather, studies show that a high sense of efficacy tends to promote a prosocial orientation, involving cooperativeness and an interest in each other's welfare.

Collective efficacy can be enhanced by "equipping people with a firm belief that they can produce valued effects by their collective action and providing them with the means to do so" (Bandura 1997). This is a group enablement process. Group efficacy becomes more than the sum of the personal efficacies of group members because there is an interaction among members and a coordination of their skills, competencies, and activities. In parallel to personal self-efficacy, the strength of individuals' belief in their collective efficacy determines the goals they are willing to set, how much effort they put into the group's endeavors, how much they are willing to persist in the face of difficulties, their morale and resilience, and their level of performance.

Building Collective Efficacy Through Group Goal Setting

Collective efficacy involves the power to produce change in the social or political environment. Social cognitive theory suggests that to build collective efficacy, individuals need to learn how to exert influence

NUTRITION EDUCATION IN ACTION 6-1

Theories Used and Potential Mediators of Behavior Change in the Treatwell 5-a-Day Worksite Program

Level of Influence	Intervention Audience	Theoretical Models	Hypotheses About Mediators of Behavior Change	Measures
Intrapersonal	· Worker	· Social cognitive theory · Health belief model	· Higher self-efficacy about dietary change is associated with increased fruit and vegetable consumption. · Knowledge of the diet–cancer link (outcome expectations: perceived risk) is associated with increased fruit and vegetable consumption.	· Self-efficacy · Knowledge (outcome expectations)
Interpersonal	· Family · Coworkers	· Social support · Social networks and ties · Social cognitive theory	· High family and coworker support for dietary change is associated with increased fruit and vegetable consumption. · High family support for dietary change is associated with increased availability of fruits and vegetables in the home. · The type of family ties will influence the strength of the relationships between family support and changing eating habits.	· Family support · Coworker support · Social norms · Availability of fruits and vegetables in the home · Type of family ties
Organizational	· Worksite	· Organizational change and development · Policy	· Worksite mean increases in fruit and vegetable consumption will be greatest where fruits and vegetables are most available and a catering policy supports the purchase of healthy foods. · Program implementation and participation will be highest where effective communication channels exist and policies permit employee change agents to participate. · Coworker support for dietary changes will be highest in worksites with high coworker cohesion and positive labor–management relations.	· Worksite characteristics
Community	· Media (national campaign) · Grocery store	· Social marketing	· Workers reporting awareness of the national campaign are more likely to increase consumption of fruits and vegetables. · Workers reporting participating in grocery store programs are more likely to report increased consumption of fruits and vegetables.	· Awareness of grocery store campaign · Participation in grocery store campaign

Source: Sorensen, G., M. K. Hunt, N. Cohen, et al. 1998. Worksite and family education for dietary change: The Treatwell 5-a-Day program. *Health Education Research* 13:577–591. Used with permission.

over community practices that affect their lives. The process for building collective efficacy is rather like a group goal-setting process: group members identify the issue of concern, set small goals to address the concern, and, when these produce tangible results, come to believe that they have the capability to change the social and political environments in which they live. This leads them to believe that they can overcome even more difficult problems and hence to set more ambitious goals. Other processes are also used. However, they all work, in part, by enhancing individuals' sense of efficacy that they can bring about tangible changes in their lives. There is evidence that skills in advocacy and community building raise both personal and collective efficacy, which can result in collective actions that may in turn change community practices and policies.

Empowerment

What is empowerment? *Empowerment*, a term that is used loosely and has many definitions, is similar to the process of group enablement of social cognitive theory. Many see it as largely a personal process in which individuals develop and use needed knowledge, competence, or confidence for making their own decisions (somewhat like self-efficacy). Some may even refer to learning to read food labels as empowerment. However, empowerment is generally described as "a social process through which individuals, communities, and organizations gain mastery over their lives, in the context of changing their social and political environment to improve quality of life" (Wallerstein 1992). That is, it is a social process of recognizing and enhancing people's abilities as a group to meet their own needs and to mobilize the necessary resources to take more control of their environment. It is about political and social power, not just personal power.

Education for Social Action

The concept of empowerment education was originally developed by Paolo Freiere of Brazil as a "pedagogy of the oppressed," or education for critical consciousness, that involves developing an understanding of root causes of problems. The central method for empowerment is *conscientizacion*, or group consciousness-raising (Friere 1970, 1973). Empowerment education is a process whereby the group members develop identity and social support for each other, specify the problems in their lives, reflect on the root causes of these problems, and develop plans of social or political action. It is thus education for social change. It emphasizes the importance of social context in food- and nutrition-related practices and shifts the viewpoint away from victim blame and toward system blame. However, the social context is not to be seen as a structural barrier to good health that needs to be changed by health promotion interventions much the way a wall needs to be torn down, but as something to be understood and transformed by people and communities through the process of empowerment (Travers 1997a).

Strategies to Strengthen Empowerment

Nutrition educators may facilitate this educational process, when appropriate, or provide technical assistance. More specifically, in this consciousness-raising process, the educator poses problems to the group participants, who draw upon their own knowledge and experiences to try to understand their lives in relation to the problem. Group members, through dialogue, come to a collective understanding of the root causes of the problem and begin to see how they can make changes in their situation. They become empowered to transform their reality through change in the social or political condition of their lives. Such an empowerment process can bring about not only *personal empowerment* but also empowerment at the *organizational level*, where the influence of the organization in broader society is enhanced, and at the *community level*, where individuals and organizations work together to bring about desired outcomes in the community (Israel et al. 1994). As the word *power* in the term *empowerment* suggests, the process is ultimately about changed power relationships between individuals within groups and between groups and social structures. Such an approach has been advocated for nutrition education (Kent 1988; Rody 1988; Travers 1997a; Arnold et al. 2001).

Projects Focusing on Empowerment

Several examples from the food and nutrition field illustrate this approach.

Senior Citizens Project

The Tenderloin Senior Organizing Project (TSOP) involved older adults who lived isolated lives in hotel residences in a crime-ridden neighborhood (Minkler 1997). Health educators used a combination of educational and organizing approaches to assist residents to identify issues of importance to them, understand the root causes of these issues in the political and social structures of the community, and develop social support and a sense of community through group discussions and tasks. The hotel residents recognized the need to work with other hotels and community groups on shared problems, such as crime. As they achieved success on this issue, including convincing the mayor to put more beat patrol officers in the neighborhood, they took on the issue of poor food availability. They established mini-markets in three hotels, a coopera-

tive breakfast program in another, and a no-cook cookbook for those not allowed to cook in their hotels. As they developed more collective efficacy and became more empowered, they took more control of the project and the health education staff decreased their roles, serving primarily as resource persons.

Parent Center

Another nutrition education program for social change involved low-income women who met weekly informally over coffee at a Parent Center (Travers 1997b). The issue of common concern to them was feeding their families on a low income. The nutrition educator posed questions that led to group dialogue and discussion, out of which emerged the group's perception that foods cost more in low-income neighborhoods. This led them to make a structured comparison study of prices for foods in their local stores and prices in stores of the same chain in middle-income neighborhoods.

- *Role of the nutrition educator.* The nutrition educator provided technical assistance on this task. When their findings showed that prices in inner-city stores were consistently higher than in middle-income neighborhoods, the women came to realize that the difficulty they had in getting adequate nutrition was partly the result of social inequities. They came to the decision to write to the stores to express their concern about inequities in pricing and quality. This resulted in the chain store lowering the prices within the low-income neighborhoods. The nutrition educator facilitated the process by obtaining a word processor and writing the letter with them. This success led to a sense of empowerment. The activity also led them to recognize that their welfare allowances were not adequate to meet their needs. The impact of this information on them personally was a relief from self-blame as they realized that their inability to purchase enough food for their families was not because of their personal inadequacies but because of government policy.
- *Parent action.* This then led them to decide to take action toward change. They wrote letters to political leaders and worked with other community groups, resulting in some increase in the welfare allowances. Finally, when some time later there was an attempt to close the Parent Center because of budget cuts, the women organized a march on city hall and got media attention, which prevented closure.

School-Based Intervention

In a more formal setting of a school, an empowerment process was used in a curriculum development project (da Cunha, Contento, & Morin 2000). In this process, the nutrition educator first met with the teachers, school food personnel, and administrators in several high-poverty schools to raise questions about the problem of poor nutrition among the students. The members of the school staff were concerned. The schools nominated a small group, made up of teachers, school food service personnel, and a parent, to meet with the nutrition educator to address their concerns. They realized that they needed to find out more about the problem, so they designed and conducted a comprehensive needs assessment among the students and their families. From this needs assessment they then designed a nutrition education curriculum to address the needs identified and helped each other in the implementation of the curriculum. The group met weekly after school on their own time for seven months. The nutrition educator used a consciousness-raising and empowerment process throughout, helping the group, through dialogue and interpretations based on their own experience and knowledge, to make their own decisions. The nutrition educator acted as a facilitator and provided technical assistance in conducting the needs assessment and developing the curriculum but did not direct the choice of content.

Youth Empowerment

Empowerment of youths was the basis of a project in which high school students operated farm stands in low-income communities (Hughes, Blalock, & Strieter 2005). The youths made changes in their communities by creating access to affordable, locally grown food and supporting local farmers and growers. At the same time, the youths learned important skills in business, finance, and working together in mature and productive ways, preparing them for the workforce.

Summary

In all the food-related cases just described, we can see that the specific issues of concern are identified by the people in the community rather than the intervention staff, that the process aims to bring about social change through the empowerment of individuals and groups, that the role of the nutrition educator is to facilitate and advocate rather than to be the expert who provides all the information, and that forming collaborations may enhance effectiveness of action. It should also be noted that collective efficacy and empowerment approaches work on a long time frame, often involving months and years, but the environmental changes brought about are more likely to be long-lasting.

Building Coalitions and Collaborations

In organizational-level interventions, working in collaboration with decision makers and policy makers is vital. This is even more true at the community level. Here, nutrition educators in most cases develop partnerships and participate in coalitions with other groups who have similar goals to bring about community changes that are supportive of the behavioral goals of the nutrition education program. Nutrition educators participate in numerous coalitions. Here are a few examples to illustrate the types of collaborations in which individual nutrition educators or programs can participate.

Community Coalitions and Partnerships: Examples

Building Breastfeeding-Friendly Communities

An example in the United States of a collaboration regarding a very specific behavior is a program wherein WIC nutritionists worked with other food assistance programs and a variety of community partners to build breastfeeding-friendly communities (Singleton et al. 2005). The aim was to increase public awareness, acceptance, and community support for breastfeeding. The program in one state included a public forum with 145 key community stakeholders to develop a blueprint for action to assist communities, families, schools and child-care centers, health care systems, policy makers, and worksites in their efforts to make breastfeeding the norm for infant feeding. The partnership also initiated a public awareness campaign and activities to advocate for changes in health care systems, the insurance industry, the business community, and educational systems to encourage breastfeeding, and advocacy for changes in the availability of resources for community organizations and families.

Working with Low-Income Audiences

Another example is a partnership between two organizations—Share Our Strength and Head Start—to improve the diets of low-income com-

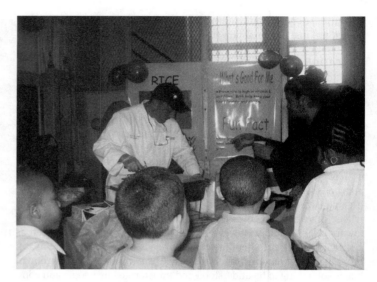

A school food chef demonstrates a new lunch recipe and provides opportunities for children to taste.

munity members. Share Our Strength is a national organization with a presence in many communities that seeks to inspire and organize individuals and businesses to share their strengths to help end hunger. Its national nutrition education program, Operation Frontline, mobilizes volunteer chefs, nutritionists, and financial planners to teach nutrition, healthy cooking, and food budgeting classes to individuals at risk of hunger. Head Start provides education and meals to low-income preschool children. Operation Frontline teaches its six-week curriculum to Head Start program parents, providing an example of a partnership between a government program and a community program to enhance the reach and effectiveness of both organizations (Jones 2005). The program has resulted in increased parental knowledge and skills.

Working in Coalitions: Benefits and Costs

The attempts of any given group to bring about social change are greatly enhanced by building coalitions with other groups who have similar goals. Coalitions and collaborations can mobilize material resources and peoples' knowledge, skills, and enthusiasms to achieve desired goals in a way that is not possible for small groups alone. There are costs as well, however. Collaborative efforts are complex, and leadership roles, decision making, social support, and social network concerns are issues that must be addressed satisfactorily for all collaborating groups involved; working these out may take time and effort. Even when coalition members are satisfied and actively involved, this does not guarantee that the coalition will be effective in achieving agreed-upon goals. Leadership and management must also be effective.

Successful Partnerships

Factors that are likely to enhance successful collaboration include the following: a shared and agreed-upon vision and mission, reached by consensus through open dialogue, negotiation, and problem solving; a unique purpose that is meaningful to members; tasks that are clear and empowering; a sense of productivity and efficiency; a skilled convener and facilitator of team building and conflict resolution; broad-based involvement in decision making; open, frequent communication, with communication feedback loops; benefits that accrue to members for participation; relationships that are based on trust, openness, and respect; power sharing; and adequate resources (Rosenthal 1998).

Nutrition Education Networks

Nutrition education networks have also come into existence in many states in the United States, with funding from the USDA and other sources. These networks are partnerships and coalitions among the Supplemental Nutrition Assistance Program, the Cooperative Extension Service, private volunteer organizations such as the American Cancer Society or American Heart Association, grocery stores, universities, and others with the aim of fostering collaboration among food assistance programs and developing and delivering consistent nutrition messages across network partnerships to low-income, Supplemental Nutrition Assistance Program (SNAP) audiences. These partnerships have used a variety of channels to reach these audiences—direct and indirect nutrition education as well as social marketing (http://www.csres.usda .gov/nea/food/fsne/fsne.html).

Nutrition education networks often work with physicians, health departments, school districts, and community-based organizations to promote healthy eating and physical activity habits in school-aged children and their parents. They have also initiated a wide range of activities to promote policy initiatives and to empower people to be advocates for healthier food and activity environments in their schools and communities. They often have worked to change organizational policies and the physical environment to help low-income families eat healthier diets, be more active, and participate in USDA nutrition assistance programs. An example is the California Nutrition Network, which sponsors a wide range of nutrition education activities (California Department of Public Health 2007).

Community-Level Interventions

Numerous community-level interventions have been conducted over the years, including early large-scale projects such as the Stanford, Minnesota and Pawtucket heart health programs (Shea & Basch 1990a, 1990b). *Community-based* interventions are those in which the community is very much involved in the design, implementation, and evaluation of the program through partnerships and coalitions. This allows for the intervention to be based on the assets of the community as well as the deep understanding members of the community have about themselves. Many recent interventions have addressed the issue of obesity (Economos & Irish-Hauser 2007; DeMattia & Denney 2008). Here are a couple of examples.

Shape Up Somerville (SUS): Eat Smart, Play Hard

SUS was a community-based participatory research project that illustrates the social ecological approach. It addressed the concerns about childhood obesity by addressing children's before school, during school, after school, home, and community environments. It is described in **Nutrition Education in Action 6-2**.

HOPE (Health Opportunities, Partnerships, Empowerment) Works

HOPE Works was a community-based participatory research project that recognized the importance of positive psychology and hope to make health and life changes. It involved low-income, ethnically diverse rural women. The model used the idea of "talking circles" in Native American communities. Community women were trained to organize and facilitate HOPE circles of 8 to 12 women from their social networks. These circles met twice a month for 6 months, where they set goals for

health and social/economic improvement and learned about healthy eating, physical activity, economic empowerment, financial literacy, and developing small businesses. The program evaluation involved surveys, pedometers, food diaries, and weight measurements. Preliminary results showed that HOPE Circle participants decreased their body mass index (BMI) compared to comparison women and significantly increased their fruit and vegetable intake and physical activity. They also started small businesses (Benedict & Campbell 2009).

Farmers' Markets

Many communities now have initiated farmers' markets where local growers can bring their produce and other farm products into cities at markets set up by the community. Supplemental Nutrition Assistance Program Electronic Benefit Transfer (EBT) cards often are accepted at these markets, making fresh local foods available to low-income residents in communities.

Physical Locality Effects

There is evidence that neighborhoods have an impact on obesity and health (Harrington & Eliot 2009; Dengel et al. 2009). Within neighborhoods are many retail food stores such as supermarkets and grocery stores, and restaurants and fast food outlets. There is an association between access to supermarkets and healthier food intakes, such as increased fruit and vegetable intakes, mostly because supermarkets tend to offer a greater variety of foods at a lower cost. Nutrition interventions within grocery stores using point-of-choice information, increased availability, increased variety, pricing, and promotional strategies have resulted in moderate improvements in healthy eating behavior such as fruit and vegetable consumption (Glanz et al. 2007).

The term *food deserts* has come to describe areas within urban centers as well as in rural areas where low-income people do not have access to fruits, vegetables, and other wholesome, healthful foods at affordable costs (Smith & Morton 2009). Researchers are using geographic information systems (GISs) to map locations of supermarkets in geographic areas to identify such deserts. Nutrition educators have worked in coalition with others to change policies so as to encourage supermarkets to locate in these deserts.

The built environment and walkability of neighborhoods have also been shown to be associated with health conditions. Walkability includes the notion of safe streets, attractive sidewalks with places of interest, and connections to places people need to go. Higher neighborhood walkability, for example, is associated with more walking, lower BMI, and lower blood pressure (Rohere, Pierce, & Dennison 2004; Rundle et al. 2008; Li et al. 2009). Again, in coalition with others, nutrition educators have worked to increase availability of safe and attractive places for people to walk.

Investment in Community-Level Actions

A number of foundations have invested grant funding to improve community empowerment and changes in policy and environment to support healthy eating and physical activity. Among them is the Robert Wood Johnson Foundation's (RWJF) Active Living and Healthy Eating (Sallis et al. 2009) and Bridging the Gap (Chaloupka & Johnston 2007) initiatives, which support research to identify promising policy and environmental strategies for increasing physical activity, promoting healthy eating, and preventing obesity (http://www.rwjf.org).

The W. F. Kellogg Foundation's national Food & Fitness Initiative within its Food and Community Program has invested locally in several communities around the United States in collaborative efforts dedicated

NUTRITION EDUCATION IN ACTION **6-2**

Shape Up Somerville (SUS)—Eat Smart, Play Hard: A Social Ecological Approach

Environmental factors at the community level may contribute to the development and maintenance of obesity. Children, in particular, have very little control over their food choices and options for physical activity. School-based programs have been developed, but school time accounts for less than 50% of children's waking hours. Shape Up Somerville was developed to change the environment to prevent obesity in elementary school children.

Program

This three-year program was directed at children in grades 1 through 3 and was designed to bring about energy balance by increasing physical activity options and availability of healthful foods within children's before-, during-, and after-school, home, and community environments. It used a multifaceted collaborative community participatory research (CBPR) approach. The community was involved in all phases: designing, implementing, and evaluating the intervention, and identifying how the data would be used to improve the health of the community. The intervention involved not only children, parents, and teachers but also food service providers, city departments, policy makers, health care providers, restaurants, and the media.

Evaluation

Three matched, culturally diverse communities were assigned to intervention and control conditions. About 1,200 children in public schools in the intervention community participated in the classroom curriculum and pre and post evaluations.

Results

- *Students:* The intervention resulted in a significant decrease in the BMI z-scores in children ($P = .001$).
- *School environment:* More fruits, vegetables, and whole-grain and low-fat milk products were available; menus and à la carte items were brought into closer compliance with guidelines; attitudes of students, parents and guardians, school faculty, and food service staff improved; and policies related to food in schools were adopted.
- *Restaurants:* About one third of restaurants actively recruited became SUS-approved restaurants, agreeing to serve smaller portions and offer healthier options. SUS approval was marketed to the community.

Components of the SUS program	
Before School • Breakfast program • Walk to school campaign	*Home* • Parent outreach and education • Family events • Child's "Health Report Card"
During School • School health office • School food service • SUS classroom curriculum — 30-minute nutrition and physical activity lesson each week — 10-minute daily "Cool Moves" • Enhanced recess • School Wellness policy development *After School* • SUS after-school curriculum • Walk from school campaign	*Community* • SUS community advisory council • Ethnic-minority group collaborations • City employee wellness campaign • Farmers' market initiative • SUS "approved" restaurants • Annual 5K family fitness fair • Media—columns and ads • City ordinances on walkability/bikeability

Sources: Economos, C. D., R. R. Hyatt, J. P. Goldberg, et al. 2007. A community intervention reduces BMI z-score in children: Shape Up Somerville first year results. *Obesity* 15:1325–1336; Economos, C. D., S. C. Folta, J. P. Goldberg, et al. 2009. A community-based restaurant initiative to increase availability of healthy menus options in Somerville, Massachusetts: Shape Up Somerville. *Prevention of Chronic Disease* 6(3). http://www.cdd.gov/pcd/issues/2009/jul/o8_0165.htm; and Goldberg, J. P., J. J. Collins, S. C. Folta, et al. 2009. Retooling food service for early elementary school in Somerville, Massachusetts: The Shape Up Somerville experience. *Prevention of Chronic Disease* 6(3):A103.

to changing the policies, practices, and systems that prevent communities from being healthy. The foundation aims to create vibrant communities that provide equitable access to affordable, healthy, locally grown food and safe and inviting places for physical activity and play (http://www.kkf.org/faf).

■ POLICY AND SYSTEMS CHANGE ACTIVITIES

Policy activities are extremely important to help make the healthful choices the easy ones. They enable changes in systems and social structures to facilitate the enactment of healthful food and physical activity behaviors. Policy complements education and environmental change (Rothschild 1999).

Relationship Among Education, Environmental Change, Policy, and Systems

Education, as we have seen, involves a combination of theory-based strategies to increase awareness, enhance motivation, and facilitate the voluntary adoption or maintenance of behaviors that are conducive to health. Some researchers note that it does not provide, on its own, direct or immediate reward or punishment (Rothschild 1999). Sometimes, the anticipated outcomes nutrition educators bring to the public's attention are far into the future, such as "If you drink milk now, you are less likely to develop osteoporosis when you are old."

Environmental change attempts to make the environment favorable for the new behavior. Changing the environment can promote voluntary changes in behavior by offering audiences the benefits people want and reducing the barriers they are concerned about, accompanied, in social marketing, by effective communications or persuasion to enhance motivation. Environmental changes reduce barriers by providing the products or services that would make enacting the behavior easier, for example, by increasing the availability of fruits and vegetables in grocery stores in the audience's community and making them more accessible through pricing incentives or the use of coupons. In this case, the anticipated outcomes or rewards are more immediate.

Policy complements these approaches and can also have an important and positive role here. Policies and regulations can ensure the performance of a desirable behavior when it would be difficult to carry out because of social pressure to conform to a different standard. For example, food policies or nutrition standards for all foods available in school could make it easier for students to eat more fruits and vegetables or drink fewer sweetened beverages, even though less healthy options might be more appealing to students and financially desirable to schools. Nutrition educators need to participate in relevant food policy decisions. This may require them to serve as advocates for healthy policies to policy makers and even lawmakers at the local or national level.

Systems changes, often linked to policy change, can be made to be more supportive of healthful action. A *system* is a group of independent but interrelated and interacting elements—individuals, institutions, and infrastructure—that form a unified whole. Examples include the school system, the transportation system, and the parks and recreation system. Thus the individuals, institutions, and infrastructure that make up the food system are involved in the interconnected activities of producing, processing, distributing, retailing, preparing, and consuming food. Systems are not static but constantly changing and evolving. Public policy, organizational policy, and other actions can bring about changes in systems. System change complements other venues for facilitating healthful action.

Organizational-Level Policy Activities

Organizational policies regarding school, worksite, and community food environments influence people's food choices and eating patterns. Thus, an important venue for nutrition education is to work with policy makers to develop or modify existing policies to make them more supportive of healthy eating and active living.

School Policies

School Food Environment

Many food-related environmental issues that influence youth food intake in schools need to be addressed by institutional policy action rather than, or in addition to, classroom education because the school food environment is challenging:

- *Food used in school fundraising.* Short of funds, many schools sell food products to raise money; these products are usually high-fat or high-sugar items such as candy, chips, or sweetened beverages.
- *Food is often used in the classroom as a reward or incentive.* Again, most often such foods tend to be high-fat and high-sugar, largely because these are liked by students.
- *Food advertising.* In schools, advertising of food occurs directly on vending machines, book covers, wall boards, hallway decorations, sports scoreboards, and in student publications and yearbooks, and indirectly through coupons to fast food outlets given for academic achievement.
- *Contracts for beverage sales.* In schools, contracts, usually for soft drinks, have been common in exchange for signing bonuses and a percentage of the profits. Beverage contracts present a nutrition education challenge because the schools must urge students to consume these beverages to guarantee contracted minimum purchases, yet nutrition guidelines would advocate for healthier options on a regular basis.

In response to these challenges, the Institute of Medicine developed recommendations for nutritional standards for foods and beverages available in the school environment outside the USDA school meals program (Institute of Medicine 2007). These include making only healthful foods and drinks available in all venues during the school day.

Local Wellness Policies

Over the years, nutrition educators have advocated that schools form school nutrition advisory councils or health councils made up of teachers, administrators, parents, students, and intervention staff to assess the overall school food environment, consider and discuss issues, and advance school-level policy that promotes a healthful food environment so as to make the healthful choice the easy choice (Kubik, Lytle, & Story 2001; Lytle et al. 2004). In the United States, such an approach has become reality. The Child Nutrition and WIC Reauthorization Act of 2004 required each local educational agency participating in a program authorized by the National School Lunch Act or the Child Nutrition Act to establish a local school wellness policy. The policy at a minimum has to include the following (Child Nutrition and WIC Reauthorization Act 2004):

- Goals for nutrition education, physical activity, and other school-based activities that are designed to promote student wellness
- Nutrition guidelines selected by the local school for all foods available on campus during the school day, with the objectives of promoting student health and reducing childhood obesity

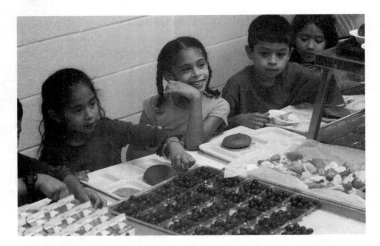

Local school wellness policies have improved the nutritional value of school lunches.

- Guidelines for reimbursable school meals that are no less restrictive than regulations and guidance of the USDA for program requirements and nutrition standards
- A plan for measuring implementation of the local wellness policy

The law requires the following participants to be involved in the wellness policy process: parents, students, representatives of the school food authority, the school board, school administrators, and the public. A nutrition educator is not specifically required to be part of the team, but can offer his or her services as a member of the public or as a parent.

Although all schools or school districts have such policies in place, the comprehensiveness of the policies differ and the degree to which they are implemented in schools also differ. In a survey of schools across the United States, changes in food service operations included the use of nutrition guidelines for à la carte foods, beverages, fundraisers, parties, and vending (Longley & Sneed 2009). Other research also shows some progress (U.S. Department of Agriculture 2005; Story, Nanney, & Schwartz 2009), but much still needs to be done and nutrition educators can help with the process in collaboration with the schools.

Workplace Policies

Many interventions in the worksite have tested a comprehensive, multilevel approach to creating an environment supportive of healthy eating by addressing organizational issues as well as the physical and social environments (Sorensen et al. 1998; Beresford et al. 2001). Health professionals are very important for educating decision makers and management about the importance of food and health issues and convincing them to take action. They also can initiate programs and provide services and technical support. However, they need to work in collaboration with both employees and management to develop policies and procedures so as to implement and institutionalize programs.

A review of such studies finds that a number of organizational factors are related to program effectiveness (Sorensen et al. 2002):

- Management commitment and supervisory support are essential. Policies need to be modified and this requires management support.
- Worker involvement in planning and implementation is just as important. This can be done through such mechanisms as an

"employee advisory board" at each site and through delivery of the intervention by peers. The employee advisory board chooses the intervention components to be implemented in the individual worksite setting, disseminates program messages and information throughout the worksite, and encourages long-term incorporation of the program into the worksite (Sorensen et al. 1990; Sorensen et al. 1992; Cousineau et al. 2008).

The more that employees are involved, the greater are the number of activities implemented (Hunt et al. 2000). Worksite management must put in place policies to permit and encourage employees to take work time to participate in these health promotion activities (Williams et al. 2007).

Community- and City-Level Food Policy Activities

Many community organizations focus on food policy. For example, the food policy council is composed of stakeholders from various segments of a state or local food system. Councils can be officially sanctioned through a government action such as an executive order or can be grassroots efforts. The primary goal of many food policy councils is to examine the operation of a local food system and provide ideas or recommendations for how it can be improved. Nutrition educators are often members of such councils to broaden the scope of the councils, in which members may be more concerned with emergency food assistance or agriculture policy in the most traditional sense (see http://www.statefoodpolicy.org).

Various food security coalitions and farm and food projects also work to analyze and develop policy initiatives to link local farmers and communities so as to rebuild and restore regional food and agriculture systems to enhance the economic livelihoods of family farms and rural communities and at the same time provide healthy and affordable food for the community (e.g., see http://www.foodsecurity.org).

Cities have also become involved in food and physical fitness policy. Some cities such as New York City have initiated regulations that require chain fast food restaurants to post calorie counts of food items on the menu board itself. Cities can also enact regulations so that mobile carts get permits to sell fresh fruits and vegetables in city streets, becoming green carts. Another example is a recommendation of the president of Manhattan borough, New York City, that one fifth of foods used in government-related venues come from local "food sheds," a term that is analogous to watersheds (Stringer 2009).

National-Level Public Policy

The main vehicle for national public policy in relation to food is through advocacy action in relation to proposed or existing legislation. These activities are described in Chapter 18.

■ STRATEGIES TO IMPROVE ENVIRONMENTAL AND POLICY SUPPORTS FOR ACTION OR BEHAVIOR CHANGE

Based on the considerations just discussed, nutrition educators can use many different kinds of activities to address environmental determinants of health actions or behavior change. In most of these activities, nutrition educators need to work in collaboration with others, such as food or service providers and decision makers. This usually involves educating decision makers or policy makers in organizations and communities about the importance of food and nutrition issues, and then building coalitions with them to develop and implement plans to enhance the opportunities for individuals to engage in identified health-promoting actions. It also means collaborating with program participants and other like-minded community groups to work toward developing or revising public policies, or even legislation, to support the behaviors or issues that are of concern to the program.

Figure 6-2 shows how nutrition education can be directed at various levels of influence using the logic model: the individual and household level; the interpersonal level; the institutional, organizational, and community level; and the social structures, policies, and systems level. The educational activities at both the individual and interpersonal levels

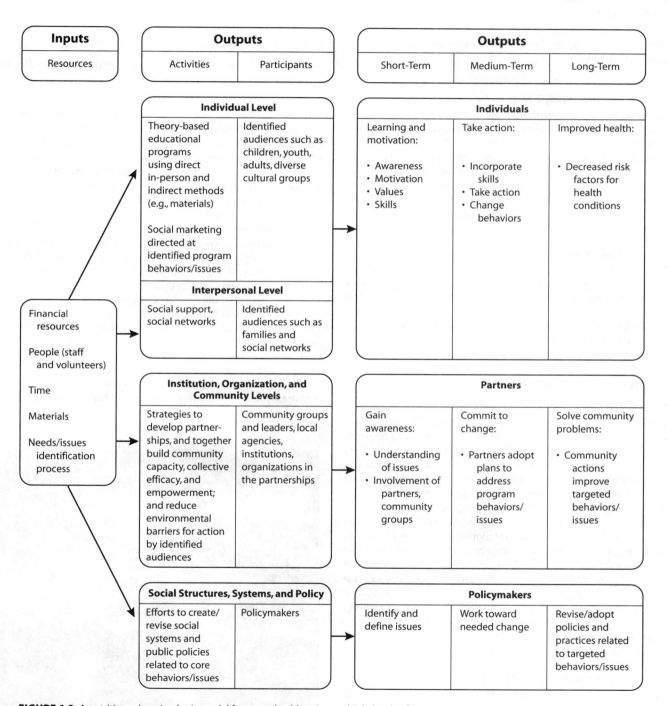

FIGURE 6-2 A nutrition education logic model framework addressing multiple levels of intervention.

Source: Based on Helen Chipman (national coordinator), Supplemental Nutrition Assistance Program Education (SNAP-Ed), NIFA/USDA, and Land Grant University System Partnership. 2006, January. Community Nutrition Education (CNE) Logic Model, Version 2: Overview. http://www.nifa.usda.gov/nea/food/fsne/logic.html. Used with permission.

address personal mediators of action or behavior change, such as beliefs, attitudes, affect, and skills, with immediate-, intermediate-, and extended outcomes for individuals. The activities at the other levels are directed at environmental determinants of behavior change and are also designed to affect individuals, but in this case by making the healthy action also the easy action through changes in policy, systems, and social structures.

Nutrition Education Activities Directed at the Interpersonal Level

Social Networks and Social Support

Enhancing Existing Social Networks

To enhance social support for the key food- and nutrition-related behavior or behaviors that have been identified as of concern to the program (e.g., increasing breastfeeding rates, increasing the consumption of fruits and vegetables), existing social networks can be called upon and expanded. For example, parent associations in schools, employee associations at workplaces, and groups that meet regularly in communities and organizations may be interested in nutrition issues. Nutrition education programs can work with these groups to make them more supportive of the targeted behaviors or practices.

Developing New Social Network Linkages

Programs frequently create social support for program participants by initiating a social support group through which new social network linkages are built. For example, a group can be developed for those in a workplace who are interested in weight control or weight acceptance. Support groups can be developed at a health center for those with HIV/AIDS, or cooking classes and behavioral change sessions can be created for participants in a program.

Organizational-Level Activities

Changing the Food Environment

Foods offered at nutrition education program sites, such as schools, workplaces, communities, soup kitchens, or food banks, can be modified to make them more supportive of the healthful behaviors identified as important by nutrition educators or by participants. In schools, this means making changes in the school meal offerings, vending machines, à la carte offerings, and food items sold in school stores.

Bringing about changes at such sites may require the use of both motivational- and action-phase activities, this time directed at the providers of food as the audience so that they are motivated to make changes in the foods offered. Professional development workshops and incentives are important here. Changes in the food offered may require changes in organizational policy and union rules so that food service staff can make the changes, which will require negotiations and advocacy. Making such food changes possible may also require changes in physical facilities at sites such as schools or other locations so that foods can actually be cooked or prepared on site. All of these actions require coalition building with groups that have authority in the relevant areas.

Pricing and Promotional Activities

Changes in the pricing of food items can be helpful in supporting healthful eating. As we have seen, large price changes are effective in increasing the sales of healthy items in organizations but are not financially sustainable over the long term. A more sustainable strategy is to raise prices slightly (5% to 10%) on more popular, high-fat, high-sugar foods

to subsidize more healthful, but higher-priced foods such as fruits and vegetables or lower-fat alternatives (sold at, say, 15% lower than otherwise) in such a way as to be revenue neutral to the organization in which the food sales occur. Attractive presentation of the foods and promotional activities can further increase the choice of these foods. Again, nutrition educators need to work with food providers to bring about such changes.

Community-Level Activities

Building Community Capacity: Facilitating Collective Efficacy and Empowerment

Collective Efficacy

The processes of enhancing collective efficacy and empowerment are somewhat similar. In the process of enhancing collective efficacy, group members, with the technical assistance of the nutrition educator, identify the issue of concern to them in the social and political environments. They can start out by setting small goals that will help to address the concern. When these are accomplished, the group members can pose even more difficult problems and set more ambitious goals. Such an approach can be effective with many age groups, particularly youth.

Empowerment strategies generally involve some sort of consciousness-raising process, whereby the educator poses problems to the group participants and asks them to draw on their own knowledge and experiences to try to understand their lives in relation to the problem. Group members, through dialogue, come to a collective understanding of the root causes of the problems and begin to see how they can make changes in their situation. They then set goals for actions that they will take to transform their reality through making changes in the social or political condition of their lives. In these settings, the role of the nutrition educator is to facilitate the process at the beginning, if needed, until the group has developed its own agendas and procedures and no longer needs the nutrition educator. Another possibility is that a group has already initiated community action and needs the nutrition educator as a resource person.

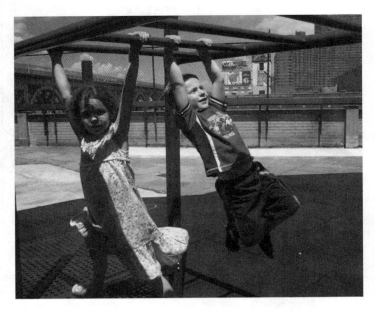

Playgrounds in a community encourage physical activity.

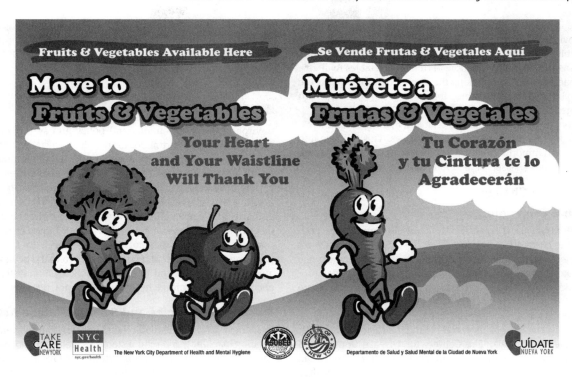

FIGURE 6-3 New York City Department of Health and Mental Hygiene: Diet.
Source: Courtesy of the New York City Department of Health and Mental Hygiene.

Community-Based Programs

Developing community-based interventions requires that nutrition educators work in collaboration or partnership with various sectors within the community, perhaps community centers, health centers, food banks, churches, community gardens, schools, restaurants, and so forth. The role of the nutrition educator can vary considerably, from being a member of the team and only providing technical expertise in the food, nutrition, and activity areas, to providing more of a coordinating or organizing role. This means that the nutrition educator must have a deep understanding of the community and respect for a diversity of backgrounds.

Informational Environment

Information provided in public forums serves several purposes. It can provide motivational (why-to) or instrumental (how-to) information on an important issue. However, the information can also help to establish social and community norms that are supportive of dietary change. For example, numerous posters about breastfeeding or eating fruits and vegetables can encourage people to see these behaviors as the social norm. They can also serve as cues to action. In addition to posters in schools, at work, or in community centers, billboards in the community can help establish norms and serve as cues to action. Promotions through other media, such as radio and magazines, can be supportive of the behavior change that is targeted by the intervention. Studies have shown that posters could increase stair use in blue- and white-collar worksites, shopping centers, and other locations (Kerr et al. 2000, 2001; Kwak et al. 2007).

The New York City Department of Health has provided posters for use in multiple settings. Two are shown in **Figure 6-3** and **Figure 6-4**: one

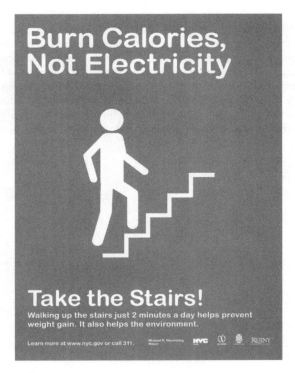

FIGURE 6-4 New York City Department of Health and Mental Hygiene: Exercise.
Source: Courtesy of the New York City Department of Health and Mental Hygiene.

poster is for use in small neighborhood grocery stores. As you can see, the graphic provides why-to, or motivational, information: "Move to Fruits & Vegetables. Your Heart and Your Waistline Will Thank You," and how-to, or instrumental, information: "Fruits & Vegetables Available Here." The second poster is about taking the stairs rather than taking the elevator and can be used in any building. It links a "green" message with a health message: "Burn Calories, Not Electricity. Take the Stairs."

Information on the number of calories on menu items in fast food restaurants has become available in some communities. This can signal to people that this is an important feature to consider and may have some impact on food choices (Bassett et al. 2008; Harnack et al. 2008).

Policy and System Changes

Organizational Food Policy

Nutrition educators can assist organizations to develop appropriate policies with respect to foods offered on site. Thus, in schools, they can work with local wellness councils made up of teachers, school food service staff, administrators, community members, and students. They can provide technical assistance to these councils to review and help evaluate the effectiveness of policies to encourage healthful food environments that address the following issues: food used in school fundraising or in the classroom as a reward or incentive, food advertising in schools, and beverage sales in schools. The Centers for Disease Control and Prevention (CDC) has developed a monitoring tool that schools can use to assess the school health environment and evaluate how they are doing (Centers for Disease Control and Prevention 2004a, 2004b). Within workplaces and other settings, vendors are usually for-profit operations. However, even here food policies can be developed so that healthful foods are more available and accessible.

Community and National Policy

Many community organizations and national organizations focus on food policy. Nutrition educators can work within them to advocate for, create, or revise policies that are supportive of the behaviors or issues that are important for nutritional health. Here, nutrition educators can provide technical assistance as well as influence. Nutrition educators also can bring their knowledge and skills to food assistance programs and public health agencies. Nutrition educators need to stay informed about policies and issues as they come up and participate, where possible and appropriate, to have a voice in how these policies will be developed and implemented. Some of these national policy activities are described in Chapter 18 of this book.

■ SUMMARY

Environmental interventions and policy and system change activities seek to enhance opportunities for people to engage in healthful food and activity behaviors. Addressing environmental determinants of people's health-related action takes many different approaches and involves a variety of venues. Nutrition educators inform, educate, and form partnerships with others—food and service providers, decision makers with authority and power, and policy makers—to address the environmental determinants that mediate the behaviors or practices targeted by nutrition programs. Thus, nutrition educators work with schools, Head Start programs, workplaces, and communities to make healthful foods available and accessible and to develop policies and system changes that encourage and reinforce healthful eating practices, as follows:

Schoolwide Policies and System Change Activities

In schools, schoolwide food-related policies about beverage availability, vending machines, and school stores, as well as school cafeteria policies, should provide students the opportunity to have easy access to healthful food choices and to see healthful food practices modeled.

Worksite Interventions

In workplaces, healthful alternatives should be made available in the cafeteria and in vending machines and should be promoted.

Making the Healthful Choice the Easy Choice

In all settings, the healthful choice should be an easy choice. Active participation of community members and worksite employees as well as leaders must be incorporated into any interventions. Indeed, community empowerment and collective efficacy are high priorities. Adopting these comprehensive approaches enhances the likelihood of improving the effectiveness of nutrition education interventions for individual and environmental change.

Questions and Activities

1. Think about one or two dietary changes you have tried to make. What factors in the environment have been helpful in supporting your change, and what factors have not been helpful? List five of each. Based on this chapter, what do you think that nutrition educators could have done to be helpful to you?

2. What would the ideal healthful food and activity environment look like to you—at work or school or in the community? What role do you think nutrition educators should play in promoting an environment that is supportive of healthful eating?

3. What is the social ecological approach to nutrition education? Describe the levels of influence in this approach and the role of nutrition educators in each.

4. Define the following terms and describe how they relate to nutrition education. Give examples:
   a. Social networks
   b. Social support
   c. Collaboration

5. What is community capacity? How can it be strengthened? What is the role of nutrition educators in the process?

6. "Local wellness policies" are required in the United States. What are these? How are nutrition educators involved?

7. If you were asked to name five things that schools could do to support healthy eating and active living, what would they be? What is the evidence for your recommendations?

8. If you were asked to name three things that worksites could do to support healthy eating and active living, what would they be? What is the evidence for your recommendations?

9. Describe "community-based participatory research." How might nutrition educators be involved?

10. What do we mean by policy in relation to diet and physical activity? How are education, environmental change, and policy related? What is the role of nutrition educators in policy making?

11. What skills do you think nutrition educators should have to be able to work in collaboration with others to bring about environments and policy that are supportive of health? What role would you like to see yourself play in these activities?

References

Abratt, R., and S. D. Goodey. 1990. Unplanned buying and in-store stimuli in supermarkets. *Managerial Decisions and Economics* 11:111–121.

American Academy of Pediatrics Committee on Environmental Health. 2009. The built environment: Designing communities to promote physical activity in children. *Pediatrics* 126(6):1591–1598.

Ammerman, A. S., C. H. Lindquist, K. N. Lohr, and J. Hersey. 2002. The efficacy of behavioral interventions to modify dietary fat and fruit and vegetable intake: A review of the evidence. *Preventive Medicine* 35(1):25–41.

Arnold, C. G., P. Ladipo, C. H. Nguyen, P. Nkinda-Chaiban, and C. M. Olson. 2001. New concepts for nutrition education in an era of welfare reform. *Journal of Nutrition Education* 33(6):341–346.

Bandura, A. 1997. *Self efficacy: The exercise of control*. New York: WH Freeman.

———. 2001. Social cognitive theory: An agentic perspective. *Annual Review of Psychology* 51:1–26.

Bassett, M. T., T. Dumanovsky, C. Huang, et al. 2008. Purchasing behavior and calorie information at fast-food chains in New York City, 2007. *American Journal of Public Health* 98(8):1457–1459.

Benedict, S., and M. K. Campbell. 2009. *HOPE Works: A successful community based project to address obesity, hope, and economic determinants of health among low income, rural, ethnically diverse women*. Paper presented at the International Society for Behavioral Nutrition and Physical Activity Annual Meeting, Portugal.

Beresford, S. A., B. Thompson, Z. Feng, A. Christianson, D. McLerran, and D. L. Patrick. 2001. Seattle 5 a Day worksite program to increase fruit and vegetable consumption. *Preventive Medicine* 32(3):230–238.

Berge J. M., M. Wall, K.W. Bauer, and D. Neumark-Sztainer. 2009. Parenting characteristics in the home environment and adolescent overweight: a latent class analysis. *Obesity* Oct 8 (Epub ahead of print).

Berkman, L. F., and T. Glass. 2000. Social integration, social networks, social support, and health. In *Social Epidemiology*, edited by L. F. Berkman and I. Kawachi. New York: Oxford Press.

Burgess-Champoux, T. L., N. Larson, D. Neumark-Sztainer, P. J. Hannan, and M. Story. 2009. Are family meal patterns associated with overall diet quality during the transition from early to middle adolescence? *Journal of Nutrition Education and Behavior* 41(2):79–86.

California Department of Public Health. 2007. Network for a Healthy California. http://www.dhs.ca.gov/ps/cdic/cpns/network.

Center for Food and Justice. 2010. *About the national Farm to School program*. http://www.farmtoschool.org/about.htm.

Centers for Disease Control and Prevention. 2004a. School Health Index: A self-assessment and planning guide. Elementary school version. Atlanta, GA: Author.

———. 2004b. School Health Index: A self-assessment and planning guide. Middle school/high school version. Atlanta, GA: Author.

Chaloupka, F. J., and L. D. Johnston. 2007. Bridging the Gap: Research informing practice and policy for healthy youth behavior. *American Journal of Preventive Medicine* 33(4 Suppl):S147–S161.

Child Nutrition and WIC Reauthorization Act. 2004, June 30. Local wellness policy. Section 204 of Public Law 108-265. Enacted by the 108th Congress of the United States of America.

Cohen, D. A. 2008. Obesity and the built environment: Changes in environmental cues cause energy imbalances. *International Journal of Obesity* 32:S137–S142.

Contento, I. R., S. S. Williams, J. L. Michela, and A. B. Franklin. 2006. Understanding the food choice process of adolescents in the context of family and friends. *Journal of Adolescent Health* 38(5):575–582.

Council of Economic Advisors. 2000. *Teens and their parents in the 21st century: An examination of trends in teen behavior and the role of parental involvement*. Washington, DC: Author.

Cousineau, T., B. Houle, J. Bromberg, K. C. Fernandez, and W. C. Kling. 2008. A pilot study of an online workplace nutrition program. *Journal of Nutrition Education and Behavior* 40:160–167.

Cullen, K. W., T. Baranowski, E. Owens, T. Marsh, L. Rittenberry, and C. de Moor. 2003. Availability, accessibility, and preferences for fruit, 100% fruit juice, and vegetables influence children's dietary behavior. *Health Education and Behavior* 30(5):615–626.

Cullen, K. W., and I. Zakeri. 2004. Fruits, vegetables, milk, and sweetened beverages consumption and access to a la carte/snack bar meals at school. *American Journal of Public Health* 94(3):463–467.

da Cunha, Z., I. R. Contento, and K. Morin. 2000. A case study of a curriculum development process in nutrition education using empowerment as organizational policy. *Ecology of Food and Nutrition* 39:417–435.

Davis, E. M., K. W. Cullen, K. B. Watson, M. Konarik, and J. Radcliffe. 2009. A Fresh Fruit and Vegetable Program improves high school students' consumption of fresh produce. *Journal of the American Dietetic Association* 109(7):1227–1231.

DeMattia, L., and S. L. Denney. 2008. Childhood obesity prevention: Successful community-based efforts. *Annals of the American Academy of Political and Social Science* 615:83–99.

Dengel, D. R., M. O. Hearst, J. H. Harmon, A. Forsythe, and L. A. Lytle. 2009. Does the built environment relate to the metabolic syndrome in adolescents? *Health Place* 15(4):946–951.

Economos, C. D., and S. Irish-Hauser. 2007. Community interventions: A brief overview and their application to the obesity epidemic. *Journal of Law and Medical Ethics* 35(1):131–137.

Edmundson, E., G. S. Parcel, H. A. Feldman, et al. 1996. The effects of the Child and Adolescent Trial for Cardiovascular Health upon psychosocial determinants of diet and physical activity behavior. *Preventive Medicine* 25(4):442–454.

Engbers, L. H., M. N. van Poppel, A. Paw, M. J. Chin, and W. van Mechelen. 2005. Worksite health promotion programs with environmental changes: A systematic review. *American Journal of Preventive Medicine* 29(1):61–70.

Feuenekes, G. I. J., C. De Graff, S. Meyboom, and W. A. Van Staveren. 1998. Food choice and fat intake of adolescents and adults: Association of intakes within social networks. 26:645–656.

French, S. A., R. W. Jeffery, M. Story, et al. 2001. Pricing and promotion effects on low-fat vending snack purchases: The CHIPS Study. *American Journal of Public Health* 91(1):112–117.

French, S. A., and G. Stables. 2003. Environmental interventions to promote vegetable and fruit consumption among youth in school settings. *Preventive Medicine* 37(6 Pt 1):593–610.

French, S. A., M. Story, R. W. Jeffery, P. Snyder, M. Eisenberg, A. Sidebottom, and D. Murray. 1997. Pricing strategy to promote fruit and vegetable purchase in high school cafeterias. *Journal of the American Dietetic Association* 97(9):1008–1010.

French, S. A., and H. Wechsler. 2004. School-based research and initiatives: Fruit and vegetable environment, policy, and pricing workshop. *Preventive Medicine* 39(Suppl 2):S101–S107.

Friere, P. 1970. *Pedagogy of the oppressed*. New York: Continuum.

———. 1973. *Education for critical consciousness*. New York: Continuum.

Fulkerson, J. A., S. A. French, M. Story, H. Nelson, and P. J. Hannan. 2004. Promotions to increase lower-fat food choices among students in secondary schools: Description and outcomes of TACOS (Trying Alternative Cafeteria Options in Schools). *Public Health Nutrition* 7(5):665–674.

Fulkerson, J. A., D. Neumark-Sztainer, P. J. Hannan, and M. Story. 2008. Family meal frequency and weight status among adolescents: Cross-sectional and 5-year longitudinal associations. *Obesity (Silver Spring)* 16(11):2529–2534.

Furst, T., M. Connors, C. A. Bisogni, J. Sobal, and L. W. Falk. 1996. Food choice: A conceptual model of the process. *Appetite* 26(3):247–265.

Gillespie, A. H., and G. W. Gillespie. 2007. Family food decision-making: An ecological systems framework. *Journal of Family and Consumer Sciences* 99(2):22–28.

Gillespie, A. H., and W. L. Johnson-Askew. 2009. Changing family food and eating practices: The family food decision-making system. *Annual Review of Behavioral Medicine* Nov 3 (Epub ahead of print).

Glanz, K., J. F. Sallis, B. E. Saelens, and L. D. Frank. 2005. Healthy nutrition environments: Concepts and measures. *American Journal of Health Promotion* 19(5):330–333, ii.

———. 2007. Nutrition Environment Measures Survey in stores (NEMS-S): Development and evaluation. *American Journal of Preventive Medicine* 32(4):282–289.

Goodman, R. M., et al. 1999. Identifying and defining the dimensions of community capacity to provide a basis for measurement. *Health Education and Behavior* 25:258–278.

Gottlieb, B. H. 1985. Social networks and social support: An overview of research, practice, and policy implications. *Health Education Quarterly* 12(1):5–22.

Green, L. W., and M. W. Kreuter. 2004. *Health promotion planning: An educational and ecological approach.* 4th ed. New York: McGraw-Hill Humanities/Social Sciences/Languages.

Hannan, P., S. A. French, M. Story, and J. A. Fulkerson. 2002. A pricing strategy to promote sales of lower fat foods in high school cafeterias: Acceptability and sensitivity analysis. *American Journal of Health Promotion* 17(1):1–6, ii.

Harnack, L. J., S. A. French, J. M. Oakes, M. T. Story, R. W. Jeffery, and S. A. Rydell. 2008. Effects of calorie labeling and value size pricing on fast food meal choices:

Results from an experimental trial. *International Journal of Behavior Nutrition and Physical Activity* 5:63.

Harrington, D. W., and S. J. Eliot. 2009. Weighing the importance of neighborhood: A multilevel exploration of the determinants of overweight and obesity. *Social Science and Medicine* 68(4):593–600.

Harrington, K. F., F. A. Franklin, S. L. Davies, R. M. Shewchuk, and M. B. Binns. 2005. Implementation of a family intervention to increase fruit and vegetable intake: The Hi5 + experience. *Health Promotion Practice* 6(2):180–189.

He, M., C. Callaghan, A. Evans, and G. Mandich. 2009. Healthy eating champions award for elementary schools. *Canadian Journal of Dietetic Practice and Research* 70(2):101–104.

Hearn, D. M., T. Baranowski, J. Baranowski, et al. 1998. Environmental influences on dietary behavior among children: Availability and accessibility of fruits and vegetables enable consumption. *Journal of Health Education* 29:26–32.

Hoelscher, D. M., P. Mitchell, J. Elder, A. Clesi, and P. Snyder. 2003. How the CATCH Eat Smart program helps implement the USDA regulations in school cafeterias. *Health Education and Behavior* 30:434–446.

Hughes, L. J., L. Blalock, and L. Strieter. 2005. Youth-oriented farm stands as a vehicle for improving food security in targeted low-income communities. *Journal of Nutrition Education and Behavior* 37(Suppl 1):S36.

Hunt, M. K., R. Lederman, S. Potter, A. Stoddard, and G. Sorensen. 2000. Results of employee involvement in planning and implementing the Treatwell 5-a-Day work-site study. *Health Education and Behavior* 27(2):223–231.

Institute of Medicine. 2007. *Nutrition standards for foods in schools: Leading the way towards healthier youth.* Washington, DC: National Academies Press.

Israel, B., B. Checkoway, A. Schulz, and M. Zimmerman. 1994. Health education and community empowerment: Conceptualizing and measuring perceptions of individual, organizational, and community control. *Health Education Quarterly* 21(2):149–170.

Israel, B. A, and K. A. Rounds. 1987. Social networks and social support: A synthesis for health educators. *Health Education and Promotion* 2:311–351.

Jones, A. S. 2005. Start by eating right: Promoting healthy eating in young children through partnerships between Share Our Strength and Head Start and other community agencies. In *National nutrition education conference.* Washington, DC: U.S. Department of Agriculture, Food and Nutrition Service.

Jordan, A. B. 2008. Overweight and obesity in America's children: Causes, consequences, solutions. *Annals of the American Academy of Political and Social Science* 615:225–243.

Kent, G. 1988. Nutrition education as an instrument of empowerment. *Journal of Nutrition Education* 20:193–195.

Kerr, J., F. Evans, and D. Carroll. 2000. Posters can prompt less active individuals to use the stairs. *Journal of Epidemiology and Community Health* 54:942–943.

Kerr, J., F. Evans, and D. Carroll. 2001. Six-month observational study of promoted stair climbing. *Preventive Medicine* 33:422–427.

Kistin, N., M. S. Abramson, and N. Dublin. 1994. Effect of peer counselors on breastfeeding initiation, exclusivity, and duration among low-income urban women. *Journal of Human Lactation* 10:11–16.

Kremers, S. P. J., G-J. de Bruijn, T. L. S. Visscher, W. van Mechelen, N. K. de Vries, and J. Brug. 2006. Environmental influences on energy-balance-related behaviors: A dual-process view. *International Journal of Behavioral Nutrition and Physical Activity* 3:9.

Kubik, M. Y., L. A. Lytle, and M. Story. 2001. A practical, theory-based approach to establishing school nutrition advisory councils. *Journal of the American Dietetic Association* 101(2):223–228.

Kwak, L., S. P. J. Kremers, M. A. van Baak, and J. Brug. 2007. A poster-based intervention to promote stair use in blue- and white-collar worksites. *Preventive Medicine* 45(2–3):177–181.

Li, F., P. Harmer, B. J. Cardinal, and N. Vongjaturapat. 2009. Built environment and changes in blood pressure in middle aged and older adults. *Preventive Medicine* 48(3):237–241.

Liquori, T., P. D. Koch, I. R. Contento, and J. Castle. 1998. The Cookshop Program: Outcome evaluation of a nutrition education program linking lunchroom food experiences with classroom cooking experiences. *Journal of Nutrition Education* 30(5):302.

Longley, C. H., and J. Sneed. 2009. Effects of federal legislation on wellness policy formation in school districts in the United States. *Journal of the American Dietetic Association* 109(1):95–101.

Luepker, R. V., C. L. Perry, S. M. McKinlay, et al. 1996. Outcomes of a field trial to improve children's dietary patterns and physical activity. The Child and Adolescent Trial for Cardiovascular Health. CATCH Collaborative Group. *Journal of the American Medical Association* 275(10):768–776.

Lytle, L. A., D. M. Murray, C. L. Perry, et al. 2004. School-based approaches to affect adolescents' diets: Results from the TEENS study. *Health Education and Behavior* 31(2):270–287.

Lytle, L. A., E. J. Stone, M. Z. Nichaman, et al. 1996. Changes in nutrient intakes of elementary school children following a school-based intervention: Results from the CATCH Study. *Preventive Medicine* 25(4):465–477.

Matson-Koffman, D. M., J. N. Brownstein, J. A. Neiner, and M. L. Greaney. 2005. A site-specific literature review of policy and environmental interventions that promote physical activity and nutrition for cardiovascular health: What works? *American Journal of Health Promotion* 19(3):167–193.

McLeroy, K. R., D. Bibeau, A. Steckler, and K. Glanz. 1988. An ecological perspective on health promotion programs. *Health Education Quarterly* 15:351–377.

Minkler, M. 1997. Community organizing among the elderly poor in San Francisco's Tenderloin district. In *Community organizing and community building for health*, edited by M. Minkler. New Brunswick, NJ: Rutgers University Press.

Ness, K., P. Elliot, and V. Wilbur. 1992. A peer educator nutrition program for seniors in a community development context. *Journal of Nutrition Education* 24:91–94.

Osganian, S. K., M. K. Ebzery, D. H. Montgomery, et al. 1996. Changes in the nutrient content of school lunches: results from the CATCH Eat Smart Food Service Intervention. *Preventive Medicine* 25:400–412.

Patterson, R. E., A. R. Kristal, K. Glanz, et al. 1997. Components of the working well trial intervention associated with adoption of healthful diets. *American Journal of Preventive Medicine* 13(4):271–276.

Perry, C. L., D. B. Bishop, G. Taylor, et al. 1998. Changing fruit and vegetable consumption among children: The 5-a-Day Power Plus program in St. Paul, Minnesota. *American Journal of Public Health* 88(4):603–609.

Perry, C. L., D. B. Bishop, G. L. Taylor, et al. 2004. A randomized school trial of environmental strategies to encourage fruit and vegetable consumption among children. *Health Education and Behavior* 31(1):65–76.

Reynolds, K. D., F. A. Franklin, D. Binkley, et al. 2000. Increasing the fruit and vegetable consumption of fourth-graders: Results from the High 5 project. *Preventive Medicine* 30(4):309–319.

Rody, N. 1988. Empowerment as organizational policy in nutrition intervention programs: A case study from the Pacific Islands. *Journal of Nutrition Education* 20:133–141.

Rohere, J., J. R. Pierce Jr., and A. Dennison. 2004. Walkability and self-rated health in primary care patients. *BMC Family Practice* 5:29.

Rosenthal, B. B. 1998. Collaboration for the nutrition field: Synthesis of selected literature. *Journal of Nutrition Education* 30(5):246–267.

Ross, N. J., M. D. Anderson, J. P. Goldberg, and B. L. Rogers. 2000. Increasing purchases of locally grown produce through worksite sales: An ecological model. *Journal of Nutrition Education* 32(6):304–313.

Rothschild, M. L. 1999. Carrots, sticks, and promises: A conceptual framework for the management of public health and social issues behaviors. *Journal of Marketing* 63:24–37.

Rundle, A., S. Fiels, Y. Park, L. Freeman, C. C. Weiss, and K. Nickerman. 2008. Personal and neighborhood socioeconomic status and indices of neighborhood walk-ability predict body mass index in New York City. *Social Science and Medicine* 67(12):1951–1958.

Sallis, J. F., T. L. McKenzie, T. L. Conway, et al. 2003. Environmental interventions for eating and physical activity: A randomized controlled trial in middle schools. *American Journal of Preventive Medicine* 24(3):209–217.

Sallis, J. F., C. T. Orleans, and D. M. Buchner. 2009. Active living research: A six-year report. *American Journal of Preventive Medicine* 36(2S):S1–S72.

Sciacca, J. P., B. L. Phipps, D. A. Dube, and M. I. Ratliff. 1995. Influences on breast-feeding by lower-income women: An incentive-based, partner-supported educational program. *Journal of the American Dietetic Association* 95(3):323–328.

Shea, S., and C. E. Basch. 1990a. A review of five major community-based cardiovascular disease prevention programs. Part I: Rationale, design, and theoretical framework. *American Journal of Health Promotion* 4(3):203–213.

———. 1990b. A review of five major community-based cardiovascular disease prevention programs. Part II: Intervention strategies, evaluation methods, and results. *American Journal of Health Promotion* 4(4):279–287.

Singh, A. S., A. Paw, M. J. Chin, et al. 2006. Design of the Dutch Obesity Intervention in Teenagers (NRG-DOiT): Systematic development, implementation and evaluation of a school-based intervention aimed at the prevention of excessive weight gain in adolescents. *BMC Public Health* 6:304.

Singh, A. S., A. Paw, M. J. Chin, J. Brug, and W. van Mechelen. 2007. Short-term effects of school-based weight gain prevention among adolescents. *Archives of Pediatric and Adolescent Medicine* 161(6):565–571.

Singleton, U., A. Williams, C. Harris, and G. G. Mason. 2005. *Building breastfeeding friendly communities with community partners*. Washington, DC: U.S. Department of Agriculture, Food and Nutrition Service.

Smith, C., and L. W. Morton. 2009. Rural food deserts: Low-income perspectives on food access in Minnesota and Iowa. *Journal of Nutrition Education and Behavior* 41(3):176–187.

Sorensen, G., J. Hsieh, M. K. Hunt, D. H. Morris, D. R. Harris, and G. Fitzgerald. 1992. Employee advisory boards as a vehicle for organizing worksite health promotion programs. *American Journal of Health Promotion* 6(6):443–450, 464.

Sorensen, G., M. K. Hunt, N. Cohen, et al. 1998. Worksite and family education for dietary change: The Treatwell 5-a-Day program. *Health Education Research* 13(4):577–591.

Sorensen, G., M. K. Hunt, D. Morris, et al. 1990. Promoting healthy eating patterns in the worksite: The Treatwell intervention model. *Health Education and Research* 5(4):505–515.

Sorensen, G., A. M. Stoddard, A. D. LaMontagne, et al. 2002. A comprehensive worksite cancer prevention intervention: Behavior change results from a randomized controlled trial (United States). *Cancer Causes and Control* 13(6):493–502.

Sorensen, G., A. Stoddard, K. Peterson, et al. 1999. Increasing fruit and vegetable consumption through worksites and families in the Treatwell 5-a-day study. *American Journal of Public Health* 89(1):54–60.

Sorensen, G., B. Thompson, K. Glanz, et al. 1996. Work site-based cancer prevention: Primary results from the Working Well Trial. *American Journal of Public Health* 86(7):939–947.

Story, M., K. M. Kaphingst, R. Robinson-O'Brien, and K. Glanz. 2008. Creating healthy food and eating environments: Policy and environmental approaches. *Annual Review of Public Health* 29:253–272.

Story, M., L. A. Lytle, A. S. Birnbaum, and C. L. Perry. 2002. Peer-led, school-based nutrition education for young adolescents: Feasibility and process evaluation of the TEENS study. *Journal of School Health* 72(3):121–127.

Story, M., M. S. Nanney, and M. B. Schwartz. 2009. Schools and obesity prevention: Creating school environments and policies to promote healthy eating and physical activity. *Milbank Quarterly* 87(1):71–100.

Stringer, S. M. 2009. *Food in the public interest: How New York City's food policy holds the key to hunger, health, jobs, and the environment*. New York: Office of the Manhattan Borough President.

Te Velde, S. J., M. Wind, C. Perez-Rodrigo, K. I. Klepp, and J. Brug. 2008. Mothers' involvement in a school-based fruit and vegetable promotion intervention is associated with increased fruit and vegetable intakes—the Pro Children study. *International Journal of Behavioral Nutrition and Physical Activity* 5:48.

Travers, K. D. 1997a. Nutrition education for social change: Critical perspective. *Journal of Nutrition Education* 29(2):57–62.

———. 1997b. Reducing inequities through participatory research and community empowerment. *Health Education and Behavior* 24(3):344–356.

U.S. Department of Agriculture. n.d. Healthy Schools: Local wellness policy requirements. http://www.fns.usda.gov/tn/healthy/wellness_policyrequirements .html.

———. 2003. *Expanded food and nutrition education program, national impact data*. Washington, DC: Author.

———. 2005. *Making it happen! School nutrition success stories*. Food and Nutrition Service FNS-374. Alexandria, VA: Food and Nutrition Service USDA, Centers for Disease Control and Prevention, U.S. Department of Health and Human Services, and U.S. Department of Education.

Ventura, A. K., and L. L. Birch. 2008. Does parenting affect children's eating and weight status? *International Journal of Behavioral Nutrition and Physical Activity* 5:15.

Wallerstein, N. 1992. Powerlessness, empowerment, and health: Implications for health promotion programs. *American Journal of Health Promotion* 6(3):197–205.

Wansink, B. 2006. *Mindless eating*. New York: Bantam Books.

Whitaker, R. C., J. A. Wright, T. D. Koepsell, A. J. Finch, and B. M. Psaty. 1994. Randomized intervention to increase children's selection of low-fat foods in school lunches. *Journal of Pediatrics* 125(4):535–540.

Williams, A. E., T. M. Vogt, V. J. Stevens, et al. 2007. Work, Weight, and Wellness: The 3W Program: A worksite obesity prevention and intervention trial. *Obesity (Silver Spring)* 15(Suppl 1):16S–26S.

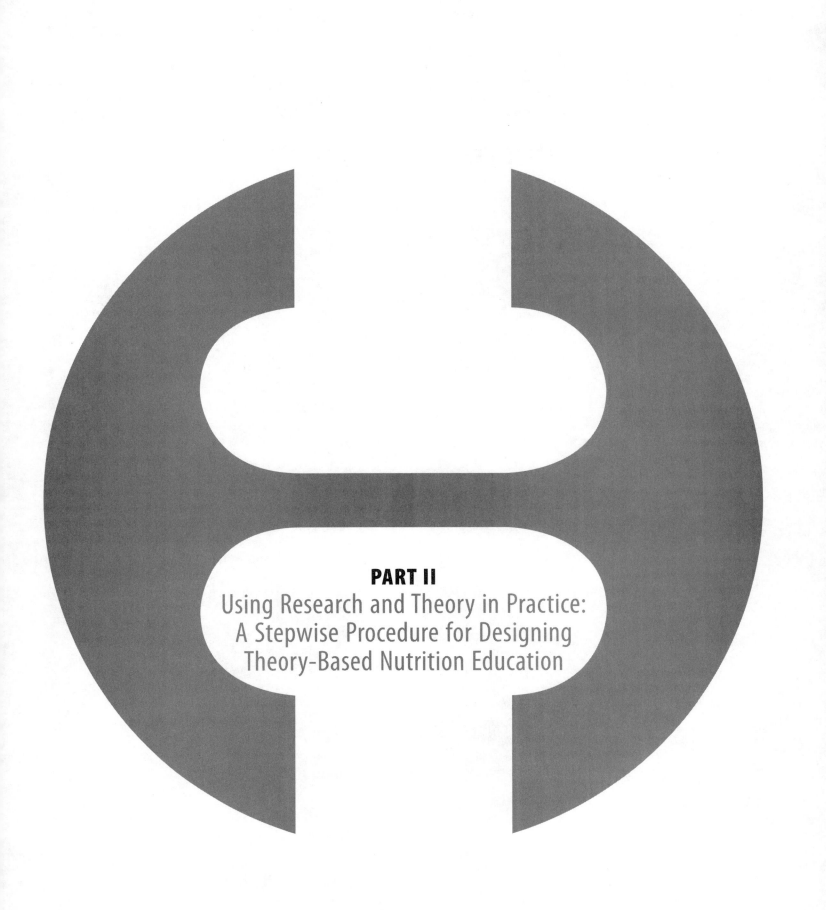

PART II
Using Research and Theory in Practice:
A Stepwise Procedure for Designing
Theory-Based Nutrition Education

CHAPTER

7

Step 1: Analyzing Food and Health Issues to Specify the Behavior or Action Focus of the Program

OVERVIEW

This chapter provides an overview of a systematic stepwise procedure for designing nutrition education that applies theory to practice. It also describes Step 1: how to conduct an analysis of health issues and needs, identify behaviors or practices contributing to the issues for given audiences, and specify the behaviors or actions that will be the focus of the program. A case study illustrates the procedure.

CHAPTER OUTLINE

- Introduction
- Overview of the Stepwise Procedure for designing theory-based nutrition education
- Step 1: analyzing health issues to specify the behavioral focus for a given audience: beginning with the end in sight
- Step 1A: identifying health issues or needs and intended audience
- Step 1B: identifying the behaviors and practices that contribute to the issue or need
- Step 1C: stating the behavioral or action goals to be the focus of the program
- Case study
- Your turn: completing the Step 1 worksheets

LEARNING OBJECTIVES

At the end of the chapter, you will be able to:

- Describe a six-step procedure for designing theory-based, behavior-focused nutrition education
- State why it is important to use a systematic process to identify the focus and targets for nutrition education
- Develop skills in conducting a needs and issues analysis: identifying the high-priority food or health issues or needs of the intended audience and the behaviors or practices that contribute to the needs or issues
- Identify appropriate information sources for these assessments
- Compare advantages and disadvantages of different methods for obtaining the assessment information

INTRODUCTION: A STEPWISE PROCEDURE FOR DESIGNING THEORY-BASED NUTRITION EDUCATION

This chapter begins a new section of the book. So far, you have learned about the theories derived from evidence that explain why individuals take the health actions they do and how they change. You have examined how nutrition education interventions can be based on these theories. But how exactly do you translate these theories into a format that is usable for guiding implementation in the real world? This is the central task of this book: using theory and evidence to design nutrition education for the typical practice settings in which most nutrition educators work.

Planning Frameworks and Behavior Change Theory

A number of planning frameworks are available for promoting health, such as the PRECEDE-PROCEED model (Green & Kreuter 2004). However, they are not designed to provide information on the specifics of how to actually design educational group sessions and interventions that use theory variables. This section of the book provides a planning framework for nutrition education—a stepwise procedure—and shows how to incorporate theory variables into the planning process.

Stepwise Procedure as a Translational and Implementation Framework

The translational and implementation framework is presented here in the form of a logic model and stepwise procedure for designing nutrition education that translates theory into practice and provides strategies for

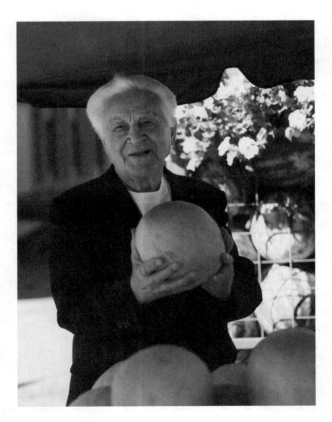

In many communities, buying produce at a farmers' market is common practice.

implementation. It is a systematic step-by-step procedure for designing behavior-focused and evidence-based nutrition education that integrates theory and research with practice at each step. In this book, this process is called the Stepwise Procedure for Designing Theory-Based Nutrition Education (abbreviated sometimes as the Stepwise Procedure). It consists of six steps.

This chapter describes an overview of the entire Stepwise Procedure and discusses Step 1. This part of the book aims to be very practical so that you will be able to apply the six-step process to any program of your choosing. Worksheets are provided for you to use for each step. This chapter introduces a case study that you will follow throughout the six steps as an example. Clearly, how nutrition educators translate theory into appropriate educational practice in real-world situations is crucial for success.

Beginning with the End in Sight

The end you must keep in sight for the design process is a ready-to-implement program that is likely to be effective for a given audience, along with a carefully designed plan to evaluate the program (**Figure 7-1**). This "program" can consist of one education session delivered to a group or a program with several components delivered at several levels of intervention, such as classroom, parents, and school environment components, or group education, supermarket environment changes, and policy. An outline of the key features of the Stepwise Procedure is shown in the form of a flowchart (**Figure 7-2**).

The first step is extremely important for designing an effective program. This step is often called a *needs assessment*, *needs analysis*, *issues analysis*, or *formative research*.

The process starts when a health issue of concern is considered serious and prevalent enough to justify the expenditure of time and resources. You also identify for whom this issue is of greatest concern.

The issues most often refer to health issues facing individuals within your intended audience, such as increased risk of developing heart disease, type 2 diabetes, or osteoporosis. Issues of concern can also refer to those related to ecological health of the food system, such as excessive greenhouse gas emissions—or carbon footprint—from excessive transportation, processing, or packaging of food. In addition, issues can refer to those related to societal issues related to food such as the impact of the food system on the fabric of rural communities or working conditions of those who work on farms.

In this step, you also identify the individual behaviors or community practices that contribute to the food or health issue for the given audience and prioritize them. From these, you select one or a few major behaviors or practices for the program to address. These can be called the *target behaviors* or *core practices*. Examples are breastfeeding, safe food handling behaviors, eating more fruits and vegetables, or eating local foods produced sustainably. These behaviors or practices are stated in terms of *changes* the program seeks to achieve.

In *Step 2*, you then identify the personal psychosocial determinants of these behaviors and practices (such as perceived benefits or sense of self-efficacy) that are relevant and of high priority for the selected core behaviors or practices in a given group and setting. You also identify modifiable environmental determinants that facilitate or impede the core behaviors. Because these identified determinants are those that can be modified by educational, advocacy, or policy means and can thus mediate changes in the target behaviors or practices, they are called *potential mediators of behavior change* in the context of nutrition education.

In *Step 3*, you select the theory you will use and clarify the educational philosophy that will guide the session or intervention; you also

FIGURE 7-1 As you begin the Stepwise Procedure, have the end in sight: You will have educational plans for your intended audience and environmental/policy support plans.

Step 5 Individual Component Case Study — Designing Activities for Mediators

Write a narrative educational plan that you will actually use to deliver your session. Think of a catchy title that will be meaningful to your audience. Make sure that activities are sequenced. For each educational activity, create a heading with a title and the mediator(s) addressed. Then write a detailed procedure for the activity. It is customary to place an overview or outline of activities and a materials list at the beginning of the teaching plan.

The Whys of Colorful Eating

Overview of Content (50–60 minutes)
1. Introduction—overview, and gain attention
2. Brainstorm and record on newsprint the benefits of eating F&V
3. Emphasize importance of different colors
4. Fill out 24-hour recall checklist to assess colorfulness of F&V intake
5. Brainstorm and use newsprint to record barriers to eating F&V
6. Brainstorm ways to overcome barriers/discuss how to make eating all the colors of the rainbow easier
7. Discuss influence of peers and provide alternate models
8. Appreciate the rainbow of fruits and vegetables by tasting F&V
9. Group values discussion
10. Pros and cons worksheet of adding F&V to your diet
11. Goal setting and wrap up

Materials
- Five to 10 different F&V, such as eggplant, blueberries, zucchini, kale, green grapes, jicama, potato, carrots, kumquat, tangerine, tomato, or strawberry
- Copies of the 24-hour recall checklist and pros/cons and goal setting worksheets
- Fruit salad or vegetables and dip
- Newsprint
- Markers
- Pencils or pens

Lesson Plan
1. Introduction—Overview and gain attention (3 minutes)
   Demonstrate the wide variety of colors that are found in F&V. Hold up F&V. Ask the following series of questions to facilitate conversation: What is the name of this food? Have you seen this food before? Are there other foods that are similar in color? Are there other foods that are similar in shape? Have you eaten this food before? Encourage participation from the entire group. Discuss why it is important to eat a variety of colors. (Address any behavior problems immediately, and talk about the importance of creating a positive and supportive environment.)

2. Benefits of F&V—Brainstorm and record on newsprint (6 minutes) (perceived benefits)
   "Now that we are familiar with how a variety of different F&V look, we are going to continue to explore what we already know about F&V. Let's make a list of some of the benefits of eating a wide range of F&V." Discussion will follow. Ensure that the following benefits of eating F&V are covered: Provides essential vitamins, minerals, fiber, and other nutrients; can increase energy; helps make hair and skin healthy; builds strong bones and muscles; and decreases risk for certain diseases.

3. Benefits of F&V—Emphasis on importance of different colors (3 minutes) (perceived benefits)
   List the following colors on newsprint: blue/purple, green, white, yellow/orange, and red. Emphasize a need for a variety of different color F&V. Different colors reflect the presence of different phytonutrients. Explain that by eating all different colors they are eating a wide range of different nutrients. Tell students that instead of needing to remember that orange color vegetables are filled with carotenoids and dark blue/purple fruits, like blueberries, are filled with resveratrol, they should remember to eat the rainbow, and they will eat all the different nutrients they need! Ask the group if there are any questions in order to clear up misconceptions.

4. Self-Assessment of Intake—24-hour recall checklist to assess colorfulness of F&V intake (9 minutes) (perceived risk)
   Distribute checklist and ask participants to think about what F&V they ate yesterday (or during the past week). Each participant should write down the F&V they ate from each color group. Discussion starters: Is there a rainbow on your plate? What colors are you missing?

5. Barriers to eating F&V—Brainstorm and record on newsprint (5 minutes) (barriers and self-efficacy)
   Make a list of the reasons why it is sometimes hard to eat all the colors of the rainbow. Ask students what prevents them from eating all the different colors. Ensure that the following topics are mentioned: lack of time, not available, my parents don't buy/cook them, and dislike taste.

6. Brainstorm Ways to Overcome Barriers—Discuss how to make eating all the colors of the rainbow easier (6 minutes) (self-efficacy)
   Based on the list of barriers, ask for suggestions on ways to overcome each barrier. For example: lack of time—pre-cut vegetables or whole fruit for a snack; dislike taste—provide culturally appropriate suggestions on how to prepare. Record on newsprint. Ask for other suggestions about how to eat a variety of foods. If there is a color that most participants seem to be lacking, this is the time to focus on that particular color.

7. Social Influences—Discuss influence of peers and provide alternate models (5 minutes) (social norms)
   What might your friends say when you choose to eat F&V or bring them as a snack? Allow for adequate discussion time. If the participants suggest that it might be seen as "uncool," provide alternate stories or media models that show F&V consumption as "cool." Make sure that the models are appropriate for the specific age, gender, and culture of the group.

8. Tasting F&V—Appreciate the rainbow of fruits and vegetables by tasting F&V (10–20 minutes) (benefits)
   Provide a rainbow fruit salad or a rainbow vegetable plate with dips for the participants to enjoy. Depending on time and facilities, allow participants to prepare the snack.

9. Group Values Discussion (5 minutes) (values clarification)
   Now that you have discussed the importance of eating a rainbow of F&V, and ate a great snack with a rainbow of colors in it, ask the participants for their thoughts now about F&V. Facilitate discussion by presenting value statements using a scale of 1–10, such as, How important is it to you to eat a rainbow of different F&V? How likely do you think it is that you will eat a rainbow of different F&V during the next week?

10. Pros and Cons of Adding F&V to your diet (5 minutes) (benefits versus barriers)
    Hand out pros and cons worksheet. Ask the participants to write at least three personal pros and three cons about eating a rainbow of different colored F&V.

11. Goal Setting and Wrap Up (8 minutes) (goal setting)
    Review the reasons why and ways to increase the colorfulness and number of F&V in diet. Encourage participants to make a clear statement about what actions they will take in the next week. For some it might be adding one F&V a day to their diet, for others it might be adding a different color F&V. Take a few minutes to fill out the worksheet. Ask participants, "Will some of you now share the goals you set for yourself?" After a participant reads his or her goal, ask if others have a similar goal. Encourage the members of the group to support each other in reaching their goals. Thank the group and include any reminders about future meetings or events.

Designing Activities for Mediators

...ucation, and nutrition education program objectives to create ...essions and environmental supports plans for environmental/

...roducts

...session you will conduct. The educational plan consists of a set ...r the session based on these objectives. You will use a matrix ...o deliver the session.

...general and specific support objectives.

...his worksheet is available at http://nutrition.jbpub.com/

...olicy Support Plan

...hool Environment Component

...d vegetables (F & V) to 2 and a half or more cups a day

...nvironmental Support Objectives

...anizational food policy	...will enhance motivation of school administrators to create healthy environment.
	The nutrition education program will provide many opportunities for youth to taste F&V.
Information environment	The school will activate school food policy council to develop guidelines for foods available in school.
	The school will make cafeteria information environment supportive of eating fruits and vegetables.

Design your environmental-policy support plan in matrix format. Write specific objectives for the supports in your theory model (Step 3). Then write the theory-based strategy you will employ to address the support and the practical activity that will operationalize the strategy.

Environmental/Policy Supports (Step 3)	Specific Support Objectives*	Strategies to Achieve Environmental Support Objectives
Decision-makers' awareness and motivation	Increase school administrators' beliefs in importance of healthful school environment (outcome expectations)	Individual meetings or presentations to staff about importance of healthful eating for learning; discussion of financial impacts, success stories
Social support	Increase social modeling by valued celebrities	Bring in local celebrities for school assembly to talk about why they choose healthy eating patterns
Food environment	School will provide many opportunities for students to taste F&V	Nutrition educators and food service staff will provide taste tests for F&V in the cafeteria
	School food service personnel will increase fruits and vegetables in meals; obtained from local farmers in a farm-to-school program	Provide professional development and manuals for food service personnel; provide information on potential vendors for local produce
Organizational food policy	Activate school food policy council to develop guidelines for foods available in school	Presentations to or conversations with school administrators, teachers, parent associations about need for school policies
	School nutrition advisory council will develop food policies	Recruitment to council: administrators, food service staff, teachers, students, parents, and others
	Develop guidelines of items in vending machines and school store	Provide technical assistance to develop guidelines for vending machine and school store items
	Vending machines will carry healthful F&V items	Vendors will supply healthful items in vending machines; develop system for monitoring compliance
	School stores will carry healthful F&V food items	Develop guidelines of items in school store (e.g., 50% will be healthful items)
Information environment	Make eating F&V normative; develop posters for cafeteria; newsletter to family	Focus group with teens; design posters with teens about eating F&V and post them

* Use your findings about the changes that could be made in your audience's environment (Step 2D) for each support to guide your writing of the specific objectives.

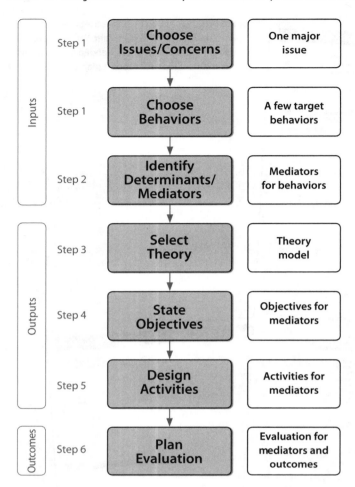

FIGURE 7-2 Flowchart of steps in designing theory-based nutrition education.

decide on the program components. In *Step 4*, you state appropriate educational objectives for each mediator. In *Step 5*, you create theory-based experiences and environmental support activities for each mediator. Designing educational strategies and practical learning experiences matched to behavioral theory constructs is at the heart of effective nutrition education. Finally, in *Step 6* you plan the evaluation. You will have achieved the end that you had in sight.

The Stepwise Procedure as Coaching

The design process may at first glance seem overly structured. You may have conducted nutrition education before and did not use such a systematic or structured approach—and the sessions went well. You wonder about the necessity of going through these steps so systematically. The best way to view this section of the book is to see it as guidance from research and evidence on refining the practice of nutrition education to enhance its effectiveness. An analogy may be useful here. A young girl is an excellent baseball player and seems to have natural talent as a pitcher. The coach carefully analyzes her moves as she pitches, giving her specific guidance on making her moves more precise and effective. He gives her specific moves to practice, which do not come naturally at first, but she practices these moves until they become second nature, making her a formidable pitcher.

In the same way a pitcher can have natural talent, you already have skills in nutrition education. This book offers coaching based on research evidence. Designing effective nutrition education sessions takes work and requires a systematic process. Try it out and use it a few times. With practice, this systematic process will become second nature and you will adapt it to your own style to design group sessions with ease and to plan appropriate environmental supports.

Nutrition Care Process and Model

The process described here may be new to you or similar to a process you have used before. Key features are similar to the Nutrition Care Process and Model of the American Dietetic Association (ADA 2008), which uses the following four steps in the clinical setting for individuals:

- Nutrition assessment and reassessment
- Nutrition diagnosis
- Nutrition intervention
- Nutrition monitoring and evaluation

Defining Terms

The terms *behaviors* and *practices* are here used interchangeably, although *practices* has a connotation of long-standing behaviors or commonly practiced behaviors in the community, such as safe food handling practices, breastfeeding, or buying produce at a farmers' market. Evidence is strong that nutrition education is more likely to be effective when it is focused on behaviors, practices, or clearly defined issues. When the focus is clear and specific, effectiveness is increased. However, there may be situations where the behaviors are very broad, such as "healthy eating" or "active living." For example, a school garden may be instituted for the stated goal of "improving children's eating habits" (very broad). However, before designing the nutrition education intervention, more immediate behaviors or practices may need to be selected, such as increasing children's fruit and vegetable intakes by familiarizing students with how food is grown and providing opportunities for youth to taste fresh produce, thereby coming to like it. Such behavioral goals may be embedded in the larger goal of improving informed decision making about food system issues. Developing a school garden also may serve non-nutrition–related goals, such as increasing the attractiveness of the campus, instilling a feeling that the school cares, and engendering a greater commitment to coming to school, and hence better academic performance. Thus, nutrition education goals may be embedded in broader goals.

The term *intended audience* is used rather than *target population* to refer to the individuals or specific subgroup of the population with whom you will be working, to convey the sense that the group members are not a "target" of educator activities so much as partners with whom you work so that together you can address needs and issues of importance.

The term *nutrition education intervention* is here used to denote any set of systematically planned educational activities or learning experiences that is provided to a group in a variety of settings, along with relevant environmental supports where appropriate. The term *intervention* is problematic to some educators because it can seem to imply that nutrition educators are intervening in people's lives, possibly against their will. It is not used in that sense here; rather, it is a convenient way to describe a range of planned activities of varying scope. Thus, the term encompasses both nutrition education of several sessions delivered by one person and programs involving many components and perhaps several media and delivered by many nutrition educators over a long time span.

■ OVERVIEW OF THE STEPWISE PROCEDURE: LINKING THEORY AND RESEARCH TO PRACTICE AT EVERY STEP

The steps of the Stepwise Procedure are summarized as follows:

Step 1. Analyzing issues and needs to state program behavioral goals: beginning with the end in sight:

- Analyze health issues of concern and audience(s) for whom these issues are relevant and important
- Identify behaviors and practices that contribute to the issues of concern: what needs to change? Prioritize these behaviors or practices
- State behavioral or action goals that will be the focus of the session or program

Step 2. Using theory and evidence to identify mediators of targeted behavior: why do people do what they do? How do they change?

- Describe the social and cultural environment of the intended audience
- Identify potential personal psychosocial mediators of the program's goals for behaviors or practices
- Identify environmental determinants that may mediate the program's goals for behaviors or practices

Step 3. Select theory or model to guide program, clarify philosophy, and choose components:

- Select a theory or create a relevant theoretical model based on mediators
- Articulate the educational philosophy underlying the intervention
- Determine the channels and components for the program

Step 4. State objectives for mediators:

- State educational objectives for the personal psychosocial mediators of the goal behaviors or actions of the program
- State change objectives for the environmental support mediators of goal behaviors or actions of the program

Step 5. Design theory-based strategies and practical activities to address mediators:

- Design educational strategies and activities for the personal psychosocial mediators of core behaviors of the program
- Design change strategies and activities for the environmental support mediators of goal behaviors of the program

Step 6. Plan the theory-based evaluation:

- Plan the outcome evaluation
- Plan the process evaluation

Note that the Stepwise Procedure places heavy emphasis on addressing *mediators* of the behaviors, actions, or practices targeted by the program. Identifying and specifying mediators are thus important activities in the design process. The centrality of mediators for behavior change intervention trials has been emphasized by researchers (Baranowski et al. 1997; Baranowski et al. 2009).

We also can lay out the Stepwise Procedure in the form of a logic model for planning purposes. This is shown in **Figure 7-3**, with Step 1

highlighted. The tasks and products for each step also are shown in this figure.

The procedural steps for designing nutrition education activities are laid out sequentially, but in reality they are closely interrelated, so you must go back and forth between steps when designing nutrition education. This is indicated by the arrows that go in both directions in Figure 7-3. In addition, at each step you need to check to see whether what you are doing is on track and appropriate. This may mean conducting focus groups or interviews, pilot testing intervention components, rewriting material, seeking new information, and so forth.

■ STEP 1: ANALYZING HEALTH ISSUES TO SPECIFY THE BEHAVIORAL FOCUS FOR A GIVEN AUDIENCE: BEGINNING WITH THE END IN SIGHT

A nutrition education activity is initiated when someone or some organization expresses an interest or a concern about some food- or nutrition-related issue. The interest may be expressed quite informally: the leader of an after-school program for middle school students may think that it would be a good idea for the group members to learn about eating more healthfully because she has observed that they skip lunch and grab some less than healthful snacks or fast food on the way to the program. She invites you to come provide a couple of sessions.

Or the concern may be based on extensive national data about the health concerns of a particular group, such as overweight in children. The tendency of nutrition educators is to rush to design activities for their sessions or program based on what they know. After all, designing and implementing exciting learning experiences, seeing the group gain new insights and respond with enthusiasm, and making a difference in people's lives are what drew you to the profession in the first place. Indeed, many people have made career changes to become nutrition educators.

Understanding your audience is crucial. However, for nutrition education to be effective and of value to the audience, you must first clarify a few questions: what exactly are the needs or issues that any given nutrition education activity should address? For whom are these issues of concern? Are they concerns of the nutrition educator or nutrition agency or are they concerns of the audience? Why are they of concern? What are the possible causes? (See **Box 7-1**.) It is extremely important to understand the intended audience as thoroughly as possible given practical and resource constraints.

Why Analyzing Health Issues Is Important

Although informal judgments of needs and issues of concern can sometimes suffice, a more systematic or formal assessment of issues and problems has the following advantages:

- Helps you better understand your audience and the context of their lives
- Takes much of the guesswork out of nutrition education design
- Provides a basis for selecting behaviors and practices that are of concern and the development of appropriate program goals and educational objectives to address them
- Makes clear the rationale for choosing particular priorities
- Makes it easier to use scarce resources appropriately
- Documents the need for funding or justifies expenditure of resources
- Provides a basis for measuring results

Inputs: Collecting Assessment Data			Outputs: Designing the Theory-Based Intervention			Outcomes: Evaluation Plan
Step 1 ←→ **Analyze issues and audiences to state program behavioral goals**	**Step 2 ←→** **Identify potential mediators to achieve program behavioral goals**	**Step 3 ←→** **Select theory, philosophy, and components**	**Step 4 ←→** **State objectives for mediators**	**Step 5 ←→** **Design theory-based strategies and activities for mediators**		**Step 6** **Plan evaluation**
Tasks • Analyze issues and select audience • Identify behaviors or patterns contributing to issue • Specify behavioral or action goals of the program	*Tasks* • Identify personal psychosocial mediators • Identify environmental support mediators	*Tasks* • Select theory or create appropriate model • Clarify philosophy (education and content) • Determine program components	*Tasks* • State educational objectives for psychosocial mediators • State change objectives for environmental support mediators	*Tasks* • Design activities to address psychosocial mediators • Design activities to address environmental support mediators • Implementation plan		*Tasks* • Design outcome evaluation plan • Determine tools to measure impact • Plan process evaluation
Product • *Description of issue of concern* • *Statement of action or behavioral goals for program*	*Product* • *List of potential mediators for action or behavior goals*	*Product* • *Theory/model for program, philosophy, and components*	*Product* • *Objectives for each mediator*	*Product* • *Educational plans for sessions linking mediators, objectives, and strategies* • *Environmental support plans*		*Product* • *Evaluation plan* • *List of indicators and measures for outcomes* • *Procedures and measures for process evaluation*

FIGURE 7-3 Stepwise Procedure for designing theory-based nutrition education: Step 1.

Such an assessment ensures that your food and nutrition education sessions or programs are directed at issues, needs, or problems that have been identified as important national or local priorities or that are perceived to be of concern or interest in the community or intended audience.

Clarifying Terms

This systematic assessment process is called by different names in different arenas. Educators talk about identifying the "sources of the curriculum"—how to select what they will teach. Program planners talk about "needs assessments" or "formative assessments." Social marketers talk about "market research," "formative research," or "front-end assessment" and consider this activity to be of crucial importance to the social marketing process. The term *needs assessment* is frequently used across many fields. This book uses the terms *needs analysis* and *issue identification*. However, the terms are used in a broader sense, encompassing the notion of analysis beyond identifying needs and problems to include identifying issues of concern or interest to the intended audience. Included here also is identification of the assets of the group or community in relation to the health issue.

Who Participates in Identifying and Analyzing Issues or Needs?

In many situations, you as the nutrition educator are the person identifying the issues or conducting the needs analysis. You may have been asked to conduct short-term nutrition education with a group such as an older adults' lunch program, a program for individuals with AIDS, or a group of low-income mothers of young children. With few resources,

the responsibility rests with one person: you. In other situations, a department, community group, or an agency is charged with providing nutrition education services, and several staff members may be involved. Examples might be a community program or other long-term project, such as a school curriculum or nutrition education activities and programs sponsored or funded by a government agency. Here, staff, along with an advisory group made up of some key individuals from the setting or community in which the nutrition education will be conducted, may be needed.

Involving Program Participants Enhances Buy-In and Effectiveness

In a comprehensive review of nutrition education programs conducted around the world from 1900 to 1970, Whitehead (1973) found that the programs that were more successful in changing behavior were those that did two things: they explicitly made behavior change a goal of the program, and they involved community stakeholders in all phases of the program, including the issues identification and needs analysis process, program planning, implementation, and evaluation. Thus, even in the situations described earlier, involving others in the needs analysis process may be beneficial.

The initiative for a new nutrition education program or for modifying an existing one can come from the top (such as the national, state, or local government, or agency and program directors), from the grassroots (such as community members or parents of school children), or from anywhere in between (such as the nutrition educator in a community organization, government agency, or corporation). Regardless of the level at which the program idea originates, it is important to involve in

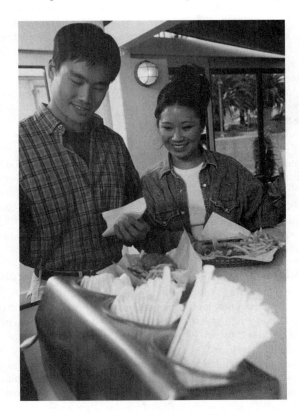

Box 7-1   **Beginning with the End in Sight**

The end to have in sight for the design process is a **ready-to-implement** educational plan for a session or program, accompanied by clearly specified supportive environmental or policy actions where appropriate, that is likely to be effective for a given audience, along with a carefully designed plan to evaluate the program.

Use the Stepwise Procedure in Figure 7-3 to develop a plan for nutrition education, whether it consists of only several educational sessions or of many components. After you have used this procedure a few times, you will become comfortable with it and will go through the procedure relatively quickly. If you are already an experienced facilitator of theory-based behavior-focused nutrition education groups, you can use the procedure more informally. It is still important, however, to address *all* steps in the process systematically, so as to clearly link theory, research, and practice at each step.

the needs analysis process appropriate levels of people who have a stake in the program, such as community members, citizen groups or students, nutrition education staff, teachers, agency heads, or school principals. The decision who to include is an important one. Researchers have found that the more individuals or groups are involved in the decision making, the greater their acceptance of, and their sense of satisfaction with, decisions made (Rogers & Shoemaker 1971; Rogers 2003).

Clarifying Roles

The functions and roles to be played by the people selected then need to be clarified. Will their role be informal? Will they constitute a committee or task force that will actually do some of the work, or will they serve as an advisory board, with staff members of an organization, nutrition educators, or others doing the actual assessment? Some members of this group may also serve later as knowledgeable informants about the needs of the intended audience. Any of these configurations are referred to as the *nutrition education team*.

Overview of Step 1

Step 1 consists of three components:

- Step 1A: Analyzing the health issues of concern and audience for whom the issues are relevant and important
- Step 1B: Identifying behaviors and practices that contribute to the issues of concern: what does the intervention want to change?
- Step 1C: Specifying behavioral or action goals that will be the focus of the session or program

■ STEP 1A: IDENTIFYING HEALTH ISSUES OR NEEDS AND INTENDED AUDIENCE

The first decision you have to make is who you want to reach and about what issue. In many cases, the intended audience or the health issue to be addressed is already determined by others, such as by the mission of the agency or organization in which the nutrition education will be

conducted or by some funding source. For example, the audience is already determined if the setting is an adolescent health clinic, a school, a Women, Infants and Children (WIC) clinic, or a senior center. Or the health issue may be determined if the setting is a heart association, a cancer society, or an HIV clinic.

Alternatively, it may be that a community expresses the desire for something of importance to them, such as a community vegetable garden and nutrition education to go with it. Or you may have been asked to provide a series of sessions to some intended audience, such as adolescent girls, or in a specific location, such as the local Y. Yet, even in these settings there are both subpopulations and a variety of issues that can be addressed. In addition, often organizations are looking for new directions. It may also be that an organization needs data to provide a rationale for selection of a new focus. Because there are obviously many populations that experience numerous health issues of concern, and resources are usually limited so that you cannot address them all, it is very important to identify a primary audience carefully and to focus on a specifically defined health, nutrition, or food issue. Use the worksheets at the end of this chapter to record your findings for Step 1A. The case study serves as an example of how to complete the worksheets.

Health Issues and Needs Identified from Scientific Research

One good place to start in identifying critical food and nutrition issues and a primary audience is to examine the nutrition science, epidemiology, and food systems literature. What does the latest scientific research suggest are important health issues facing the nation or a particular

Helping teenagers learn to substitute healthier snack alternatives for French fries and chips is just one example of a nutrition education activity.

group? What are some key concerns about ecological or community issues with respect to the food system? For which populations or groups are these nutritional and food-related concerns most urgent?

Health Issues

Health concerns can be described in terms of food-related issues or nutritional problems, such as rates of cardiovascular disease, cancer, hypertension, or diabetes, malnutrition in infants, breastfeeding, childhood obesity, or bone health. These can be identified through literature reviews, health surveys, national mortality and morbidity data, including indicators of health or rates of disease, or through data about specific populations.

Nutrition science research based on experimental, clinical, epidemiological, or field studies is constantly generating data on the relationship between diet and health. Consequently, the nutrition profession has expectations about what nutrition education should address. For example, scientific research or expert panels may have determined that a nutrition-related issue is of national concern, such as childhood obesity, bone health in adolescents, or diabetes in the public at large. Epidemiological data may indicate that the mortality or morbidity resulting from disease is high in a particular population (e.g., a community is known to have a high rate of hypertension or diabetes). These data can cause concern for health professionals or nutrition experts and engender a sense of need for action.

Health of the Food System

For programs that focus on food education, the choice of focus of an intervention may be based on concern about food system issues, such as concern about the carbon footprint of a group's current dietary patterns or whether the current food system is sustainable in the long term. Needs analysis information might include research data on the energy used for different food packaging and transportation practices, nature of the local food supply, or food safety. Epidemiological data may provide information on the prevalence of farmers' markets, small and medium-sized farms, and community-supported agriculture farms in the local area.

Societal Concerns Related to Food

For some nutrition education programs, a choice of focus might be based on a concern about the impact of food system practices on social systems and communities, or whether food production labor and trade practices are fair, described in terms of impacts on farmers and local communities. Assessment data might thus include information about the availability of foods produced through fair trade practices or institutional policies with respect to purchasing and serving such foods.

Health Issues and Needs Identified by National Policy

What are the stated national food, health, and nutrition goals of the country? Each country has developed nutrition, health, and food policy documents to guide government programs and provide information to the public. The choice of issues to address in a nutrition education intervention can be based on such policy initiatives. In the United States, nutrition recommendations based on the results of these and other surveys are spelled out from time to time in various government documents such as *Healthy People 2010*, the *Dietary Guidelines for Americans*, MyPyramid, *Physical Activity Guidelines for Americans*, and so forth. Private voluntary health organizations, such as cancer societies or heart associations, also publish guidelines for the public that can be used as a basis for choice of an issue for an intervention program. The specific

health needs of the population to be reached by the intervention also can by identified through review of various government surveys, such as the National Health and Nutrition Examination Survey (NHANES) or Continuing Survey of Food Intake of Individuals (CSFII) in the United States.

Concerns about the food system becoming and remaining sustainable are described in various government documents, policy documents of food system research institutes and organizations, and publications of world health and agricultural organizations. You can consult these and other documents as you design your nutrition education sessions or program.

Health Issues and Needs Specific to the Intended Audience

Obtaining information about the intended audience is extremely important and can come from objective or subjective data sources.

Epidemiological and Empirical Information (Objective Data)

If the intended audience has already been designated based on specific requests or on the mission of an agency or organization, you may be able to obtain information about food and health status of a specific intended audience directly from previously collected data in local databases (e.g., city or county health data) or existing records. For example, data may show that the given group is at nutritional risk (e.g., for hypertension). In many situations, however, the information will be inferred either from general surveys or from indirect indicators. For example, the older adults who are likely to participate in your program may have high rates of obesity or diabetes because national surveys indicate that such nutritional problems are common among older adults in general.

Health Issues and Needs as Stated by the Intended Audience (Subjective Data)

Just as important as the actual, objective food and nutritional issues identified by science research or national policy documents are the food and health issues and needs as perceived by the intended audience. Individuals are the experts on their own lives, so it is important to understand what they perceive as issues and dilemmas. What food- or nutrition-related issues are they concerned about? What other health needs or competing, non-health-related concerns do they have? If at all possible, the nutrition educator should obtain information directly from the intended audience through focus group discussions, in-depth interviews of key informants, or surveys.

Balancing Objective and Subjective Data

The issues or needs as seen from the point of view of the group or intended audience may or may not be the same as the objective nutritional problem or issue of concern. An example is the town of Kerelia in Finland, where the heart disease rate was one of the highest in the world. When the citizens heard the statistics, they were very concerned and requested the government to do something about it. Here objective data and subjective perceptions converged. But sometimes a community or group may have concerns that are different from those of the nutrition professional. For example, parents of a child in a child-care facility may be mostly concerned about the cost and hours of the facility, whereas a nutritionist may be mostly concerned that the facility provides tasty and healthful food for the children.

Nutrition education programs sometimes fail because they do not pay enough attention to the participants' *own* perception of their food and health issues and needs (and existing strengths). In conducting assessments, then, whether formally or informally, include discussions with individuals or small groups and *listen carefully*. You may find that potential participants have important insights into their condition and useful ideas about possible solutions if they are encouraged to share them with you.

Note: These data are for health issues and *not* for food-related behaviors.

Health Issues and Needs Stated as Priorities by Organizations or Funding Sources

You may need to consider some administrative issues as you choose the nutrition education focus. You may work for an agency or organization, or the nutrition education sessions you have been asked to design will be conducted in, or for, an agency or organization that has its own priorities. Examples might be an after-school program, extension program, public health department, or senior center. Thus, information on the general administrative needs of the sponsoring agency may also be necessary before you plan and implement a nutrition education program. You can ask questions such as the following:

- How will the nutrition education program enhance the overall mission of the organization or funder?
- What are the expectations of the organization or funding source about the nutrition education component? What factors within the organization will facilitate or hinder the design and implementation of your nutrition education program? For example, will the nutrition education component compete with other components for funds? For facilities?
- How much do other personnel expect to become involved with the nutrition education sessions or program you design?

Prioritize Health Issues

Whether the needs analysis has been comprehensive or brief, you, or the nutrition education team, will probably have gathered information on more issues than you have the time or resources to address. Thus, you must prioritize and focus. In addition, the information from all the various sources should be balanced. For example, the perceptions of the intended audience may be at odds with the issues of professional concern based on scientific findings and epidemiological data. These differing interests have to be balanced as you select an issue or need to address that is appropriate to a given nutrition education session or program.

Choice of *issue or need* to address can be based on the following (as suggested by Green & Kreuter 2004):

- Which of these issues or needs are categorized as local, regional, or national priorities?
- Which issues, if appropriately addressed, are likely to have the greatest impact on the outcomes desired?
- Which issues or needs are most amenable to intervention by educational means?
- Which issues or needs are considered by the intended audience to be most important?
- Which issues or needs are considered by the sponsoring agency or funding source to be most important?

Select the Audience

Choice of *intended audience* is usually made in conjunction with the data on food and health issues. For the given food or health issues se-

lected, the choice of audience can be based on greatest need or interest using criteria such as the following:

- Size of the population for whom the issues are a problem or of concern (e.g., childhood obesity affects millions)
- The severity or incidence of the nutritional condition or food system situation (e.g., diabetes is severe and is found in high incidence in certain populations)
- Those who are most ready for change

Product from Step 1A: Statement of Health Issues or Needs and Intended Audience

Using the criteria listed, prioritize health conditions, food-related concerns, and group interests to identify the major issues and the intended audience that the intervention will address. Use the Step 1A worksheet to help you in this process. Examples of issues and audiences are childhood overweight prevention, osteoporosis prevention among community adults, or heart disease prevention among women. See **Nutrition Education in Action 7-1** for some specific examples.

■ STEP 1B: IDENTIFYING THE BEHAVIORS AND PRACTICES THAT CONTRIBUTE TO THE HEALTH ISSUE

Information about the health status or the food-related concerns of a group does not provide a sufficient basis for an educational intervention. You need to know the diet-related behaviors and practices contributing to the food- and nutrition-related problems because *these behaviors* are the focus of nutrition education, as shown in the Figure 7-2 flowchart and in the Figure 7-3 Stepwise Procedure graphic. The extensiveness of the information you want, as well as the degree of accuracy you need, depends very much on the nature and duration of your intervention.

If you are providing only one or two sessions with a given audience, it is still important to collect behavioral information, but a simple questionnaire that you design may be sufficient. If the intervention is with a group that you will be working with for some time, and formal evaluation data will be needed for the agency or funder, you will want to use some more formal instruments that are available or adapt them for your use.

The next step, then, is to identify which behaviors, actions, or dietary practices may have contributed to the food- and health-related issues of concern that you have identified for the intended audience. The Step 1B worksheet can help you with this process.

Review of the Relevant Nutrition Research Literature

The nutrition research literature is a good place to start looking for information regarding the primary audience you have selected and the key needs or issues that you have identified. Here you are seeking data on food-related *behaviors*, *actions*, or *practices* that have been shown to have impacts on the specific health or food issues you identified. The degree of specificity of the information may vary for each issue and population. But it is important to have specific information if it is available.

For example, which food practices of the family or social environment contribute to the high incidence of overweight in this particular group of school-aged children? Too many sweetened beverages? Too little physical activity? Or both? Which behaviors of the identified primary audience lead to the audience's high serum cholesterol levels? Do people eat high-fat foods too often or do the food preparation methods add fat to

NUTRITION EDUCATION IN ACTION **7-1**

Choice of Focus for Nutrition Education: Examples of Issues, Audiences, and Behaviors

Food or Health Issues and Audience	Behavioral Focus
Diabetes health: It's in Your Hands: a community-based approach (audience) to diabetes self-management (issue)	Diet (fruit and vegetable and fat intakes), exercise, medications, blood glucose monitoring, and foot care (*JNEB* 2007, O6)
Using science education to move middle schoolers (audience) toward more healthful food and activity choices (issue): an outcome evaluation of *Choice, Control, & Change*	Increasing fruit and vegetable intake and physical activity and decreasing intakes of sweetened beverages, packaged snacks, fast food, and TV leisure screen time (*JNEB* 2007, O15)
"What's Cooking?": culinary nutrition education (issue: cooking skills) in the supermarket (audience: moms)	Fruit and vegetable intake, cooking at home (*JNEB* 2007, 07)
Garden-based learning experiences for sixth-grade students (audience) to increase vegetable intake (issue)	Frequency and variety of vegetables consumed (*JNEB* 2005, O25)
Promotion of the healthy traditional Latino diet (issue) among youth ages 8 to 12 years (audience)	More beans, fruits, and vegetables and fewer high-sugar and high-fat foods (*JNEB* 2005, O23)
Overcoming "picky eating" (issue) in preschoolers (audience)	Increasing familiarity with 13 novel foods (*JNEB* 2005, O17)
Promoting healthful eating through youth-operated farm stands (issue) in low-income communities (audience)	Increased access to affordable, high-quality, locally grown produce (environmental support), and increased redemption of food stamps and consumption of local produce (*JNEB* 2005, O26, O27)
Improving the school food environment with the use of local foods (issue) by food service directors (audience)	Use of foods from local producers through a Farm to School program
Improving child feeding practices and physical activity behaviors of preschoolers (issue) through a newsletter intervention with parents (audience)	Child feeding practices of parents (pressure to eat, restriction, perceived responsibility, and monitoring of child's eating) and physical activity behaviors in children (time spent playing outdoors, active play, and watching television) (*JNEB* 2005, O75)
Food safety education (issue) for persons living with HIV/AIDS (audience)	Appropriate food handling and cooking behaviors; personal behaviors such as hand washing
A health-centered curriculum (issue) for community adults (audience)	Increased pleasurable and healthy eating, enjoyment of physically active living, and body-size acceptance of self and others (*JNEB* 2004, O47)
Incorporating physical activity in nutrition education classes for adult limited-resource audiences (audience) through use of walking DVD programs. Obesity prevention (issue)	Intentional walking for physical activity (*JNEB* 2009, S25:P20)
Bring Some Fruit to School Program to improve health (issue) in elementary school children (Italy) (audience)	Increased intakes of fruits, vegetables, legumes, fish, and fewer sweetened drinks and packaged snacks (*JNEB* 2009, S23:P15)

Sources: Journal for Nutrition Education and Behavior 2004;36(Suppl.1); *Journal for Nutrition Education and Behavior* 2005;37(Suppl. 1); *Journal for Nutrition Education and Behavior* 2007;39(Suppl. 1); and *Journal for Nutrition Education and Behavior* 2009;41(Suppl. 1).

foods (e.g., frying foods), or both? Which behaviors contribute to the low vitamin C status? Are people eating too few vegetables and fruits in their diets or are they cooking vegetables in such a way as to destroy the vitamin C, or both? Which healthful behaviors and practices are already being practiced by the group (i.e., what are the group's assets)?

Perhaps they already practice a number of behaviors that are healthful, such as a high consumption of beans and whole grains, and can be encouraged to do more.

Review of Monitoring Data or Consumer Surveys

Reviewing monitoring data or consumer surveys can also provide valuable information. For example, if adolescents are the intended audience that you have selected, and overweight prevention is the key health issue identified for the focus of your nutrition education program or sessions, then you will want to review existing consumer surveys, national or local monitoring data, or surveys of food purchasing practices for information on behaviors that might contribute to the issue of overweight.

Even if it is not possible to obtain information directly from the group, knowledge about the food practices and habits of people similar to the intended group is extremely helpful. This information search may yield the finding, for example, that frequent consumption of high-fat fast foods and sweetened drinks and low intakes of fruits and vegetables are contributing behaviors to overweight in similar adolescents.

Information from the Intended Audience

Surveys

If it is possible to survey the primary audience, you should do so because questionnaires that ask about specific dietary practices provide you with specific information that is extremely useful. For example, people often have misconceptions about the amount of fat or amount of fruits and vegetables in their diets (Bogers et al. 2004).

Informal surveys using short checklists to find out about behaviors and practices of your audience may be sufficient for your purposes. If you need to be more systematic, you may need to use more formal instruments. Some of the kinds of data you can collect are listed here, along with methods for assessing them. An example of an instrument is given in **Table 7-1**.

- *Food purchasing behaviors or practices.* Specific shopping practices, such as using a shopping list, doing comparison shopping, or using coupons can be obtained from surveys and interviews (Hersey et al. 2001).
- *Intake of specific foods or food items.* Food frequency questionnaires can be comprehensive (Willett et al. 1987; Block et al. 1992) or can be short and targeted to the behaviors of interest, in which case they often are called *checklists* or *screeners* (such as screeners for fruits and vegetables, high-fat foods, or local foods) (Thompson & Byers 1994; Block et al. 2000; Yaroch, Resnicow, & Khan 2000; Townsend et al. 2003; McPherson et al. 2000; McClelland et al. 2001). For nutrition education in most practice settings, short food intake checklists are sufficient.
- *Specific observable behaviors.* Examples are using skim milk instead of whole milk, taking the skin off chicken when eating chicken, or eating whole-grain bread instead of white bread. These behaviors can be assessed using questionnaires such as the Kristal Food Habits Questionnaire (Shannon et al. 1997).

TABLE 7-1	**Food Behavior Checklist for Limited-Resources Audiences**

Scores of 1 to 5 = Never, Sometimes, Often, Usually, Always. Scores for those items with yes/no responses are shown in parentheses.

Fruit and vegetable items

Do you eat more than one kind of fruit daily?	____
During the past week, did you have citrus fruit (such as orange or grapefruit) or citrus juice? (yes = 2; no = 1)	____
Do you eat more than one kind of vegetable daily?	____
How many servings of vegetables do you eat each day?	____
Do you eat two or more servings of vegetables at your main meal?	____
Do you eat fruits or vegetables as snacks?	____
How many servings of fruit do you eat each day?	____

Milk items

Do you drink milk daily?	____
During the past week, did you have milk as a beverage or on cereal?	____

Fat and cholesterol items

During the past week, did you have fish? (yes = 2; no = 1)	____
Do you take the skin off chicken?	____

Diet quality

When shopping, do you use the Nutrition Facts label to choose foods?	____
Do you drink regular soft drinks?	____
Do you buy Kool-Aid, Gatorade, Sunny Delight, or other fruit drink/punch?	____
Would you describe your diet as excellent (5), very good (4), good (3), fair (2), or poor (1)?	____

Food security

Do you run out of food before the end of the month?	____

Source: Reprinted from *Journal of Nutrition Education and Behavior,* Vol 35, M. S. Townsend, L. L. Kaiser, L. H. Allen, A. Block Joy, and S. P. Murphy. "Selecting Items for a Food Behavior Checklist for a Limited-Resource Audience," pages 69–82. Copyright 2003, with permission from the Society for Nutrition Education.

Food safety behaviors belong in this category and can also be assessed; examples are cooking foods adequately, practicing personal hygiene, and keeping foods at a safe temperature (Meideros et al. 2001).

- *Eating patterns.* Examples are whether the audience eats breakfast, or fruit as a snack, or three meals a day. You can devise an instrument to fit your purposes.
- *Quality of diet.* Sometimes a single question can be used, such as "How would you describe the quality of your diet?" Alternatively, it can be judged from analysis of MyPyramid servings or other instruments.

Interviews

If at all possible, talk to the intended audience about their behaviors and practices. Behavioral data can be obtained through individual interviews, focus groups, or intercept interviews as people leave a food store. Pay special attention to culture-specific foods and practices.

Observations

Observations are difficult to do but can be very informative. They can be quite informal, such as observing what children eat in school or what teenagers purchase in the school neighborhood after school.

Prioritize the Behaviors or Practices That Contribute to the Issue or Need

Again, you or the nutrition education team probably have gathered information on more behaviors or practices than you have the time or resources to address, so you have to prioritize and focus. For example, the behaviors could be as follows: low intake of fruits and vegetables, high intake of high-calorie foods and snacks, sedentary behaviors, and high consumption of sweetened drinks and low consumption of milk and dairy products. These may be more behaviors than you can address in your program, given time and resource constraints, if you wish to have a meaningful impact on behavior. (You could provide informational talks on all of these topics to raise awareness of the issues, but that does not mean the lectures will have an impact on attitudes or action.) Rate the behaviors or practices on the basis of the criteria described below (Rogers 2003; Green & Kreuter 2004) and use the Step 1B worksheet to record your ratings.

The criteria for rating the behaviors are discussed in the following subsections.

1. How Important Is It to Change This Behavior or Engage in a New Practice?

Each of the behaviors or practices of concern you have identified should be rated in terms of importance based on its *prevalence* in the population and the *strength of its contribution* to the health condition or food-related issue identified. This can be done by asking the following questions: do these behaviors occur frequently in the population identified? Do these behaviors clearly and significantly contribute to the health condition or food-related issue that you have identified as of concern for your selected group or population?

Prevalence information can be obtained from national or local monitoring data. The strength of the evidence linking the behaviors to the health condition or food issue can be evaluated based on a review of the relevant nutrition science literature. For example, several behaviors have been shown to be of high prevalence and to be strongly linked to cardiovascular risk: a diet high in saturated fat and a diet low in fruits and vegetables. Sedentary behavior is also highly prevalent and highly linked to risk of overweight, but only moderately related to cardiovascular and cancer risk. Breastfeeding is of low prevalence but is highly linked with healthy outcomes for the baby.

2. How Modifiable Is the Behavior or Practice by Educational Methods?

For each of the behaviors identified, ask: how amenable to change or modification is the behavior? A given behavior may be a very important contributor to the health or food system issue identified, but it is not a suitable target for a nutrition education intervention unless there is reasonable evidence that it is changeable by educational means. This judgment can be based on evidence from the scientific and professional nutrition education, health education, and health promotion literature that such behaviors have responded previously to interventions.

Criteria for Determining Modifiability

You also can use criteria from the Diffusion of Innovations literature to select the behaviors to focus on in the program (Rogers & Shoemaker 1971; Rogers 2003). Studies in this area have found that the likelihood of people accepting or adopting an innovation (in this case, a diet- or physical activity–related behavior) is influenced by a number of features of the innovation or behavior. You can use these findings as criteria for the changeability of the behaviors you have identified as potential targets of the program:

- *Relative advantage:* Is the new behavior seen by the intended audience as better than the one it will replace?
- *Complexity:* Is the new behavior easy to understand, act on, and adopt? How many substeps may be involved?
- *Compatibility:* How compatible is the new behavior with existing practices, values, and cultural norms of the primary group or intended audience?
- *Trialability:* Can the behavior be tried out before making a long-term commitment to act upon it or to adopt it?
- *Observability:* Are the positive results of the behavior change easily visible to the intended audience?

3. How Feasible in Practice?

How feasible will it be for you to design an intervention that can address the behavior or practice, based on considerations of available resources and the potential duration and intensity possible for the intervention? How much time and resources will you be able to devote to the intervention? How long a program can you offer? Will that be sufficient to show change?

4. How Desirable to Intended Audience?

It is extremely important to obtain substantial subjective information from the intended audience. How desirable is it to the intended audi-

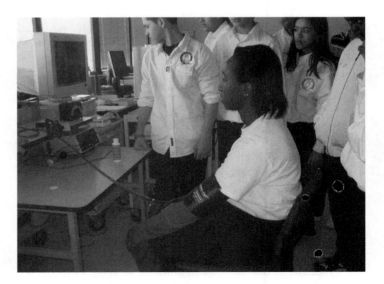

Students learn about blood pressure and how it relates to their diet.

ence to take this action or to adopt this particular recommended dietary behavior? Do *they* see the behavior as realistic? Effective? Practical? Easy to do?

Practical Method for Prioritizing Behaviors or Practices

The information that you have collected so far should now permit you to identify the specific food- and diet-related behaviors or practices that will be the focus of your nutrition education intervention or program. You can prioritize informally, but it is best to be systematic about selecting priority behaviors to address. Some kind of rating system can be devised to evaluate each behavior on all of these criteria. See Step 1B Worksheet as an example. Filling out this worksheet can help you systematically review the data and make a judgment about choice of behavioral focus. If a team is involved, it may be most useful if each member first completes such a rating scheme and then the team meets to discuss the choices. This process encourages an informed and reasoned discussion of the evidence to make a sound decision.

Focusing Is Important

The Step 1B worksheet asks you to identify up to five behaviors or practices that are of concern or of importance. From these you will select the behaviors that will be the focus of your nutrition education

program (we suggest one to three). How many and which behaviors you select will depend largely on the intensity and duration possible for the program: how many sessions or components comprise the program and how long will each session or component last? What are the resources and personnel available?

Sometimes one or two behaviors may be closely related to each other and can be addressed together. For example, eating more fruits and vegetables and eating fewer high-fat foods might be addressed together because an increase in fruits and vegetables in the diet may substitute for high-fat foods (e.g., fruits instead of high-fat desserts). For the issue of childhood overweight prevention, the behaviors identified as relevant may be eating more fruits and vegetables, eating more low-fat foods, drinking fewer sweetened drinks, and decreasing sedentary behavior. For the issue of eating more local foods, the behaviors may be buying more local foods and cooking more local foods. For each example, you may not have the time and resources to address all the behaviors, so select those that you *can* address.

Some Examples

Nutrition Education in Action 7-2 provides some examples of how the nutrition education issues, audiences, and behaviors have been stated for the Supplemental Nutrition Assistance Program–Education component (SNAP-Ed) and the Team Nutrition program.

NUTRITION EDUCATION IN ACTION **7-2**

Examples of Core Behavior Goals of Nutrition Education Programs and Their Rationales

Supplemental Nutrition Assistance Program–Education (SNAP-Ed)

Although there are many important nutrition-related issues that affect the SNAP–eligible audience, the Food and Nutrition Service of the U.S. Department of Agriculture (USDA) encourages states to focus their Supplemental Nutrition Assistance Program–Education (SNAP-Ed) program efforts on the following behavior outcomes:

- Eat fruits and vegetables, whole grains, and fat-free or low-fat milk or milk products every day.
- Be physically active every day as part of a healthy lifestyle.
- Balance calorie intake from foods and beverages with calories expended.

These behaviors are associated with a reduced risk of some forms of cancer, type 2 diabetes, and coronary heart disease. It is appropriate to focus on these behavior outcomes for SNAP-Ed because low-income individuals often experience a disproportionate share of diet-related problems that are risk factors for the major diseases contributing to poor health, disability, and premature death.

Team Nutrition

The USDA's Team Nutrition promotes comprehensive, behavior-based nutrition education to enable children to make healthy eating and

physical activity choices. Social cognitive theory is the foundation of efforts to help children understand how eating and physical activity affect the way they grow, learn, play, and feel today as well as the relationship of their choices to lifelong health. These efforts are designed to increase their understanding that healthy eating and physical activity are fun and that skills developed today will assist them in enjoying healthy eating and physical activity in later years.

All program materials encourage students to make food and physical activity choices for a healthy lifestyle. The focus is on five behavior outcomes:

- Eat a variety of foods
- Eat more fruits, vegetables, and grains
- Eat lower-fat foods more often
- Get your calcium-rich foods
- Be physically active

Sources: Food and Nutrition Service, U.S. Department of Agriculture. 2009. *Supplemental Nutrition Assistance Program guiding principles.* http://www.fns.usda .gov/snap/nutrition_education/default.htm; and Food and Nutrition Service, U.S. Department of Agriculture. n.d. About Team Nutrition. http://www.fns.usda.gov/tn/ about.

STEP 1C: STATING THE BEHAVIORAL OR ACTION GOALS TO BE THE FOCUS OF THE PROGRAM

From the set of identified behaviors or practices of concern, select and finalize those that the program or sessions will address and state them in terms of targeted core behaviors or program behavioral goals.

These goals should describe the purpose or desired *behavioral* or *action outcomes* for the program, or even individual sessions. As noted previously, evidence suggests that nutrition education is more likely to be effective if it focuses on *specific* behaviors or community practices. Thus, state the program goals in terms of behaviors or practices. The scope of the behavioral goal or goals reflects the duration, intensity, and extensiveness of the program. Examples of behavioral goals are to increase fruit and vegetable consumption among adolescents, increase calcium-rich food consumption of women in the WIC program, increase participation in the farmers' market Supplemental Nutrition Assistance Program Electronic Benefit Transfer (EBT) card program, increase the choice of more healthful snacks and beverages by elementary school students, increase the proportion of women with type 2 diabetes who practice effective food management skills, and increase the number of people who participate in community-supported agriculture.

Specificity of Behavioral Goals

Some nutrition educators like to state program behavioral or action goals in terms of very specific behavioral objectives, specifying the exact changes desired, such as the following: adolescents will eat two or more cups of fruits and vegetables a day, or the proportion of women breast-feeding for at least four weeks will increase from 20% to 40%. In this book, both levels of specificity are referred to as *behavioral goals* for two reasons. First, writing "behavioral objectives" in addition to "behavioral goals" adds another step in an already long process. Second, the term *behavioral objectives* has other meanings in the educational field, as you shall see in Chapter 10; thus, there may be confusion about what the term means. The choice of specificity depends on the purposes of your program. If you will be measuring specific behavioral outcomes in your evaluation, you need to state your behavioral outcomes in specific terms.

For example, a behavioral goal can be stated generally as follows: to increase fruit and vegetable intake among adolescents. You could state

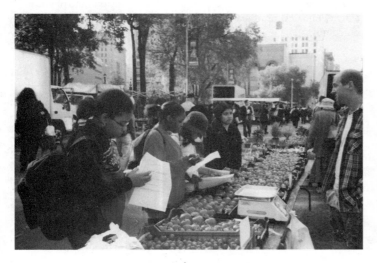

Students can find out the cost of tomatoes as part of a scavenger hunt.

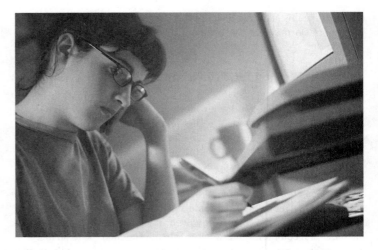

Nutrition education research can be gathered at town or university libraries.

the goal more specifically: adolescents in seventh and eighth grades will increase their fruit and vegetable intake to 2.5 cups or more a day. Use the Step 1C worksheet to state your program's behavioral goals.

Nutrition Education in Action 7-3 provides some examples of how the nutrition education focus and issues, audiences, and behaviors have been stated for some social marketing and Web-based programs.

PAUSE

It is important at this point to resist a strong desire to launch into designing the food and nutrition education program given what you already know about the participants. Even knowledge about the specific behaviors leading to a given health condition may not be sufficient. In one study, the diets of low-income families in Brazil were found to be deficient in protein (the nutritional status problem), and the families were not using soybeans as part of the diet. Because soybeans are produced in Brazil and are a good source of protein, a nutrition education campaign was developed directed at increasing consumption of these beans (Wright, Horner, & Charini 1982). When it met with very little success, families were then interviewed about *why* they did not eat soybeans. Among the reasons were dislike of the taste of soybeans, unfamiliarity, lack of interest, unavailability of soybeans, and lack of knowledge about preparation methods. Only when such information was available was it possible to design and test several more appropriate approaches. Such considerations, then, lead to another set of factors that must be assessed when you wish your nutrition education efforts to be successful: the determinants of mediators of action or behavior change; these are described in the next chapter.

CASE STUDY

A case study is presented to illustrate the design process. This case study is used throughout the next several chapters for each of the steps. Here it begins with Step 1 of the nutrition education design process.

The case involves a university-affiliated organization that works with children and youth. Thus, the general audience is already determined. The mission of the organization is to provide health services to youth and their families in the community. The community is ethnically and economically diverse. The agency has provided general health services in schools, but it has not developed a nutrition education program

---

NUTRITION EDUCATION IN ACTION 7-3

Examples of Behavioral Goals of Nutrition Education Programs

Sisters Together: Move More, Eat Better

Sisters Together is a national initiative of the Weight-Control Information Network (WIN) designed to encourage black women ages 18 and older to maintain a healthy weight by becoming more physically active and eating healthier foods.

Sisters Together works with national and local newspapers, magazines, radio stations, schools, and consumer and professional organizations to raise awareness among black women about the health benefits of regular physical activity and healthy eating. This effort is timely because recent statistics indicate that nearly 80% of black women are overweight or obese.

Pick a Better Snack

Pick a Better Snack is a social marketing campaign in Iowa directed at low-income families and children. The objectives are to:

- Increase awareness of the campaign's logo and supporting messages
- Improve attitudes about eating fruits and vegetables as snacks

- Increase fruit and vegetable consumption among low-income children and their families

We Can!

We Can! (Ways to Enhance Children's Activity and Nutrition) is a national education program designed for parents and caregivers to help children 8 to 13 years old stay at a healthy weight. Parents and caregivers are the primary influencers for this age group. We Can! offers parents and families tips and fun activities to:

- Encourage healthy eating
- Increase physical activity
- Reduce sedentary or screen time

Sources: Weight-Control Information Network. Sisters Together: Move More, Eat Better. http://win.niddk.nih.gov/sisters/index.htm; Iowa Department of Public Health, Iowa Department of Education. Pick a better snack and act. http://www.idph.state.ia.us/Pickabettersnack; and U.S. Department of Health and Human Services, National Institutes of Health. We Can! http://www.nhlbi.nih.gov/health/public/heart/obesity/wecan.

---

before. Agency directors think that it will be important to use some of its funds to develop a nutrition education program for youth in the schools it serves because they believe, from their experience, that the diets of youth need improving. However, they do not have any specific data on their youth in relation to nutrition or what kind of program should be developed. Thus, the organization needs to find out the major nutrition-related health issues and problems that face the youth in their community and to develop a nutrition education program that addresses these issues.

In Step 1 of the Stepwise Procedure, we first analyze the health issues and needs of this audience, and then the behaviors or practices that youth engage in that contribute to these health issues or concerns. From this analysis we can identify a few behaviors or practices that the program will encourage to address the health issues. These recommended practices or behaviors become the behavioral goals of the program.

Thus, in the case study, we conduct all the steps described in this chapter with the following results:

Step 1A. Analyze the health issues of the given audience. The major health issue identified is obesity in the youth, bringing with it risk for chronic disease.

Step 1B. Identify the high-priority behaviors or practices that contribute to the health issues. The behaviors contributing to the health issue are: eating too few fruits and vegeta-

bles; drinking too many sweetened drinks; eating too many highly processed, energy dense snacks; eating out at fast food restaurants; and sedentary behavior.

Step 1C. State the program's behavioral or action goals for the audience. The behavioral goals describe the desired behavioral outcomes for the program as follows:

- Increase fruit and vegetable intakes to 2.5 or more cups a day
- Increase physical activity to 10,000 steps or more per day
- Decrease intake of highly processed, energy dense snacks to 150 calories or less per day
- Decrease intake of sugar-sweetened beverages to less than 8 oz per day

We decide to call the program "Taking Control: Eating Well and Being Fit." In the next chapter we will explore the determinants or potential mediators of these behavioral goals.

■ YOUR TURN: COMPLETING THE STEP 1 WORKSHEETS

The worksheets that have been described throughout the chapter can be found at the end of this chapter. Use them as you start the design process for a hypothetical or real nutrition education program.

Questions and Activities

1. What do you see as the advantages and disadvantages of using a systematic process for designing theory- and evidence-based nutrition education?

2. Why is it important to do a thorough assessment of the needs, interests, and concerns of the intended audience?

3. On what basis would you select the issues or problems you would address in a nutrition education program?

4. As mentioned earlier in the book, nutrition education is more likely to be effective if it focuses on behaviors and practices. What does that mean for the needs analysis process?

5. How would you select which behaviors or practices your program should address for your intended audience? That is, what criteria would you use and why?

6. If you have provided nutrition education sessions before, which of the steps from the Stepwise Procedure did you use, whether consciously or unconsciously? Do you think the steps are really needed? Why or why not?

References

Agricultural Research Service, U.S. Department of Agriculture. 2000. *Continuing survey of food intakes by individuals 1994–1996 (CSFII 1994–1996)*. Washington, DC: Author.

American Dietetic Association. 2008. Nutrition Care Process and Model Part I: The 2008 update. *Journal of the American Dietetic Association* 108:1113–1117.

Baranowski, T., E. Cerin, and J. Baranowski. 2009. Steps in the design, development, and formative evaluation of obesity prevention–related behavior change. *International Journal of Behavioral Nutrition and Physical Activity* 6:6.

Baranowski, T., L. S. Lin, D. W. Wetter, K. Resnicow, and M. D. Hearn. 1997. Theory as mediating variables: Why aren't community interventions working as desired? *Annals of Epidemiology* 7:589–595.

Block, G., C. Gillespie, E. H. Rosenbaum, and C. Jenson. 2000. A rapid food screener to assess fat and fruit and vegetable intake. *American Journal of Preventive Medicine* 18:284–288.

Block, G., F. E. Thompson, A. M. Hartman, F. A. Larkin, and K. E. Guire. 1992. Comparison of two dietary questionnaires validated against multiple dietary records collected during a 1-year period. *Journal of the American Dietetic Association* 92:686–693.

Bogers, R. P., J. Brug, P. van Assema, and P. C. Dagnelie. 2004. Explaining fruit and vegetable consumption: The theory of planned behavior and misconception of personal intake levels. *Appetite* 42:157–166.

Green, L. W., and M. M. Kreuter. 2004. *Health promotion planning: An educational and ecological approach*. 4th ed. New York: McGraw-Hill.

Hersey, J., J. Anliker, C. Miller, et al. 2001. Food shopping practices are associated with dietary quality in low-income households. *Journal of Nutrition Education and Behavior* 33:S16–S26.

McClelland, J. W., D. P. Keenan, J. Lewis, et al. 2001. Review of evaluation tools used to assess the impact of nutrition education on dietary intake and quality, weight management practices, and physical activity of low-income audiences. *Journal of Nutrition Education* 33:S35–S48.

McNeal, J. U. 1992. *Kids as customers: A handbook of marketing to children*. New York: Lexington Books.

McPherson, R. C., D. M. Hoelscher, M. Alexander, K. S. Scanlon, and M. K. Serdula. 2000. Dietary assessment methods among school-aged children. *Preventive Medicine* 31:S11–S33.

Medeiros, L., V. Hillers, P. Kendall, and A. Mason. 2001. Evaluation of food safety education for consumers. *Journal of Nutrition Education* 33:S27–S34.

Rogers, E. M. 2003. *Diffusion of innovations*. 4th ed. New York: Free Press.

Rogers, E. M., and F. F. Shoemaker. 1971. *Communication of innovations: A cross-cultural approach*. New York: Free Press.

Shannon, J., A. R. Kristal, S. J. Curry, and S. A. Beresford. 1997. Application of a behavioral approach to measuring dietary change: The fat and fiber-related diet behavior questionnaire. *Cancer Epidemiology, Biomarkers and Prevention* 6:355–361.

Thompson, F. E., and T. Byers. 1994. Dietary assessment resource manual. *Journal of Nutrition* 124(11 Suppl):2245S–2317S.

Townsend, M. S., L. L. Kaiser, L. H. Allen, A. Block Joy, and S. P. Murphy. 2003. Selecting items for a food behavior checklist for a limited-resources audience. *Journal of Nutrition Education and Behavior* 35:69–82.

Whitehead, F. 1973. Nutrition education research. *World Review of Nutrition and Dietetics* 17:91–149.

Willett, W. C., R. D. Reynolds, S. Cottrell-Hoehner, L. Sampson, and M. L. Browne. 1987. Validation of a semi-quantitative food frequency questionnaire: Comparison with a 1-year diet record. *Journal of the American Dietetic Association* 87:43–47.

Wright, M., M. R. Horner, and L. H. Charini. 1982. Approaches for increasing soybean use by low-income Brazilian families. *Journal of Nutrition Education* 14(3):105–107.

Yaroch, A. L., K. Resnicow, and L. K. Khan. 2000. Validity and reliability of qualitative dietary fat index questionnaires: A review. *Journal of the American Dietetic Association* 100(2):240–244.

Before you design any nutrition education intervention, whether it is a few sessions or a larger program with several components, it is important to determine your intervention focus and identify your intended primary audience. When those have been determined, you will need detailed information on the behaviors and practices that contribute to the issue or problem you have selected as your intervention focus. Step 1 worksheets will help you conduct assessments to obtain the information you will need.

Think of yourself as a detective as you work through these worksheets. You are trying to find out as much as you can to determine which core behaviors or behavioral goals will be the targets for your educational sessions.

The information you collect may be quite extensive, depending on the scope and duration of your intervention, and will vary by category. Cite information sources (e.g., journal article, government report, observation, interview) used in the worksheet in a bibliography at the end of this step.

At the end of the Step 1 worksheets, you should have products for Steps 1A, 1B, and 1C as follows:

Step 1A: Health issues or needs (one or two) and primary intended audience for the nutrition education intervention. Examples are "overweight in teenagers" or "low rates of breastfeeding in a low-income audience."

Step 1B: High-priority behaviors contributing to the selected issues. A set of one to a few nutrition-related behaviors or community practices that contribute to the health issue(s) that you identified.

Step 1C: Statement of the program's behavioral or action goals. The behavioral or action goals describe the purpose or behavioral outcomes for the program in terms of behaviors or community practices.

Use these worksheets as guides to help you identify program behavioral goals. Cite information sources in the text and add references to the bibliography at the end of the step. Electronic versions of these worksheets are available at http://nutrition.jbpub.com/ education/2e/. If you are unable to access the worksheets electronically, you can write onto this blank worksheet or create a text document that uses the same flow of information.

> **NOTE:** The program described in this case study is a multi-component program, and each box in this step has been completed comprehensively. If the program you create is smaller (e.g., one or two lessons), you will still complete each box but in less detail, as the amount of detail needed for each box is dependent upon the scope and duration of the program.

Step 1A: Issues and intended audience

Describe the demographics of your audience (e.g., age, subgroup, ethnicity) and the location of the site.

The organization initiating the program is a university affiliated non-profit organization that provides health services to youth and families in the community.

This program will focus on students who attend a large middle school that services the 7th and 8th graders for the entire city. There are approximately 1750 students in the school. Parents of students in the school and school community members will also be indirectly impacted.

Per the last census, the community in which the intervention will be taking place is ethnically diverse: 55% of the population is white, 30% black or African American, 10% Hispanic, and 5% from other races. The median household income is $32,000, and the median family income is approximately $40,000. Roughly 20% of the population is below the poverty level.[1] The demographics of the students and their parents mirror those of the community at large.[2]

The school where the intervention program will be implemented currently provides health care services to the students and their families. There is a clinic within the school that offers basic medical services, such as wellness exams and treatment for common disease and conditions. The clinic also has a dental unit that provides dental cleanings and cavity fillings. The clinic is a source of pride for the school and the community, and there has been recent interest in adding nutrition-related programs that would help promote wellness and prevent certain conditions, like obesity. There is a lot of support from faculty, parents, and the general community for this expansion. However, the school does not have the expertise to do it alone, so we will help them conduct a needs assessment, develop an appropriate program, and plan the evaluation.

Analyze the priority health issues for your audience.

Research. What does scientific research suggest as the major health issues for this audience?

Overweight and obesity:

- Rates have doubled in U.S. children in the past two decades. 14% of 6- to 19-year olds are now estimated to be overweight and 14% are "at risk for overweight."[3,4]

- Rates are highest and rising the fastest among African American, Hispanic, Asian American, and Native American adolescents living in low-income communities.[3]

- Childhood overweight is associated with both immediate (e.g., increased cholesterol levels, risk of type 2 diabetes) and long-term consequences (e.g., cardiovascular disease, type 2 diabetes, metabolic syndrome).[5,6]

- Overweight adolescents have a 70% chance of becoming overweight or obese adults.[7]

- Childhood overweight also carries with it immediate social consequences since overweight children often experience rejection by peers, psychological distress, dissatisfaction with their bodies, and low self-esteem.[8,9]

Metabolic syndrome (MetS):

- It is estimated that ~9.2% of all adolescents (12–19 years old) have MetS based on pediatric standards developed from ATP III.[10]

- This rate is higher among overweight or obese adolescents. One in three could be classified as having MetS, and two thirds have at least one metabolic abnormality.[6,10] Biomarkers of an increased risk of adverse cardiovascular outcomes are already present in these youngsters.[6]

- MetS puts adolescents at risk for long- and short-term complications associated with heart disease and diabetes.

Asthma:

- On average, in a classroom of 30 students, about 3 are likely to have asthma. It is estimated that approximately 5.6 million children and adolescents (5–17 years old) have asthma.[11]

- Asthma is one of the leading causes of school absenteeism.[12]

- Asthma may prevent students from engaging in physical activity because of fears of an attack.

+

Policy. What do governmental guidelines recommend as priority health issues?

Overweight and obesity:

- Various governmental organizations at the federal, state, and local levels have made calls to action for childhood obesity/obesity prevention. At the federal level, the Office of the Surgeon General[7] has issued a statement naming obesity as a priority, and the Department of Health and Human Services listed obesity as one of it target health priorities in *Healthy People 2010*.[13] At the local level, some municipalities require that BMIs are taken and provided to parents as part of the report card.

Metabolic syndrome (MetS):

- *Healthy People 2010* lists diabetes, heart disease, and obesity as focus areas.[13] These conditions are all associated with MetS.

Asthma:

- Respiratory disease, including asthma, is focus of *Healthy People 2010*.[13]

+

+

Audience. What are specific health issues and needs related to the intended audience (from objective and subjective data)?

- The city health department study demonstrated that the rates of overweight/risk for overweight among the city's children and adolescents are higher than the national rates. However, rates of asthma and anemia are lower than national rates.[14]

- Adolescents consider "weight" to be an important issue. Adolescents also think about other health conditions like diabetes, asthma, and food allergies. These issues are most important to students who have the condition or have a close friend or young family member with the condition.[15]

+

Organization. What does the organization and/or funding source state as key health priorities to address?

- The program funder is a university-affiliated organization whose mission is to provide nutrition education and services to the pediatric population and their families in the community. Addressing overweight prevention has been selected by the agency as its priority area for education and service.

- Promoting health—physical and mental—and the development of healthy habits is part of the mission of the school.[15]

Determine one or two priority health issues for the program to address. From the issues you identified, prioritize based on greatest need, whether education can help, the importance to the audience, and importance to the organization.

> In this population, overweight/obesity is the issue of greatest need because it has the ability to impact the most students. Education and environmental change are appropriate ways to address it. Additionally, addressing it is important to students, parents, and other community members who comprise the program's audience. It also is of importance to the funding group. In addition, obesity and metabolic syndrome are closely related. Therefore, addressing obesity may indirectly impact the issue of metabolic syndrome.

Step 1B: Contributing behaviors or practices

Identify the behaviors or practices that contribute to the priority health issues.

Nutrition research literature		Monitoring data or consumer surveys		Information from intended audience
General diet: • It is suggested that consuming a diet high in fruits, vegetables, and unprocessed grains is beneficial for health. Specific behaviors: • Fruits and vegetables: Fruits and vegetables have high water and fiber content, which increase volume. They are low in calories and energy density. Eating fruits and vegetables can contribute a sense of fullness and help people maintain their weight.[16] • Added sugars: High intakes of added sweeteners make it difficult for most people to maintain their weight. Ludwig et al.[17] show that consumption of sugar sweetened beverages is an independent risk factor for obesity in children aged 11–12 years. For every additional serving of sugar-sweetened drink consumed, the odds of becoming obese increase by 60%. Another study links soft drink consumption to excess energy intake and weight gain among adolescents.[18] • Increased sedentary behavior: Watching television and computer usage increase the odds of being overweight.[19-22]	+	General diet: • Among children aged 6–11 years, trends show increases in intakes of soft drinks, fruit drinks, and candy and decreases in milk and certain vegetables. Intakes of discretionary fat and added sugars were much higher than recommended.[23] Specific behaviors: • Fruits and vegetables: Only 30% of youths eat the recommended amount of fruits and only 36% eat the recommended servings of vegetables (including fried potatoes).[24] • Added sugars: Adolescents, on average, get 11% of all their calories from carbonated beverages, fruit-flavored and part-juice drinks, and sports drinks. This equals 15 teaspoons of sugar per day from these drinks.[25] • Fast food: Those who regularly eat fast food have higher intakes of calories, fat, sodium, and carbonated soft drinks and lower intakes of fruits and vegetables.[26] • Increased sedentary behavior: Only 35% of adolescents meet physical activity recommendations. Only 54% attend PE class 1 or more days a week while 35% watch 3 or more hours of television during the school week.[27]	+	From surveys of and interviews with the intended audience,[15] the following information arose: • Fruits and vegetables: These students eat on average only 2 servings of fruits and vegetables each day, mostly fruits. • Added sugars: They drink two 16-ounce bottles of sugar-sweetened beverages each day. • Packaged snacks: They eat an average of 3 packaged sweet and salty snacks every day, such as cookies, baked goods, and potato chips. • Fast food: They eat at fast food places four times a week, usually with friends or family. • Increased sedentary behavior: Students all live close to school, so they walk to school (a few blocks) but do not walk much otherwise. Some do go to the park and play basketball with friends. On average, they watch television about 3–4 hours a day. Those who have computers at home average an hour each day playing videogames.

List the top behaviors or practices that contribute to the priority health issues. Then rate each issue on importance, modifiability, feasibility, and desirability.

Behavior/practice	Importance for health issue	Modifiable*	Feasible	Desirable to audience
1. Eating too few fruits and vegetables	5	5	4	3
2. Drinking too many sweetened drinks	5	4	5	2
3. Eating too many high-fat, high-sugar, highly processed snacks	5	4	5	3
4. Eating out at fast food restaurants	5	4	3	2
5. Sedentary behavior	5	4	5	3

*Consider complexity, relative advantage, compatibility, and observability of behavior.

Step 1C: Behavioral goals

Choose one or a few behavioral goals from the list above to be the focus of your program. State the selected behavioral goals and provide justification for the selection of your focus behavior.

Four of the above behaviors that contribute to childhood overweight will be addressed by this program through the following behavioral goals:

- Increase intake of fruits and vegetables (youth to aim for 2.5 or more cups a day)
- Decrease daily intake of sugar-sweetened beverages to less than 8 oz
- Decrease calories from high-fat, high-sugar snacks to 150 or less per day
- Increase physical activity to 10,000 steps per day

These behaviors are priorities in terms of importance, modifiability, feasibility, and desirability to audience. First, data have shown that children and adolescents do not meet recommended intakes of fruits and vegetables, foods that are correlated with reduced risk of cardiovascular disease/some types of cancer and that also may assist with weight maintenance. Second, this group consumes much more than the recommended amounts of sweetened beverages, which contributes to excess calories and is related to dental caries. Third, the group consumes large amounts of high-fat, high-sugar snacks. Although these snacks are extremely palatable, the large amount of calories in these foods can lead to weight gain. Additionally, many of these snacks are highly processed with substances (e.g., added sugars, trans-fats, salt) that are associated with preventable chronic diseases, including heart disease. Fourth, physical activity helps maintain energy balance and keep muscle strength and cardiovascular fitness. The amount of physical activity decreases after childhood, making them more sedentary, and a sedentary lifestyle is related to overweight.

NOTE: The remainder of this case study will focus on only one of the four target behaviors: increasing intake of fruits and vegetables.

References

1. Any Town Middle School. Middle school enrollment demographics. Any Town, USA: Author; 2009.

2. Ogden CL, Carroll MD, Curtin LR, McDowell MA, Tabak CJ, Flegal KM. Prevalence of overweight and obesity in the United States, 1999–2004. *JAMA*. Apr 5, 2006;295(13):1549–1555.

3. Ogden CL, Carroll MD, Flegal KM. High body mass index for age among US children and adolescents, 2003–2006. *JAMA*. May 28, 2008;299(20):2401–2405.

4. Cook S, Weitzman M, Auinger P, Nguyen M, Dietz WH. Prevalence of a metabolic syndrome phenotype in adolescents: findings from the third National Health and Nutrition Examination Survey, 1988–1994. *Arch Pediatr Adolesc Med*. Aug 2003;157(8):821–827.

5. Weiss R, Dziura J, Burgert TS, et al. Obesity and the metabolic syndrome in children and adolescents. *N Engl J Med*. Jun 3, 2004;350(23):2362–2374.

6. U.S. Department of Health and Human Services. *The surgeon general's call to action to prevent and decrease overweight and obesity*. Washington, DC: Author; 2001.

7. Institute of Medicine. *Food marketing to children: threat or opportunity?* Washington, DC: National Academies Press; 2005.

8. Wadden TA, Stunkard AJ. Social and psychological consequences of obesity. *Ann Intern Med*. Dec 1985;103(6(Pt 2)):1062–1067.

9. American Heart Association National Center. Metabolic Syndrome—Statistics. http://docs.google.com/gview?a=v&q=cache: 98hCjmbvYxUJ:www.americanheart.org/downloadable/heart/1197995069526FS15META08.pdf+metabolic+syndrome+and+children +rates&hl=en&gl=us.

10. American Lung Association Epidemiology and Statistics Unit Research and Program Services. *Trends in asthma morbidity and mortality*. Washington, DC: Author; 2009.

11. Akinbami LJ. *The state of childhood asthma, United States, 1980–2005*. Hyattsville, MD: National Center for Health Statistics; 2006.

12. U.S. Department of Health and Human Services. *Healthy People 2010: Understanding and improving health*. Washington, DC: Government Printing Office; 2000.

13. Any Town Health Department. Town health statistics. Any Town, USA: Author; 2008.

14. University-Town Partnership. Intervention needs assessment findings: Survey and interview results, 2009.

15. U.S. Census Bureau. Census data: Any Town, Any State. http://quickfacts.census.gov/qfd/states.

16. Centers for Disease Control and Prevention. *Can eating fruits and vegetables help people to manage their weight?* Washington, DC: Author; 2000.

17. Ludwig DS, Peterson KE, Gortmaker SL. Relation between consumption of sugar-sweetened drinks and childhood obesity: a prospective, observational analysis. *Lancet*. Feb 17, 2001;357(9255):505–508.

18. Tam CS, Garnett SP, Cowell CT, Campbell K, Cabrera G, Baur LA. Soft drink consumption and excess weight gain in Australian school students: results from the Nepean study. *Int J Obes (Lond)*. Jul 2006;30(7):1091–1093.

19. Michela JL, Contento IR. Cognitive, motivational, social, and environmental influences on children's food choices. *Health Psychol*. 1986;5(3):209–230.

20. Contento IR, Michela JL. Nutrition and food choice behavior among children and adolescents. In: Goreczny AJ, Hersen M, eds. *Handbook of pediatric and adolescent health psychology*. Boston: Allyn and Bacon; 1998:249–273.

21. Gortmaker SL, Peterson K, Wiecha J, et al. Reducing obesity via a school-based interdisciplinary intervention among youth: Planet Health. *Archives of Pediatric and Adolescent Medicine*. Apr 1999;153(4):409–418.

22. Robinson TN. Reducing children's television viewing to prevent obesity: a randomized controlled trial. *JAMA*. Oct 1999;282(16):1561–1567.

23. Enns CW, Mickle SJ, Goldman JD. Trends in food and nutrient intakes by children in the United States. *Family Economics and Nutrition Review*. 2002;14(2):56–68.

24. Munoz KA, Krebs-Smith SM, Ballard-Barbash R, Cleveland LE. Food intakes of U.S. children and adolescents compared with recommendations. *Pediatrics*. Sep 1997;100(3 Pt 1):323–329.

25. Agricultural Research Service U.S. Department of Agriculture. Continuing food intake by individuals 1994–1996 (CSFII 1994–1996). Washington, DC: Author; 2000.

26. Paeratakul S, Ferdinand DP, Champagne CM, Ryan DH, Bray GA. Fast-food consumption among US adults and children: dietary and nutrient intake profile. *J Am Dietet Assn*. Oct 2003;103(10):1332–1338.

27. National Center for Chronic Disease Prevention and Health Promotion. Data and statistics: YRBSS: Youth Risk Behavior Surveillance System. http://www.cdc.gov/HealthyYouth/yrbs/index.htm.

Before you design any nutrition education intervention, whether it is a few sessions or a larger program with several components, it is important to determine your intervention focus and identify your intended primary audience. When those have been determined, you will need detailed information on the behaviors and practices that contribute to the issue or problem you have selected as your intervention focus. Step 1 worksheets will help you conduct assessments to obtain the information you will need.

Think of yourself as a detective as you work through these worksheets. You are trying to find out as much as you can to determine which core behaviors or behavioral goals will be the targets for your educational sessions.

The information you collect may be quite extensive, depending on the scope and duration of your intervention, and will vary by category. Cite information sources (e.g., journal article, government report, observation, interview) used in the worksheet in a bibliography at the end of this step.

At the end of the Step 1 worksheets, you should have products for Steps 1A, 1B, and 1C as follows:

Step 1A: Health issues or needs (one or two) and primary intended audience for the nutrition education intervention. Examples are "overweight in teenagers" or "low rates of breastfeeding in a low-income audience."

Step 1B: High-priority behaviors contributing to the selected issues. A set of one to a few nutrition-related behaviors or community practices that contribute to the health issue(s) that you identified.

Step 1C: Statement of the program's behavioral or action goals. The behavioral or action goals describe the purpose or behavioral outcomes for the program in terms of behaviors or community practices.

Use these worksheets as guides to help you identify program behavioral goals. Cite information sources in the text and add references to the bibliography at the end of the step. Electronic versions of these worksheets are available at http://nutrition.jbpub.com/education/2e/. If you are unable to access the worksheets electronically, you can write onto this blank worksheet or create a text document that uses the same flow of information.

Step 1A: Issues and intended audience

Describe the demographics of your audience (e.g., age, subgroup, ethnicity) and the location of the site.

Analyze the priority health issues for your audience.

Research. What does scientific research suggest as the major health issues for this audience?

+

Policy. What do governmental guidelines recommend as priority health issues?

+

Audience. What are specific health issues and needs related to the intended audience (from objective and subjective data)?

+

Organization. What does the organization and/or funding source state as key health priorities to address?

Determine one or two priority health issues for the program to address. From the issues you identified, prioritize based on greatest need, whether education can help, the importance to the audience, and importance to the organization.

Step 1B: Contributing behaviors or practices

Identify the behaviors or practices that contribute to the priority health issues.

Nutrition research literature	Monitoring data or consumer surveys	Information from intended audience

+

+

List the top behaviors or practices that contribute to the priority health issues. Then rate each issue on importance, modifiability, feasibility, and desirability.

Behavior/practice	Importance for health issue	Modifiable*	Feasible	Desirable to audience
1.				
2.				
3.				
4.				
5.				

*Consider complexity, relative advantage, compatibility, and observability of behavior.

Step 1C: Behavioral goals

Choose one or a few behavioral goals from the list above to be the focus of your program. State the selected behavioral goals and provide justification for the selection of your focus behaviors or community practices.

References

CHAPTER

8

Step 2: Identifying Potential Mediators of Program Behavioral Goals and Actions

OVERVIEW

This chapter describes how to use theory and research to identify personal psychosocial determinants and environmental factors that are potential mediators of the actions or behavior changes targeted by the program for the intended audience.

CHAPTER OUTLINE

- Getting to know your audience and their environments
- Step 2A: describing generally the social and cultural context that influences perceptions and attitudes
- Step 2B: identifying relevant individual and community strengths or assets
- Step 2C: identifying potential person-related mediators
- Step 2D: identifying environmental and policy factors
- Step 2E: other audience characteristics and program resource considerations for delivering the intervention
- Case study
- Your turn: completing the Step 2 worksheets

LEARNING OBJECTIVES

After completing this chapter, you will be able to:

- Appreciate the importance of thoroughly understanding the intended audience
- Develop skills in identifying the personal psychosocial factors that are potential mediators of the program's targeted behaviors, as well as the environmental factors that impede or support these behaviors for this audience
- Compare the advantages and disadvantages of different methods for obtaining the assessment information

■ GETTING TO KNOW YOUR AUDIENCE AND THEIR ENVIRONMENTS

Understanding the interests, motivations, cultural values, and concerns of a given audience is very challenging because individuals' food and physical activity behaviors involve many complex, and often conflicting, beliefs and emotions that are embedded in many aspects of their life histories and current life situations. But understand these you must if you are to design learning experiences that are meaningful and effective for the intended audience. Social marketing places a high priority on this type of assessment, calling it *formative research*.

Figure 8-1 shows that Step 2 is about identifying the determinants of behavior and mediators of change. In this step, you seek to understand

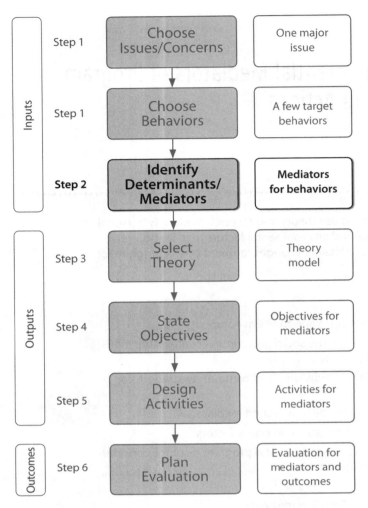

FIGURE 8-1 Flowchart of steps in designing theory-based nutrition education: Step 2.

your audience in depth. Think of yourself as a detective, aiming to identify the determinants or mediators of the behavior goals or the health-promoting actions or behavior changes that you selected for the program in Step 1.

The Stepwise Procedure (**Figure 8-2**) graphic highlights the tasks and products for Step 2. A worksheet is provided at the end of the chapter for you to use as you proceed through this chapter; the case study serves as an example of how to complete the worksheets.

Why Do People Do What They Do? What Would Help Them Take Action or Change?

Influences on people's food and activity behaviors and community practices are legion and can be quite powerful. Helping people make changes means that you need to understand these numerous influences for your audience. You cannot be effective without knowing why people do what they do and how they change.

Social and Cultural Contexts

The social and cultural contexts of people's lives, their religious beliefs, their ethnic origins, and lifestyles all influence their perceptions about

their current and desired food and activity behaviors. These influences provide the context within which psychosocial mediators operate. (This issue is discussed in greater detail in Chapter 4.) It has been found that psychosocial variables from theory help explain health behavior within the context of culture (Liou & Contento 2001). For example, for those who live in a collectivist culture where the basic social unit is the group or family, not the individual, perceived benefits of taking action (outcome expectations) might not be stated as impact on personal health, but "by keeping ourselves strong and healthy, we are better able to take care of others in our families and in our communities." Or for women of young children, the perceived benefits of a dietary behavior may be in terms of the health of their children rather than their own health. Consequently, it is important to know about people's perceptions based on their cultural context, life stage, and family situation before you explore the personal psychosocial mediators in depth.

Psychosocial Mediators

These potential mediators of behavior change can be placed into two major categories: person-related or personal psychosocial mediators (such as beliefs, attitudes, feelings, identities, or self-confidence in making changes), and environment-related factors. These potential personal and environmental mediators are the primary targets of nutrition education.

Theory Provides Guidance

Let theory guide you as to what you should assess for your intended audience. You cannot ask questions about everything in their lives—that would be very time-consuming and unnecessary. According to theory, you should ask about the potential *mediators* of action or behavior change. This is important because the specific personal and environmental mediators that you identify will become the primary targets of the educational strategies and learning experiences that you will design. Theory can thus provide an important and efficient framework for conducting the needs analysis, just as it does for conducting the nutrition education intervention itself. Knowledge of theory enables you to conduct a more thorough, accurate, and complete analysis (Baranoski et al. 2009).

If you have identified more than one behavior, practice, or issue, the potential mediators of each of these may have to be assessed separately. For example, there is evidence that the motivations and barriers may be different for actions involving *adding* foods to the diet (such as fruits and vegetables) compared with those of *reducing* the amount in the diet, such as eating fewer high-fat foods or drinking fewer sweetened beverages. The kinds of mediators may also differ between food-related behaviors and physical activity behaviors. Thus, the determinants that may mediate behavior change may be quite different for each of the following target behaviors if they are chosen: eating more fruits and vegetables, eating fewer high-energy snacks, and reducing sedentary behaviors. Clearly, limiting the number of behaviors or practices to address makes the nutrition education sessions or program easier to conduct and more likely to be effective.

Step 2 consists of five components:

- *Step 2A:* Describing generally the social and cultural context that influences perceptions
- *Step 2B:* Identifying individual and community assets in relation to program behavioral goals or actions
- *Step 2C:* Identifying personal mediators of action or behavior change

Inputs: Collecting Assessment Data			Outputs: Designing the Theory-Based Intervention			Outcomes: Evaluation Plan
Step 1 ⟷ **Analyze issues and audiences to state program behavioral goals**	Step 2 ⟷ **Identify potential mediators to achieve program behavioral goals**	Step 3 ⟷ **Select theory, philosophy, and components**	Step 4 ⟷ **State objectives for mediators**	Step 5 ⟷ **Design theory-based strategies and activities for mediators**		Step 6 **Plan evaluation**
Tasks • Analyze issues and select audience • Identify behaviors or patterns contributing to issue • Specify behavioral or action goals of the program	*Tasks* • Identify personal psychosocial mediators • Identify environmental support mediators	*Tasks* • Select theory or create appropriate model • Clarify philosophy (education and content) • Determine program components	*Tasks* • State educational objectives for psychosocial mediators • State change objectives for environmental support mediators	*Tasks* • Design activities to address psychosocial mediators • Design activities to address environmental support mediators • Implementation plan		*Tasks* • Design outcome evaluation plan • Determine tools to measure impact • Plan process evaluation
Product • *Description of issue of concern* • *Statement of action or behavioral goals for program*	*Product* • *List of potential mediators for action or behavior goals*	*Product* • *Theory/model for program, philosophy, and components*	*Product* • *Objectives for each mediator*	*Product* • *Educational plans for sessions linking mediators, objectives, and strategies* • *Environmental support plans*		*Product* • *Evaluation plan* • *List of indicators and measures for outcomes* • *Procedures and measures for process evaluation*

FIGURE 8-2 Stepwise Procedure for designing theory-based nutrition education: Step 2.

• *Step 2D:* Identifying environmental supports for action or behavior change
• *Step 2E:* Other audience characteristics and resource considerations

■ STEP 2A: DESCRIBING GENERALLY THE SOCIAL AND CULTURAL CONTEXT THAT INFLUENCES PERCEPTIONS AND ATTITUDES

To find out about the beliefs, feelings and motivations, and skills that the intended audience may have as a result of their social situations and cultural context, you might ask some of the following questions:

• *General cultural beliefs:* What are some general cultural beliefs that influence their eating and activity patterns? What is the community's sense of time and space?
• *Religious beliefs:* Do they have religious beliefs that influence their eating patterns?
• *Lifestyle and work style:* How do they perceive their lifestyle (work, family, recreation, social life) as influencing their willingness and ability to make healthy food and activity choices?
• *Life stage and life trajectories:* What life stage are they in at this time? Are they in their child-rearing stage? Retired? How does that influence their perceptions, food choices, and other dietary behaviors? What previous life experiences, life trajectories, or life stage considerations are important to them at this point?

■ STEP 2B: IDENTIFYING RELEVANT INDIVIDUAL AND COMMUNITY STRENGTHS OR ASSETS

The groups and communities with whom nutrition educators work already have practices, beliefs, and attitudes that are health-promoting. You can build on these. So, it is important to learn about them.

• *Behaviors and practices.* What is the intended audience already doing that is healthy? For example, what current diet-related practices are health enhancing? How can you build on these to achieve the health outcomes and behavioral goals of your program?

What are some potential person-related mediators or beliefs and attitudes that are already assets in terms of the behaviors targeted by the program? What personal or cultural beliefs and attitudes does the intended audience possess that make positive contributions to nutritional health or the sustainability of the food system? What do they already know about the issues of concern? What knowledge and skills do they already possess to address the concerns? What community support systems are supportive of healthy eating, active living, and sustainable food systems?
• *Environmental factors that already facilitate the targeted actions or behaviors.* What are the strengths of the community in terms of environmental infrastructure or activities that are conducive to health? What resources are available, such as healthy food stores, farmers' markets, or food pantries? What nutrition education services are already available? What health-promoting city or regional policies are already in place that would support the

behavioral goals of your program? What do audience members say they would like their environments to be like?

■ STEP 2C: IDENTIFYING POTENTIAL PERSON-RELATED MEDIATORS

After understanding some general background factors about your audience, you can seek to understand the audience more specifically. Where, then, to begin? What shall you ask about? This is where theory can be of assistance: it provides a framework for asking questions. As mentioned in earlier chapters, behavior change can be seen as occurring in two phases: a motivational, pre-action phase, where the emphasis is on beliefs and feelings, and an action phase, where the emphasis is on knowledge and skills. Some mediators are more important than others in each phase. You can thus ask questions that are related to each of the phases of behavior change. The answers are crucial for determining educational objectives in Step 4 and for designing educational strategies in Step 5.

Identifying Potential Motivators of Action or Behavior Change

As noted earlier, theory provides a framework for asking questions. You can systematically ask about the potential influences or mediators of change based on theory variables or constructs. You might want to consider assessing some or all of the mediators listed below, depending on which theory you use to structure the intervention. The centrality of mediators in nutrition education is emphasized by research evidence (Baranowski et al. 1997; Baranowski et al. 2009).

If you have already chosen an existing theory or have created an intervention model based on theory and evidence, then you need to assess only those mediators or theory constructs that are part of your model.

If you are not yet sure which model is appropriate, then you should collect the information on a variety of mediators of behavior change or theory constructs such as those listed here. Information on them will be usable for whatever model you create for the intervention (Shaikh et al. 2008). Ask the audience about specific potential factors that would motivate them to take action.

Questions About Potential Mediators of Motivation

Here is a list of potential motivation-related mediators of the behavioral goals of your program. For each of these mediators assess *potential motivations* for engaging in the program-specified behavior(s):

- *Perceived risk (perceived severity and perceived susceptibility).* What are their beliefs regarding the severity of the health issue identified and their perception of their personal susceptibility or vulnerability to it? For example, how likely do they think it is that they will develop heart disease? Hip fractures? Or that their children will become obese?
- *Perceived benefits (positive outcome expectations).* What expectations do participants have about how certain behaviors are related to the health condition? Because these behaviors may reduce the risk for the health issue or improve health, you can ask, how do they see the goal behaviors as reducing the risk of disease? What would be the benefits of increasing their intakes of fruits and vegetables?
- *Perceived barriers (negative outcome expectations).* What barriers do the intended audience see for engaging in the behavior? What costs? In social marketing language, what must they exchange or sacrifice for the benefits they will experience?

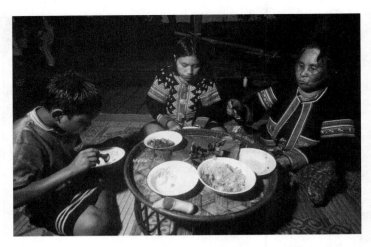

Cultural identity and acculturation are factors in food choices.

- *Culture-specific health and food beliefs.* What are the specific culturally based health beliefs that will influence whether the intended audience will engage in the identified behaviors, such as culture-specific perceived benefits and barriers?
- *Attitude (cognitive).* What are the intended audience's attitudes toward the behaviors that are advocated by the program? What would motivate them to change? Attitudes or motivations depend on beliefs and outcome expectations (listed previously).
- *Attitudes (affective): feelings or affect.* What feelings do they anticipate they will have about engaging in the targeted behavior? Will they have anticipated regret about not taking action?
- *Values.* What values do the intended audience have that might influence whether they will consider taking action on the needs or issues identified?
- *Food preferences and enjoyment (positive outcome expectations).* What are the participants' food preferences, likes, and dislikes? We know that taste is one of the most important mediators of food choices. How do they judge the program's recommended behavior(s) in terms of foods they will eat? Will these foods be enjoyable? Satisfying? Filling?
- *Social norms or felt group pressure.* Do participants believe that their culture or specific individuals or groups important to them think they should or should not perform the particular behaviors or practices recommended by your program? How much are they motivated to comply with these expectations of how they should behave?
- *Social roles.* What are participants' conceptions of behaviors that are appropriate or desirable for people holding their particular position in their group or society? For example, what are their perceptions about whether women in their station in life should breastfeed or bottle-feed?
- *Cultural and ethnic identities.* What are participants' ethnic and cultural identities? If they are immigrants, what is their degree of acculturation? It has been found that degree of acculturation is a better gauge of attitudes and practices in terms of diet than length of stay is (Liou & Contento 2001). (See **Box 8-1**.)
- *Self-identities.* What are their self-identities? For example, do they see themselves as health-conscious consumers, "green" consumers, vegetarians, or other identities?

Box 8-1 **Considering Acculturation of Intended Audiences**

Audiences of nutrition education programs are very diverse, coming from a variety of ethnic, cultural, and social backgrounds. Many have come from a variety of countries of origin. Some schools report that their students speak some 50 or more different languages. Not all individuals from the same country of origin are alike. Indeed the differences within groups may be as great as between groups. Individuals may be at different levels of acculturation, including differences in the degree to which they have adopted mainstream American foods and food practices. This is important to find out so that your nutrition education program is appropriate for your audience. The following short acculturation questionnaire may help you understand your audience better.

	(1) Only Spanish/Chinese/Arabic, etc.	(2)	(3) Both equally	(4)	(5) Only American/English
What language do you speak?					
What language do you think in?					
What types of food do you prefer to eat?					
What foods do you usually eat at home?					
What are your favorite types of restaurants?					
When you select friends, what ethnic background do you prefer?					
When you select health professionals, what ethnic background do you prefer?					

Sources: Liou, D., and I. R. Contento. 2001. Usefulness of psychosocial theory variables in explaining fat-related dietary behavior in Chinese Americans: Associations with degree of acculturation. *Journal of Nutrition Education* 33:322–331. And modified from Suinn, R. F., K. Rickard-Figueroa, S. Lew, and P. Vigil. 1987. The Suinn-Lew Asian self-identity acculturation scale: an initial report. *Educational and Psychological Measurement* 47:401–407.

- *Perceived behavioral control or personal sense of control or agency.* To what extent do participants believe that they have some control over their behaviors, their health, and their environment? That they can take charge?
- *Perceived self-efficacy.* What are the participants' perceptions of their ability to carry out desirable health actions? For example, although participants may believe that eating fewer rich desserts will lead to the weight loss they desire, they may not feel confident that they can resist eating rich desserts.
- *Stage of motivational readiness to take action.* Overall, at what stage are they with respect to motivational readiness to take action—pre-action or ready to take action? More specifically, are they in the precontemplation, contemplation, deciding, action, or maintenance stage?

Such information on the motivations of the intended audience is vital for developing sessions, programs, and media campaigns for helping them understand and appreciate why to take action. However, such information may not be enough to plan a successful program. Participants must also have access to the knowledge and skills needed to carry out the advocated behaviors. Determining whether they do is the next step.

The public does not, of course, use the words from the theory just listed; they use different terms for mediator. **Table 8-1** presents an example of the wording used by middle schoolers to describe why they chose goals to eat more healthfully. The words of the youth are mapped on to theory constructs.

Identifying Potential Facilitators of Action or Behavior Change

Behavioral Capabilities

Behavioral capabilities are the food- and nutrition-specific knowledge and cognitive, affective, and behavioral skills that people need in order to be able to act on their motivations to eat healthfully. Such knowledge and skills are important for people to act appropriately on their motivations. For example, during earlier decades in the United States, many people thought that eating large quantities of red meat was vital to getting enough protein in the diet. They were motivated to eat healthfully, but their knowledge about what constitutes healthful eating was not correct.

Thus, before conducting an educational intervention, you must find out whether the participants have the necessary nutrition informa-

TABLE 8-1	**Examples of Middle School Youth's Descriptions of Their Motivations and Skills for Choosing Healthful Behavioral Goals, Mapped onto Theory Mediators**

Youths' Descriptions of Motivations	Mediators from Theory
I want to stay healthy.	Outcome expectations
So I can lose weight.	
So I can get strong and smarter.	
Because you get better eyesight and better skin.	
Because all I did was drink soda and I got bumps on my face.	
I don't walk enough.	Self-assessment
I eat too much junk food.	
I usually eat at fast food restaurants.	
I don't drink a lot of water.	
I want to know how many steps I walk per day.	Self-monitoring
I want to see what would happen to my body.	
I know I can achieve this goal and be successful.	Self-efficacy
I want to prove that I can stop eating potato chips.	
The doctor said to eat healthy food and fruits; she said I don't eat enough.	Perceived social norms
My mom thinks I don't drink enough water.	
It's important.	Values
It is a goal I want to accomplish.	
Because it's easier. It's easy to follow.	Barriers
I like to walk. I love vegetables.	Feelings/affective attitudes

Source: Petrillo-Myers, M., H. Lee, P. Koch, and I. R. Contento. 2009. Middle school students' reasons for selecting specific obesity risk reduction goals: Mapping to potential mediators from theory. *Journal of Nutrition Education and Behavior* 41(4S):O38.

tion and food-related skills to act upon their motivations. Assess the following:

- *Food- and nutrition-related knowledge to carry out targeted behavior (how-to knowledge).* For example, do they know how many servings of fruits and vegetables they should eat? Which foods are high in saturated fat? The nutritional value of favorite snacks? What information would they like to learn about?
- *Food- and nutrition-related behavioral skills.* Examples are label reading, food safety practices, cooking skills, menu modification skills, breastfeeding, and choosing local foods. What skills do *they* think they will need to take action? What skills would they like to acquire?
- *Critical thinking skills.* Can they discuss the advantages and disadvantages of different kinds of foods and food practices (e.g.,

traditional, organic, local, genetically modified)? Breastfeeding versus bottle-feeding? Weight-loss diets?
- *Misconceptions.* What are their misconceptions?

Self-Regulation Skills

What self-regulation skills do they currently have to take charge of their behaviors?

- *Ability to make action plans; goal-setting and self-monitoring skills.* How do they usually make changes? Have they made action plans before? How useful were these plans for them?
- *Emotion-coping skills.* Do they cope with stress by eating food? Do they have specific difficulties in certain situations? Do they have the emotion-coping skills to handle stress more appropriately so as not to use food as a stress reducer?
- *Reward structures.* What are the reward structures for people's behaviors?

It is important to ask the intended audience about *potential* knowledge and skills they think they will need to overcome barriers and enact the targeted behaviors or practices.

Methods of Assessing Potential Personal Mediators of Behavior Change

Indirect Methods

You can find out about the attitudes, beliefs, and other person-related variables listed earlier indirectly through a review of the relevant stud-

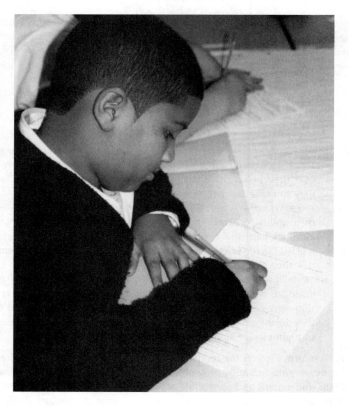

Questionnaires provide an excellent window into one's motivations and barriers for nutritious eating.

TABLE 8-2	Tool to Assess Psychosocial Indicators of Fruit and Vegetable Intake in Limited-Resources Audiences
Mediator/Theory Construct	**Items**
Perceived benefits[a]	I feel that I am helping my body by eating more fruits and vegetables.
	I may develop health problems if I do not eat fruits and vegetables.
Perceived barriers	I feel that fruit is too expensive.
	I feel that fruit is not always available.
	I feel that fruit is time-consuming to prepare.
	I feel that fruit is not liked by my family.
	I feel that fruit is not tasty.
	(Similar items for vegetables)
Perceived control[a]	In your household, who is in charge of what foods to buy?
	In your household, who is in charge of how to prepare the food?
Self-efficacy[a]	I feel that I can plan meals or snacks with more fruit during the next week.
	I feel that I can eat fruits or vegetables as snacks.
	I feel that I can add extra vegetables to casseroles and stews.
	I can eat two or more servings of vegetables at dinner.
Social support[b]	Are there other people encouraging you to buy, prepare, and eat fruits and vegetables?
	(My children, partner, mother, father, other)
Perceived norms[a]	People in my family think I should eat more fruits and vegetables.
	My doctor (or WIC nutritionist) tells me to eat more fruits and vegetables.
Intention: readiness to eat more fruits and vegetables[c]	I am not thinking about eating more fruit (coded as 1; precontemplation).
	I am thinking about eating more fruit (coded as 2; contemplation).
	I am definitely planning to eat more fruit in the next month (coded as 3; preparation).
	I am trying to eat more fruit now (coded as 4; action).
	I am already eating two or more servings of fruit a day (coded as 5; maintenance).
	(Similar items for vegetables)
Diet quality	How would you describe your diet? (5-point scale: Very poor to very good)

Note: Only selected items of this assessment tool are shown.

[a] Scores of 1 to 3 range from disagree (1), neither agree or disagree (2), to agree (3).

[b] Instructions to client: "Check as many as apply." Coding: no = 0 = no support; yes = 1 = support by one person; yes = 2 = support by > 2 persons.

[c] Instructions to client: "Check one."

Source: Townsend, M. S., and L. L. Kaiser. 2005. Development of a tool to assess psychosocial indicators of fruit and vegetables intake for two federal programs. *Journal of Nutrition Education and Behavior* 37:170–184. Used with permission of the Society for Nutrition Education.

ies on motivation to act and the dietary change process; monitoring data for the intended audience or similar population (e.g., adolescents, postmenopausal women, African American men); government and industry opinion surveys of people's beliefs and attitudes; food marketing surveys; studies of population segmentation by psychographic variables; or existing records for the group. A review of measures used in nutrition education programs for various population groups is provided by Contento, Randell, and Basch (2002).

Direct Methods

It is best to obtain information directly from the intended audience, if possible. You can administer surveys or brief questionnaires, using existing instruments or intervention-specific instruments that you design. **Table 8-2** is an example of an instrument that has been validated for use with low-income audiences and assesses motivational readiness to take action. **Table 8-3** shows an instrument validated to ask specifically about self-efficacy in relation to the behavior of fat intake.

TABLE 8-3	A Self-Efficacy Measure for Fat Intake Behaviors of Low-Income Women	
Item	**Domain**	
I can stick to low-fat foods on a regular basis . . .		
When nervous	Negative affect/feelings	
When angry		
When upset about events in my life		
When happy	Positive affect/feelings	
At a party		
When eating out at a restaurant with others		
When lots of high-fat foods are available	Availability	
When someone offers me high-fat foods		

Source: Chang, M. W., S. Nitzke, R. L. Brown, L. C. Baumann, and L. Oakley. 2003. Development and validation of a self-efficacy measure for fat intake behaviors of low-income women. *Journal of Nutrition Education and Behavior* 35:302–307. Used with permission of the Society for Nutrition Education.

Talking personally with the group is highly desirable. You can conduct focus group interviews, in-depth individual interviews of individuals from the intended audience or key informants, or intercept interviews as individuals leave stores, clinics, or service centers. Use the Step 2 worksheets as a guide for recording your answers.

Nutrition Education in Action 8-1 contains examples of open-ended questions for use with young adults, and **Nutrition Education in Action 8-2** describes the outcomes of in-depth interviews with community members. **Table 8-4** summarizes the advantages and disadvantages of a variety of methods to gather assessment data.

■ STEP 2D: IDENTIFYING ENVIRONMENTAL AND POLICY FACTORS

Identifying the environmental conditions that either facilitate or impede healthful dietary practices is very important. It grounds your educational activities in the real world of your audience. You can use the information in two major ways: (1) to plan educational activities that take into account the realities of the participants' lives, for example, in terms of their time and resources; and/or (2) to embark on partnerships with providers of food or services or with community organizations to facilitate and enlarge the audience's opportunities for action.

Identifying Potential Environmental Supports for Action

To design appropriate educational activities, you need information about various aspects of the environment that may affect the behaviors or ac-

---

NUTRITION EDUCATION IN ACTION 8-1

Open-Ended Questions

The following questions were used for assessing the opinions on fruits and vegetables of ethnically diverse young adults (ages 16–25) in a community program:

- *How many fruits and vegetables do you believe you need to eat each day? Why or why not?* Responses varied, with a majority indicating between two and five servings a day. "Good for the body" or health-related answers were the top reasons to eat fruits and vegetables each day.
- *If you learned the following facts (list provided) about fruits and vegetables, which would most likely cause you to eat more fruits and vegetables?* The top two facts selected from the list were "eating fruits and vegetables gives me healthy and beautiful teeth, gums, skin, and hair" and "eating fruits and vegetables helps reduce my risk of developing a chronic disease such as cancer, heart disease, or stroke."
- *What would encourage you to eat more fruits and vegetables?* Freshness, increased availability and selection, and health were the top reasons mentioned.
- *How important is it to you to eat fruits and vegetables?* Seventy-one percent said that it was "very important," and 21% said it was "somewhat important."

- *Do you eat fruits and vegetables in the cafeteria? Why or why not?* Seventy-five percent indicated that they ate fruits and vegetables in the cafeteria for reasons of taste or health. Those who did not cited the lack of freshness and availability.
- *When you buy beverages from vending machines, which ones do you usually choose?* Cola, water, and non-cola-flavored soda were the more frequent choices. Only 5% indicated usually purchasing fruit juice. Thirty-nine percent indicated that they would purchase 100% fruit juice if it were available in the vending machine.
- *When are you most willing to eat more fruits and vegetables? Breakfast, lunch, between meals, dinner, or dessert?* Responses were divided between all times, with slightly more respondents favoring fruits and vegetables for lunch.
- *How would you prefer to receive nutrition information?* Taste tests, brochures, posters, classes, staff at the campus health clinic, radio, and television were the top preferred methods for the target audience to receive nutrition information.

Source: California Project LEAN, California Department of Health Services. 2004. *Community-based social marketing: The California Project LEAN experience.* Sacramento, CA: Author. http://www.californiaprojectlean.org.

NUTRITION EDUCATION IN ACTION 8-2

Wellness IN the Rockies (WIN the Rockies): A Research, Education, and Outreach Project that Seeks to Address Obesity Innovatively and Effectively

The Focus of the Program

Overall project goals are to enhance the well-being of individuals by improving their attitudes and behaviors related to food, physical activity, and body image; and to help build communities' capacities to foster and sustain these changes.

Assessment

Prior to developing the various nutrition education programs of this project, program staff gathered narratives or life stories related to physical activity, food and eating, and body image from extensive interviews and focus group discussions with 103 adults. The narratives were tape recorded. Key quotations were identified and grouped into 146 narrative thematic codes using grounded theory.

Values

Values emerged as an important theme. A major finding of relevance here is that being productive, working hard, and not wasting resources were important values. Thus, physical activity should be productive or serve some purpose, such as mowing the lawn or doing other chores. Going to the gym to exercise or just going for a walk was not seen as productive. These activities were a "waste" of time compared with

activities in which work was being accomplished or compared with other things that they might be doing with their families or communities.

In the same way, wasting food was seen as violating an important value of not wasting resources. That value led to the importance of cleaning one's plate and not squandering food.

The Power of Others

The study also found that other people have profound and often lifelong impacts on individuals' feelings about their body and physical abilities. These feelings in turn can contribute to their sense of identity and influence their lifestyles and their long-term health. Thus, individuals need to create social environments that nurture others, particularly youth, rather than be critical and hurtful. Respecting diverse body sizes becomes highly important.

Sources: Pelican, S., F. Vanden Heede, B. Holmes, et al. 2005. The power of others to shape our identity: Body image, physical abilities, and body weight. *Family and Consumer Sciences Research Journal* 34:57–80; Wardlaw, M. K. 2005. New you/health for every body: Helping adults adopt a health-centered approach to well-being. *Journal of Nutrition Education and Behavior* 37:S103–106; and Pelican, S., F. Vanden Heede, and B. Holmes. 2005. *Let their voices be heard: Quotations from life stories related to physical activity, food and eating, and body image.* Chicago, IL: Discovery Association Publishing House.

---

tions targeted by the program and that may be important for planning appropriate nutrition education activities, such as the following.

Social Environment

- *Family and cultural support.* What degree of family and community support is there for the targeted behaviors? What is the general life situation of members of the target group? Find out about the family or household structures of the group; for example, are they mostly single parents? Who is responsible for buying food and for preparing it? Do they eat with others whose needs must be considered, such as children or partners? How could support be increased?
- *Social networks and support.* What is the size and quality of their social networks? Do they receive support from their social networks to maintain the desired behavior after it has been adopted? Are work arrangements conducive to the new behaviors being enacted on a long-term basis? Also inquire about *potential* social supports: how could you, or the nutrition education program, help them develop better social supports for enacting the targeted healthful behaviors? Is the intended audience interested in working with others to change their food environment? If so, what exactly would they like to do? Does the group have collective efficacy skills to advocate for themselves?

- *Community capacity and empowerment skills.* Is the group interested in advocacy to improve their food environment? If so, what experiences have they had before in working with groups to change their environment? What skills do they have in organizing groups, building coalitions, and planning and executing advocacy? What skills would they like to acquire?

Food Availability and the Built Environment

- *Availability and accessibility of food needed to enact the target behaviors.* Find out whether the foods the intended audience will need to enact the targeted behaviors or practices are available and accessible to them. Are these foods available and accessible in their workplaces or school cafeteria or the local grocery store? For example, are fruits and vegetables or local or minimally processed and packaged foods easily accessible? Where do most people seem to be eating? If you are working in coalition with others about food sustainability issues, you might want to survey how many farmers' markets are available and accessible to your intended audience and whether they accept Supplemental Nutrition Assistance Program electronic benefit cards.
- *State of the built environment.* Is the built environment conducive to active living? You or your team can draw a map of the community showing the location and type of grocery stores, fast food

TABLE 8-4	Advantages and Disadvantages of Various Methods of Issue Identification and Needs Analysis	
	Advantages	**Disadvantages**
Review of research or survey literature	Quick, inexpensive, nonthreatening	Information not specific to intended audience
National survey and monitoring data, opinion polls	Quick, inexpensive, nonthreatening	Information not specific to intended audience
Review of existing records of intended audience	Information specific to intended audience; quick, inexpensive, nonthreatening to intended group	Limited to quality of data, scope of data
Surveys of intended audience		
Telephone	Information specific to group; chance for detailed insight into perceived and real needs	Expensive; extensive training needed for interviewers; leaves out people with no phones or unlisted numbers
Group administered	Quick, inexpensive; information specific to intended audience	Survey instrument must be designed and tested
Mailed survey	Information specific to intended audience; chance for more honest answers	Eliminates low-literacy individuals; responses less open-ended than in-person interviews; moderately expensive; time delay in getting information; may get low response rate
Individual interviews		
Informal	Information specific to intended audience; inexpensive	Not systematic
Formal in-person interviews	Information specific to intended audience; comprehensive insight into intended audience	Expensive; extensive training needed for interviewers; time-consuming
Group meetings		
Group discussion	Relatively low cost, quick	People attending may not be representative; not enough time for people to express their thoughts or needs publicly
Focus groups	Provides detailed information on beliefs, emotions, and attitudes	Expensive; training needed for interviewers
Observation	Accurate information on behaviors	Expensive; can be intrusive; can alter the behavior being observed if observation is known

outlets, restaurants, farmers' markets, and parks. If that is not possible, at least walk around the neighborhood and see what is there. Is good-quality, fresh produce available? What kind of restaurants and food vendors are around? How walkable are the streets in the neighborhood? Are there safe and attractive parks nearby?

Resources and Economic Environment

- *Financial resources.* What resources does the group have for healthful eating and active living? Do members of the intended audience have enough money to afford the foods targeted in the intervention? Do they have access to food assistance programs? Are prices of foods in their neighborhood supportive of the targeted behaviors?
- *Transportation.* Do they have easily accessible transportation to and from grocery stores?
- *Practical constraints.* Do they have cooking facilities or refrigerators? What are the time constraints of the intended audience?

- *Economic realities.* What are the causes of the "problems behind the problems" in terms of the social and economic realities of people's lives?

Such information will assist you to develop a nutrition education program that is realistic for the intended audience. For example, if people work two jobs and have little time to prepare food, educational activities need to take this into consideration. You may also need to direct people to other nutrition services and resources that may be available to them.

Information Environment

- *Media messages.* Ask about what media they use, and the frequency and intensity of their use of these media (such as viewing TV or reading magazines). What media images are important to them?
- *Information environment of intervention setting.* What is the information environment of the setting in which the intervention

itself will take place (such as the school or community centers)? How may it be changed to be more supportive of the targeted behaviors?

Policy Environment

Investigate institutional, community, or government policies that may affect the behavioral goals of your program.

- *Policies related to food and activity in workplaces that might impede or facilitate the healthful behaviors targeted by your program.* Are employees given time off to participate in health promotion activities? What policies need to be modified or enacted?
- *Local wellness policies in schools.* How well are they being implemented? Is the wellness committee meeting regularly? Are the appropriate and required stakeholders on it? Does the food served conform to policy? What kinds of food are used in school fundraising, in the classroom as rewards, and in celebrations? What foods are displayed in cafeterias and hallways? What yet needs to be done?
- *Policies related to food and activity at the community level that might impede or facilitate the healthful behaviors targeted by your program.* What policies need to be modified or enacted?
- *Public policies related to food and activity that might impede or facilitate the healthful behaviors targeted by your program.* What policies need to be modified or enacted?

Identifying Partners to Provide Environmental and Policy Supports for Program Behavioral Goals

Promoting environmental supports for action is important when it is possible, given the resources and the goals, duration, and scope of the program. You will most likely need first to educate decision makers who are direct providers of foods or services and those who have policy-making roles in various settings. When such people or groups are convinced of the importance of your program goals, you can then work in coalition with them to bring about environmental supports for action.

Identifying Decision Makers and Policy Makers in Organizations and Communities

In this substep, you want to identify the potential organizations or agencies with whom you can partner to increase opportunities for your audience to be able to take the actions that are the focus of the program. Here are some potential partners:

- Principals and school superintendents
- Food service providers in schools and workplaces
- Public health agencies (local, state, and national)
- Hospitals and school health services personnel
- State and local Cooperative Extension Service personnel
- Chefs and restaurant owners
- Supermarkets and local grocery stores
- Farmers and farmers' markets
- Gardening associations
- Sustainable food systems organizations
- Community organizations related to food and nutrition, such as food recovery programs, food banks, soup kitchens, and food security and hunger organizations

Conducting Environmental and Policy Analyses

With partnerships or coalitions in place, you and the partners can determine the assessment activities you will conduct. Data concerning potential environmental and policy mediators can be obtained from quantitative and qualitative methods such as the following: literature review of similar settings; review of policy documents, existing data, surveys, checklists, environmental health index assessments; observation of availability of food and active living opportunities in settings that are relevant to the behavioral goals of your program (grocery stores, farmers' markets, workplace, school, and so forth); focus group discussions; and interviews of key informants.

Example of Summary of Assessment Information

Table 8-5 provides a summary of what might be found from such an assessment process.

■ STEP 2E: OTHER AUDIENCE CHARACTERISTICS AND PROGRAM RESOURCE CONSIDERATIONS FOR DELIVERING THE INTERVENTION

Identifying Relevant Audience Characteristics

This is the time to find out some relevant specifics about the audience or primary group: cultural background considerations, educational level, academic skills, the physical and cognitive developmental level of children, preferred learning styles and instructional formats, and special needs. More specifically, find out about the following (if relevant):

- *Educational level.* What grade are they in (for children)? How much schooling have they completed (for adults)? Where?
- *Physical and cognitive developmental levels/abilities (children only).* At what stage is their physical and cognitive development?
- *Literacy/numeracy skills.* How well can your audience read? What are their math skills?
- *Preferred learning styles or instructional formats.* Which do they prefer: lectures, reading, discussion, activities, group work, or field projects? Any predominant learning style: imaginative, analytic, common sense, and dynamic? (See Chapter 15.)

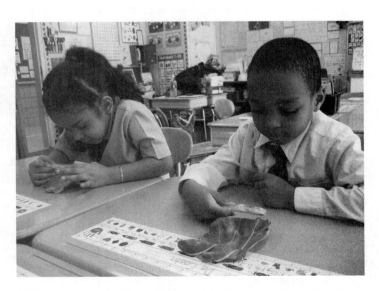

Children can examine different foods in a scientific way in order to become familiar with them.

TABLE 8-5 **Summary of Identification of Potential Mediators of the Targeted Behavior for the Case Study Example: Increase Intake of Fruits and Vegetables Among Middle-School Adolescents**

Food Practices or Behaviors to Be Targeted	Potential Personal Mediators of Targeted Behaviors		Potential Environmental Mediators of Targeted Behaviors
	Motivational Mediators	Behavior Change Mediators	
Current practice: Low intake of F&V *Targeted behavior:* Intake of four or more cups of F&V per day	Sense of threat/awareness of risk • *Current:* Low • *Potential motivators:* Personalizing the risks	Self-efficacy • *Current:* Not familiar with different F&V; unwilling to venture • *Potential:* Exposure to new foods; easy to incorporate	Availability and accessibility • *Current:* Students do not eat the F&V offered • *Potential:* In partnership with school food service, develop salad bars at reasonable cost to students
	Outcome expectancies/barriers • *Current:* Taste bad, inconvenient, go bad quickly • *Potential motivators:* If taste good, etc.; immediate benefits for health (skin, eyes), for performance of activities they value	Food/nutrition skills • *Current:* Need skills to choose and prepare F&V snacks • *Potential:* Making learning skills fun; tips for making F&V convenient	Social support • *Current:* No support for F&V among other teens • *Potential:* Train peer educators; find celebrity role models
	Social norm • *Current:* Friends do not eat vegetables; unaware of media influence • *Potential motivators:* Make veggies cool; make aware of media influence on food choices	Self-regulation skills • *Current:* Impulse eating; low SR skills • *Potential:* Learn goal setting and self-monitoring	Information environment • *Current:* No role models of teens eating F&V; few ads • *Potential:* Provide posters, newsletters, etc.

Note: F&V = fruits and vegetables; SR = self-regulation.

- *Special needs.* Are there learning disabilities or physical disabilities that you should consider? If you will be working with an adult group, will children be present? Can child care be provided?
- *Emotional needs.* What is going on emotionally in the lives of your audience? How will this influence their ability to hear your message?
- *Social needs.* How well does your group know each other? Does the intended audience have high community cohesion?

Practical and Program Resource Considerations

Practical and resource considerations may dictate the duration and intensity of the program that are possible, whatever the merits of nutrition education identified in the previous assessments. Ask questions such as the following: What resources will be available for the nutrition education intervention in monetary terms? How long a program is possible or considered desirable? One session or many? One component or many? What space and equipment are available? What other resources will be available? What is the nature of the facilities and the setting? What channels are possible given these constraints? Will the program involve group sessions, audiovisual or print media, health fairs, media campaigns, all of them, or other channels?

When planning group sessions, here are some practical details to consider:

- *Time.* How much time do you have for your sessions? How much time will you have for setup and cleanup?
- *Space available and its arrangement.* What is the physical space like? How can you change the space to meet your needs? What space restrictions are you working within?
- *Equipment available.* What equipment (audiovisual, cooking, etc.) is available to you? What could you bring if you needed to?
- *General administrative/facilities support.* How helpful are your key contact persons in terms of troubleshooting, providing supplies, helping with promotion, and providing technical assistance during your sessions? For example, will the classroom teacher remain in the room and help with classroom control? Will the senior center director remain in the room and help with technical problems if they come up?

■ CASE STUDY

In our Step 1 assessment in Chapter 7, we chose "Taking Control: Eating Well and Being Fit" as the title of the program and identified the four behavioral goals for our audience:

- Increase intake of fruits and vegetables
- Reduce consumption of sweetened beverages

- Reduce intake of packaged highly processed, energy dense snacks
- Increase physical activity

In designing the full program, we would need to identify the motivators and facilitators of change separately for all four behaviors because it is unlikely that these would be the same for all behaviors. For example, the motivators and facilitators for eating more fruits and vegetables would likely be different from those for decreasing consumption of sweetened beverages. Therefore, for reasons of space, in Step 2 of the case study we focus on only one of the four behaviors—eating more fruits and vegetable. Thus, we conduct a comprehensive analysis to identify only those determinants of behavior that can potentially mediate an increase in the behavior of eating more fruits and vegetables for this audience.

This comprehensive analysis includes obtaining information on the following:

- Description of the sociocultural environment in which the audience lives
- List of current behaviors, practices, policies, and environmental factors that are assets for the audience to be able to achieve the program's behavioral or action goals
- List of audience's specific motivational mediators and skills, derived from theory, that would help them to achieve the program's behavioral or action goals
- List of potential actions for the program to take to provide environmental and policy supports for the audience's achievement of the program's behavioral or action goals
- Description of audience characteristics and resource considerations that help in planning the practical aspects of the sessions or program

The results of this comprehensive analysis are described in detail in the case study.

■ YOUR TURN: COMPLETING THE STEP 2 WORKSHEETS

In Step 1, you selected one or two high-priority food and/or health issues and a high-priority primary audience. You also identified some key behavioral outcomes that will be the focus of the intervention. In this chapter, you record your assessment results on the Step 2 Worksheets and identify key relevant potential mediators of the actions or behaviors that are the focus of the program. These key mediators of behavior change are the targets of your educational strategies.

After completing Steps 1 and 2 you should have statements regarding the following:

- *Health issue(s) and intended audience for the program.* For example, "obesity in children" or "osteoporosis among adult women."
- *High-priority target health-promoting actions or changes in behavior (one or a few) or a set of related behaviors or community practices that will be the focus of the intervention or program.* These are the behavioral goal(s) or targeted behaviors or practices of the program. For example, improved food safety behaviors among low-income women.
- *Personal and environmental determinants that are potential mediators of the target behavior changes or practices.* This list can, and indeed should, be quite long (e.g., 8 to 10 items). You will prioritize them later, in Step 3, based on evidence and on the theory or model you select to guide the intervention. They then become the basis for writing educational and support objectives that will guide the development of your program.

Mediators as the Bridge Between Theory and Nutrition Education Practice

Although a comprehensive process of selecting the behavioral focus of the intervention and identifying the specific mediators that will be the targets of educational strategies may seem time-consuming and even tedious, it is probably the most critical step in creating effective nutrition education learning experiences in practice settings. Besides providing you with helpful data, an audience assessment can be a useful tool in establishing a rapport with audience participants. If done thoughtfully, a good assessment of health issues and their causes for an audience may even reveal preconceptions you may have had about the participants, as well as your own attitudes about teaching and learning. Nutrition education is most successful when both group participants and educators can communicate openly, honestly, and with respect for each other as individuals. A comprehensive analysis and assessment process helps to establish this relationship.

Questions and Activities

1. In the last chapter, you identified food and nutrition issues of concern for a given audience and the behaviors or practices that contribute to them. You also identified the behaviors or practices that will be the focus of your program. Why is it important to identify the potential mediators of these behaviors and practices?

2. Name and briefly describe the two major categories of potential mediators of healthful action or behavior change.

3. Summarize several methods for assessing potential personal mediators of behavior change. Which methods for which potential mediators do you think will be useful for an audience you have in mind or will be working with? Why? Give their relative advantages and disadvantages.

4. How can nutrition educators use information about potential environmental influences on behavior in nutrition education programs? How can they assess such influences for a given audience? Describe several methods of assessment and their relative advantages and disadvantages.

5. List five audience characteristics that are important to know before you deliver your nutrition education program.

References

Baranowski, T., E. Cerin, and J. Baranowski. 2009. Steps in the design, development, and formative evaluation of obesity prevention–related behavior change. *International Journal of Behavioral Nutrition and Physical Activity* 6:6.

Baranowski, T., L. S. Lin, D. W. Wetter, K. Resnicow, and M. D. Hearn. 1997. Theory as mediating variables: Why aren't community interventions working as desired? *Annals of Epidemiology* 7:589–595.

Contento, I. R., J. S. Randell, and C. E. Basch. 2002. Review and analysis of evaluation measures used in nutrition education intervention research. *Journal of Nutrition Education and Behavior* 34:2–25.

Liou, D., and I. R. Contento. 2001. Usefulness of psychosocial variables in explaining fat-related dietary behavior in Chinese Americans: Association with degree of acculturation. *Journal of Nutrition Education and Behavior* 33:322–331.

Shaikh, A. R., A. L. Yaroch, L. Nebeling, M. C. Yeh, and K. Resnicow. 2008. Psychosocial predictors of fruit and vegetable consumption in adults: a review of the literature. *American Journal of Preventive Medicine* 34(6):535–543.

In Step 2, you will find out as much as possible about why audience members make the food and activity choices they do as well as what might motivate, facilitate, and support them to take on the goal behaviors. Theory provides you with the framework to ask the questions and organize the answers.

At the end of the Step 2 worksheets, you should have the following products for Steps 2A, 2B, 2C, 2D, and 2E:

Step 2A: Description of the sociocultural environment in which your audience lives.

Step 2B: List of current behaviors, practices, policies, and environmental factors that are *assets* for the audience's achievement of the program goal behaviors.

Step 2C: List of thoughts, feelings, and skills that are rooted in theory and potentially mediate the audience's motivation for and ability to achieve the program goal behaviors.

Step 2D: List of potential actions for the program to take to provide environment and policy supports for the audience's achievement of the program goal behaviors.

Step 2E: Description of audience characteristics and list of resource considerations that will help you plan the practical aspects of your program.

Use these worksheets as guides to help you identify the personal mediators and environmental determinants of change. Cite information sources in the text and add references to the bibliography at the end of the step. Electronic versions of these worksheets are available at http://nutrition.jbpub.com/education/2e/. If you are unable to access the worksheets electronically, you can write onto this blank worksheet or create a text document that uses the same flow of information.

NOTE: This part of the case study focuses on only one of the program's goal behaviors: increasing intake of fruits and vegetables. If you create a program with multiple goal behaviors, you will need to complete Steps 2B, 2C, and 2D separately for each behavior.

Step 2A: Audience's sociocultural environment

Describe the social and cultural environment of the audience with respect to your goal behaviors. Consider the following questions: What is their life stage (e.g., teen, senior, mother), and how does this stage influence their eating and activity patterns? What is their living situation, and how does this influence their eating and activity patterns? What are the cultural beliefs that influence their eating and activity patterns? How does their lifestyle (e.g., work, family, recreation, social obligations) influence their ability to make healthy food and activity choices? How do their religious beliefs influence their eating and activity patterns?

The primary participants are adolescents who are in the 7th and 8th grades. This is an age when students may be experiencing great physical and emotional changes. Additionally, this is an age when they want and are given more individual freedom. They are strongly influenced by their friends/peers and less influenced by their parents.

By middle school, students are able to understand the consequences of their actions and make choices accordingly. So, while preferences are the major determinant of food choices for young children, adolescents become increasingly able to align their food choice behaviors with their goals. By middle school, children are able to integrate motivations and cognitions in a self-regulatory process for a variety of food choice criteria, including not only taste and convenience but also in terms of health and weight concern issues.[1,2]

All of the students live with a parent or other adult caregiver. Sixty percent report having input on household groceries, and 60% have regular responsibilities at home ranging from chores to taking care of younger siblings.[3]

The students report that they are as busy or busier than the average middle school student. Outside of school, 40% are involved with organized sports, and 50% take part in after-school activities associated with the school (e.g., baseball, art club, yearbook).[3]

Eating out at local diners and fast food spots with friends after school is a "status" symbol.[1] National data shows that by adolescence children are spending $4 billion per year on foods and snacks for themselves.[4]

The demographics of the students and the community in which they live are diverse,[3] and no primary cultural or religious belief that influences food choice stands out.

Step 2B: Individual and community assets

Identify existing behaviors, practices, environmental factors, and policies that support your goal behaviors.

Individual behaviors and community practices that support your program's behavioral goals	Environmental factors and policies that support your program's behavioral goals
• Although, at this time, the average student is not engaged in practices that promote the adoption of the goal behaviors, there are a number of students (~20%) who regularly reach one or more of the behavioral goals.[1]	• Promoting health—physical and mental—and the development of healthy habits are parts of the mission of the school.[5] • The school has a fledgling School Wellness Council.[1] • There is a tradition of peer leadership (e.g., all conflict mediation includes a peer as one of the mediators), and some of the students who are looked at as leaders already reach one or more of the behavioral goals.[1]

+

Step 2C: Potential personal mediators

Find out about your audience's thoughts and feelings related to the motivational mediators listed below from psychosocial theories.

Potential motivating mediators from theory	Audience's thoughts and feelings in relation to each mediator, specific to achieving your goal behaviors
Perceived risk or sense of concern	Need increased awareness of the risks associated with eating too few fruits and vegetables.
Perceived benefits (i.e., positive outcome expectations)	Want to know specific benefits in eating fruits and vegetables—pleasant taste, a role in keeping the body healthy, role in maintaining healthy weight, and provision of energy.
Perceived barriers (i.e., negative outcome expectations)	Want to figure out solutions to specific barriers to eating more fruits and vegetables—cost, time to prepare, availability, and not liking the taste.
Affective attitudes (i.e., feelings about the behavior)	Need to build positive attitudes about eating fruits and vegetables by gaining appreciation for the taste of fruits and vegetables and by understanding that benefits outweigh barriers.
Perceived behavioral control/self-efficacy	Want to believe that eating fruits and vegetables is something that is under their control—something that they can make happen.
Social norms (i.e., what others think participants should do)	It would be desirable that students believe that their peers think they should eat more fruits and vegetables.
Descriptive norms (i.e., beliefs of others about the behavior)	It would be important for students to believe that their peers regularly eat fruits and vegetables and think that doing so is "cool."
Other	*Stage of Readiness to Change*—The group is thinking about changing. They need to be more motivated to actually start to work towards the goal behavior.

Find out about your audience's knowledge, skills, and other factors from theory listed below.

Facilitating mediators from theory	Audience's knowledge and skills in relation to each mediator, specific to achieving your goal behaviors
Food and nutrition knowledge	Students need to understand more about fruit and vegetable serving sizes and recommendations.
Food and nutrition skills related to the targeted behavior	Students would like to improve their food preparation and selection skills as related to fruits and vegetables.
Critical thinking skills	Students want to be able to evaluate the benefits of different fruits and vegetables.
Self-efficacy	Students need to increase their perception of their ability and confidence to find, purchase, and/or prepare fruits and vegetables.
Goal setting (making action plans)	Students need to identify a specific number of fruits and vegetables they want to eat each day and set clear and feasible plans for achieving that number.
Self-assessment/self-monitoring skills	Students need to learn skills to assess their fruits and vegetables intakes compared to recommendations, make plans for eating recommended amounts, and monitor how they are doing.
Reinforcements	Students should receive positive or encouraging comments during and after eating fruits and vegetables.
Others	

Step 2D: Environmental/policy supports

Find out how you could change the environmental and policy supports listed below to facilitate your intended audience in performing your goal behaviors.

Environmental and policy supports	How each environmental and policy support could be changed, specific to achieving your goal behaviors
Decision-makers' awareness and motivation	Increase the awareness of parents and school staff about the importance of a healthy school environment that promotes fruits and vegetables and motivate them to make the necessary changes.
Social environment (e.g., family, networks, support)	Create a social norm where eating fruits and vegetables is the norm among students, staff, and family members.
Food environment (e.g., availability, accessibility)	Create a food environment that makes affordable fruits and vegetables easily available and accessible.
Built environment (e.g., walkable streets, parks)	Make fruits and vegetables more convenient (e.g., have bowls of free fruit in the lunch room).
Organizational food policy	Make fruits and vegetables less expensive and more accessible alternatives to other snacks in the cafeteria and other sites around the school that sell food.
Information environment (e.g., media watched/read, setting)	Messages about eating fruits and vegetables (e.g., sharing their benefits, removing misconceptions).
Policy activities at the community and national levels	A school policy that would make fruits and vegetables affordable and accessible.

Step 2E: Audience and resources

Add details about your audience that are important for delivering your program.

Audience trait	Description
Educational level or schooling	Participants are in the 7th and 8th grades at the city middle school. Eighty-one percent of the city's adult population has completed high school or has high school equivalency, and 35% have a college degree or higher. It is assumed that the parents of the students have similar educational attainment.[6]
Physical and cognitive developmental level and ability (children only)	The average student participant is at the expected level for physical and cognitive abilities. City test scores indicate that the average student is at grade level for math and reading.[5] When thinking about health and making choices, middle school students are able to integrate motivations and cognitions in a self-regulatory process for a variety of food choice criteria, including not only taste and convenience but also in terms of health and weight concern issues.[3,4]
Literacy and numeracy skills	Participants, on average, read at a 7th-grade level and can add, subtract, multiply, and divide with whole numbers and fractions.
Preferred learning style	Per student comments and discussions with school faculty, students like group work and interactive styles of learning. The school stresses group and hands-on work throughout the curriculum.
Special needs	There are no specific special needs that need to be met.
Emotional needs	There are no specific emotional needs that need to be met.
Social needs	There are no special social needs.

Describe the resources available for your program.

Program resources	Available resources
Time	The school has offered access to students in their health education classes. The curriculum will take place two days a week for a consecutive 5 weeks.
Space	The regular classroom teachers will be leading lessons in usual assigned rooms.
Equipment	The program will have access to standard classroom equipment, including markers, dry erase board, overhead projectors, and television with VCRs. Some classrooms have SmartBoards. Most copying will need to occur off premise.
General administrative support	The school is supportive and will assign the teachers who will be leading the lessons.

References

1. Michela JL, Contento IR. Cognitive, motivational, social, and environmental influences on children's food choices. *Health Psychol.* 1986;5(3):209–230.

2. Contento IR, Michela JL. Nutrition and food choice behavior among children and adolescents. In: Goreczny AJ, Hersen M, eds. *Handbook of pediatric and adolescent health psychology.* Boston: Allyn and Bacon; 1998:249–273.

3. University–Town Partnership. Intervention needs assessment findings: Survey and interview results, 2009.

4. McNeal JU. *Kids as consumers: A handbook of marketing to children.* New York: Lexington Books; 1992.

5. Any Town Middle School. Middle school enrollment demographics. Any Town, USA; 2009.

6. U.S. Census Bureau. Census Data: Any Town, Any State. http://quickfacts.census.gov/qfd/states.

In Step 2, you will find out as much as possible about why audience members make the food and activity choices they do as well as what might motivate, facilitate, and support them to take on the goal behaviors. Theory provides you with the framework to ask the questions and organize the answers.

At the end of the Step 2 worksheets, you should have the following products for Steps 2A, 2B, 2C, 2D, and 2E:

Step 2A: Description of the sociocultural environment in which your audience lives.

Step 2B: List of current behaviors, practices, policies, and environmental factors that are *assets* for the audience's achievement of the program goal behaviors.

Step 2C: List of thoughts, feelings, and skills that are rooted in theory that potentially mediate the audience's motivation for and ability to achieve the program's goal behaviors or community practices.

Step 2D: List of potential actions for the program to take to provide environment and policy supports for the audience's achievement of the program goal behaviors.

Step 2E: Description of audience characteristics and list of resource considerations that will help you plan the practical aspects of your program.

Use these worksheets as guides to help you identify the personal mediators and environmental determinants of change. Cite information sources in the text and add references to the bibliography at the end of the step. Electronic versions of these worksheets are available at http://nutrition.jbpub.com/education/2e/. If you are unable to access the worksheets electronically, you can write onto this blank worksheet or create a text document that uses the same flow of information.

■■■■■■■■■■■ **Step 2A: Audience's sociocultural environment** ■■■■■■■■■■■

Describe the social and cultural environment of the audience with respect to your goal behaviors. Consider the following questions: What is their life stage (e.g., teen, senior, mother), and how does this stage influence their eating and activity patterns? What is their living situation, and how does this influence their eating and activity patterns? What are the cultural beliefs that influence their eating and activity patterns? How does their lifestyle (e.g., work, family, recreation, social obligations) influence their ability to make healthy food and activity choices? How do their religious beliefs influence their eating and activity patterns?

Step 2B: Individual and community assets

Identify existing behaviors, practices, environmental factors, and policies that support your goal behaviors.

Individual behaviors and community practices that support your program's behavioral goals	Environmental factors and policies that support your program's behavioral goals

+

Step 2C: Potential personal mediators

Find out about your audience's thoughts and feelings related to the motivational mediators listed below from psychosocial theories.

Potential motivating mediators from theory	Audience's thoughts and feelings in relation to each mediator, specific to achieving your goal behaviors
Perceived risk or sense of concern	
Perceived benefits (i.e., positive outcome expectations)	
Perceived barriers (i.e., negative outcome expectations)	
Affective attitudes (i.e., feelings about the behavior)	
Perceived behavioral control/self-efficacy	
Social norms (i.e., what others think participants should do)	
Descriptive norms (i.e., beliefs of others about the behavior)	
Other	

Find out about your audience's knowledge, skills, and other factors from theory listed below.

Facilitating mediators from theory	Audience's knowledge and skills in relation to each mediator, specific to achieving your goal behaviors
Food and nutrition knowledge	
Food and nutrition skills related to the targeted behavior	
Critical thinking skills	
Self-efficacy	
Goal setting (making action plans)	
Self-assessment/self-monitoring skills	
Reinforcements	
Others	

Step 2D: Environmental/policy supports

Find out how you could change the environmental and policy supports listed below to facilitate your intended audience in performing your goal behaviors.

Environmental and policy supports	How each environmental and policy support could be changed, specific to achieving your goal behaviors
Decision makers' awareness and motivation	
Social environment (e.g., family, networks, support)	
Food environment (e.g., availability, accessibility)	
Built environment (e.g., walkable streets, parks)	
Organizational food policy	
Information environment (e.g., media watched/read, setting)	
Policy activities at the community and national levels	

Step 2E: Audience and resources

Add details about your audience that are important for delivering your program.

Audience trait	Description
Educational level or schooling	
Physical and cognitive developmental level and ability (children only)	
Literacy and numeracy skills	
Preferred learning style	
Special needs	
Emotional needs	
Social needs	

Describe the resources available for your program.

Program resources	Available resources
Time	
Space	
Equipment	
General administrative support	

References

CHAPTER 9

Step 3: Selecting Theory, Educational Philosophy, and Program Components

■ INTRODUCTION: PRELIMINARY PLANNING

Having a thorough understanding of the intended audiences, including the health issues that face them, the behaviors or practices that contribute to the health issues, and their motivations, skills, and environmental context, is an important first step in designing nutrition education. However, before rushing to do what you like to do best based on this understanding, such as preparing presentations or designing exciting activities for a group, you still have some preliminary planning to do. You need to think through carefully how best to address the health issues identified, given the behaviors or practices that contribute to them and the influences on these behaviors and mediators of change. **Figure 9-1** reminds us where we are in the design process, and **Figure 9-2** summarizes the tasks and products for Step 3. A worksheet is provided at the end of

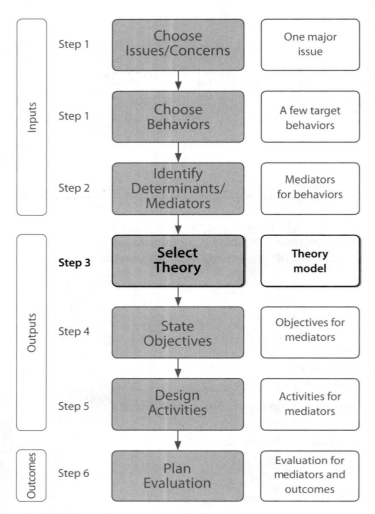

FIGURE 9-1 Flowchart of steps in designing theory-based nutrition education: Step 3.

the chapter for you to use as you proceed through this chapter; the case study serves as an example of how to complete the worksheets.

In this preliminary planning step, you will

- Select the theory or create the conceptual model that will guide your program
- Articulate your philosophy about nutrition education
- Clarify your perspectives on nutrition content and issues
- Determine how many and which components your program will have

After you have completed this preliminary planning step, you can write educational objectives directed at the relevant mediators of change that you have identified and design appropriate theory-based educational strategies and activities directed at these mediators.

■ SELECTING A THEORY OR MODEL

From Step 2, you now have a long list of people's beliefs, motivations, and skills in relation to the behavioral goal of your program. These are the potential mediators of change to achieve the behavioral goals. These

are also the direct targets of your nutrition education activities. However, a list by itself is not sufficient. Theory helps you organize that list into a meaningful set of related predictors of behavior change suitable for nutrition education. It provides a mental map for what to address and how to do so. Clearly laying out the theory or conceptual model for the intervention or program before you begin is crucial.

Consider the following in choosing your theory:

- *Audience stage of readiness to take action.* Based on what you found out, is the intended audience mostly those who are not yet aware or motivated to take action or are they already motivated and need skills and other resources to act on their motivations? Thus, will the program aim to increase awareness, promote active deliberation, and enhance motivation to take action? Or will it focus on building skills and the ability to take action? Will it aim to do both?
- *Individual and environmental components.* Given the duration and scope of the intervention that is feasible based on practical constraints and resource considerations, will your program consist of only in-person sessions or will it be possible for your program to work in partnership with others to promote environmental and policy supports for action? That is, will the program be able to address both personal and environmental mediators of behavior?
- *The strength of the evidence for the theory constructs (mediators of behavior) used with the intended audience for the behaviors that you have selected as the focus of the program.* Information on the nature of the evidence for various theories was explored in the first part of this book in a general way. It is helpful, however, to have specific evidence for the behavior and audience you have selected. Examples might be specific evidence from the research literature of specific mediators that are effective for increasing fruit and vegetable consumption among pregnant women or eating more calcium-rich foods among adolescents.

Because developing educational strategies directed at each of the mediators requires much time, energy, and other resources on your part, as well as time commitment and effort on the part of the intended audience, you want to choose carefully the theory you use and those theory constructs that are most likely to serve as the mediators in your program. Below we discuss how theory may be useful in the different phases and components of the nutrition education intervention.

Theories Especially Useful for the Motivational Phase of Nutrition Education

If your intended audience is mostly unaware or unengaged in the behaviors or practices that are the goals of the program, your educational goal will likely be to increase awareness, promote active contemplation, enhance motivation, assist the audience in understanding and resolving any ambivalences, activate decision making, and facilitate the formation of intentions to take action. Beliefs and attitudes, including feelings and emotions, are at the heart of the motivation to act, as you saw earlier in the book. This is a deliberative phase for individuals. The emphasis in nutrition education here is on *why to* take action. Examples may be public health or health communication campaigns or motivational sessions or materials.

The following theories provide the most guidance on designing messages and activities that increase awareness and enhance motivation. The outcome desired is the formation of an intention to act, based on active contemplation and a deliberative decision-making process. Individuals

Inputs: Collecting Assessment Data			Outputs: Designing the Theory-Based Intervention			Outcomes: Evaluation Plan
Step 1 ⟵⟶ **Analyze issues and audiences to state program behavioral goals**	**Step 2** ⟵⟶ **Identify potential mediators to achieve program behavioral goals**	**Step 3** ⟵⟶ **Select theory, philosophy, and components**	**Step 4** ⟵⟶ **State objectives for mediators**	**Step 5** ⟵⟶ **Design theory-based strategies and activities for mediators**	**Step 6** **Plan evaluation**	
Tasks • Analyze issues and select audience • Identify behaviors or patterns contributing to issue • Specify behavioral or action goals of the program	*Tasks* • Identify personal psychosocial mediators • Identify environmental support mediators	*Tasks* • Select theory or create appropriate model • Clarify philosophy (education and content) • Determine program components	*Tasks* • State educational objectives for psychosocial mediators • State change objectives for environmental support mediators	*Tasks* • Design activities to address psychosocial mediators • Design activities to address environmental support mediators • Implementation plan	*Tasks* • Design outcome evaluation plan • Determine tools to measure impact • Plan process evaluation	
Product • Description of issue of concern • Statement of action or behavioral goals for program	*Product* • List of potential mediators for action or behavior goals	*Product* • Theory/model for program, philosophy, and components	*Product* • Objectives for each mediator	*Product* • Educational plans for sessions linking mediators, objectives, and strategies • Environmental support plans	*Product* • Evaluation plan • List of indicators and measures for outcomes • Procedures and measures for process evaluation	

FIGURE 9-2 Stepwise Procedure for designing theory-based nutrition education: Step 3.

can, of course, choose not to act, and their decision needs to be respected. They will take action when they choose to do so and are ready.

- *Psychosocial theories that focus on personal decision-making and motivational factors* such as the health belief model; precaution adoption process model; the theory of planned behavior and its extensions that include considerations of affect or feelings, values, self-identities, and personal norms; or attitude-change theories or health communications using the elaboration likelihood model
- *Models of food choice* that address food preferences and enjoyment, emotions and mood, and physiological impacts of food on the body
- *Models from grounded theory and interpretative research with this intended audience or applicable to this audience* with an emphasis on personal and cultural meanings and values and self-identities

Theories Especially Useful for the Action Phase of Nutrition Education

Translating intentions into action is difficult for all people, and assisting individuals to do so is a major task of nutrition education. Here, the emphasis is on facilitating individuals' ability to take food-related actions or change their dietary behaviors. Individuals with strong intentions will form implementation intentions or begin making simple plans of action. Those with weak intentions may need some reminders and cues to action. Food- and nutrition-specific knowledge and skills are important, including food choice and food preparation skills. Critical

evaluation skills may be important, where appropriate. The emphasis is on information and skills for *how to* take action.

In addition, self-regulation skills or skills in being able to take charge of their own behaviors and exercising choice (including goal-setting and self-monitoring skills) are important for individuals to be able to act on their chosen motivations and intentions and to express personal agency. The following theories provide the most guidance in action-planning and self-regulation skills:

- *Social cognitive theory* with its emphasis on self-efficacy and self-regulation (Bandura 1997, 2001, 2004)
- *Self-efficacy and self-regulation theories* (including the health action process approach), which describe how people set implementation or goal intentions, make plans for attaining the goals, and maintain goal commitments (Schwarzer 1992; Gollwitzer 1999; Bagozzi & Edwards 1999; Abraham & Sheeran 2000; Sniehotta, Scholz, & Schwarzer 2005)

Theories Useful for Both Motivational Phase and Action Phase Nutrition Education

In most instances, nutrition education seeks to include both motivational and action phase activities—both why-to and how-to education. This can occur at varying levels of depth and breadth. That is, one can begin with motivational activities and conclude with how-to activities in one session. Each of these components would, of course, be brief in this instance. Or the activities can be spread over several sessions and even between components so that health communications through the

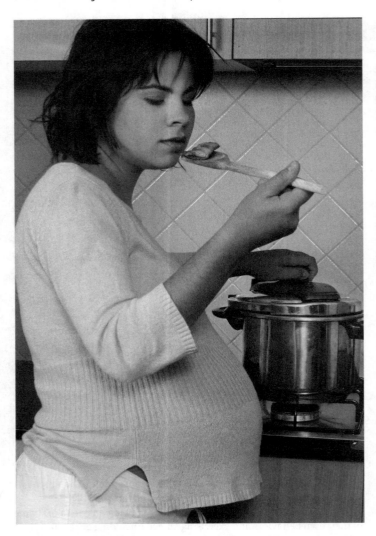

A pregnant woman's health goals may include preparing and eating meals with the proper nutrients for two.

mass media, emphasizing motivational messages, can be accompanied by group sessions that focus on how-to skills.

- *The extended theory of planned behavior* is useful here, with its strong emphasis on motivation, accompanied by setting behavioral intentions or goals and developing implementation plans.
- *Social cognitive theory* provides extensive guidance on translating motivation into action through goal-setting and self-regulation practices, as well as on how individuals and their environments interact, mutually influencing each other. Often nutrition education interventions use social cognitive theory without the environmental component. This is not a true use of the theory but is a widespread practice.
- *The health action process approach* also provides guidance for both phases of health education.
- *The transtheoretical model* describes processes of change for all stages and suggests that procedures or strategies for change can be based on these processes.

Integrated Models or Polytheoretical Models

The various theories have many mediators in common so that they overlap each other. Consequently, several integrated models have been developed that combine constructs from several theories (Kok et al. 1996; Fishbein 2000; Institute of Medicine [IOM] 2002).

Constructs in common that have been shown to be important *motivators* of food- and nutrition-related behavior or mediators of dietary change are the following:

- Outcome expectations (including perceived benefits and barriers or pros and cons of change)
- Attitudes or affect (feelings)
- Perception of risk/threat of current behavior (in some theories)
- Food preferences and enjoyment based on sensory-affective factors
- Perceived social and personal norms
- Self-efficacy or perceived control in performing the targeted behaviors

Constructs in common that have been shown in many studies to be important for *facilitating the ability to act* are as follows:

- Self-efficacy
- Perceived behavioral control or personal agency
- Self-regulation skills, including goal setting and self-monitoring
- Behavioral capabilities or food- and nutrition-specific knowledge and skills to enact goals, including food preparation or physical activity skills, and critical evaluation skills where relevant

General Model of Determinants of Health Behavior Change

A general or polytheoretical model of the determinants of behavior change is shown in **Figure 9-3**. It was developed by a committee of the Institute of Medicine that included the key researchers who originated the health belief model, theory of planned behavior, and social cognitive theory, among others (IOM 2002). It combines the basic constructs of theory of planned behavior (attitudes, social norms, and perceived behavioral control) and perceived risk from the health belief model with the emphasis on skills and environmental constraints from social cognitive theory. The model acknowledges the importance of environmental barriers or supports but does not elaborate on them.

The Health Action Process Approach (HAPA) Model

The HAPA model is shown in Chapter 5, Figure 5-2 (Schwarzer 1992; Sniehotta et al. 2005). This model incorporates perceived risk from the health belief model with outcome expectations and self-efficacy variables from social cognitive theory that are also in common to many theories. It incorporates a time dimension, with a pre-action motivational phase and an action phase. It points out that self-efficacy is needed at all phases of change: making an intention, developing action plans, and in initiating and maintaining action. The model also acknowledges the importance of environmental barriers or supports but does not elaborate on them.

An Integrative Framework for Translating Theory into Effective Nutrition Education Practice: Linking Mediators to Education

The framework shown in **Figure 9-4** is the translational and implementation model that is used in this book: it focuses on the use of theory to design the "outputs" section of the logic model. It translates behavioral

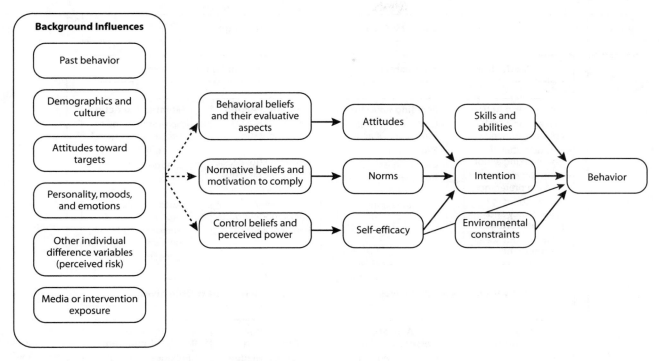

FIGURE 9-3 General model of determinants of health behavior change.

Source: Institute of Medicine. 2002. *Speaking of health: Assessing health communication strategies for diverse populations.* Washington, DC: National Academies Press. Used with permission from the National Academies Press, National Academy of Science.

theory into a format that is suitable for conducting nutrition education in practice settings.

The constructs in common among several theories have been used to build the integrative framework for nutrition education interventions shown in Figure 9-4. The framework suggests that dietary change can be thought of as occurring in sub-four phases: considering action, deciding on action, initiating action, and maintaining action. It proposes that nutrition education intervention objectives are different for each phase. The integrative framework links mediators of change from theory, phases of change, and nutrition education objectives for intervention. An environmental support component also is very important. Useful theories for each phase also are listed.

- *Considering action* involves mediators of motivation for dietary change from theory such as perception of risk, outcome expectations, attitudes based on beliefs and feelings about taking action, sensory affective aspects of food, social norms, and self-efficacy.
  The objective of the nutrition education program in this motivational phase is to increase awareness and enhance motivation.
- *Deciding on action* involves cost-benefit analyses, resolving ambivalences, and experiencing cues to action.
  The objective of the nutrition education program is to activate decision making.
- *Initiating action* involves several mediators or procedures of change from theory: action plans or implementation plans, behavioral capabilities (learning-relevant diet-related knowledge and skills), social modeling, and self-efficacy.
  The objective of the nutrition education program is to facilitate the ability to act.

- *Maintaining action* requires self-regulation (self-direction) skills including planning and self-monitoring skills, emotion-coping skills, and perceived personal agency or autonomous motivation based on competence, autonomy, and sense of relatedness to others. Developing personal food policies is very helpful.
  The objective of the nutrition education program is to strengthen self-regulation skills.
- *Environmental supports for action* are based on concepts in common from research using the social ecological approach: social factors such as social support, institutional/community actions including community capacity building for collective efficacy, physical factors such as food availability and accessibility/built environment, and social systems, structures, and policy.
  The objective of the nutrition education program is to work in collaboration with decision makers and policy makers at many levels to increase environmental and policy supports for action.

Constructing Your Intervention Theory Model

After you have chosen your theory or combined theory constructs as demonstrated earlier, create an intervention model specific to your particular audience. That is, operationalize the theory for your particular audience. Decide whether you will address all the mediators in the theory or only some. Evidence from ongoing research can suggest which specific theory constructs are most likely to serve as mediators of the behavior in an educational program for your particular audience. Also consider the length of your program and resources available as to how many and which mediators you will address. In creating your intervention model, you must specify the exact outcome expectations, values, attitudes, affect, and self-efficacy issues (or other constructs you intend to address) and the supportive environmental changes you seek

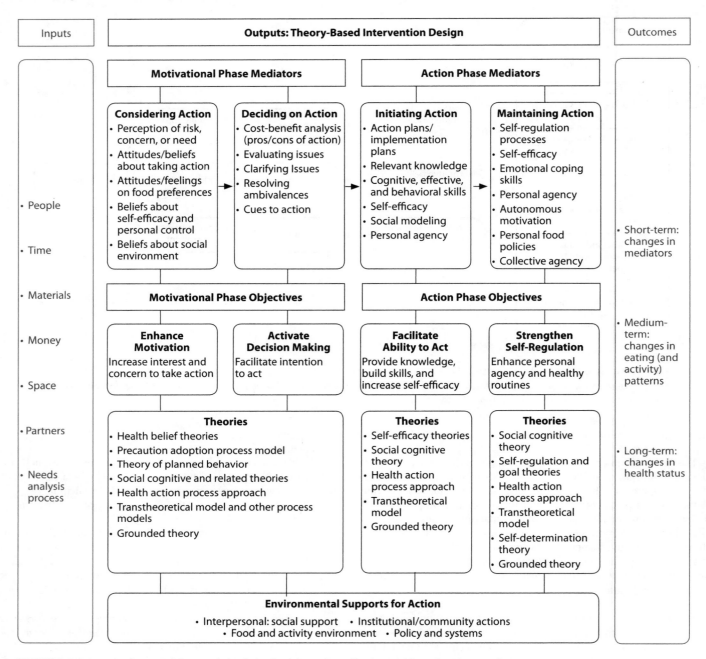

FIGURE 9-4 Integrative framework for translating behavioral theory into effective nutrition education practice.

to bring about. Drawing a diagram to illustrate the relationships among constructs can be very helpful. State your theory and draw a diagram of your model in the Step 3 worksheet.

■ ARTICULATING A PHILOSOPHY OF NUTRITION EDUCATION FOR THE PROGRAM

Regardless of the theory you have selected, your choice of *approach* to designing nutrition education sessions or programs and how you translate behavioral theory into educational practice are very much influenced by your perspective or philosophy of nutrition education, so you

should clarify this philosophy before you begin. As a nutrition educator with considerable background in the natural sciences, you might not think of yourself as using philosophy in your work, but you do.

For example, Chapter 1 described many reasons it is almost impossible for nutrition education to be value free even if it wants to be. Hence the view of nutritionist Jean Mayer (1986) seems appropriate: that nutrition education has the value-laden goal of improving the health and well-being of individuals and communities. Indeed, nutrition education, along with health education, allied health professions, social work, and similar professions, is often described as a "helping" profession. There is, of course, a dilemma for nutrition educators here because there is a tension between the act of helping on the part of nutrition educators and human agency or self-determination on the part of participants. For those in the nutrition professions, then, a philosophy about "helping" is particularly important.

Who Is Responsible for the Problem or the Solution?

One way to approach these issues, proposed by Brickman and colleagues (1982), is to think about who is responsible for the problem (that is, who is to blame for the current condition, such as a person's type 2 diabetes or obesity) and who is responsible for the solution in a given situation (that is, who is to control future events) and therefore what "helping" or "educating" means.

Brickman's Model of Helping

Based on these attributions of responsibility, Brickman and associates propose four models of helping (**Table 9-1**):

- *Medical model.* Individuals are not responsible for problems or solutions. This philosophical perspective is called the medical model because in this instance neither the individual's health condition, such as hypertension, nor its solution is seen as the individual's responsibility. Individuals are *in need of treatment* by professionals, using medication or drugs, perhaps. Many professionals and group participants like the medical approach because it seems to promise a quick solution and permits people to accept assistance without being blamed for their condition. It may be a suitable model for certain situations or conditions, especially emergencies related to a medical condition such as diabetes. However, the medical model is a special case of the more general approach of paternalism. In this approach, the nutritionists are the experts, the dominant figures, who have the information—and hence power—and tend to take control of decisions, leaving little room for the autonomy of the audience members (Achterberg & Trenkner 1990). Education using this model can be coercive because participants may not be told about acceptable alternatives and given a choice about which actions, if any, they wish to take. Even if benign, this approach can create dependency on the part of participants.
- *Moral model.* Individuals are responsible for both problems and solutions. This philosophical perspective is at the other end of

the spectrum from the medical model. Here, the individuals are considered to have full personal responsibility for having created their problems and also for solving them. They are considered to have considerable personal control. They are primarily *in need of motivation*. This is a widely accepted perspective. In a free society with freedom of choice, and in a food system that offers 50,000 food items in the typical supermarket, individuals are considered to have control over their own food intake. Hence, their health conditions are the result of their own choices and actions. The role of nutrition educators in this model is to increase interest and enhance motivation. However, this approach can result in "person blame," in which people are blamed for their conditions, such as heart disease. It becomes easy to ignore the fact that genetic factors affect health, as do powerful environmental forces and social conditions that shape and reinforce behavior, and resource considerations that limit choices for some.

- *Enlightenment model.* Individuals are responsible for problems but are not responsible for solutions. In this philosophical perspective, individuals recognize and accept that their lifestyles and health behaviors have led to problematic consequences (weight gain, hypertension, or type 2 diabetes) but feel that they cannot do much about it. They need to be enlightened about the true nature of their problem(s) and are primarily *in need of enlightenment and discipline*, which can often be supplied by some outside force. Thus, those in Overeaters Anonymous believe that they are responsible for their overeating or weight problems but need an outside authority or support group to help them gain control over their behavior and their lives.
- *Compensatory model.* Individuals are not responsible for problems but are responsible for solutions. Here, individuals are not blamed for their current condition or problems but are held responsible for solving these problems. They have to compensate or cope with the particular problems they have. In this philosophical perspective, individuals are seen as suffering problems that are not of their own making, but which instead result from the failure of their social environment to provide them with the goods and services to which they are entitled, such as accessibility to nutritious, wholesome food or to education. Individuals are thus primarily *in need of power*. The role of the nutrition educator is to mobilize resources for them and/or to assist them to acquire the skills of collective efficacy or empowerment to deal effectively with the environment to obtain what they need.

Of these perspectives, Brickman and colleagues prefer the compensatory model because it is the only one that resolves the dilemma faced by nutrition educators: it justifies the act of helping or assisting (because individuals are not responsible for their problems) but still leaves the individuals with active control over their lives (because they are responsible for using this help to find a solution if they wish). They also point out that it is important that the health professional (nutrition educator) and the intended audience have the same expectations and subscribe to the same philosophical perspective in terms of the particular intervention. At the least, they should be aware of each others' philosophical perspectives and resolve any differences in expectation.

Who Makes the Decisions About Solutions?: Active Participation and Joint Decision Making

So, what then are the relative responsibilities of the nutrition educator and the participants in making decisions about dietary change?

TABLE 9-1	**Models of Helping and Coping**	
Self Responsible for the Problem	**Self Responsible for the Solution**	
	High	**Low**
High	Moral model (need motivation)	Enlightenment model (need discipline)
Low	Compensatory model (need power)	Medical model (need treatment)

Source: Based on Brickman, P., V. C. Rabinowitz, J. Karuza, D. Coates, E. Cohn, and L. Kidder. 1982. Models of helping and coping. *American Psychologist* 37:368–384.

TABLE 9-2	Decision-Making Roles of Nutrition Educator and Group Participants	
Nutrition Educator Responsibility	Participant Responsibility	
	Yes	No
Yes	Active participation	Authoritative guidance
No	Independent decision making	No decision making occurs

Source: Modified from Roter, D. 1987. An exploration of health education's responsibility for a partnership model of client–provider relations. *Patient Education and Counseling* 9:25–31.

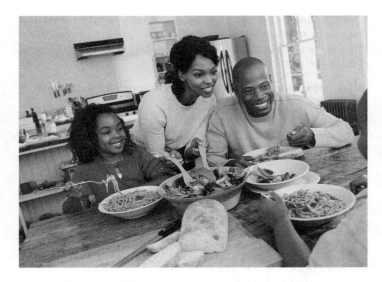

Our eating behaviors are influenced by a variety of factors.

Roter's Decision-Making Model

Roter's decision-making model is shown in **Table 9-2**. It was proposed to describe the relationships between clients and health providers, such as physicians, but applies more generally (Roter 1987). In this decision-making model, *authoritative guidance* is equivalent to the medical model in Table 9-1, and *independent decision making* is equivalent to the moral model. When no one takes responsibility for a health issue, no decision is made. However, this model proposes that there can be an active partnership between the educator and group members in which both are involved in *joint decision making* to arrive at mutually agreed-upon goals (Achterberg & Trenkner 1990; Parham 1990; Charles, Gafni, & Whelan 1999).

Humans Have Free Will

Others emphasize the fact that humans have agency or free will. People act, not just react (Bandura 2001). This free will, or the capacity to choose, gives human beings their unique place in the world and their human dignity. This makes behaviors hard to predict because behaviors have many rational and irrational determinants. Individuals should have "the freedom to choose their own motivations, beliefs and objectives in living; and the freedom to select among alternatives that can, or might, bring about those objectives" (Achterberg & Trenkner 1990). Nutrition educators can engage in a dialogue with individuals about ways of living that they find most worthwhile, exploring questions such as "Will losing weight help me to achieve the goals that I have set for myself? Is being physically fit the most important purpose in life?" Buchanan proposes that the nutrition educator and participants should be "fully engaged in mutual dialogue, deliberation, and debate with the aim of finding ways that we can work together to make this a better world" (Buchanan 2004, p. 152).

Self-Determination Theory

Self-determination theory suggests a similar approach (Deci & Ryan 2000, 2008). This theory proposes that achievement of goal-directed behavior, and indeed of psychological development and well-being, is very much dependent on people's inherent need for autonomy, competence, and relatedness. Nutrition education that provides support for individuals' experience of autonomy, positive feedback in situations where individuals feel they are responsible for their competent actions,

and a secure base of relatedness between educator and participants can lead to intrinsic motivation and integrated self-regulation or self-determination.

Applying to Practice

In practice, groups include those who need motivation, those who need power or skills, and those who need both. Thus, joint decision making and mutual participation in the process of change proceed best through a two-phase sequence in which motivation is first facilitated and supported by the nutrition educator or nutrition education program. This is a time to build trust, whereby feelings and expectations are expressed and motivations are developed. In the second phase, skills are provided at a time when they are helpful so that individuals can choose actions for change, internalize them, and then maintain the actions by themselves (Kolbe et al. 1981; Achterberg & Trenkner 1990). Although the model of joint decision making and active participation was developed to describe one-on-one interactions, it can be applied to groups. In this case, joint decision making comes from (1) a thorough understanding of the group

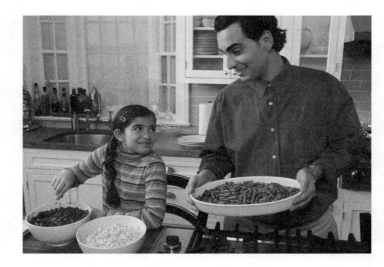

Preparing and cooking food with others reinforces nutritional goals.

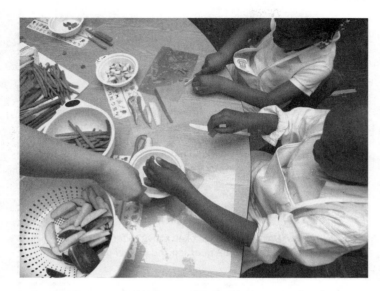

Cooking can be an important feature in nutrition education for young children, such as seen here at a CookShop program.

as the program is being designed, involving the group in the assessment process; and (2) designing session activities that are interactive so that the audience's prior knowledge, feelings, and expectations can be incorporated and on-site corrections can be made to the education or lesson plan, if necessary, to suit the situation on the ground.

Two-Phase Process

This two-phase process is similar to the two phases for conducting group nutrition education proposed in this text, whereby in the early phase the emphasis is on encouraging active deliberation and motivation, and in the later phase the emphasis is on empowerment through acquisition of relevant food and nutrition knowledge and skills and behavioral self-regulation skills, accompanied, where appropriate, by collective efficacy and advocacy skills to take action on the environment. Nutrition education provides the structure and educational resources to assist individuals as they seek to become motivated, willing, and able to take action, but individuals choose the goals that are important for them at any given time and ways to achieve the goals. That is, the nutrition educator has a role, and the individuals have a role.

Other Considerations

"Life Is Open-Ended"

Achterberg and Trenkner (1990) provide thoughtful perspectives about nutrition education that are useful to consider at this time. One is that "life is open-ended," meaning that change is always possible. Thus, nutrition educators should not give up on any group or individual. Maybe not now, but perhaps sometime later, the nutrition education messages and activities you have provided will become meaningful and acted upon. This also means that you can encourage the intended audience members to view change as always possible, if and when they choose to change. Maybe not now, but sometime in the future they may be in a better place to take action. This approach also is a central tenet of chaos theory (described in Chapter 3): nutrition educators thus should still design theory-based interventions, but they cannot tell when the messages and activities will coalesce in the minds of group participants.

"Life Is Difficult"

Life can be difficult, for both the intended audience and for you. You have to accept that your intended audience members have many issues and concerns in life, and nutrition may not be a high priority at the time of your nutrition education activity. You also have to accept that nutrition education is difficult and that you experience many professional dilemmas for which there are no easy solutions.

Nutrition Education in Action 9-1 provides the statements of the philosophies and perspectives of one particular program as an illustration. The philosophy and perspectives of the case study intervention are shown at the end of the chapter.

■ CLARIFYING THE PROGRAM'S PERSPECTIVES ON NUTRITION CONTENT

All nutrition educators have a point of view about the content of nutrition education. This book takes the stance that the *content* of nutrition education is broad, focusing on behaviors that are conducive to the health and well-being of individuals, their communities, and their food systems. This scope is similar to that stated by the Society for Nutrition Education in its mission and vision statements: "healthy, sustainable food choices" and "healthy people in healthy communities."

You, or the nutrition education planning team, also need to clarify your own or the organization's stand on substantive issues related to the scope and content of the educational intervention that you are designing, both in broad terms and in specific ones. Now is the time to consider how the intervention will treat the issues in your program, such as the following:

- *Food production issues.* Will you consider how food is grown, processed, and transported in your recommendations regarding foods to eat? When you encourage a group to increase their fruit and vegetable intake, will you suggest any particular source? For example, will you recommend fruits and vegetables from all sources—fresh, frozen, canned, local, flown in from another country? If you will be working with a school or workplace to increase the number and variety of fruits and vegetables offered, will you be concerned about the source of these, such as whether they are from local farmers or whether they are organic? These considerations influence your messages as well as any environmental component that you may design, such as a farm-to-school component.

- *All-foods fit.* Will you take the stance that there are no "good foods" or "bad foods," that is, that all foods fit into a healthful diet? Or will you take the stance that although all foods fit, some foods are more nutritious than others and use a "sometimes foods" and "anytime foods" approach, or some other approach?

- *Whole foods versus fortified and processed foods.* What will be your stance on using fortified foods (e.g., highly processed cereal fortified with vitamins) to obtain nutrients or on eating whole foods (e.g., whole-grain cereals)? Calcium tablets or calcium-containing foods?

- *Weight.* Will you encourage health at every size or will you encourage weight control or weight loss along with healthy eating?

- *Breastfeeding.* Will you favor breastfeeding or bottle-feeding, or will you promote both as equally acceptable nutritional alternatives? This will influence your design of educational content.

- *Supplements.* Will you recommend dietary supplements or not?

NUTRITION EDUCATION IN ACTION **9-1**

The Wellness IN the Rockies (WIN the Rockies) Project

Project Description and Philosophy

Project: WIN the Rockies is a research, education, and outreach project that seeks to address obesity innovatively and effectively.

Philosophy: People have responsibilities for their own health, but communities need to create environments that foster good health and provide healthy options.

Mission: To assist communities in educating people to:

- Value health
- Respect body-size differences
- Enjoy the benefits of self-acceptance
- Enjoy healthful and pleasurable eating

Components for Adults, Children, and Patients

Adults

- *A New You: Health for Every Body.* Ten 1-hour sessions for small groups that can be mixed, combined, or taught independently.

- *Cook Once: Eat for Two Weeks.* A family mealtime program that can be used in a class setting or as a do-it-yourself program. It involves recipes and food purchasing directions.
- *WIN Steps.* A community walking program.

Children

- *WIN Kids Lessons.* Thirteen lessons for youth that address food and eating, physical activity, and respect for body-size differences.
- *WIN Kids Fun Days.* A collection of 40 activities for youth.
- *WIN the Rockies Jeopardy.* A question and answer game for youth.

Patients

- *Goal-setting forms.* Health improvement goals for adult patients in consultation with their health care providers.

Source: University of Idaho, Montana State University, and University of Wyoming. 2005. A community-based research, intervention, and outreach project to improve health in Idaho, Montana, and Wyoming. http://www.uwyo.edu/wintherockies.

- *Sweetened beverages.* What will the intervention recommend about drinking sweetened beverages, particularly if it is a school-based intervention that involves school meals or school food policy?
- *Genetically engineered foods.* What is your stance on genetically engineered foods? What will you say in your educational sessions? Will you be concerned about this issue when you choose foods for your environmental component, if you will have one?

■ CLARIFYING THE PROGRAM'S PERSPECTIVES ON USE OF EDUCATIONAL MATERIALS FROM A VARIETY OF SOURCES

Nutrition education interventions are often not well funded and therefore cannot afford to develop and print their own high-quality educational materials. Instead, they use educational materials from a variety of sources. These often are of high quality and visually appealing. These sources may be from nonprofit voluntary organizations such as heart associations or cancer societies, or from the food industry or other businesses. You and your team should carefully discuss the pros and cons of using materials from other sources and decide your policy regarding the use of such materials. You might want to consider the following guidelines for good practice that were established by the International Organization of Consumers Unions (1990):

- *Accuracy.* Information must be consistent with established fact or best evidence. It should be appropriately referenced so that it can be easily verified.
- *Objectivity.* All major or relevant points of view are fairly presented. If the issue is controversial, arguments in favor must be balanced by arguments against. The sponsor bias should be clearly stated, and reference to opposing views should be made.

- *Completeness.* The materials contain all relevant information and do not deceive or mislead by omission—and not just by commission.
- *Nondiscriminatory.* The text and illustrations are free of any reference or characteristics that could be considered derogatory or that stereotype a particular group.
- *Noncommercial.* Sponsored material that is specifically designated as being for educational use should be clearly presented as such. Promotional materials should not be presented as "educational." There should be no implied or explicit sales message or exhortation to buy a product or service. Corporate identification should be used to identify the sponsor of the material and provide contacts for further information, but text and illustrations should be free of the sponsor's brand names, trademarks, and so forth.

■ ARTICULATING YOUR NEEDS AND APPROACH AS A NUTRITION EDUCATOR

You may also want to think about the following about yourself:

- Your skill level and experience in teaching, conducting workshops, designing health fairs, developing materials, and so forth; professional experience, such as in Cooperative Extension Service; level of understanding of nutrition and food and food systems issues (one or several courses in nutrition, graduate work).
- Preferred style of providing sessions for groups, such as lectures, discussion, hands-on activities, group work, field projects, food demonstrations, or cooking with groups.
- Personal priorities and motivations for being a nutrition educator. Why do you want to educate people about nutrition? What made you want to enter the field?

If you will be designing and/or delivering the nutrition education as a team, you may want to discuss these issues openly so that you can integrate team members' individual preferences and skills into the educational plan and create activities that use your complementary skills.

■ SELECTING THE PROGRAM COMPONENTS OR CHANNELS

You are now ready to select how many and which program components you will design. Your choice will depend heavily on the scope of the intervention possible given the resources available identified in your findings from Steps 1 and 2. Your choice of theory is also influenced by these considerations. The "program" may thus consist of only a few sessions or of many components that involve many channels, such as group sessions, health fairs, lunch room signage, a Web component, or a media campaign.

Theory Variables You Will Address

Assume that you (and your nutrition education team members) have chosen social cognitive theory as your theoretical framework as most suitable for the behavioral goals of your program. Thus, you want the program to address the personal and environmental mediators of the behaviors targeted in your program. Because this theory is an extremely complex theory if used in its entirety, and because of the scope that is possible based on the resources you have available to you, you have decided that the intervention model will focus on only the following key personal potential mediating variables: physical outcome expectations (benefits, including taste), social outcome expectations (social norms), and self-evaluative expectations, along with self-efficacy as a motivational variable, and goal-setting and behavioral capabilities (food- and nutrition-related knowledge and skills) as variables that facilitate action. You wish to include some modest environmental changes as well.

Box 9-1 summarizes the key elements that contribute to the effectiveness of nutrition education interventions, as determined by reviews of studies. You should consider these as you choose your channels and components.

Selecting How Many and Which Components

Your nutrition education program may consist of only several group sessions with a particular audience. If you are considering other components, answers to the following questions may be helpful:

1. *What types of components or what channels are usually used in programs with this audience for the goal behaviors of your program that you identified in Step 1?* Review the research evidence and literature on evaluated, or even nonevaluated, programs. Look into programs produced by various government and other professional organizations. For programs with children and youth, the primary components are usually those directed toward school curricula, the school environment, the school food service, after-school programs, family, peers, and relevant community institutions such as the Girl and Boy Scouts to which youth may belong. With adults, the primary sites for nutrition education are workplaces, community agencies, Cooperative Extension Program sites, outpatient clinics, and churches. In these sites, program components are usually directed at the primary audience (e.g., employees, attendees of an organization's activities, such as a congregation) and their families.

2. *What intervention duration will be available to you to achieve action or change?* Note: Based on the evidence, adequate duration and intensity are required for changes in behavior or health actions to occur. Some studies suggest that as many as 30 to 50 hours may be needed (Connell, Turner, & Mason 1985).

3. *What resources will you have to develop the program? What is the time frame available?*
   - *Personnel and skills:* How many nutrition education personnel will be available for this program? What skills do you collectively possess? For development of the program, you need skills in creating exciting activities for the audience, artistic skills to develop attractive materials, and desktop publishing abilities. To the extent possible, use resources that are already available. However, you still need to adapt materials for your own sessions and program. For delivery of the program, you need skills in working with groups or in providing professional development regarding your project for others who will work with you, such as teachers or community leaders. If you plan on evaluating the program, you also need skills in evaluation. This text seeks to help you acquire or hone these skills.
   - *Time:* You will need to allow time to develop the program, no matter how short or long it is: time for writing lessons,

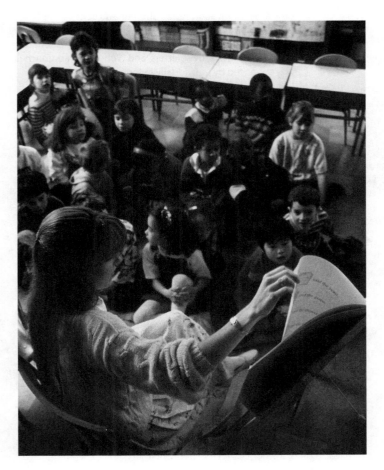

Encourage students to write down their health goals then share students' responses with the entire class.

Box 9-1 **Elements of Effectiveness for Nutrition Education**

General

- Nutrition education is more likely to be effective when it focuses on specific food choice behaviors or diet-related practices.
- Nutrition education interventions are more likely to be effective when they employ educational strategies that are directly relevant to the behavioral focus and are derived from appropriate theory and prior research evidence.

Communications and Educational Strategies for Enhancing Awareness and Motivation

- Addressing the motivators that have personal meaning for the particular population group is of primary importance.
- Taking into account the group's stage of motivational readiness to take action and adopt dietary change may improve effectiveness.
- Use of personalized self-assessment of nutritional status or food-related behaviors and feedback in comparison with recommendations can enhance motivation.
- Direct experience with food can enhance enjoyment of healthy food, motivation to act, and self-efficacy.
- Active participation is important.
- The effectiveness of communications through nonpersonal media such as letters, newsletters, and Web-based approaches can be enhanced by individually tailoring the messages.
- Mass media health campaigns can increase awareness of issues, affect beliefs and attitudes, and increase knowledge of targeted behaviors.
- A variety of nontraditional channels show promise.

Strategies for Facilitating the Ability to Take Action and Maintain Behavioral Change

- Use of a systematic goal-setting and self-regulation (or self-directed action) process that fosters people's agency is most likely to be effective in facilitating individuals' ability to take action and maintain change. In this process, individuals are provided opportunities to conduct accurate self-assessments and compare them with recommendations; learn of effective behaviors for healthful and enjoyable eating (and physical activity); choose among alternatives to set their own goals; learn the cognitive, affective, and behavioral skills needed to achieve their goals; monitor their progress toward goal attainment; and experience a sense of agency or self-influence and control.
- Sufficient attention to the complexity of food-specific issues is important.
- Adequate duration and intensity of the intervention are needed for changes in health actions to take place.
- Use of small groups is likely to improve the effectiveness of nutrition education interventions.

- Cultural appropriateness or sensitivity, along with behavioral theory, can enhance effectiveness.
- Long-term maintenance of behavior change is enhanced with continued experience of the new way of eating to increase familiarity and enjoyment, and opportunity to develop personal food-related routines or policies.

Environmental Interventions

- Social support such as family and peer involvement is important in all population groups and should be incorporated.
- Collaborating with policy makers, service providers, organizations, community leaders, and agencies is important for promoting healthful food environments in schools, workplaces, and communities.
- Enhancing community capacity and facilitating collective efficacy or agency to create environments that provide healthy options are likely to enhance individuals' ability to take action.
- Delivering nutrition education through multiple venues and directed at multiple levels of influence enhances dietary change.

Nutrition Educator Factors

- The credibility and trustworthiness of the nutrition educator enhance audiences' willingness to respond to, and accept, the message. Open-mindedness and fairness engender a safe learning environment.
- Being organized is key to being effective. This allows for wise use of time and increased participant interest and engagement as well as enhanced credibility for the nutrition educator.
- The educator's ability to adapt to the situation on the ground is important for implementation of the intervention.
- Sensitivity to the audience is crucial to the effectiveness of nutrition education. This includes being appropriate in terms of developmental level and age-related concerns as well as sensitivity in terms of the culture and resources of the audience.

Sources: Contento, I. R., G. I. Balch, S. K. Maloney, et al. 1995. The effectiveness of nutrition education and implications for nutrition education policy, programs, and research. *Journal of Nutrition Education* 127:279–418; Ammerman, A. S., C. H. Lindquist, K. N. Lohr, and J. Hersey. 2002. The efficacy of behavioral interventions to modify dietary fat and fruit and vegetable intake: A review of the evidence. *Preventive Medicine* 35(1):25–41; Pomerleau, J., K. Lock, C. Knai, and M. McKee. 2005. Interventions designed to increase adults' fruit and vegetable intake can be effective: A systematic review of the literature. *Journal of Nutrition* 135:2486–2495; and Shaya, F. T., D. Flores, C. M. Gbaryor, and J. Wang. 2008. School-based obesity interventions: A literature review. *Journal of School Health* 78:189–196.

developing handouts, creating needed artwork, pilot testing (if your program is more than a one-time event), and developing evaluation instruments. In terms of implementation, you also need to be clear about how much time will be available to you in the setting in which you intend to conduct the program. In schools, it is difficult to get more than six or seven 45-minute periods of class time. In community settings, attendance at more than three to six sessions is difficult to achieve. The time frame determines how many goals and objectives you can write and how many activities you can conduct.

- *Money:* You need money for the handouts, student or participant activity sheets, and other materials that you develop. In schools, you usually also need money for binders for students and manuals and honoraria for teachers. In nutrition education, money for food is always an important consideration. It is effective to bring samples of what you are talking about or food items to taste, or items to cook, if food preparation is being considered. This usually means that you also need to supply plates and utensils for the group. If you use mass mailing, there are costs for mailing and postage and other media costs.

4. *What collaborations will you include?* Many nutrition education programs need to involve collaborations with other people and organizations to accomplish nutrition education goals. You need to seek these out: school district superintendents or principals, school food service directors, public health agencies, parent–teacher organizations, workplaces, community leaders and organizations, churches and other religious institutions, or existing task forces or coalitions.

5. *What products will you need to produce?* Whether for one session or for a more extensive program, you need to develop the materials you will use in the program. Even for one session with

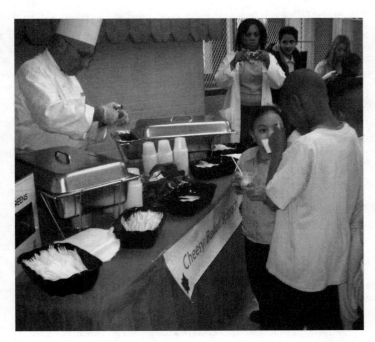

School food services can provide opportunities for children to taste and enjoy new vegetables.

adults, you need to produce an education plan plus all the materials you will use, such as newsprint on an easel and markers, slides, worksheets, or handouts. To the extent possible, use existing materials. For school-based programs you will need a manual that includes the classroom component activities or curriculum; student activity worksheets and homework; and perhaps computer-based activities or videotapes, recipes for classroom food activities, or rewards. You may also need a teacher professional development manual. For environmental support activities, you may need to help school food service staff develop recipes. You may also need to develop school food service training manuals and cafeteria posters. For community-based programs, many of the same products may be needed.

For workplace or community-based programs, you will need a manual that includes the lesson plans of group session activities, brochures, handouts, worksheets, and other materials. These materials all need to be designed to look catchy, inviting, professional, coherent, and appropriate to the audience as well as true to the goals and objectives of the program. The previous considerations of personnel, time, and money help you decide how many of these materials you will be able to produce and who will produce them. Examples of program components and products are shown in **Table 9-3**.

■ CONCLUSIONS

Based on these considerations, you need to decide which components to incorporate into your program.

Workplace Interventions

For a workplace intervention, will you plan group sessions only, or will you use other channels as well, such as health fairs, lunchroom food item signage, and a media campaign? Will you be able to facilitate changes in what is available in the cafeteria and/or vending machines? Will you be able to include a physical activity component? Will you be able to offer a family component?

School-Based Interventions

For a school-based program, will you design a student classroom curriculum only? Or will you include food-tasting activities in the cafeteria, posters, and health fairs as well? For changes in the environmental determinants, will you be able to work with the school food service director to make changes in school meals? Will you be able to initiate or support a food or health policy council? Will you involve the parents? If so, how—through newsletters or activities to be taken home and activities to be done by students and family together? Will you organize family nights? **Box 9-2** shows an example of the types of components recommended for a comprehensive school-based program to promote healthful eating habits.

Community-Based Interventions

For a community-based program, will you design group nutrition education sessions for participants only at community sites? Will you include a mass media campaign, including Web-based activities; health fairs; billboards; and other community activities? Will you be able to capitalize on opportunities to collaborate with others to make vouchers available for participants at supermarkets and farmers' markets? Can you go further and collaborate with supermarkets or restaurants to place

TABLE 9-3   **Potential Program Components and Implementation Products: Examples**

Program Components	Potential Program Products
School-based programs	
Classroom component: N-session program	Classroom curriculum or manual of lessons/activities for the N sessions
	Student activity sheets and homework
	Audiotapes and videotapes
	Computer and website activities
	Incentives and rewards
	Snack preparation and taste-testing recipes
Teacher professional development sessions: 2	Teacher professional development manual
Family involvement component:	
• Educational sessions	Family educational session manual for sessions
• Other activities	Family educational session materials
	Family activities done by family and youth at home
	Newsletters and other mailed information
	Recipes and tip sheets for family activities
	Family fun nights protocols
School environment (through collaborations)	
· School food service changes	School food service professional development manuals; menu modification manual
· School food policies	School food environment assessment tools
	School Wellness Policy councils' recruitment and activity protocols
	School Wellness Policy manuals
· School informational environment	Classroom and cafeteria posters
Workplace programs	
Worksite educational component	
· Kickoff event	Protocol for kickoff activities
· Educational session	Manual of lessons/activities for the sessions
	Activity sheets, handouts
· Activities	Health fair protocol
	Food demonstration protocol
	Cholesterol screening equipment and education protocol
	Nutrition quizzes
· Information distribution	Brochures and self-assessment with feedback materials
Worksite environment component (through collaborations)	Worksite food environment assessment tools
	Employee councils' recruitment and activity protocols
· Worksite food service offerings	Recommended menu offerings/modification manual
· Catering policies	Catering policy document
· Information environment	Nutrition information in cafeterias (signage) and vending machines
Family component	Family newsletters, activity sheets, recipes, tip sheets
Community programs	
Community educational component: N sessions	Manual with protocol for sessions/activities for the N sessions
	Activity sheets, handouts
	Snack preparation and taste-testing recipes
	Cooking classes: protocols for teaching skills, recipes
	Incentives and rewards
Social marketing component	Social marketing materials
Farmers' market component: N tours	Manual with protocol for farmers' markets tours
	Recipes and handouts

$\mathcal{B}$ox 9-2   Guidelines for School Health Programs to Promote Healthful Eating

Based on the available scientific literature, national nutrition policy documents, and current practice, the Centers for Disease Control and Prevention provides the following broad recommendations for ensuring a quality nutrition program within a comprehensive school health program:

- *Policy:* Adopt a coordinated school nutrition policy that promotes healthy eating through classroom lessons and a supportive school environment.
- *Curriculum for nutrition education:* Implement nutrition education from preschool through secondary school as part of a sequential, comprehensive school health education curriculum designed to help students adopt healthy eating behaviors.
- *Instruction for students:* Provide nutrition education through developmentally appropriate, culturally relevant, fun, participatory activities that involve social learning strategies.
- *Integration of school food service and nutrition education:* Coordinate school food service with nutrition education

and other components of the comprehensive school health program to reinforce messages on healthy eating.

- *Professional development for staff:* Provide staff involved in nutrition education with adequate preservice and in-service professional development that focuses on teaching strategies for behavioral change.
- *Family and community involvement:* Involve family members and the community in supporting and reinforcing nutrition education.
- *Program evaluation:* Regularly evaluate the effectiveness of the school health program in promoting healthy eating and change the program as appropriate to increase its effectiveness.

Source: Centers for Disease Control and Prevention. 1996. Guidelines for school health programs to promote lifelong healthy eating. *Morbidity and Mortality Weekly Report* 45(RR-9):1–41.

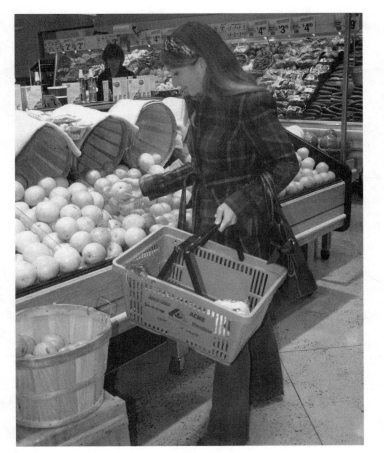

Visually appealing produce displays in grocery stores can sway shoppers.

signage on certain healthful items and even negotiate reduction in the prices on them?

■ CASE STUDY

In this step the case study for the ongoing hypothetical program to promote more healthful eating and physical activity by middle school adolescents presents the *theory*, *educational philosophy*, and *components* for "Taking Control: Eating Well and Being Fit." Use it as an example to help you think through your philosophy, select your theoretical framework to design your own nutrition education sessions or program, and select the components you will incorporate.

Recall that four behavioral goals were chosen for the program "Taking Control: Eating Well and Being Fit": increase intake of fruits and vegetables; reduce consumption of sweetened beverages; reduce intake of packaged, highly processed energy dense snacks; and increase physical activity.

The theory chosen is social cognitive theory, and the educational philosophy is laid out in the case study as is the approach to nutrition content. The program will recommend eating whole, less processed foods obtained from local sources to the extent possible and consistent with youths' resources and access.

Based on the findings from Steps 1 and 2, we have chosen three components to address these behavioral goals: a classroom curriculum, a parent component, and an environmental change component involving changes in school meals, food policies, and school food and information environment. The logic model within the case study program shows these three components and the products we will produce for each component as we design the intervention:

- The classroom curriculum component consists of 10 sessions: an introductory lesson, two on each of the behavioral goals, and a concluding lesson.

- The family component consists of two group sessions, one on fruits and vegetables and one on sweetened beverages, plus two newsletters, one on packaged, processed, high-calorie snacks and one on physical activity.
- The environmental support component consists of changes in school meals, schoolwide food policy, social support, and school information environment.

■ YOUR TURN: COMPLETING THE STEP 3 WORKSHEETS

Review the information on mediators that you obtained in Step 2. You and/or your planning team should now select the theory you will use to design the nutrition education intervention and create the specific intervention model. Now is also the time to clarify the philosophical perspective of the program in terms of educational approach and food and nutrition content. You should also determine the number of components and which channels or venues you will use.

At this point, you do not need to plan the details of activities for these various venues and channels. That will come in the next few chapters. Here, you need only decide which components and channels you will incorporate so that you can write goals and objectives and design appropriate activities for each of these components.

Questions and Activities

1. Describe at least three criteria that nutrition educators can use to select which theory to use for a given nutrition education program or session. Show how you would use these to select a theory for your program.

2. What are the advantages and disadvantages of using integrated or polytheoretical models for intervention purposes? Under what circumstances can you see yourself using the integrative model from the Institute of Medicine or the health action process approach model?

3. How is theory translated into educational practice according to the integrative framework for translating theory into effective nutrition education practice?

4. List, and briefly describe, three theory constructs in common to several theories that are useful in interventions that focus on increasing awareness and enhancing motivation. How might these constructs be used in developing your intervention model?

5. List, and briefly describe, three constructs in common to theories that are useful in interventions that focus on facilitating the ability to take action. How might these constructs be used in developing your intervention model?

6. Compare, contrast, and critique the medical, moral, enlightenment, compensatory, and joint decision-making models for helping people, indicating when and how each of them might be used in nutrition education, or even if they should be used.

7. Think carefully through your program for your intended audience: which philosophical model of helping will guide your approach?

8. What factors should you consider as you select components for your program?

References

Abraham, C., and P. Sheeran. Understanding and changing health behavior: From health beliefs to self-regulation. In *Understanding and changing health behavior: From health beliefs to self-regulation*, edited by P. Norman, C. Abraham, and M. Conner. Amsterdam: Harwood Academic Publishers.

Achterberg, C., and L. L. Trenkner. 1990. Developing a working philosophy of nutrition education. *Journal of Nutrition Education* 22:189–193.

Bagozzi, R. P., and E. A. Edwards. 1999. Goal striving and the implementation of goal intentions in the regulation of body weight. *Psychology and Health* 13:593–621.

Bandura, A. 1997. *Self-efficacy: The exercise of control.* New York: WH Freeman.

———. 2001. Social cognitive theory: An agentic perspective. *Annual Review of Psychology* 51:1–26.

———. 2004. Health promotion by social cognitive means. *Health Education and Behavior* 31 (2):143–164.

Brickman, P., V. C. Rabinowitz, J. Karuza, D. Coates, E. Cohn, and L. Kidder. 1982. Models of helping and coping. *American Psychologist* 37:368–385.

Buchanan, D. 2004. Two models for defining the relationship between theory and practice in nutrition education: Is the scientific method meeting our needs? *Journal of Nutrition Education and Behavior* 36:146–154.

Charles, C., A. Gafni, and T. Whelan. 1999. Decision-making in the physician–patient encounter: Revisiting the shared treatment decision-making model. *Social Science & Medicine* 49:656–661.

Connell D. B., R. R. Turner, and F. F. Mason. 1985. Summary of findings of the school health education evaluation: Health promotion effectiveness, implementation, and costs. *Journal of School Health* 55(8):316–321.

Deci, E. L., and R. M. Ryan. 2000. The "what" and "why" of goal pursuits: Human needs and the self-determination of behavior. *Psychological Inquiry* 11(4):227–268.

———. 2008. Facilitating optimal motivation and psychological well-being across life's domains. *Canadian Psychology* 49:14–23.

Fishbein, M. 2000. The role of theory in HIV prevention. *AIDS Care* 12(3):273–278.

Gollwitzer, P. M. 1999. Implementation intentions—strong effects of simple plans. *American Psychologist* 54:493–503.

Institute of Medicine. 2002. *Speaking of health: Assessing health communication strategies for diverse populations.* Washington, DC: National Academies Press.

International Organization of Consumers Unions. 1990. Code of good practice. In *IOCU code of good practice and guidelines for business sponsored educational materials used in schools.* Policy statement. London: Author.

Kok, G., H. Schaalma, H. De Vries, G. Parcel, and T. Paulussen. 1996. Social psychology and health. *European Review of Social Psychology* 7:241–282.

Kolbe, L. J., D. C. Iverson, W. K. Marshal, G. Hochbaum, and G. Christensen. 1981. Propositions for an alternate and complementary health education paradigm. *Health Education* 12(3):24–30.

Mayer, J. 1986. Social responsibilities of nutritionists. *Journal of Nutrition* 116:714–717.

Parham, E. 1990. Applying a philosophy of nutrition education to weight control. *Journal of Nutrition Education* 22:194–197.

Prochaska, J. O., and W. F. Velicer. 1997. The transtheoretical model of health behavior change. *American Journal of Health Promotion* 12:38–48.

Roter, D. L. 1987. An exploration of health education's responsibility for a partnership model of client–provider relations. *Patient Education and Counseling* 9:25–31.

Schwarzer, R. 1992. Self-efficacy in the adoption and maintenance of health behaviors: Theoretical approaches and a new model. In *Self-efficacy: Thought control of action*, edited by R. Schwarzer. London: Hemisphere.

Sniehotta, F. F., U. R. Scholz, and R. Schwarzer. 2005. Bridging the intention-behavior gap: Planning, self-efficacy, and action control in the adoption and maintenance of physical exercise. *Psychology and Health* 20:143–160.

In Step 3, you lay out the theoretical and philosophical basis for your nutrition education program. Additionally, you identify the components that will make up your program.

At the end of the Step 3 worksheets, you should have the following products:

Step 3A: Program theoretical model

Step 3B: Statement of personal philosophy of nutrition education

Step 3C: Statement of personal perspective on nutrition content and issues

Step 3D: List of program components

Use the provided worksheets as a guide to help you select your theory model and describe your program's philosophy. Electronic versions of these worksheets are available at http://nutrition.jbpub.com/education/2e/. If you are unable to access the worksheets electronically, you can write onto this blank worksheet or create a text document that uses the same flow of information.

Step 3A: Theoretical model for program

State the theoretical model you will be using for your program. Then draw a diagram of the model you selected, including the mediators you will address and how they relate to one another and your target behavior. Use the data you included in Steps 2C and 2D to guide your theory model selection.

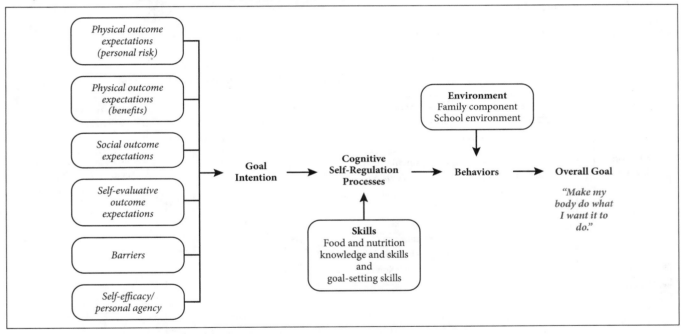

Step 3B: Philosophy of nutrition education

Describe your philosophy of nutrition education.

This program believes that youth have responsibilities for their health and the power to make healthful food and activity choices, but that they need the necessary understanding, motivation, and tools to take charge in today's difficult environment. The program also believes that it is the responsibility of the school and home to provide an environment that is supportive and makes healthful options available. The philosophy is that regardless of how the teens acquired their eating patterns, they need motivation to act and a sense of agency. It also recognizes that individuals need skills and environmental support, thus suggesting a compensatory model.

The program's aim is to assist youths to increase awareness of their own behaviors and of environmental forces influencing their choices and to enhance their ability to make healthful food choices and overcome environmental barriers. Activities will provide them with tools to take charge of their own eating and activity patterns through goal-setting and self-regulation processes. The aim will be carried out through a program directed at personal mediators that includes two phases: a phase that encourages analysis of self and environment, understanding, deliberation, and motivation and a phase that focuses on skills to take action. The program will also include an environmental component to provide support and increase options for the behaviors identified.

Step 3C: Perspectives on nutrition content and issues

Provide your perspective on nutrition content and issues relevant to your program goals.

It also is the position of this program to encourage youth to eat foods that are minimally processed, naturally nutrient dense, and fresh and local to the extent feasible given resource and availability constraints. Also, the issue of weight will not be addressed directly; instead, healthful eating and activity patterns will be emphasized.

Step 3D: Program components

List and/or diagram the components that will make up your program.

The program will consist of three components:
- A classroom curriculum component
- A parent component
- Changes in the school environment to increase options for healthful eating

LOGIC MODEL FRAMEWORK FOR COMPONENTS OF CASE STUDY

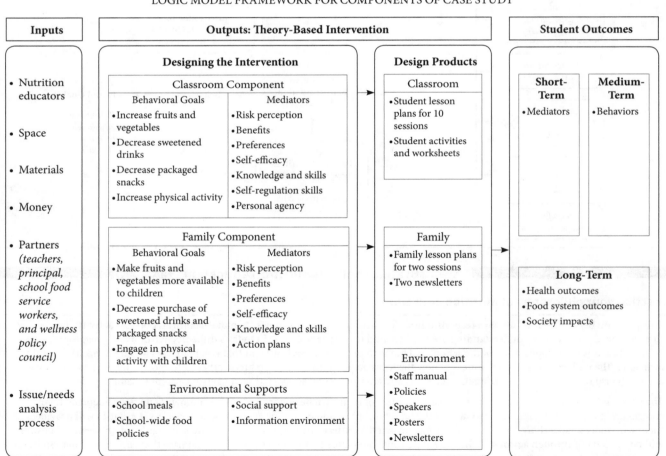

In Step 3, you lay out the theoretical and philosophical basis for your nutrition education program. Additionally, you identify the components that will make up your program.

At the end of the Step 3 worksheets, you should have the following products:

Step 3A: Program theoretical model

Step 3B: Statement of personal philosophy of nutrition education

Step 3C: Statement of personal perspective on nutrition content and issues

Step 3D: List of program components

Use the provided worksheets as a guide to help you select your theory model and describe your program's philosophy. Electronic versions of these worksheets are available at http://nutrition.jbpub.com/education/2e/. If you are unable to access the worksheets electronically, you can write onto this blank worksheet or create a text document that uses the same flow of information.

Step 3A: Theoretical model for program

State the theoretical model you will be using for your program. Then draw a diagram of the model you selected, including the mediators you will address and how they relate to one another and your target behavior. Use the data you included in Steps 2C and 2D to guide your theory model selection.

Step 3B: Philosophy of nutrition education

Describe your philosophy of nutrition education.

Step 3C: Perspectives on nutrition content and issues

Provide your perspective on nutrition content and issues relevant to your program goals.

Step 3D: Program components

List and/or diagram the components that will make up your program.

CHAPTER

10

Step 4: Translating Behavioral Theory into Educational and Support Objectives

OVERVIEW

This chapter describes key issues in translating behavioral theory into educational objectives and environmental support objectives and provides guidance on how to do so.

CHAPTER OUTLINE

- Introduction
- Determining nutrition education program objectives to achieve targeted actions or behaviors
- Writing educational objectives for educational sessions to address potential personal mediators of behaviors
- Writing environmental support objectives for the targeted behaviors
- Case study
- Your turn: completing the Step 4 worksheets

LEARNING OBJECTIVES

At the end of the chapter, you will be able to:

- Appreciate the importance of writing objectives for nutrition education sessions and programs
- Describe how to translate behavioral theory into educational objectives
- Write nutrition education program educational objectives to achieve the behavioral goals of the session or program
- Write general and specific educational objectives to guide specific learning experiences or activities within each session or component
- Write support objectives to guide activities to promote a supportive environment for action

■ INTRODUCTION: TRANSLATING BEHAVIORAL THEORY INTO NUTRITION EDUCATION PRACTICE

You have spent some time getting to know your audience: the food and health issues they face, the food and activity behaviors and practices they could take that would help to address these health issues, and their potential motivations for making these changes and the skills they need. That is a first step. The question is now: how exactly shall you structure the educational sessions or program to assist the intended audience to achieve the changes they want? Here, focusing on what you wish to accomplish and articulating your objectives are crucial. **Figure 10-1** shows where we are in the design process.

Consider the following scenario. A middle school has invited a nutrition educator to speak at a school assembly of several health classes (about 100 students) about "the importance of good nutrition." The nutrition educator designs a 45-minute presentation that consists of

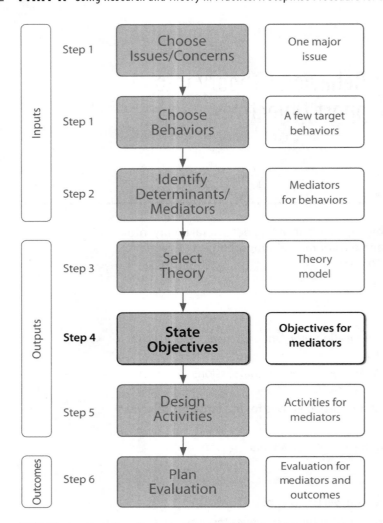

FIGURE 10-1 Flowchart of steps in designing theory-based nutrition education: Step 4.

computer slides. Starting with a description of what teens typically eat, she discusses the components of a healthy diet, covering the major recommendations of the government's guidelines, and then talks about the importance of eating more fruits and vegetables and how to add them to the diet; of eating fewer high-energy-dense, high-fat, high-sugar foods; the importance of regular meals during the day and of selecting healthy snacks and portion sizes; and the importance of being physically active and how to be more active.

She begins to notice that the teens are getting restless. When she ends, one teen approaches, very worried, and says, "This isn't going to be on the final exam, is it? That was a lot of information and I couldn't write it all down." Another says, "I got rather confused and couldn't follow everything you said, so I'm not sure what I should be eating."

Later she tells a colleague about her experience. Her colleague asks her, "What was the overall educational objective of your talk? What did you hope to accomplish?" The nutrition educator is rather surprised. "I didn't have a specific objective," she says. "This was the only time they were going to hear about nutrition in their health class this year, so I just wanted to make sure they got lots of information so that

they could make wise choices." What is going on here? The nutrition educator did not clearly think through the goal for the session or the specific educational objectives. She rambled on, providing a good deal of interesting information but no clear, identifiable message. So, it is not surprising that the teens would leave with no clear understanding of what to do to eat well. A clear behavioral goal and several specific educational objectives would have helped to focus the presentation and enhance the ability of the youth to make healthy choices. Sometimes less is more—when it is well focused.

Even in situations where you think objectives are not needed, such as in facilitated group dialogues or discussions where the sessions are conducted in a flexible way so as to allow you to follow group interests to some degree, objectives and educational plans are still important for providing a map for how to proceed. Without a clear plan, discussions can ramble, and no clear message comes through. Participants often leave such sessions frustrated.

In Step 4, you convert behavioral theory into a format that is needed to guide the design of the program: specifying objectives. These include general *nutrition education program objectives* to guide the entire program and *educational and support objectives* directed at the mediators of behavior that are part of your theory model to achieve the program's targeted behavioral goals. You will go back and forth between this step and the next because in the next step you select educational strategies and design practical learning experiences that address these mediators of behavior change. The tasks and products for Step 4 are highlighted in the logic model graphic in **Figure 10-2**.

Converting Theory into Program, Educational, and Support Objectives

Many different terms are used with somewhat similar meanings: goals, objectives, performance objectives, performance indicators, behavioral objectives, educational standards, nutrition competencies, and so forth. Nutrition educators need not be rigid about which terms to use. This text uses the term *goals* to refer *only* to the *behavioral* goals for the program that you established in Step 1. *Objectives* have the below meanings in this text.

Nutrition Education Program Objectives

Nutrition education program objectives are general statements of how to achieve the behavioral goals of the nutrition education program. Such focusing is necessary whether for a program of several months' duration involving many components or for one or two sessions.

Educational Objectives

Educational objectives provide a road map on how to proceed. They describe how to address the behavioral goals through educational means. These are written for each individual educational session.

Educational objectives are based on theory variables. Educational objectives in the context of nutrition education are ways to convert and operationalize mediators of health behavior change into educational strategies. They are stated in learner terms. That is, in terms of what the learner gets out of the intervention or what the learner can think, feel, or be able to do as a result of the educational experience.

- *General educational objectives* provide overall guidance for the development of activities of a given session or a series of sessions on the same issue or behavior.
- *Specific educational objectives* guide the development of each of the activities within a given session.

Inputs: Collecting Assessment Data			Outputs: Designing the Theory-Based Intervention		Outcomes: Evaluation Plan
Step 1 ⟵⟶ **Analyze issues and audiences to state program behavioral goals**	**Step 2** ⟵⟶ **Identify potential mediators to achieve program behavioral goals**	**Step 3** ⟵⟶ **Select theory, philosophy, and components**	**Step 4** ⟵⟶ **State objectives for mediators**	**Step 5** ⟵⟶ **Design theory-based strategies and activities for mediators**	**Step 6** **Plan evaluation**
Tasks • Analyze issues and select audience • Identify behaviors or patterns contributing to issue • Specify behavioral or action goals of the program	*Tasks* • Identify personal psychosocial mediators • Identify environmental support mediators	*Tasks* • Select theory or create appropriate model • Clarify philosophy (education and content) • Determine program components	*Tasks* • State educational objectives for psychosocial mediators • State change objectives for environmental support mediators	*Tasks* • Design activities to address psychosocial mediators • Design activities to address environmental support mediators • Implementation plan	*Tasks* • Design outcome evaluation plan • Determine tools to measure impact • Plan process evaluation
Product • *Description of issue of concern* • *Statement of action or behavioral goals for program*	*Product* • *List of potential mediators for action or behavior goals*	*Product* • *Theory/model for program, philosophy, and components*	*Product* • *Objectives for each mediator*	*Product* • *Educational plans for sessions linking mediators, objectives, and strategies* • *Environmental support plans*	*Product* • *Evaluation plan* • *List of indicators and measures for outcomes* • *Procedures and measures for process evaluation*

FIGURE 10-2 Stepwise Procedure for designing theory-based nutrition education: Step 4.

Environmental Support Objectives

Environmental support objectives are those actions that the program takes, often in collaboration with other partners, to promote supportive environmental changes and policies that will increase the opportunities for participants to take action.

- *General support objectives* provide overall guidance for the development of activities for a given environmental or policy component.
- *Specific support objectives* guide the development of each of the activities within a given component.

Note: This chapter describes how to write all of these objectives. However, in this chapter's worksheets on Step 4, you determine only the objectives that will guide the entire nutrition education program. In the next three chapters, you write the general and specific educational and support objectives at the same time as you create your activities and develop your educational plan (or lesson plan) and your environmental and policy support plan.

■ DETERMINING NUTRITION EDUCATION PROGRAM OBJECTIVES TO ACHIEVE TARGETED ACTIONS OR BEHAVIORS

To achieve the behavioral goals of the program, write nutrition education program objectives that guide the creation of your *educational* activities within and among program components. Think about environmental support objectives, where feasible, to support the educational objectives to achieve the program outcomes.

To illustrate, consider the case study of middle school teens presented in these chapters, where there are several *behavioral goals* or *desired behavioral outcomes*:

- Youth will increase their intake of fruits and vegetables.
- Youth will decrease the amount of sweetened beverages they consume each day.
- Youth will decrease the number of packaged, processed, high-calorie snacks they consume each day.
- Youth will increase their walking to 10,000 steps a day and participate actively, when possible, in gym or other school-sponsored physical activities.

The *nutrition education program objectives across all the components* to achieve the behavioral outcomes of this case study could be that the program will do the following:

- Increase awareness in youth of the importance of food and activity choices to improve energy balance and enhance motivation to make healthy choices through a school curriculum and school-wide activities
- Facilitate the ability to act by providing opportunities to gain relevant food and nutrition knowledge and practice food-related skills and self-regulation skills through a school curriculum
- Increase opportunities for youth to engage in healthful eating at school and home through an educational component with parents and environmental and policy initiatives in the school

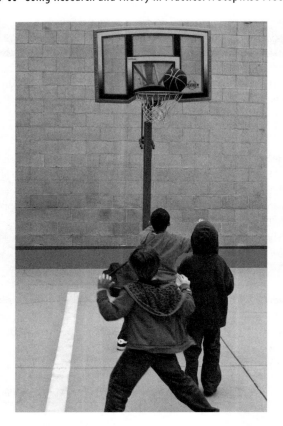

School-sponsored physical activity, such as an informal basketball game, is a fun way for students to meet their exercise requirements.

General and specific educational and environmental support objectives are then written to achieve these general educational program objectives. See the case study at the end of the chapter.

■ WRITING EDUCATIONAL OBJECTIVES FOR EDUCATIONAL SESSIONS TO ADDRESS POTENTIAL PERSONAL MEDIATORS OF BEHAVIORS

Program components, such as educational sessions, that are directed at personal psychosocial mediators of the target behaviors focus on addressing personal motivational mediators and decision-making processes in pre-action phase activities, and on cognitive self-regulation or self-influence skills for action and maintenance phase education. Personal mediators are those that rest within the individual and have the potential of being influenced by educational or learning experiences. These potential mediators include perceived risk, attitudes, affect/feelings, perceived benefits and barriers, outcome expectations, values, perceived responsibility, self-identify, self-efficacy, social norms, and goal-setting skills.

The mediators that you will address in your program are those that are part of the model that you created in Step 3 to guide your program based on theory and evidence. Select those mediators that can be realistically addressed in the sessions or program to enhance motivation or increase behavioral skills, or both, given the time and resources you have available. Most nutrition educators have the tendency to try to cover too much.

Considerations in Writing Educational Objectives

For each personal mediator of behavior change in your theory, write one or more educational objectives to guide the design of educational activities to address that mediator. These objectives provide ways to convert mediators to a form that is useful for guiding the design of learning activities.

Learning Objectives and Educational Objectives: A Clarification of Terms

The objectives are expressed in terms of the learner or participant and are thus often called *learning objectives*. This term is often used interchangeably with *educational objectives* because learning is what the participant does, and educating is what you do to encourage learning. Both terms refer to the same activity with the same desired outcomes. Both terms are used in this text, but *educational objectives* is favored to remind you of what you must do as a nutrition educator to facilitate learning.

Objectives Are About Ends, Not Means

Objectives are used to describe ends intended by the program, not the means to get there. They state what the program or individual will have achieved at the end of the program. They should *not* be a statement of what the *nutrition educator* will do, such as "demonstrate a food preparation technique" or "show a film," or even what the intended audience member will do, such as "discuss" or "make a salad." Instead, learning objectives are statements of what the *participant* needs to know, feel, or be able to do differently in terms of the specific mediators of behavior in order to achieve the behavioral goals.

Educational/Learning Objectives Use Concrete Verbs

Learning objectives state exactly what the learner will be able to do; are measurable; and are related to achievement in terms of a particular personal mediator of action or behavior change, such as self-efficacy, perceived benefits, perceived behavior control, goal setting, and so forth. Specific educational objectives have the following form: "At the end of the session/program, participants will be able to . . ." followed by a verb such as *describe, state, identify, translate, judge*, and so forth.

General Educational Objectives

Based on the theory you have chosen, identify the three to six major mediators that you think you have time to cover and that evidence suggests will contribute to increasing the group's motivation and ability to enact the goal behaviors. Write general educational objectives directed at these mediators.

Case Study Example

Here is an example of general educational objectives from the case study, where the behavioral goal is that youth will increase their consumption of fruits and vegetables. These objectives will guide educational activities across two sessions.

Potential Mediators	General Educational Objectives *At the end of the sessions, youth will be able to:*
Outcome expectations	Demonstrate understanding and appreciation of the importance of eating a variety of fruits and vegetables (F&V)
Perceived threat	Evaluate their own intake of F&V compared to recommendations

Potential Mediators	General Educational Objectives *At the end of the sessions, youth will be able to:*
Self-efficacy	Demonstrate increased self-efficacy in eating a variety of F&V each day
Behavioral capability	Demonstrate increased knowledge and skills in incorporating F&V into their daily food patterns
Goal setting	Prepare action plans using goal-setting and decision-making skills to increase their consumption of F&V

Specific Educational Objectives

You then write *specific* learning objectives that will guide the development of *specific* educational activities to achieve the general educational objectives. These specific learning objectives guide the design of *each* of the specific educational activities or learning experiences within individual sessions or program components as identified by the general educational objectives. There will be many of these, depending on the length of each session and the extensiveness of the program component.

Case Study Example

Specific educational objectives in the case study are written to guide the learning experiences within each session. They are linked to the mediators that are part of the theory selected and the information obtained in Step 2. See the case study for details. They take the following format:

Potential Personal Mediators of Behavior from Theory	Potential Mediators of Change: Findings from Step 2	Specific Learning Objectives for Each Personal Mediator
	Audiences' thoughts and feelings for each mediator (from Step 2)	At the end of the session, participants will be able to:
Outcome expectations (perceived benefits)	Students will eat F&V if they taste good, make them look good, help them build strong bones	State specific health and personal benefits for eating F&V

Objectives in Practice

In practice, you will probably go back and forth between general and specific objectives, and between objectives and educational activities. As you come up with exciting and relevant activities, you should think carefully about their purpose (specific objectives) in achieving the behavioral goals of the program and how they relate to the general educational objectives. If they do not serve any of the identified larger purposes, you should drop the activities, no matter how exciting. However, at this point you may want to rethink your general objectives. Perhaps they need to be changed to accommodate the specific objectives and activities because you consider them important to achieving the behavioral goal.

Writing Educational Objectives for Head, Heart, and Hand

People are more likely to take action or make changes in their lives if they participate in activities that engage their heads, hearts, and hands. Thus, the effectiveness of nutrition education is improved if nutrition

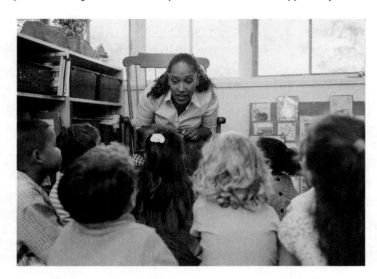

In classroom settings, school- and teacher-provided resources will shape what types of programs nutrition educators can design.

educators design learning experiences that fully engage participants by providing opportunities for thinking (head), feeling (hearts), and doing (hands).

Indeed, educators categorize "learning" tasks, and hence educational objectives, as falling into these three areas of the human experience, calling them the cognitive, affective, and psychomotor domains (Bloom et al. 1956; Marzano & Kendall 2007; Gronland & Brookhart 2008):

- *Cognitive domain* objectives aim to promote abilities in thought, understanding, and cognitive skills.
- *Affective domain* objectives aim to promote changes in attitude, feeling, or emotion.
- *Psychomotor domain* objectives aim to promote improvement in physical or manipulative skills.

Thus, you should check that your objectives address all three domains of learning.

Writing Educational Objectives That Reflect Desired Levels of Attainment of Skills

Within each domain, learning tasks are considered to range in a graded sequence from simple to complex. Nutrition educators should ensure that their objectives are set at the appropriate level of complexity for any given task and, as important, that any given session or program includes objectives for more complex understandings and attitudes, as well as the simple ones.

Table 10-1, Table 10-2, and **Table 10-3** provide detailed outlines of the learning tasks in the cognitive, affective, and psychomotor domains and a list of verbs that you can use as you write educational objectives in each of these domains.

Cognitive (Knowing or Thinking) Domain

Human beings are thinking beings. Just about everything people do involves them thinking about it and interpreting it in some way. Educational objectives can range from simple recall of facts to highly original and creative ways of combining and synthesizing new ideas. Bloom

TABLE 10-1   Cognitive Domain: Levels of Thinking

Levels of Thinking (Levels of Complexity of Learning Tasks)	Description	Useful Verbs
Knowledge	Recalling information as it is learned	List, recall, name, define, state, label, tell, record
Comprehension	Reporting information in a way other than how it was learned to show understanding	Describe, recognize, explain, discuss, identify, report, review, locate, translate
Application	Applying learned information to a new context	Apply, demonstrate, use, interpret, illustrate, modify, operate, predict, dramatize, sketch
Analysis	Taking learned information apart into components so that its organizational structure may be understood	Analyze, calculate, test, compare, contrast, criticize, diagram, distinguish, differentiate, appraise, debate, relate, examine, inspect, categorize
Synthesis	Putting together parts and elements into a unified organization or whole, with emphasis on creating new meaning or structure	Compose, create, plan, propose, design, formulate, arrange, construct, organize, manage, prepare, relate
Evaluation	Making judgments about the value of something using appropriate criteria	Evaluate, rate, compare, value, revise, judge, select, measure, estimate, conclude, justify, criticize

Sources: Adapted from Bloom, B. S. 1956. *Taxonomy of educational objectives. Handbook I: Cognitive domain.* New York: David McKay; and Cruikshank, K. A. 2000. *Taxonomy for learning, teaching, and assessing: A revision of Bloom's taxonomy of educational objectives.* Boston: Allyn & Bacon.

TABLE 10-2   The Affective Domain: Levels of Affective Engagement

Levels of Engagement and Integration	Description: Stages Within Level	Useful Verbs
Receiving: Paying attention	1. Awareness with no position taken 2. Willingness to receive or attend to information 3. Will not avoid stimulus	Answers, chooses, describes, follows, locates, names, points to, selects
Responding: Active participation	1. Complying with expectations of educator 2. Stating or defending own position 3. Beginning of own emotional response with satisfaction (Opinions/position formation)	Answers, assists, aids, helps, complies, conforms, discusses, labels, tells, reads, performs, reports, writes, recites, selects
Valuing: Behavior based on positive regard for something	1. Tentative acceptance with readiness to reevaluate 2. Conviction 3. Commitment to the behavior or action; beginning to internalize own viewpoint (No longer motivated primarily by value to comply with others; beginning to internalize own viewpoint)	Completes, demonstrates, explains, initiates, joins, proposes, reports, shares, studies, works
Organization: Behaving according to a set of principles	1. Conceptualizing one's important values and understanding that they may be different from those of others 2. Building an internally consistent value system for guiding behavior by resolving conflicts and creating a unique value system (Developing one's own values or policies to guide action)	Adheres, alters, arranges, combines, defends, explains, generalizes, integrates modifies, orders, organizes, relates, synthesizes
Internalizing values: Behaving according to a consistent worldview	1. Integration of value into one's consistent, total worldview that guides behavior 2. Person's behavior is consistent, predictable, and characterized by the values (Person has developed a consistent and recognizable way of life guided by a set of values)	Acts, discriminates, displays, influences, modifies, performs, practices, proposes, qualifies, questions, revises, solves, verifies

Sources: Adapted from Krathwohl, D. R., B. S. Bloom, and B. B. Masia. 1964. *Taxonomy of educational objectives. Handbook II: Affective domain.* New York: Longman; and Gronland, N. E., and S. M. Brookhart. 2008. *Gronland's writing instructional objectives* (8th ed.). Upper Saddle River, NJ: Prentice Hall.

TABLE 10-3	Psychomotor Domain: Levels of Psychomotor Skills	
Levels of Performance and Skill	**Description**	**Verbs to Use**
Observing	Observes skilled performance	Observes, watches
Imitating	Follows instructions under supervision	Imitates, mimics
Practicing	Completes entire sequence repeatedly till routine	Practices, carries out
Adopting	Adapts or modifies to improve outcome further	Adapts, modifies, revises

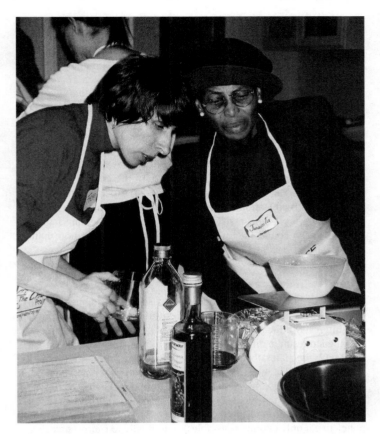

Cookbooks, friends, family, and community centers can all be used as sources for finding and learning new recipes.

and colleagues (1956) developed a taxonomy or classification system of cognitive domain objectives commonly used in education. It describes six levels of understandings that an educational experience or strategy can aim for developing in learners, beginning with *knowledge* and then moving through *comprehension* to the ability to *apply* information to new decision-making situations and the ability to *analyze* and *synthesize* information, and finally ending with *evaluation*, or wisdom regarding taking action on food and nutrition matters. Table 10-1 describes these levels.

The Cognitive Domain and Nutrition Education

In terms of theory-based nutrition education, every mediator you select for your sessions can be addressed with any of these levels of understanding, as you wish. Do you want the group participants to know something or understand something? Do you want them to be able to apply the information or to analyze it? Do you want them to be able to evaluate the information? Depending on the findings of the needs analysis in Step 2 with respect to the difficulty of the behavior change and the motivations and skills of the target group, you may seek to bring about measurable changes in understanding at different levels of difficulty or complexity: You also may set the objectives at ever higher levels, going from the simple to the more complex, during a session or over several sessions.

1. *Knowledge: Recalling information very much as it was learned.* At the lowest level of learning, this involves recall and memory. When you set objectives at this level, it means that you will design learning activities that will result in group participants being able to remember or recall specific pieces of information, terminology, and facts such as which foods are in which food groups or which foods are sources of which nutrients.

2. *Comprehension: Reporting the information in a way other than how it was learned to show that is has been understood.* This level represents the beginnings of understanding. It means that individuals are able to make sense of the information and to paraphrase it in their own words. The individuals may even be able to extrapolate the information to new but related ideas and implications, making simple inferences. For example, when you set educational objectives at this level, you are aiming for group participants to be able to understand general disease risk information and apply it to themselves, or to understand the benefits of eating fruits and vegetables.

3. *Application: Use of learned information in new and concrete situations or to solve a problem.* At this level of learning, individuals are able to carry over information, principles, concepts, or theories learned in one context to a completely new one. When you set objectives for the session at this level, you are aiming for group participants, after learning how to set goals to increase their consumption of fruits and vegetables, to be able to apply goal-setting principles to a new behavior, such as eating more foods high in calcium.

4. *Analysis: Taking information apart so that its organizational structure can be understood.* This level involves breaking information into its components to identify the elements, the interactions between them, and the organizing principles or structures. It also involves distinguishing fact from opinion, and relevant from extraneous issues or events. For example, when you set educational objectives at this level you may be aiming for group participants to be able to compare and contrast the impacts of low-fat and low-carbohydrate diets on weight and health, or to debate the pros and cons of breastfeeding versus bottle-feeding.

5. *Synthesis: Putting information together in a unique or novel way.* At this level, individuals are able to reassemble information and experiences into a unified framework to create new meaning or to

think about the situation in a new way. When you set objectives at this level, you are expecting the intended audience to be able to use what they are learning and experiencing in the program in a new way to affect their food practices and eating experiences.

6. *Evaluation: Judging the value of something for a particular purpose.* Here individuals are able to make judgments about the worth of information and experiences based on well-accepted external criteria (such as relevance to stated purposes) or on internal criteria (organization and meaning). These criteria may be given to, or created by, individuals themselves. Objectives at this level include elements of all the previous levels, as well as conscious value judgments based on the criteria. Setting the objectives at this level means that you are expecting the intended nutrition education audience to be able to evaluate the merits of different ways to assist children to learn good eating habits or to reach sound judgment regarding food and nutrition matters based on evidence.

Affective (Feelings) Domain

Humans are not only thinking beings but also feeling beings. The affective domain is associated with feelings, attitudes, values, appreciation, and interests. Educational strategies in the affective domain may be designed to result in different levels of the participants' affective engagement with the material and commitment to taking action regarding food and nutrition. The levels begin, at the lowest level, with awareness or willingness to *receive or attend to* a message, and move through *responding* to it, *valuing* the message to the point of commitment to it, *organizing* their life around the message (e.g., developing a personal food policy to eat only organic vegetables), and finally to *characterization* of themselves by their commitment to the value system (e.g., becoming known to be a vegetarian). Table 10-2 describes these levels.

The Affective Domain in Nutrition Education

For nutrition education to be effective, the intended audience must not only understand the message or information but also value it, feel it, believe it to be relevant, and feel it important to them. The affective domain objectives focus on a process of affective engagement and internalization. It categorizes into levels the inner growth that occurs as individuals become aware of, and later adopt, the attitudes and principles that assist in forming value judgments that guide their actions. Krathwohl, Bloom, and Masia (1964) identified five levels.

In terms of theory-based nutrition education, every mediator you select for your sessions can be addressed at any of these levels of engagement, as you choose. As you design your sessions, think about the level of affective engagement you wish for your audience. For example, do you want the group to just *receive* your message or do you want the group to be actively engaged and to *value* it? Do you want them to value the message enough to *make a commitment*? A general strategy is for the session (or several sessions) to provide opportunities for the group to move from lesser degrees of affective engagement and commitment to greater degrees of commitment. Therefore, the objectives will be set at ever-higher levels, during a session or over several sessions, in the classification scheme described here.

1. *Receiving: Paying attention.* At this level, the participants are willing to listen to the nutrition educator or other forms of communication and become aware of the ideas communicated. From a purely passive role, they may advance to willingness to attend to the communication despite distractions or competing stimuli.

When you set objectives at this level, it means that you expect participants to be willing to listen to a message, such as the importance of eating fruits and vegetables, but that is about all.

2. *Responding: Active participation.* This level involves willingness to participate in something, although not necessarily with enthusiasm at first. From obedient participation (perhaps a health professional has insisted that participants attend these nutrition education sessions), individuals may advance to voluntary response and, indeed, to a pleasurable feeling or satisfaction in participation.

If you set educational objectives at this level, it means that you expect that individuals will move from being onlookers during group nutrition education activities toward participating in these activities and finding that they enjoy them. Or objectives may be set even higher, expecting individuals to move from complying with the expectations of the educator, to starting to develop their own positions and taking responsibility for themselves. Objectives at this level take the form of aiming for changes in attitudes, motivations, and self-efficacy.

3. *Valuing: Consistent behavior reflecting positive regard for something.* At this level, the issue or behavior is considered to have worth. This sense of worth ranges from acceptance of the value to a deep enough commitment to the value that it is reflected in observable behavior. Behavior reflects a belief or an attitude. Thus, this level is characterized by motivated behavior in which individuals' commitments guide their behaviors. This is the level that is most appropriate for nutrition education.

When you set objectives at this level, it means that you aim for the learning activities that you design to increase participants' value for the targeted behavioral goal or issue so much that they are willing to take action. At the lower end, this may mean tentative behavior in keeping with advice from others, with readiness to reevaluate. At the upper end, individuals develop conviction about the behavior or issue, resulting in commitment. They have less need to be motivated by the need to comply with others and have begun to internalize their own viewpoints and values as a basis of action. For example, stating your educational objective at this level means that you intend for individuals to move from ambivalence, to deciding to eat more fruits and vegetables each day, and then to actually doing so.

4. *Organization: Behaving according to a set of principles.* Here individuals have established a conscious basis for making choices. They understand that there are other values beside their own. Objectives at the organization level are concerned with assisting individuals to bring together different values, resolve conflicts among them, and begin to build an internally consistent value system—a set of criteria—for guiding behavior. Individuals are aware of the basis of their own attitudes and values and are able to defend them. They begin to develop their own personal food policies.

If you set educational objectives at this level, it means that you intend for your learning experiences or activities to lead individuals now to use health, or ecological concerns, social justice issues, or personal, social, or cultural values, as a *consistent* criterion for making choices about food- and nutrition-related issues. They may develop personal food (and activity) policies to guide their choices.

5. *Internalizing values: Behaving according to a consistent worldview.* At this level, values are integrated into some kind of internally

consistent worldview so that the person is recognized by these values. The individual has developed a characteristic lifestyle.

If you set objectives at this level, it means that you expect that the educational activities or learning experiences you design will lead participants to a change in worldview and a lifestyle consistent with that worldview. For example, you expect that as a result of your educational activities, the individual will practice a new way of eating so consistently that he or she becomes known as a vegetarian, as an ecologically conscious, or "green," consumer, or as a health-conscious parent.

Note on "Behaviors" in the Context of Educational Objectives

As you can see, individuals achieving objectives set at the valuing level of the affective domain begin to demonstrate observable behaviors that reflect these values. Thus, educational objectives to achieve food- and nutrition-related *behavioral* goals will normally be set at the valuing level of the affective taxonomy.

Long-term or more intense nutrition education may be able to assist individuals to understand and internalize their values to the extent of establishing a conscious and ongoing basis for making choices, such as developing their own personal food policies. There is often miscommunication between nutritionists and educators regarding terminology, which you need to be aware of. Educators often refer to all objectives as "behavioral objectives." When nutritionists talk about objectives to facilitate behavior change, educators talk about educational (or "behavioral") objectives in the affective domain at the valuing level or above. This chapter keeps these two sets of terminology separate. Thus, according to our scheme, program behavioral goals are achieved through educational objectives set at the valuing level or above.

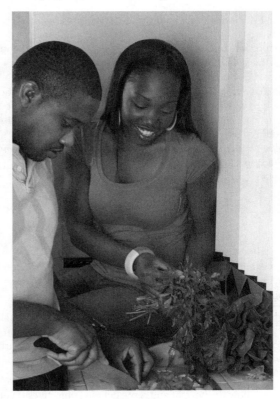

Healthy cooking habits can be formed at any age.

Psychomotor Domain

The emphasis in the psychomotor domain is on the development of psychomotor skills, even though some degree of understanding and varying degrees of emotion may also be involved. This domain involves a graded sequence from simple to complex. At the lowest level, participants *observe* a more experienced person perform the activity (e.g., preparing a recipe), and then are able to *imitate* it, and then *practice* it so that conscious effort is no longer necessary and it has become somewhat habitual in nature; finally, the individuals may be able to *adapt* the activity:

1. *Observing.* When objectives are set at this level, individuals observe a more experienced person performing the skill. Sometimes, the reading of directions, as in a recipe, can substitute for this experience. However, usually reading is supplemented with direct observation, such as watching someone preparing a salad or recipe.
2. *Imitating.* When objectives are set at this level, you provide opportunities for individuals to follow directions and sequences under close supervision. It may require conscious effort on the part of individuals to carry out the actions in sequence.
3. *Practicing.* When objectives are set at this level, you provide opportunities for the entire sequence to be performed repeatedly so that conscious effort is no longer required. The actions become more or less habitual, and you can say that the individuals have acquired the skill. Perhaps the individuals have learned to prepare recipes with vegetables in them or to modify recipes to make them lower in fat.
4. *Adapting.* Objectives at this level involve the ability to adapt or modify the actions to improve the outcome even further. This may mean the ability to adapt learned recipes to individual or family tastes.

Overall

Educational objectives help specify which kinds of strategies should be designed: ones in the cognitive domain only? The affective domain only? Or both? Will you have the opportunity to assist individuals to develop psychomotor skills as well? In reality, most activities in the food and nutrition area will involve both the cognitive (knowing) and affective (feeling) domains. It may be possible to address the psychomotor domain by including food preparation.

In the cognitive/knowing domain, educational strategies should attempt to assist the intended audience to do more difficult learning tasks, such as application or evaluation, and not just the easier tasks, such as recalling information. In the affective/feeling domain, it is preferable to design activities that actively engage participants and assist them to actively contemplate and value the message to the point of being willing to try the recommendations. Too often, objectives are set to achieve the lower levels of audience engagement, such as just listening and receiving the message (through lectures, for example). **Box 10-1** contains examples of learning objectives directed at mediators of behavior within the three domains.

Note on Writing Detailed Specific Objectives

In the educational world, writing specific "behavioral" objectives is based on the premise that learning results in an *observable* response to a specific stimulus. That is, the achievement of each objective needs to be demonstrated by a specific observable action; hence educational objectives often are referred to as "behavioral objectives" (Bloom et al.

Box 10-1   Examples of Learning Objectives Directed at Mediators of Behavior Within the Three Domains

In each example, the objective is preceded by the following phrase: "At the end of the program (or session), the participants will be able to . . ."

Motivational Mediators

1. *Concern for the problem or issue.* Demonstrate appreciation of their own susceptibility to heart disease (by naming people in their family who have died of heart disease and discussing how that made them feel).
   Affective domain: Responding level.

2. *Perceived risks.* Demonstrate the understanding that a diet high in fat increases their risk of heart disease (by correctly answering a questionnaire at the end of the program or session).
   Cognitive domain: Comprehension level. *Affective domain:* Responding level.

3. *Outcome expectations/perceived benefits.* Demonstrate the understanding that a diet high in fruits and vegetables reduces their risk of heart disease and cancer (by correctly answering a questionnaire at the end of the program or session).
   Cognitive domain: Comprehension level. *Affective domain:* Responding level.

4. *Values.* Appreciate the importance of overcoming psychological barriers to eating a lower-fat diet (by orally describing one barrier and listing one action the learner will take in the next week to overcome that barrier).
   Cognitive domain: Comprehension level. *Affective domain:* Valuing level.

5. *Self-efficacy.* Demonstrate belief in their ability to prepare foods lower in fat (by proposing to bring in a lower-fat recipe to share with the group next session).
   Cognitive domain: Comprehension level. *Affective domain:* Valuing level.

6. *Social influence.* Appreciate the role of peers in influencing food choices (by noting one instance in which the participant did not eat what peers ate and describing how that made the participant feel).
   Cognitive domain: Comprehension level. *Affective domain:* Valuing level.

Action Mediators: Facilitating the Ability to Take Action

1. *Knowledge.* Understand the dietary advice for reducing risk of cancer (by listing three of the relevant dietary guidelines without looking at materials).
   Cognitive domain: Comprehension level.

2. *Skills.*
   a. *Cognitive.* Demonstrate ability to apply the recommendations from MyPyramid (by comparing own 24-hour dietary intake to recommendations and describing implications for self).
      Cognitive domain: Evaluation level.
   b. *Affective.* Demonstrate resistance to peer pressure to eat high-fat foods (by eating a salad at lunch and not the high-fat choice of peers, and appropriately explaining/defending own choice).
      Cognitive domain: Evaluation level. *Affective domain:* Organization level.
   c. *Behavioral capability.* Demonstrate ability to stir-fry vegetables (by imitating demonstration in class by preparing identical dish at home).
      Cognitive domain: Comprehension level. *Psychomotor domain:* Imitation level.
   d. *Self-regulation skills.* Engage in systematic planning to change their own diet (by identifying a behavior that they wish to change, developing an action plan to make the change, self-monitoring the change, and sharing with the group their progress in attaining the goal).
      Cognitive domain: Evaluation level. *Affective domain:* Valuing level.
      Demonstrate satisfaction in achieving a personal dietary change goal (by rewarding self with seeing a movie).
      Affective domain: Valuing level.

3. *Social support.* Demonstrate ability to share feelings about chosen diet with friends and family and to seek support from them (by asking family to support their own macrobiotic eating pattern).
   Cognitive domain: Comprehension level. *Affective domain:* Valuing level.

1956; Krathwohl et al. 1964; Cruikshank 2000; Gronland & Brookhart 2008). The following elements are usually included:

1. The observable action expected of the learner
2. The conditions under which the observable action is to be demonstrated

Thus, specific objectives will usually take the following form:

Given _____ [*name of the condition or stimulus*], the learner (participant) will _____ [*name of the desired observable action*].

For example, "Given information on the government's food pyramid for healthy eating, the participant will be able to place foods into the correct food groups."

3. The degree of mastery required is often added as a third element. In this case, the objective might be "Given information on the government's food pyramid for healthy eating, the participant will be able to place 12 foods into the correct food groups with 80% accuracy."

You can follow this format and write detailed objectives if you wish. However, for nutrition education purposes, it is not necessary to follow this format slavishly. In addition, you may not need to write out the specific learning domains and levels for each educational objective. However, it is *very* important to be aware of, and to target, the different domains and levels in each session or throughout the program to ensure that nutrition education activities are directed at a range of levels of difficulty and that head, heart, and hand are all engaged.

■ WRITING ENVIRONMENTAL SUPPORT OBJECTIVES FOR THE TARGETED BEHAVIORS

Environmental mediators are those influences on the selected behaviors that reside outside the individual that may mediate change. From the environmental factors that may potentially mediate the goal behaviors identified in Step 2, select those that you will be able to target realistically in the intervention to increase environmental support, given your available time and resources.

In most instances, achievement of environmental support objectives involves educating and working in partnership with food or service providers, policy makers, or individuals and organizations that have decision-making authority over the environmental factors that you have identified as potentially relevant mediators of change. These might include school food service directors, school principals and superintendents, grocery store managers, parent–teacher organizations, farmers, food assistance programs, community leaders and organizations, departments of health, departments of parks or transportation, or other nonprofit organizations interested in food, physical activity, and health.

Writing General Environmental Support Objectives

First, write *general* environmental support objectives for changes in the environment to increase the opportunities of the intended audience to engage in the program goal behavior or behaviors. For the case study, these might include the following:

- The school food service will provide attractive and appealing fruits and vegetables in the school meals and other food venues, such as taste testing in the cafeteria.
- Schools will implement policies that ensure that vending machines and school stores carry water and healthy items, and not sweetened beverages or packaged snacks.
- Parents will decrease the availability of sweetened drinks and packaged snacks for their children at home and increase the accessibility of fruits and vegetables.

Writing Objectives for Interpersonal-Level Environmental Supports

Social support can be an important environmental mediator of individuals' eating patterns. If your program is to be in a worksite, or a community center or outpatient clinic, your objectives may be "to create social support groups for those in the program" or "to create a buddy system to support daily walking for health."

Children's willingness and ability to take recommended action is very much influenced by parental or family actions. Hence a parent/family component can be planned to assist them to be more supportive of their children's attempts to eat healthfully. Parents or family are external to the students. At the same time, they represent a new audience for whom general and specific educational objectives will need to be written in a process similar to that for the students described earlier.

In the case study, a parent component has as its behavioral goals: "Parents will make a variety of fruits and vegetables available and accessible to their children, decrease their purchases of sweetened drinks and packaged high-calorie snacks, and engage in physical activity with their children." General *educational* objectives of the parent component are then written for each of the parental support behaviors.

See the case study for details of behavioral goals, general educational objectives for the parent/family component, and the specific educational objectives for one session.

Writing Objectives for Potential Organizational- or Community-Level Environmental Supports

To promote environments that facilitate the enactment of the actions, behaviors, or practices targeted by the program, you need to increase the awareness of key decision makers and policy makers regarding the importance of the health, food, nutrition, or physical activity issue that the program is seeking to address and work in collaboration with them to achieve the behaviors that will contribute to health.

School Example

Using the case study as an example, this means you seek changes in the school environment to make it more supportive of the behaviors targeted by the program. Some support objectives might be the following:

- *Food environment:* School will provide many opportunities for students to taste fruits and vegetables in the cafeteria and other venues.
- *Policy:* School stores will replace high-calorie packaged snacks with healthier options.
- *Social environment:* School will increase social modeling of healthful eating by valued celebrities.
- *Information environment:* School will develop and display posters of teens eating healthful foods.

See the case study for details of the specific objectives for the school environment component.

Community Example

The objectives also can be stated more specifically, such as a community collaborative or partnership during the next four years will do the following:

Community support for:

- Support Wellness Policy Council activities so that 70% of schools will conduct a school assessment using the School Health Index or similar tool
- Close streets adjacent to 50% of schools that lack adequate gyms or playgrounds between 3 and 7 pm.
- Facilitate enforcement of existing regulations to reduce low-nutrient, high-calorie vending machine food in 50% of schools

Community-based activities:

- Create four new walking paths in the community
- Double the number of sites where city-financed exercise classes will be held
- Display walking prompts in stairwells of 70% of area organizations

■ CASE STUDY

This chapter continues the case study of nutrition education for adolescents as an example as you complete your worksheets. Recall that four behavioral goals were chosen for the program "Taking Control: Eating Well and Being Fit": increase intake of fruits and vegetables; reduce consumption of sweetened beverages; reduce intake of packaged, highly energy dense, processed snacks; and increase physical activity.

In Step 3, you chose three components: classroom curriculum, parent/family support, and school environment and policy changes. A logic model showing the three components and the design products for each is shown for the case study in Chapter 9.

The case study intervention consists of the following features within the three components. They are listed here; the details of both the actual *objectives* and *activities* for each component are described together in Chapter 11.

The classroom component:

- The program's *behavioral goals* for the adolescents.
- *Classroom curriculum*, consisting of 10 sessions: an introductory lesson, two on each of the four behavioral goals, and a concluding lesson. However, for space reasons, the case study henceforth focuses on only one behavioral goal: encouraging youth to eat more fruits and vegetables.
- For each session or lesson, the *general* educational objectives to address potential personal psychosocial mediators of the behaviors, based on the theory model created for the program.
- For each session or lesson, the *specific* educational (learning) objectives for each of the potential mediators from theory. For each of these specific educational objectives, we will create educational activities for the case study in Step 5 and add information on the *domain* in which the educational activities should occur and the *anticipated level* of cognitive difficulty or affective engagement for the group for each activity within each domain. (See Chapter 11 for details.)

For the parental/family component:

- Behavioral goals for parents.

- Family component, consisting of two group sessions, one on fruits and vegetables and one on sweetened beverages, plus two newsletters, one on packaged high-calorie snacks and one on physical activity. For space reasons, the case study henceforth focuses on only one family/parent workshop.
- *General* educational objectives for the session.
- *Specific* educational objectives for each of the mediators addressed in the session.

For the school environmental support component:

- Environmental support component, consisting of changes in school meals, schoolwide food policy, social support, and school information environment
- *General* environmental support objectives for the component
- *Specific* environmental support objectives:
  - Objectives for decision makers
  - Objectives for the food environment
  - Objectives for food policy
  - Objectives for the school social support and information environment

Note: Although this chapter describes how to write all these different kinds of objectives, the objectives themselves are stated in Chapter 11 and are written out along with the activities created to achieve the objectives.

■ YOUR TURN: COMPLETING THE STEP 4 WORKSHEETS

Use the Step 4 worksheet to write your own *program* objectives for a hypothetical or real intervention. These program level educational objectives and environmental support objectives will guide the development of nutrition education strategies and environmental support activities to be delivered through a variety of channels. You can write these in conjunction with Step 5, where you design appropriate activities based on these objectives.

Questions and Activities

1. Describe briefly three reasons why it is important to write educational objectives for nutrition education, no matter how brief.
2. What are learning objectives? Describe carefully the relationship between learning objectives for a program or session and the potential mediators of behavior or practices.
3. Objectives are often described as being written in the *cognitive*, *affective*, and *psychomotor* domains of learning. What do these terms mean? How do they guide learning?
4. For practice, select three potential mediators of the behavior of increasing the intake of calcium-rich foods among teenage girls and state *general* educational/learning objectives directed at each. Write one for each domain of learning.
5. For practice, write *specific* educational/learning objectives for the following potential mediators of the behavior of increasing the intake of calcium-rich foods among teenage girls. For each objective, indicate the learning domain and level:
   - Outcome expectations/perceived benefits
   - Perceived self-efficacy
   - Personal action goals

References

Bloom, B. S., M. D. Engelhart, E. J. Furst, W. H. Hill, and D. R. Krathwohl. 1956. *Taxonomy of educational objectives. Handbook I: The cognitive domain.* New York: David McKay.

Cruikshank, K. A. 2000. *Taxonomy for learning, teaching, and assessing: A revision of Bloom's taxonomy of educational objectives.* Boston: Allyn & Bacon.

Gronland, N. E., and S. M. Brookhart. 2008. *Gronland's writing instructional objectives.* 8th ed. Upper Saddle River, NJ: Prentice Hall.

Krathwohl, D. R., B. S. Bloom, and B. B. Masia. 1964. *Taxonomy of educational objectives: The classification of educational goals. Handbook II: Affective domain.* New York: David McKay.

Marzano, R. J., and J. S. Kendall. 2007. *The new taxonomy of educational objectives,* 2nd ed. Thousand Oaks, CA: Sage Publications

In Step 4, you translate behavioral theory into the program objectives that you need to guide the design of educational experiences and environmental-policy support activities. These objectives are directed at potential mediators of change.

At the end of the Step 4 worksheets, you will have the following product:

> **Step 4:** Several sets of objectives for your program that cut across all components.

Use the worksheets as a guide to help you write educational and support objectives rooted in your theory model from Step 3. Electronic versions of these worksheets are available at http://nutrition.jbpub.com/education/2e/. If you are unable to access the worksheet electronically, you can write onto this blank worksheet or create a text document that uses the same flow of information.

> **NOTE:** This part of the case study focuses on only one of the program's goal behaviors: increasing intake of fruits and vegetables. If you create a program with multiple goal behaviors, you will need to complete this worksheet for each of the behaviors.

Step 4: Nutrition education program objectives for all components

Determine the nutrition education program objectives that will cut across all program components to achieve the program behavioral goals for each of the three categories below.

Motivational objectives	Action objectives
Increase awareness in youth about the importance of fruits and vegetables in the diet. Enhance the students' motivation to eat fruits and vegetables through a school curriculum and school-wide activities.	Facilitate the ability to act by providing opportunities to gain relevant food and nutrition knowledge and practice food and nutrition experiences. Enhance their self-regulation skills related to fruit and vegetable intake.

Environmental-policy support objectives
Educate decision makers and work with them to increase opportunities for youth to eat more fruits and vegetables at school through policy initiatives at the school. Educate parents to increase opportunities for youth to eat more fruits and vegetables through a parent education component.

In Step 4, you translate behavioral theory into the program objectives that you need to guide the design of educational experiences and environmental-policy support activities. These objectives are directed at potential mediators of change.

At the end of the Step 4 worksheets, you will have the following product:

Step 4: Several sets of objectives for your program that cut across all components.

Use the provided worksheets as a guide to help you write educational and support objectives rooted in your theory model from Step 3. Electronic versions of these worksheets are available at http://nutrition.jbpub.com/education/2e/. If you are unable to access the worksheet electronically, you can write onto this blank worksheet or create a text document that uses the same flow of information.

Step 4: Nutrition education program objectives for all components

Determine the nutrition education program objectives that will cut across all program components to achieve the program behavioral goals for each of the three categories below.

Motivational objectives

Action objectives

Environmental-policy support objectives

CHAPTER 11

Step 5: Translating Behavioral Theory into Educational Strategies: A Focus on Enhancing Motivation for Action

OVERVIEW

This chapter and the next focus on selecting theory-based strategies and creating practical educational activities to achieve educational objectives and on sequencing the strategies into educational plans ready for implementation within groups or through other channels. The focus of *this* chapter is on designing activities to address potential mediators that increase awareness, promote contemplation, and enhance motivation. The information in Chapters 3 and 4 will help you with this step in the design process.

CHAPTER OUTLINE

- Introduction
- Getting started
- Gaining audience interest and engagement
- Translating behavioral theory into educational practice
- Designing theory-derived educational strategies for motivators of action or change
- Organizing and sequencing educational strategies and activities for implementation: the educational plan
- Case study
- Your turn: completing the Step 5 worksheets

LEARNING OBJECTIVES

At the end of the chapter, you will be able to:

- Describe the kinds of theory-based strategies to address potential mediators of target behaviors that focus on increasing awareness, promoting contemplation, and enhancing motivation
- Design specific educational activities or learning experiences to make practical the theory-based educational strategies
- Recognize the importance of using a systematic instructional design process for designing and sequencing educational strategies
- Sequence the educational objectives and strategies to create an educational plan or lesson plan
- Demonstrate skill in creating an educational plan or lesson plan

■ INTRODUCTION

A nutrition educator new to a community center has learned that the women who use the nutrition services there tend to eat fast food items high in saturated fat and calories and not many vegetables. She decides to have a session on helping the women value the importance of adding more fruits and vegetables to their diet.

She lectures on the government's food pyramid, the different food groups in it, and the number of servings from each group that the women should have. She then focuses on the vegetables group, the nutrients in some popular ones, and the number of servings they should eat. When she later sees the women at a local coffee shop, she observes the women ordering their usual items. None of them ordered any fruits or vegetables. What is going on here? The nutrition educator selected a valid affective objective—to help participants value eating fruits and vegetables; in essence, she aimed to encourage positive attitudes. She also had a behavioral goal—eating more fruits and vegetables. However, the educational format she used—a lecture—was highly didactic and cognitive, and inappropriate to the objective. It is a common practice for nutrition educators to focus solely on traditional cognitive activities when in fact they are trying to accomplish affective and behavioral change objectives. When directed to affective and behavioral objectives, the instructional content should emphasize motivational factors—mediators from theory—such as beliefs, attitudes, feelings, personal and cultural values, peer pressure, and community norms as well as knowledge and skills, and the strategies should be active and engaging.

The End in Sight Is Here: The Educational Plan

Recall that at the beginning of the Stepwise Procedure in Chapter 7 we said that the end we wanted to have in sight was a set of educational plans for your intended audience and accompanying environment and policy support plans (Figure 7-1). The Stepwise Procedure now has brought us to that end.

In Step 5, you are ready to design activities to address the potential personal and environmental mediators of program behavioral goals that you have selected as part of your theory framework. Your program may consist of only a few group sessions or several components as you determined in Step 3. For group sessions, the activities you design are then arranged in a sequence to create an educational plan (or lesson plan) for each session. If your program involves an environmental or policy component, you will develop a plan for how to increase environmental or policy support for the behavioral goals of your program. As you can see in **Figure 11-1** and **Figure 11-2**, the products of this step are a series of educational plans (or lesson plans) for group sessions with your intended audience linking mediators, objectives, and strategies, as well as environmental support plans for one or more components, if your program has more than one component.

An *educational plan* is a plan for arranging in an appropriate sequence the educational activities that you will conduct with any group, in nonformal as well as formal settings. Educational plans, in modified form, also guide educational content and activities conducted through other channels (e.g., newsletters, posters). They are similar to the notion of "messages" in social marketing approaches. These educational strategies and learning activities are designed to address the mediators of behavior change that you selected in Step 3.

Because designing such activities-filled plans is at the heart of nutrition education, we devote three chapters to Step 5. The kinds of activities that nutrition educators might create for group sessions are so numerous that we separated them into two categories—those based on mediators of motivation and those designed to facilitate action. In this chapter

we focus on designing activities that are theory-based, engaging, and motivating to the intended audience, thus increasing their interest and commitment to take action on the behaviors targeted by your program. In Chapter 12 we focus on designing activities that will facilitate the ability of group participants to take action. In Chapter 13, we focus on ways to enhance environmental and policy supports for action. These chapters are based on the integrative conceptual framework for translating behavioral theory into effective nutrition education practice presented in Chapter 9 (Figure 9-4).

Any given educational plan for groups can consist of activities that are primarily motivational or primarily skill-building, or both depending on the objectives that you select. However, in most cases, a given educational plan for group sessions or a given piece of printed or visual material will address both motivational objectives and skills-building objectives.

To cover the large number of useful strategies available to nutrition educators, this chapter focuses on how to design theory-based strategies and practical activities that operationalize mediators from theory that are likely to be effective in motivating your audience to want to take action. The relationships among mediators, objectives, and strategies are shown in **Figure 11-3**. Chapter 12 focuses on strategies to assist the group to take action. In designing your sessions or program, you will most likely go

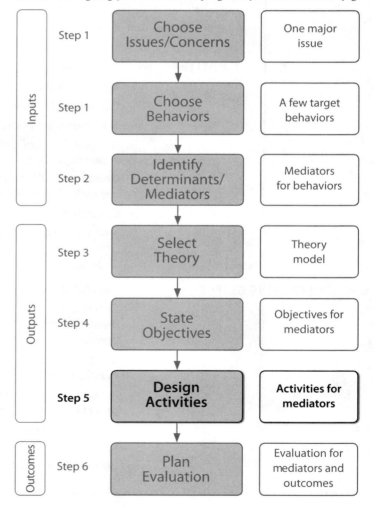

FIGURE 11-1 Flowchart of steps in designing theory-based nutrition education: Step 5.

Inputs: Collecting Assessment Data			Outputs: Designing the Theory-Based Intervention			Outcomes: Evaluation Plan
Step 1 ⟷ **Analyze issues and audiences to state program behavioral goals**	**Step 2** ⟷ **Identify potential mediators to achieve program behavioral goals**	**Step 3** ⟷ **Select theory, philosophy, and components**	**Step 4** ⟷ **State objectives for mediators**	**Step 5** ⟷ **Design theory-based strategies and activities for mediators**		**Step 6** Plan evaluation
Tasks • Analyze issues and select audience • Identify behaviors or patterns contributing to issue • Specify behavioral or action goals of the program	*Tasks* • Identify personal psychosocial mediators • Identify environmental support mediators	*Tasks* • Select theory or create appropriate model • Clarify philosophy (education and content) • Determine program components	*Tasks* • State educational objectives for psychosocial mediators • State change objectives for environmental support mediators	*Tasks* • Design activities to address psychosocial mediators • Design activities to address environmental support mediators • Implementation plan		*Tasks* • Design outcome evaluation plan • Determine tools to measure impact • Plan process evaluation
Product • *Description of issue of concern* • *Statement of action or behavioral goals for program*	*Product* • *List of potential mediators for action or behavior goals*	*Product* • *Theory/model for program, philosophy, and components*	*Product* • *Objectives for each mediator*	***Product*** • *Educational plans for sessions linking mediators, objectives, and strategies* • *Environmental support plans*		*Product* • *Evaluation plan* • *List of indicators and measures for outcomes* • *Procedures and measures for process evaluation*

FIGURE 11-2 Stepwise Procedure for designing theory-based nutrition education: Step 5.

back and forth among these various strategies and between strategies in this chapter and those described in Chapter 12.

Again, although most educational plans will focus on both motivational why-to activities and skills-building how-to activities, for purposes of illustration, an educational plan that focuses on activities to operationalize motivational mediators is shown in the case study in this chapter, and an educational plan that focuses on facilitating the ability to take action is shown in the case study in Chapter 12.

■ GETTING STARTED

Many nutrition educators find this step to be the most creative and enjoyable part of nutrition education planning: designing messages and activities that are theory based and engaging, fun, and relevant to the intended audience. This is the time to brainstorm numerous ideas for translating objectives into activities! These activities need to be based on a thorough understanding of the audience. If you are designing these sessions with a colleague or a group, it is usually helpful if one of you brings in ideas for some tentative activities for the session(s) and the others provide feedback and brainstorm. You may designate one person to do the actual writing of the lesson plans/educational plans, or you may all take turns writing the lessons.

■ GAINING AUDIENCE INTEREST AND ENGAGEMENT

Information Versus Learning Experiences

Influential educators such as Dewey (1929) and Tyler (1949) make a clear distinction between content presentations and actual learning experiences. *A learning experience is the interaction between learners and external con-* *ditions through which learning takes place.* Learning takes place through the active behavior of learners. Education is what nutrition educators do; learning is what the program participants experience and accomplish. Mere educator intentions, however, will not result in learning. Mere presentation of information may not result in learning. The dynamic engagement of the participants with the content is essential. This is the basis of all good education and is emphasized in learner-centered education.

What Is Learning?

Learning does *not* mean simply learning of facts and figures, or cognitive information and skills such as the number of calories in a teaspoon of sugar or how to read a food label. It means an *interaction between learners (program participants) and the activities educators have designed* that results in active contemplation about issues, changes in how participants view the world, an examination of their values, and changes in their expectations, attitudes, and feelings about food and nutrition, and, indeed, in their actions. Learning takes place through many venues—formal, nonformal, and informal—and individuals are all learners throughout life.

This is where the true challenge of nutrition education design rests. It calls on you not only to have a firm grasp of food and nutrition content, but also to design creative, productive, and meaningful experiences to address mediators of behavior to bring about specified goals and objectives. This involves creative risk taking on the one hand and careful organization on the other hand.

Learning Experiences and Educational Activities

Nutrition educators design the educational strategies that provide learning experiences for participants. Hence, the two terms are often used

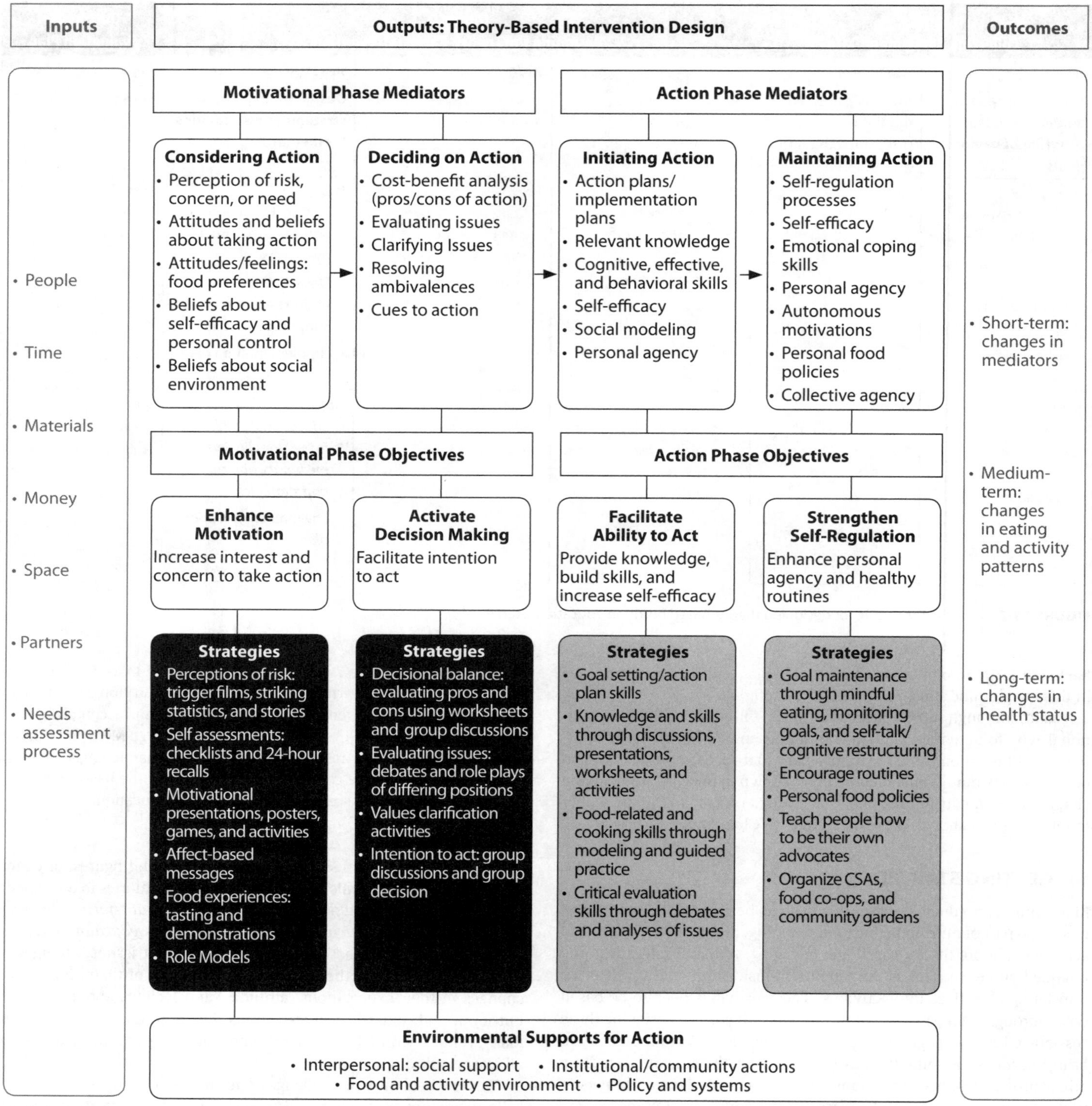

Inputs	Outputs: Theory-Based Intervention Design				Outcomes

Motivational Phase Mediators

Considering Action
- Perception of risk, concern, or need
- Attitudes and beliefs about taking action
- Attitudes/feelings: food preferences
- Beliefs about self-efficacy and personal control
- Beliefs about social environment

Deciding on Action
- Cost-benefit analysis (pros/cons of action)
- Evaluating issues
- Clarifying Issues
- Resolving ambivalences
- Cues to action

Action Phase Mediators

Initiating Action
- Action plans/implementation plans
- Relevant knowledge
- Cognitive, effective, and behavioral skills
- Self-efficacy
- Social modeling
- Personal agency

Maintaining Action
- Self-regulation processes
- Self-efficacy
- Emotional coping skills
- Personal agency
- Autonomous motivations
- Personal food policies
- Collective agency

Inputs:
- People
- Time
- Materials
- Money
- Space
- Partners
- Needs assessment process

Outcomes:
- Short-term: changes in mediators
- Medium-term: changes in eating and activity patterns
- Long-term: changes in health status

Motivational Phase Objectives

Enhance Motivation
Increase interest and concern to take action

Activate Decision Making
Facilitate intention to act

Action Phase Objectives

Facilitate Ability to Act
Provide knowledge, build skills, and increase self-efficacy

Strengthen Self-Regulation
Enhance personal agency and healthy routines

Strategies
- Perceptions of risk: trigger films, striking statistics, and stories
- Self assessments: checklists and 24-hour recalls
- Motivational presentations, posters, games, and activities
- Affect-based messages
- Food experiences: tasting and demonstrations
- Role Models

Strategies
- Decisional balance: evaluating pros and cons using worksheets and group discussions
- Evaluating issues: debates and role plays of differing positions
- Values clarification activities
- Intention to act: group discussions and group decision

Strategies
- Goal setting/action plan skills
- Knowledge and skills through discussions, presentations, worksheets, and activities
- Food-related and cooking skills through modeling and guided practice
- Critical evaluation skills through debates and analyses of issues

Strategies
- Goal maintenance through mindful eating, monitoring goals, and self-talk/cognitive restructuring
- Encourage routines
- Personal food policies
- Teach people how to be their own advocates
- Organize CSAs, food co-ops, and community gardens

Environmental Supports for Action
- Interpersonal: social support
- Institutional/community actions
- Food and activity environment
- Policy and systems

FIGURE 11-3 Integrative framework for translating behavioral theory into nutrition education strategies: Motivational phase educational strategies and activities.

interchangeably. This book uses the term *theory-based educational strategies* to describe ways to operationalize constructs of psychosocial theory describing mediators of behavior change for educational and instructional purposes. *Educational activities* or *learning experiences* are the numerous ways in which strategies are carried out in practice. These are techniques or procedures you use.

Thus, the *theory construct* of perceived threat for osteoporosis may be a potential motivational mediator of eating more calcium-rich foods to reduce the threat. The *strategy* chosen may be "confrontation of the audience with the risks." The *educational activities* or *learning experiences* might involve showing trigger films, pictures, charts, and striking national or local statistics; telling personal stories; or having the audience identify those in their families who have osteoporosis and describe their experiences.

Creating Opportunities for Active Participation and Learning

As you design activities, keep in mind that generally people remember:

- 10% of what they read
- 20% of what they hear
- 30% of what they see
- 50% of what they hear and see
- 70% of what they say and write
- 90% of what they both say and do

It is important to remember what you learned in Step 2 about your audience in terms of their preferred learning styles.

Hands-On Activities

A major way to encourage active participation is the use of *hands-on activities*. Hands-on activities enhance motivation by giving participants a sense of involvement with the learning at hand. For example, label reading can be taught in a hands-on way when participants handle real food packages, containers, and cans (empty) to determine healthful choices. Such an activity is much more motivating than simply lecturing to participants about "how to read a food label."

When conducting demonstrations, it is effective to have audience members come up to perform some aspects of the demonstration activities (e.g., spooning out the amount of fat in various fast foods) or to participate in a drama presented to the others. This not only provides active participation for some members, but also encourages peer social norms.

Role Playing

Another example of active participation is *role playing*, in which the person enacts the role of someone else by improvising rather than reading a script. Role playing attitudes counter to their own can be a powerful technique in facilitating deliberation and change in individuals' views of themselves, of other people, and of an advocated viewpoint or behavior.

Discussions

You can also engage learners in *discussion* among themselves in dyads, triads, or small groups about such topics as why it is so hard to get children to eat vegetables, why they have a hard time carrying out their intentions to eat more healthfully, what are some ideas for

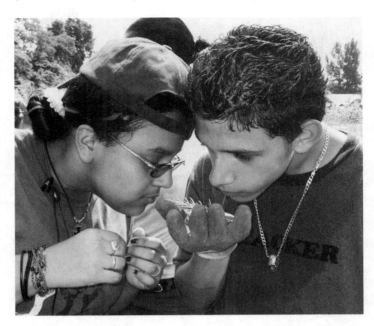

Identifying different herbs is an engaging, hands-on activity.

healthful meals in minutes, or how to make food choices in a manner that promotes local farms. Such an approach encourages cooperative learning. Research on cooperative learning indicates that when people participate in small-group activities, they are more likely to deliberate on the issues, examine their own attitudes, and desire to learn more (Johnson & Johnson 1987).

Facilitated Discussion

Facilitated discussion is a commonly used approach to group sessions that fosters active participation. Facilitated discussion is based on dialogue and exchange between the nutrition educator as facilitator of the group and group participants. It avoids lecturing, instead focusing on open-ended questions, active listening, and respect for the ideas of everyone in the group to promote active participation and weave a meaningful learning experience for all. It can include the kinds of cooperative learning discussed earlier. All these methods are described in greater detail in Chapter 15. Special consideration should be given to low-income audiences as you design activities for the challenges facing them (described in **Box 11-1**).

■ TRANSLATING BEHAVIORAL THEORY INTO EDUCATIONAL PRACTICE: STRATEGIES AND PLANS

The major task in translating theory into practice is to design, sequence, and deliver theory-based educational strategies in such a way as to achieve the behavioral goals and educational objectives you have selected.

Chapter 1 defines nutrition education as a combination of educational strategies, accompanied by environmental supports and policy, designed to facilitate the voluntary adoption and maintenance of behaviors conducive to health. This means that nutrition education consists of a set of learning activities that are systematically designed and organized with a purpose in mind.

Box 11-1 **Special Challenge of Nutrition Education with Low-Resources Audiences in Low-Income Neighborhoods**

Adopting healthful eating patterns is difficult for most people. It is especially difficult for low-resources individuals for a variety of reasons. Some of the reasons identified in studies include the following:

- Financial limitations caused by low resources
- Lack of time because many work long hours
- Lack of availability of quality healthful foods at affordable prices in neighborhood
- Family customs and habits

Low-income consumers want to ensure that no one in the family goes hungry. They thus strive to get enough food energy for all at low cost. An economic analysis of diets has found an inverse relationship between the energy density of foods, defined as available energy per unit weight (kilocalories per gram), and energy cost (dollars per kilocalorie). This means that diets based on refined grains, added sugars, and added fats cost less than the diets recommended by nutrition educators that are based on lean meats, fish, fresh vegetables, and fruits. On a *calorie per dollar* basis, bread, cookies, and even chocolate are cheaper than fruits and vegetables. One study found that adding fat and sweets to the diet *lowered* overall adjusted diet costs, whereas adding fruits and vegetables *increased* overall adjusted diet costs.

Nutrition educators must keep these economic considerations in mind when working with low-resources audiences. Institutional- and policy-level activities are also essential to complement group-level activities.

Sources: Palmieri, D., G. W. Auld, T. Taylor, P. Kendall, and J. Anderson. 1998. Multiple perspectives on nutrition education needs of low-income Hispanics. *Journal of Community Health* 23(4):301–316; and Drewnowski, A. 2004. Obesity and the food environment: Dietary energy density and diet costs. *American Journal of Preventive Medicine* 27(3, Suppl. 1):154–162.

Defining Terms

Designing nutrition education thus presents the challenge of selecting and organizing a logical and productive sequence for the educational strategies or learning experiences:

- *The education plan* for the educational strategies is referred to as a lesson plan, activity plan, educational plan, curriculum, or program.
- *Instruction* is the means or method for making the plan operational.
- *The curriculum or program* is the *what*, and instruction is the *how*. In this case, the *what* are the *mediators* of behavior change—the theory constructs—that the program addresses, and the *how* are

the educational *strategies* you use to operationalize mediators and the *activities* that translate the strategies into *learning experiences*.

- *Constructing an instructional framework* to deliver the educational strategies requires two activities:
  1. Designing the strategies that are based on theory constructs and operationalizing them
  2. Organizing and sequencing the strategies appropriately to enhance learning

The following sections provide a brief overview of these two activities, and then the remainder of the chapter is devoted to describing in great detail how to conduct these activities.

Designing Educational Strategies to Address Potential Mediators of Behavior Change

Educational strategies are ways to operationalize theory constructs so that educational means can be used to address potential mediators of behavior change.

These strategies can be used in delivering nutrition education through a variety of channels and are based on the evidence reviewed earlier in this book and on ongoing research (Contento et al. 1995; Lytle & Achterberg 1995; Ammerman et al. 2002; Baranowski et al. 2003; Pomerleau et al. 2005; Doak et al. 2006; Shaya et al. 2008; Baranowski, Cerin, & Baranowski 2009).

Strategies Described Here Are Derived from Many Theories

The strategies presented in this chapter are ways to operationalize the mediators from all the theories that are described in Part I of this book. *You will select from among these educational strategies only those that address the mediators of change designated by the theory you have selected or the conceptual model you have created for the intervention in Step 3.* That is, some strategies are relevant if you plan to use the health belief model, others if you plan to use the theory of planned behavior, and still others if you are using social cognitive theory. There are many overlaps among theories, so many of these strategies will operationalize several theories.

You will probably use many of them if you have selected the integrative model, health action process approach model, or conceptual framework for nutrition education described in Chapter 9. The integrative framework for translating behavioral theory into effective nutrition education strategies as depicted in Figure 11-3 shows the specific educational strategies and activities derived from theory that can be used to address the nutrition education program goals and potential mediators of behavior change.

Kinds of Strategies

The strategies from theory that are most useful in the *motivational phase* are described in this chapter; those most useful in the *action phase* are described in the next chapter.

People, of course, are integrated wholes—thinking, feeling, and action are not linearly organized but closely interconnected. For example, learning new skills, such as cooking, may help people act on their motivations; at the same time, the new skills may increase self-efficacy, which is likely to enhance motivation. Furthermore, the immediate social environment, such as family and friends, may provide social support for change but may also prove to be a barrier to change. In addition, individuals who are already in attendance at groups you have planned are probably the more interested and concerned ones. However, it is often the case that individuals attend sessions because others have suggested or required that they attend or because they think they are ready to make changes but are not. Hence, assisting them to review and reflect on their motivations is still useful and important.

Organizing and Sequencing Educational Strategies: Instructional Design

Instruction is the deliberate arrangement of events in the individual's environment to make learning happen and also to make it effective (Gagne et al. 2004). A *theory of instruction* is thus about how to select and arrange *events of instruction* or *sequence of activities* to provide support for the internal processes of learning.

The instructional design principles of Gagne (1965, 1985; Gagne et al. 2004) and a step model of health communications (McGuire 1984) can help you think about the sequencing of strategies. Gagne's theory of instruction has been widely used to design instruction using a variety of media (e.g., oral, written, computer-based, Web-based) for a variety of audiences (e.g., children, adults). Later, this chapter describes how to sequence educational strategies according to Gagne's instructional design principles. The end result is one or a series of educational plans or lesson plans. One such educational plan is provided in the case study in this chapter, and another educational plan in Chapter 12.

■ DESIGNING THEORY-DERIVED EDUCATIONAL STRATEGIES FOR MOTIVATORS OF ACTION OR CHANGE

Enhancing motivation focuses on "what's in it for me?" It requires nutrition educators to select educational strategies that operationalize theory constructs that are potential *motivational mediators* of action or behavior change derived from theory and nutrition education research evidence, such as beliefs and attitudes.

These strategies assist individuals to become aware of critical food-related issues; better understand their own needs, wants, feelings, motivations, and factors that seem to control their behaviors; actively contemplate the issues; resolve ambivalences; and then choose to take action—or not to do so—given their life circumstances. At the end of this process, if they intend to make a change, nutrition educators can use strategies that operationalize *action mediators* derived from theory, such as implementation intentions or action plans, to carry out the change by addressing mediators of behavior change, the subject of the next chapter.

It is important to remember that individuals make changes in their behavior only when they see the need to change, when the contemplated change touches other deeper values they have, and when they want to change. In addition, biological predispositions and powerful environmental forces make it difficult to change, so the role of education needs to be placed in context.

Summary of Strategies and Activities

Table 11-1 shows how theory-based strategies are derived from mediators of change and how they shape the educational activities or learning experiences used in nutrition education. From among the strategies, choose those that are part of the theory you selected in Step 3 and appropriate for your targeted behavior and intended audience. Not all strategies are appropriate for all situations. Your assessment in Step 2 will guide your choices.

In addition, do not attempt to accomplish too much in your sessions. People can usually process only small amounts of information at a time, so provide only what is relevant and needed to achieve the objectives. The rule of thumb is, plan to cover half as much in twice the time as you think it will take!

Educational Strategies and Activities for Theory Construct of Risk Perceptions

Several theories propose that a sense of concern about an issue or a perception of personal risk is important for individuals to be in a state of readiness to act, such as the health belief model, precaution adoption process model, social cognitive theory, and the health action process approach. Research suggest that, although such perceived risk or concern is not the most immediate or direct mediator of behavior, it often is a necessary and important first step. The strategies discussed here are similar to those designed to address the consciousness-raising and dramatic relief/emotional arousal processes of change in the transtheoretical model (see Chapter 5).

Provide Personalized Self-Assessments

- *Self-assessments can be motivating.* Self-assessment of food-related behaviors that is personalized and compared with recommendations can be an effective motivational activity as a starting point for nutrition education. People love to find out about themselves! Accurate self-assessment is key: people are often not aware of their own dietary intake status and do not perceive a need to change. Knowing about their actual behaviors can help them become more interested in deliberation of issues, and more motivated. Such personalized feedback may also counteract the tendency to be optimistically biased and encourage individuals to consider changes in their dietary behaviors based on their true risk.
- *Checklists.* Individuals can complete checklists that provide information specific to the intervention's behavioral goals, such as how many fruits and vegetables they are actually consuming, the number of sweetened beverages or milk products consumed in a day, or how many times they eat breakfast in a week.

  In the Best Bones Forever! campaign created by the Centers for Disease Control and Prevention (http://www.bestbonesforever. gov), girls can complete a "How Strong Are Your Bone Health Habits?" quiz online to find out how they are doing in terms of diet and physical activity related to bone health, or a "Are You As Bone-Health Savvy As You Think?" to find out how much they know about bone health. The website is colorful and motivating, and the quizzes are engaging. The participant gets a score and recommendations for what to do. **Nutrition Education in Action 11-1** reproduces the "Are You As Bone-Health Savvy As You Think?" quiz.

  Checklists can also be devised to see how "green" individuals' food shopping practices are (based, perhaps, on where the food comes from or its degree of packaging). Or a checklist, with a scoring system, can be devised for positive behaviors that contribute to nutritional well-being. Group members can also complete short instruments that provide them with information on their own stage of readiness to make changes in their diet.
- *Health risk appraisals.* Health risk appraisals are examples of self-assessments. As noted before, personal feedback must be accompanied by information on effective actions that individuals can take to deal with the threat or by information on potentially better alternative behaviors.

TABLE 11-1	Linking Theory, Strategies, and Educational Activities	

Potential Mediator of Behavior Change (Theory Construct)	Theory-Based Strategies for Potential Mediators of Behavior Change	Practical Educational Activities, Learning Experiences, Content, or Messages
Perceived risk	Confrontation with risks • Increase salience of issues or concern about problems • Convey threat or use fear communications (TTM: Consciousness-raising and dramatic relief)	Trigger films, pictures, charts, striking national or local statistics, personal stories, role plays, demonstration Clear image of threat (e.g., film clips on effect of high-saturated-fat diet in clogging arteries) Demonstration using plastic tube clogged with fat and colored water to show blockage
Awareness	Self-assessment: Provide personalized self-assessments to counter optimistic bias (TTM: Self-reevaluation)	Self-assessment checklists; food or activity records or recalls
Outcome expectations	Information about outcome expectations (why-to information) • Persuasive communications about positive outcomes • Information on response efficacy or effectiveness of taking action	Presentations, visuals, demonstrations of scientific evidence regarding dietary practices and health or disease risk; nutrient–health relationships (antioxidants for eye health; nutrients and bone health) Motivational activities
Perceived benefits	Information about perceived benefits of taking action or motivators with personal meaning for the intended audience (why-to information)	Messages or educational activities that provide scientific arguments for the desired action or practice to emphasize "what's in it for me?" Personal health benefits Other personal, family, or community benefits
Attitudes/affect	Reflection on affect/feelings	Attitude statements and discussion; learner-centered activities; emotion-based messaging
Self-efficacy and perceived barriers	Decrease perception of barriers or negative outcomes	Brainstorming; discussion of barriers and ways to overcome them
Food preferences	Direct experience with healthful food	Food tastings, demonstrations, cooking
Social norms	Awareness of social norms and social expectations	View print and TV ads; discuss impact of others
Habit	Bring to consciousness automatic behaviors, habits, or routines	Checklists of current practices; self-observation tool
Behavioral intention	Decisional balance: Analysis of pros and cons of action, and choice among actions Values clarification: Resolving resistance and ambivalences Anticipated regret Group decision and public commitment (TTM: Self-liberation)	Worksheets or discussions to analyze pros and cons of action; choices Values clarification worksheets for individuals, or group activities Imagery activities Group discussion followed by group decision on goals for action, and public commitment

Note: TTM = transtheoretical model.

- *24-hour food recalls as educational activity.* Here, ask the group to complete a 24-hour food intake recall, and then have members individually compare their intakes with the food pyramid recommendations. Or you can analyze the intakes of the group and use the average data as the starting point for nutrition education. For example, you can collect such data during your needs analysis process in Step 1, calculate the averages, and display them in a handout or slide when you meet with the group. This is particu-

larly useful if the group is a low-literacy audience. When time permits and the level of education enables people to do so, have people analyze their own data: self-analysis is preferable.
- *Physical activity.* In the area of physical activity, information from pedometers or physical activity can be very motivating.
- *Community self-assessments.* Self-assessments can be modified to involve assessment of relevant community or organizational behaviors and practices. Members of an organization or community

---

NUTRITION EDUCATION IN ACTION **11-1**

The Best Bones Forever Quiz: A Motivational Self-Assessment

Are You as Bone-Health Savvy as You Think?

Yeah, you're smart about school, guys, and the real scoop on all the hot bands. But do you know enough about powerful bones? Take this quiz to see how much you really know. If you score high enough, you just might win a cyber trophy.

1. You're babysitting your little sister, and you have to make a healthy dinner with vegetables. What should a bone-smart babysitter pick?
   a. French fries—Potatoes are a vegetable, right?
   b. Broccoli—With low-fat cheese for even more calcium.
   c. Skip the vegetable, Mom will never know.
   d. Lima beans—Your sister can't stand them.
2. Mom and Dad are away! You could drink soda all day, but for strong bones you . . .
   a. Slurp up the soda anyway.
   b. Drink fruit punch.
   c. Go for fat-free or low-fat milk and orange juice with added calcium.
   d. Drink diet soda.
3. It has been storming for days, and you're tired of being shut in. What is the best way to get some weight-bearing physical activity?
   a. Forget it and catch up on TV reruns.
   b. Find a comfy chair and chat on the phone.
   c. Do some stretches while watching movies. At least it's some activity.
   d. Clear some space and jump rope.

4. You're eating out with friends after a basketball game. Everyone orders chicken tenders and soda, but for healthy bones you order . . .
   a. Chicken tenders and soda too—why be difficult?
   b. Chicken tenders and low-fat milk—a yummy way to get calcium.
   c. Nothing—there's no healthy fast food.
5. Your best pal won't drink milk or eat yogurt or cheese, either. But calcium is important for strong bones. What can you do?
   a. It is really none of your business.
   b. There aren't any other foods with calcium.
   c. Tell her about other foods with calcium like broccoli and orange juice with added calcium.
   d. Who needs calcium? Isn't weight-bearing physical activity enough?
6. It's Saturday and you're playing basketball with friends when it starts to rain! What should a powerful girl do?
   a. Tell your friends they might as well go home.
   b. Get out your board games.
   c. Pick a few CDs and make up dance routines.

Those taking the quiz may submit it to receive their score to see how they stack up.

Source: Centers for Disease Control and Prevention. 2009. Best Bones Forever! http://www.bestbonesforever.gov/fun/quizzes.cfm.

---

can do an assessment about food-related practices and resources to provide themselves with a true picture of the extent of risk or the severity of an issue in the community. For example, children can first do a 24-hour food recall on themselves in terms of the packaging they disposed of at each eating occasion. Then, they can do a study in their schools to investigate how much packaging their school throws out after each lunch, from which they can calculate the amount disposed of by all schools in their city or in the United States.

Increase Awareness of Risks and Concerns: Why-to Knowledge

Information on Perceived Risk Can Be Attention-Getting

Research evidence suggests that a moderate sense of threat may be important, particularly on some issues such as food safety behaviors, but it is an empirical question whether fear will be useful for your particular audience and, if so, what the optimal level of threat might be. You must determine this information from your activities in Step 1. It has been suggested that fear may be useful for taking precautions against future problems but is counterproductive in dealing with existing problems.

Risk Information Should Be Accompanied by Actions to Reduce Risk

When using the risk perception approach, the first part of the message is designed to create a motivation to avoid risk or danger. In group settings, trigger films, pictures, charts, striking national or local statistics, personal stories, and other consciousness-raising strategies can be used to bring to life and make relevant issues of concern based on scientific evidence, such as the increase in obesity rates, breastfeeding rates, increasing portion sizes, bone loss, and metabolic syndrome in adolescents. Such activities can also be used to bring other issues to awareness, such as the rate of loss of farm land, how much of school lunches is thrown away daily, or the amount of disposable service materials (e.g., paper plates, sporks) that is thrown away each day from the school (students could also do a study to find out). Visuals are especially powerful, such as pictures or actual food products (packages only), to show the portion sizes of various food products and beverages served in movie theaters, fast food outlets, and elsewhere. Media campaigns are especially useful here.

The second part of the message should be designed to show that people can take specific actions that will reduce the threat or danger and should provide exact instructions for when, how, and where to take action.

Educational Strategies and Activities for Theory Construct of Outcome Expectations or Perceived Benefits

Increase Perception of Positive Outcomes or Perceived Benefits of Taking Action: Why-to Knowledge

As an attention-getter at the beginning of a session or series of sessions, or as part of a media campaign, the benefits of action should be presented in a way that is brief, catchy, and memorable. When benefits are explored in greater detail later in the instructional sequence, more food and nutrition data can be presented and explored.

A major task in promoting contemplation and enhancing motivation is to design activities that focus on beliefs about the potential desirable outcomes or benefits of the given behaviors. Such beliefs are powerful motivators of behavior because they are the basis of cognitive or injunctive attitudes, and thus have an impact on attitudes, intentions, and the formation of goals. In many situations, a focus on benefits is the best way to gain the attention of the intended audience. This mediator is common to the health belief model, theory of planned behavior, social cognitive theory and integrated models, among others.

Benefits Are Reasons for Taking Action

Information about desirable outcomes is usually stated in the form of reasons for the action. These reasons are of two kinds: benefits based on scientific or other kinds of evidence for the effectiveness of taking action, which this book has referred to as *why-to knowledge*, and benefits that are of personal importance to individuals. Here is the time to present the scientific studies and data that make a case for a role of diet in health, weight control, disease prevention, or bone health. For those nutrition educators interested in food sustainability issues, this is the time to talk about the benefits of eating locally and so forth. Here is also the time to explore benefits of a personal nature.

Benefits Should Be Personally Meaningful to the Audience

- *Striking information.* Perceived benefits are more effective when presented through striking statistics or personally relevant data, such as the benefits of breastfeeding in reducing infections in infants and hence visits to the doctor when working with pregnant women.
- *Attention-getting graphics.* The anticipated benefits or positive outcomes of recommended skills and behaviors can also be communicated by use of such methods as films, posters, games, role plays, or showing excerpts from magazines popular with the intended audience. Use of vivid and personal material is more likely to be effective.
- *Lunch is cool example.* In one study, an attempt to increase consumption of the school lunch was accomplished by communicating the message that eating school lunch was "cool" and by linking it with something perceived as positive—sports: a Training Table program highlighted how nutritious foods boost athletic performance. Activities must be fun, engaging, and involve active participation to the extent possible.

Benefits Differ for Diverse Groups

The relative importance of different perceived benefits, or reasons for action, may differ depending on the behavior and the group or audi-

ence. For example, for the behavior of eating fruits and vegetables, being cool may be important for teenagers, and creating clear skin may be important for young women; improving the health of the baby may be important for pregnant women, whereas reducing cancer risk may be important for men. Immediate benefits usually carry more weight than benefits in the future, particularly for teenagers. Thus, the messages about benefits or positive anticipated outcomes of action must be based on those that are personally meaningful to the specific group.

Use of the Elaboration Likelihood Method (ELM) of Communication

A focus on positive outcomes for taking action is especially useful for mass media campaigns. Here the elaboration likelihood method (ELM) of communication can be especially useful (Petty & Cacioppo 1986). As discussed in Chapter 4, this method proposes that individuals differ in their *ability* and *motivation* to process educational messages thoughtfully. Hence, nutrition education messages need to take into account the recipients' ability to process the messages and encourage their motivation to do so. Simply providing more arguments may not increase effectiveness; it is the quality of the arguments that is important.

- To increase participants' *ability* to process messages, make your messages straightforward and clear, repeat or reinforce them, and present them with a minimum of distractions.
- To address the issue of *motivation* to process messages, make messages unexpected or novel, memorable, culturally appropriate, and most important, *personally relevant*, stressing positive outcomes important to the intended audience.

Messages can involve humor, warmth, or other attributes that are appropriate for a given audience. The messages can be expressed in terms of what participants will gain from taking action as well as what they will lose by *not* taking action. These principles apply whether the messages are delivered through mass media, brochures, newsletters, or in a group setting.

The VERB campaign, created by the Centers for Disease Control and Prevention (CDC) for children ages 9 to13, was designed to increase physical activity through targeted advertising, promotions, and events for tweens. The CDC developed a variety of VERB materials to help organizations that work with children connect VERB to their programs, classes, and activities. It is an excellent example of a campaign that was based on making the outcomes meaningful for teens, based on research regarding potential motivators (see **Nutrition Education in Action 11-2**). So, although the rationale for the program was that there are health risks to inactivity and health benefits to being active, those were not the motivators (or expected outcomes) used with participating youth.

Decrease Perception of Negative Outcomes or Barriers to Taking Action

Nutrition education seeks not only to increase the perceptions of benefits but also to decrease the perceptions of barriers to taking action.

- *Group identification of barriers.* You can assist the group to share and understand the difficulties and identify their (or their family members') barriers to healthful eating practices. This can be done by having the group identify barriers verbally and listing them on newsprint, and then asking the group to brainstorm ways of overcoming these barriers. You can facilitate and add your own suggestions. This is a useful strategy for all age groups. This is the time to address and, if appropriate, change individuals' miscon-

NUTRITION EDUCATION IN ACTION **11-2**

VERB: A Physical Activity Campaign for Tweens

The VERB campaign, created by the Centers for Disease Control and Prevention (CDC 2006), worked to increase physical activity through targeted advertising, promotions, and events for tweens. The CDC also developed a variety of VERB materials to help organizations that work with children connect VERB to their programs, classes, and activities.

- *The VERB vision:* All youth leading healthy lifestyles.
- *The VERB mission:* To increase and maintain physical activity among tweens (youth ages 9–13 years).
- *Campaign audiences:* The main audience for the campaign was tweens. Other important audiences were parents and adult influencers, including teachers, youth leaders, physical education and health professionals, pediatricians, healthcare providers, and coaches.

Teens could go on the website for ideas for physical activity and participate in all kinds of online activities with other teens. Parents were also urged to participate.

Rationale for Campaign

The underlying rationale for the campaign had to do with risks to children of inactivity and the benefits of being physically active, such as strengthening muscles, bones, and joints; controlling weight; and improving overall health. Physical activity also helps to develop skills that can benefit children for life, including goal setting and achievement, getting along with others, leadership, and teamwork. Other research shows that physical activity can help increase concentration, reduce anxiety and stress, and increase self-esteem—all of which may have a positive effect on students' scholastic achievement. These important benefits of being physically active are *not,* of course, particularly meaningful to the tween audience.

What Moves Tweens

Meaningful motivators for this age group were based on VERB research findings: children this age respond to the spirit of adventure, discovery, and finding their own thing. So, adults can help tweens discover new activities that they enjoy:

- Give away small prizes such as stickers, pins, or water bottles to reward tweens for being active. Prizes serve as great incentives for kids.
- Design activities with input from the kids. They will be more inclined to participate because they want to, not because they have to, do something.
- Some tweens prefer activities with a competitive edge, whereas others simply like playing a game with friends. Find out their preferences. All tweens will experience the rewards of being active if it is enjoyable for them.
- Tweens, especially girls, like social interaction with friends. It

makes playing actively more fun and offers opportunities for peer recognition and praise.
- Praise kids just for trying something new and getting active. Your encouragement means a lot to them.

Campaign Outcomes

After one year, the VERB campaign had

- Narrowed the gap in physical activity between girls and boys
- Resulted in lower-income tweens becoming more physically active, despite greater barriers to being active
- Reached extraordinarily high awareness levels among tweens (74% nationally and 84% in high-dose communities) and very high understanding (90% nationally) of the campaign's core messages to be physically active and have fun

More specifically, evaluation measures demonstrated significant increases in physical activity as a direct result of VERB in the following key groups (Huhman et al. 2005):

Children 9–10 Years Old (8.6 million national population)

- 34% increase in free-time physical activity sessions nationally
- 32% decline in the number of sedentary 9- to 10-year-olds in high-dose communities

Girls (10 million national population)

- 27% increase in free-time physical activity sessions nationally
- 37% decline among least active in high-dose communities

Tweens from Lower- (<$25,000; 4.5 million national population) to Lower-Middle-Income ($25,000–50,000; 6 million national population) Households

- 25% increase in free-time physical activity sessions nationally among lower-middle-income households
- 31% decline among least active from lower-income households in high-dose markets
- 38% decline among least active from lower-middle-income households in high-dose communities

These analyses included children from all racial/ethnic groups. Older tweens, boys, and tweens from middle- to higher-income households also showed some increases in physical activity, but those increases were not statistically significant.

The active campaign ended, but the materials are available.

Sources: Centers for Disease Control and Prevention. 2006. Youth media campaign: VERB. http://www.cdc.gov/youthcampaign; Huhman, M., L. D. Potter, F. L. Wong, et al. 2005. Effects of a mass media campaign to increase physical activity among children: Year 1 results of the VERB campaign. *Pediatrics* 116:277–284; and Wong F. L., M. Greenwell, S. Gates, and J. M. Berkowitz. 2008. It's What You Do! Reflections on the VERB Campaign. *American Journal of Preventive Medicine* 34(6S):S175–S182.

ceptions about their ability to act. For example, for the barrier of the cost of fruits and vegetables, suggestions can be made about buying in season. For the barrier that fruits and vegetables easily go bad, suggestions can be made about how to store them to reduce spoilage, or to buy other forms, such as frozen or canned.

- *Misconceptions as barriers.* Misconceptions can also be factual in nature, such as the belief that eating calcium-rich foods can increase "hardening of the arteries."

Educational Strategies and Activities for the Theory Construct of Self-Efficacy

Enhance Self-Efficacy: Make the Desired Actions Easy to Understand and Do

Self-efficacy is important for both motivation and taking action. In the motivational phase of nutrition education, perceived barriers are closely related to, and often mirror, self-efficacy and perceived behavioral control. That is, as barriers are overcome, self-efficacy increases, and as self-efficacy increases, perceived barriers decrease. In this phase of nutrition education, therefore, *increasing self-efficacy is about reducing the perceived difficulty of taking action.* Here the focus is on making the behavior that is the target of the intervention easy to understand and carry out. This mediator is common to almost all psychosocial models of health behavior.

- *Group brainstorming.* In a group setting, you can elicit from the group tips on overcoming the perception of barriers and write them up on newsprint. Individuals who have been successful in engaging in the targeted behavior can share their experiences. Using examples of valued social models enacting the behavior, such as sports figures or successful breastfeeding moms, is also an effective strategy. In using social models, the audience must see that the outcomes of the behavior are clearly beneficial to the model.

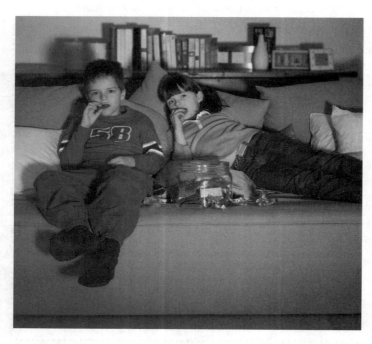

Consider all of the messages that children receive about food and where they get those messages.

In one example with inner-city teens, nutrition educators led the group through calculations that showed that packaged snacks from vending machines and their local stores actually cost more than making their own simple snacks or even fruit that could easily be carried around. They then had the teens assemble simple snacks from basic ingredients that they liked, such as raisins and nuts. The nutrition educators also calculated the time it took to make or assemble the snacks, showing how time did not have to be a barrier.

- *Media messages.* Educational strategies to increase self-efficacy can also involve mass media messages. An interesting mass media campaign to increase fruit and vegetable intake involved billboards in the community, along with flyers, that had on them a drawing of a specific fruit or vegetable accompanied by a relevant message. For example, a drawing of a banana was accompanied by the message "Peel. Eat. How easy is that?" (Iowa Department of Public Health 2005).

Educational Strategies and Activities for the Theory Construct of Affective Attitudes (Feelings)

Increase Reflection on Attitudes and Feelings About Program Goal Behaviors or Practices

Beliefs about the outcomes of behavior constitute the cognitive component of attitudes and are a major motivator of behavioral intention, as you have seen. However, the affective component of attitudes, reflecting feelings, is also a powerful motivator, if not a more powerful one when it comes to food and physical activity. Nutrition education can assist individuals to understand their own feelings and emotions about food- and nutrition-related behaviors so that they can make changes where necessary to serve their own interests in improving health.

- *Positive educational experiences.* Positive attitudes and feelings often come about from positive educational experiences such as tasting and preparing food. However, they can also arise from having group members explore their feelings, not just their thoughts, about the behaviors central to your program. This can be done through a process of attitudes clarification.
- *Attitudes clarification activity.* Present some attitude statements and ask the group to discuss them or to explore them individually. You can also use the strategy of forming an attitude line. For example, you can verbalize an attitude statement such as the following ones and have participants line up from "Strongly Agree" to "Strongly Disagree." Alternatively, the four corners of the room can be used as "attitude corners": Strongly Agree, Agree, Disagree, and Strongly Disagree. Whatever the format, individuals should be encouraged to discuss their response with their peers. Examples of attitude statements are as follows:

> Exclusively breastfeeding is best for my baby.
>
> Healthful foods take too long to prepare.
>
> People should have more willpower when they make food choices.
>
> Eating food from local farms is very important for the health of the planet.

Build on Personal Meanings

Personal meanings are important. For example, it has been found that adolescents often use eating certain foods, such as junk foods, as a way to express their independence and personal will, challenge parental authority, and test boundaries. Many women see food as an enemy. Build on the personal meanings that you identified in Step 2.

- *Group discussion.* Lead a facilitated dialogue or a set of learner-centered activities to explore the personal and functional meanings that individuals give to food and eating.
- *Written activity.* Use worksheets with engaging and challenging questions to allow participants to explore their feelings individually and privately. Provide opportunities to share if appropriate for your group. If not, ask them to take home and think about what they wrote and what they might want to do with it.

Affect/Feelings: Reflection on Potential Anticipated Regret

Anticipated regret or worry about the consequences of acting or failing to act has been shown to be a motivator of preventive health behavior.

- *Visualization activity.* Individuals can be stimulated to visualize or imagine how they will feel about themselves after they have made the decision to act or not to act. Will they regret their choice?

Provide Direct Experience with Food to Enhance Enjoyment of Healthful Foods

Study after study shows that taste is a powerful determinant of food choice. Taste is in some ways an anticipated outcome of eating a food, but it also has an important physiological component. To emphasize the tastiness of healthful foods, nutrition educators should design activities that include tasting foods prepared in a healthful and delicious way.

Cooking or Food Preparation

Although active participation in general (such as group activities, checklists, or self-appraisals) is important in enhancing motivation and self-efficacy, hands-on food-related activities are important enough to be considered a special category (Liquori et al. 1998; Ammerman et al. 2002). Cooking or food preparation can provide vivid and motivating experiences when participants are physically involved in the activities (that is, not just watching a food demonstration). An example is the Cookshop Program, in which students were actively involved in cooking in classrooms (and eating what they cooked) (Liquori et al. 1998; Levy & Auld 2004). Classes in which students cooked were compared

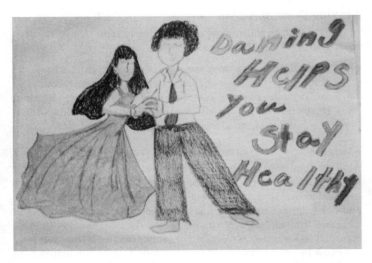

Drawing personal beliefs is a vivid example of personal motivators.

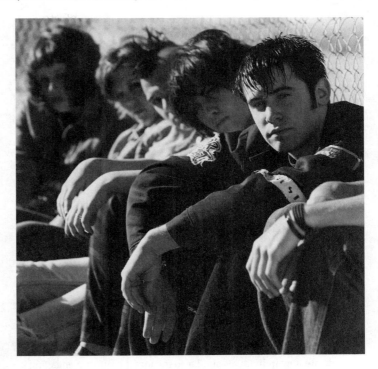

Sometimes teenage rebellion can be a factor in dietary decision making.

with classes that involved active hands-on activities but did not include preparing food. Although both groups increased in knowledge, only the group that cooked changed its behavior to eat more of the whole grains and vegetables that were offered in the school lunch.

Educational Strategies and Activities Derived from the Theory Construct of Social and Descriptive Norms

Increase Awareness of Social Norms and Descriptive Norms

Social norms or social expectations (injunctive norms) and descriptive norms (experiential norms) also are important mediators of behavior, as you have seen. You can design activities in which groups or intended audience members can be made aware of the influence of social norms on their behaviors.

- *Analyze television and print ads.* For example, mothers in the Women, Infants and Children (WIC) program can be provided with activities that analyze TV and print ads about women as mothers feeding their children and can be asked to share their feelings about the ads. Schoolchildren can be asked to conduct a survey of Saturday morning food ads, analyze them, and design an ad campaign they think would be effective in increasing the consumption of fruits and vegetables.
- *Analyze and reflect on social expectations (social norms).* You can assist the groups to identify what important others think they should be doing, such as their spouses', partners', or mothers' approval or disapproval of breastfeeding (injunctive norms), or their doctors' approval that they are eating foods lower in salt for their hypertension.
- *Analyze and reflect on attitudes and behaviors of others (descriptive norms).* Group members can analyze the many other social sources of influences on food choice, such as when eating at work,

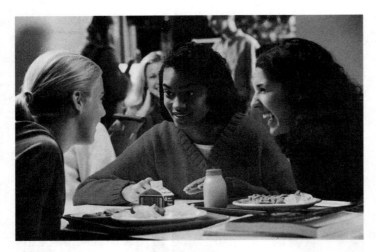

The influence of peers affects the eating patterns of adolescents.

in the cafeteria, and at home, or eating out with friends. That is, what do members of their social networks feel and do about the program targeted behaviors?

- *Social modeling.* Materials, films, and statistics can be used to indicate how individuals similar to the target group are engaging in the healthful behaviors, such as other WIC women breastfeeding, other teenagers drinking water instead of sweetened beverages, and so forth (descriptive norms).

  You can use sports figures for adolescents, either in person or through other channels such as videos or brochures. You can discuss your own experiences or that of other credible social models. When designing mass media communications, whether visual or print, you can use messages from important people with whom audience members identify. Posters can be designed that show attractive people like themselves (e.g., other schoolchildren or other WIC mothers) enjoying eating the particular foods being emphasized in the intervention.

- *Peer educators.* You can use peer educators to deliver the nutrition education, as has been done effectively in programs with adolescents, families, and older adults.

Educational Strategies for the Theory Construct of Beliefs About the Self

Clarify Self-Representation and Self-Evaluative Beliefs

Self-representations such as self-identity or social identity can be explored.

- *Self-evaluative activities.* You can use written reflection activities for individuals to explore such issues as "I think of myself as a health-conscious consumer," "I think of myself as someone who is concerned about environmental issues," "I think of myself as a good mother," and so forth. In a group where conditions are safe (see Chapter 15), these activities can be done as a group. You can also use the strategy of self-reevaluation from the transtheoretical model (TTM) to help individuals assess their images of themselves and rethink these images in positive terms.

- *Personal responsibilities and moral obligations.* Develop discussion questions or activities to explore individuals' perceptions about their responsibilities and moral obligations, both personal

and social (e.g., as a mother, a spouse, a citizen), in relation to the focus issue of your nutrition education session or program.

- *Personal ideals.* Help individuals explore ideal-self versus actual-self discrepancies by devising messages or activities to help individuals become aware of their ideals, where they come from, and how realistic or healthful they are. Individuals can then make decisions about how to handle this awareness. In similar fashion, ought-to-be self versus actual-self discrepancies can be explored through activities that bring to awareness sources of the "oughts," such as being a good mother or being thin, and how to handle them. Active methods of self-exploration and understanding, debates of pros and cons, and discussions are likely to be the most effective strategies, although films and written materials can also be helpful if used appropriately.

Educational Strategies and Activities Derived from the Theory Construct of Habits and Routines

Bring to Consciousness Automatic Behaviors, Habits, or Routines

Many of people's behaviors appear to occur without much thought. Indeed, habit or routines are important motivators of behavior. As you have seen, this results from the frequent pairing of foods and situations in which they are consumed. Nutrition education activities can bring to awareness such attitude–situation cues so that individuals can choose to change behaviors if they wish.

- *Awareness of current routines and habits.* You can devise activities to assist individuals to identify cues that seem to trigger behavior directly and unknowingly (such as the smell of baked products or the sight of ice cream) or to identify the chain of events leading to eating a second helping so that individuals will be conscious of what they are doing.

- *Replacing routines.* Nutrition education activities can be designed to bring the less positive routines (e.g., eating high-calorie snacks) to consciousness so that they can be considered and replaced by more positive routines or habits. Because these more positive behaviors may require more effort (e.g., cutting up fruits and vegetables), tip sheets, checklists, or activities can be designed to assist individuals to develop the new routines.

Provide Cues to Action

In many instances, individuals are motivated to some degree but need reminders to take action.

- *Physical cues.* Refrigerator magnets, bookmarks, grocery bags, and pencils with messages on them can provide cues to action. Mass media messages can also be very useful. Billboard messages can serve this role. You can also use more intensive methods, such as telephone calls, email messages, or mailed reminders.

Example

A nutrition intervention at a college campus based on social cognitive theory illustrates how a variety of the strategies described here were used to increase students' awareness, attitudes, outcome expectations, and behavior-related how-to knowledge to increase the behaviors of increased fruit and vegetable intake and decreased fat intake. The program, called Right Bite, is discussed in **Nutrition Education in Action 11-3**. Note the many theory variables that were addressed and the activities used to address them.

NUTRITION EDUCATION IN ACTION **11-3**

The Right Bite: A Nutrition Education Program for College Students Using Social Cognitive Theory

Right Bite Components	Description	Individual Responsible for Implementation	Social Cognitive Theory Constructs
Small group presentations	Nutrition education to small student groups. About 10 different presentations were prepared.	Peer educators	Outcome expectations
Personal follow-up (diet analysis)	One-on-one nutrition assessment and evaluation.	Peer educators	Outcome expectations; behavioral knowledge
Poster campaign	Campus role models such as the president of the college and well-known faculty members were featured in posters throughout campus.	Students in nutrition department	Outcome expectations; reinforcement; situation
Dorm contests	Healthy eating scavenger hunt.	Peer educators	Reinforcement; situation
Information tables at high-traffic areas	Nutrition information presented informally. Tables were supervised by peer educators.	Peer educators	Reinforcement
Brochure racks in dorms	Selected nutrition and exercise information was offered at dorms. Peer educators were responsible for replenishing supplies.	Peer educators	Behavioral knowledge; reinforcement
"Dear Foody" column in the campus newsletter	Brief newspaper column giving quick nutrition tips. Addressed topics of interest or concern to students.	Graduate assistant	Outcome expectations; impediments
Point-of-purchase information in campus cafeteria and vending machines	Specific nutrition analysis information about food choices.	Graduate assistant and cafeteria employees	Reinforcement
Website	Presented general program and nutrition information.	Graduate assistant	Reinforcement; impediments
Cafeteria tours	Offered specific tips on developing a healthy eating style.	Peer educators	Outcome expectations; impediments
Right Bite video	Student role models illustrated benefits of healthy eating style. Addressed most barriers identified through student focus groups during the first year of implementation.	Students in the university communication department	Impediments

Source: Evans, M. E., and M. K. Sawyer-Morse. 2002. The Right Bite Program: A theory-based nutrition intervention at a minority college campus. *Journal of the American Dietetic Association* 102(Suppl):589–593. Used with permission of the American Dietetic Association.

Designing Education Strategies and Activities to Address Behavioral Intentions

After the nutrition education activities have provided individuals with the opportunity to become more aware of their personal wants, feelings, and behaviors, to understand their own motivations and the factors that seem to control their behaviors, and to deliberate on the issues, you should now provide them with the opportunity to resolve any ambivalences that they have and to make a decision to take action, or not to do so, given their life circumstances.

Individuals' attitudes and their beliefs about the outcomes of a behavior are numerous and may often conflict and compete. Ambivalence reflects the coexistence within individuals of both positive and negative beliefs about outcomes for the same behavior (e.g., eating chocolate is both delicious and fattening), as well as numerous conflicting feelings or attitudes. Individuals can pursue many alternative wishes or actions,

and they will have to select among them. This is especially true for food choices and dietary behaviors.

The following sections describe several strategies that you may find useful to activate decision making, assist individuals to resolve ambivalences, and facilitate the formation of a behavioral intention or a goal intention. These strategies involve both cognitive and affective domains. In general they involve individuals' evaluations of the feasibility and desirability of the action or practice. Several of these strategies are similar to the transtheoretical model's strategies for self-reevaluation and self-liberation.

Provide Opportunity to Analyze the Pros and Cons of Action: Decisional Balance

- *Evaluating costs and benefits of taking action.* Nutrition educators can provide opportunities for individuals to analyze all the benefits or pros of taking action and the cons or costs of taking action through worksheets or discussions. Individuals should also examine the reverse—that is, what they will lose by *not* taking action. This can be done using a pros and cons grid similar to the following:

	Pros	Cons
If I don't take given action		
If I do take given action		

Participants can then make a decision as to whether to take action.

- *Choices among several alternatives.* Individuals do not make decisions about taking action in a vacuum. Any given action is an alternative among several potential actions: for example, eating fruit for dessert or eating cheesecake, breastfeeding or bottle-feeding, and going running or working or watching television. Worksheets thus should help individuals evaluate and make choices among alternative behaviors competing for their time and attention.

Assist Groups to Clarify Their Values

Values are an important basis for action. As you have seen, individuals are motivated to take action if the action will lead to outcomes or goals they value. Short-term goals are instrumental values, such as taste, losing weight, looking attractive, or being liked by friends. These are the outcome expectations discussed earlier.

However, people also make choices based on larger, end-state values, such as self-respect, sense of accomplishment, equality, social recognition, pleasure, true friendship, an exciting life, a world of beauty, inner harmony, freedom, happiness, mature love, wisdom, a worthwhile life, and so forth (Rokeach 1973; Buchanan 2000). For some individuals, these values are much more important than short-term, instrumental values. Again, individuals need to clarify for themselves how their current behaviors relate to these larger values and what changing these behaviors would mean to them in terms of these values.

Several activities can be used to assist people to clarify their values.

- *Value statements.* You can present some value statements and ask participants to discuss or explore them in dyads and triads.
- *Visual imagery.* One powerful activity that will help participants understand and process their feelings is to assemble pictures from magazines, photographs taken in the community, or drawings showing people engaging in different food- or health-related activities such as shopping for food, going to a farmers' market, preparing food, breastfeeding, eating at fast food restaurants, weighing themselves, or running. Show these pictures to participants and have them either write down or verbally report the feelings evoked by each picture. The answers can be coded, tallied, and reported back to the group as a whole to discuss. Participants may be surprised at their own feelings in response to the pictures as well as those of others. The next phase is to explore why particular emotions or feelings came up and to develop some understanding of these feelings, especially the problematic ones. The group can then come up with some ways to explain the problems depicted or implied by the pictures and to solve them. The Freiere *conscientizacion* process involves this process (Freiere 1970, 1973).

Resolving Resistance and Ambivalence

To be effective, nutrition education strategies and messages need to enhance positive thoughts, feelings, and a sense of empowerment to take actions in recipients. Inevitably, however, group participants or message recipients may resist what is being said. Resistance to change can be useful because it contributes to human consistency and prevents people from constantly swinging from one opinion or behavior to another. Manoff (1985) points out that potential cognitive and emotional "resistance points" of the audience, or their barriers to taking action, must be known and understood by nutrition educators. Nutrition educators should not try to talk people out of their resistance (it will not work anyway) but instead respect their position, express understanding, suggest alternative ways to think about the issue, and help them make choices.

That is, the effectiveness of nutrition education is improved if the potential internal dialogues of the audience disagreeing with the message are acknowledged, empathy with them is expressed, counterarguments are provided where appropriate or reassurance is given that the doubts do not interfere with taking action, and a way is provided for people to be able to comfortably give up the resistance or to state they are not ready to take action or do not wish to take action. This does not imply manipulation of the audience. On the contrary, it means understanding the social, cultural, religious beliefs and practices, economic conditions, and political realities of the audience and making the nutrition message relevant and actionable.

Addressing Ambivalence and Resistance

Nutrition educators need to assist individuals to resolve their ambivalences and objections, but not in a defensive way. The task is to present the other side in a neutral, professional tone. Here, sample dialogue that aims to dispel doubts is given for three examples of internal dialogues or objections of program participants:

Internal dialogue of group participant or message recipient: "My grandfather ate a high-fat diet and smoked all his life and didn't get heart disease, so why should I worry?"

Nutrition educator: "Some of you may have had a grandfather or grandmother who ate unhealthy diets and smoked and yet lived to a ripe old age. However, that grandparent was lucky. You may or may not be so lucky. If that grandparent had 50 friends and half of them practiced poor health habits (as your grandparent did) and the other half ate healthful foods, exercised, and did not smoke, on the average the latter group would live longer, healthier lives. Taking care of yourself lowers your risk of developing chronic diseases such as cancer, heart disease, and stroke."

Internal dialogue: "My mother is always bugging me about doing the right thing to control my diabetes. I hate being told what to do—I'm just not going to do it!"

Nutrition educator: Teenagers are often angry at their parents, and counterargument would not be listened to. Using an acknowledging approach, the communication with newly diagnosed teenage diabetics might go like this: "I am sure that for many of you, your mothers tend to nag you about taking care of your diabetes. But controlling your diabetes is not your mother's job—it's yours. Consider following your doctor's instructions, but not for your mother's sake. Do it for yourself. You are worth it. Your mother means well; you need only to reassure her that you've got it under control, and that her way of showing concern is not helpful."

Internal dialogue: "What you say I should do is so difficult. I'm feeling powerless."

Nutrition educator: What persons like this need is encouragement. Try a reassuring communication: "What I've recommended to you need not be accomplished in one day. Even the highest slopes can only be climbed one step at a time. Making changes to eat more ecologically is no different. You can't change the ways things are all at once. Think about one small step you are ready to change—today. For example, you may decide that you will bring your own bag to the grocery store to carry back your groceries rather than have the store put groceries in plastic bags. When you feel good about your progress, you can move on to the next action."

Other internal dialogues of program participants might include the following:

- "What you are saying is so complicated you are making me feel incompetent!"
- "You can talk all you want about eating more fruits and vegetables, but stores in my neighborhood don't carry many of them, and they're expensive."
- "Often I don't do all I'm supposed to do for my hypertension, and nothing bad happens, so I'm not going to take all this too seriously."
- "My mother never breastfed me and I turned out all right. Also, none of my friends are breastfeeding, so why should I breastfeed my infant?"

Formation of behavioral intentions is best facilitated if you know the specific potential internal dialogues, ambivalences, and objections most commonly occurring in a given group, talk about them and resolve them in a presentation, or provide opportunities for the group members to discuss them openly and resolve them in the group discussion.

Group Decision Making and Public Commitment

Individuals are more likely to follow through with a specific action or behavior pattern if their attitudes and commitments are made public than if they are kept private, particularly if their peers hold them accountable for fulfilling their commitments. To the extent that individuals, acting in the absence of coercion, make a commitment in front of others to take action, they come to see themselves as believers in that kind of activity. In addition, taking a stand publicly makes the action less likely to be denied or forgotten and more resistant to challenge in subsequent situations when the behavior can be enacted (Halverson & Pallack 1978).

Group Decision Studies of Kurt Lewin

As a result of his research on such issues as group dynamics and social influence, social psychologist Lewin concludes that commitment to an action is greater when social influence or the social support of the group is involved. During World War II, when food rationing and conservation were important concerns, Lewin conducted a series of experiments to change food habits (Lewin 1943; Radke & Caso 1948). He compared several methods with a "group decision" method in which group dis-

cussion was followed by the group setting definite goals for action. These goals could be set up by the group for the group as a whole or by each individual in the group setting. Either way, a public decision was made to try the targeted behavior, through a show of hands or verbal statements. No attempt was made to force a decision, and neither were high-pressure sales techniques used.

- *Study with stay-at-home women.* In one study with homemakers, the target behavior was using organ meats such as hearts, lungs, liver, and kidneys instead of the more common cuts of meat. In the control group (or lecture condition), a nutritionist discussed the advantages of using organ meats—low cost, nutritional value, and importance to the war effort. The information was provided in an enthusiastic but formal lecture format, with no group interaction. Recipes for "delicious dishes" were handed out.

  In the group decision situation, the nutritionist very briefly discussed similar information as for the lecture situation. The group then exchanged views on potential barriers to using organ meats (e.g., their families might not like kidneys, kidneys smell bad during cooking). The nutritionist made suggestions from time to time for dealing with these barriers, but only after group members themselves had expressed their concerns and discussed with each other ways to overcome the barriers. Group members then publicly voted on their decision to serve organ meats during the following week. In follow-up interviews in the women's homes seven days later, it was found that only 10% of the women in the lecture condition reported serving one of the three targeted organ meats, whereas 52% of the women in the group decision method condition reported trying one of these meats.
- *Study with college students.* In the second study, a request for change (via an announcement) was compared with group decision for increasing the intake of whole-wheat bread by male college students in dormitory settings.
- *Mothers of infants.* A third study compared individual instruction with group decision for getting mothers to give their babies the proper amount of cod liver oil and orange juice. These two comparisons also demonstrated that the group decision method was substantially more effective in changing behavior than the other methods were.

Family Heart Study

The group decision method of Lewin was used with success more recently in the Family Heart Study (Carmody et al. 1986), which was designed to reduce the risk of cardiovascular disease. About 200 families met monthly in small groups of 8 to 12 families over a five-year period. At each meeting, the nutritionist was present and provided some educational activities. However, much of the time was devoted to group members sharing successes and problems and then making a group decision and public commitment for actions that families would take during the coming month.

Summary

These studies indicate that a process wherein groups of peers mutually share concerns, ask for public commitments from each other, and then hold each other accountable for fulfilling their commitments to the group can exert a powerful effect on individuals' self-image, commitment, and action taking. Nutrition educators can encourage such group decision and public commitment to assist individuals to bridge the intention–behavior gap.

Intention Formation

Educational strategies can assist individuals to evaluate the desirability and feasibility of taking a particular action or making a particular behavior change and then make a decision. If they decide to take action, their decision is then their behavioral intention or goal intention.

- *Clear statement of intention of goal.* It is best to assist individuals to clearly state their behavioral intention, preferably in writing (e.g., through a commitment form, contract, pledge). Alternatively, they can make the commitment orally in the group. As discussed earlier, when group participants make public commitments, they hold each other accountable and also provide social support to each other to fulfill their commitments.

   In the context of a nutrition education program, this intention is usually the program's behavioral goal. If the program's behavioral goal is quite specific, such as for program participants to eat four or more cups of fruits and vegetables daily, the behavioral intention is stated as "I intend to eat four or more cups of fruits and vegetables daily." If the program's goal is quite broad, such as healthy eating, then individuals will choose actions they want to take to achieve the goal and express their personal, individualized goal. How to assist individuals to translate these intentions into action is the subject of the next chapter.

■ ORGANIZING AND SEQUENCING EDUCATIONAL STRATEGIES AND ACTIVITIES FOR IMPLEMENTATION: THE EDUCATIONAL OR LESSON PLAN

As noted earlier, instruction can be seen as the deliberate arrangement of events in the individual's environment to make learning happen and to make it effective (Gagne et al. 2004). A theory of instruction is thus about how to select and arrange educational activities *events of instruction* to provide support for the internal processes of learning. Such a theory provides nutrition educators with practical guidance on how to arrange educational strategies within a session or over several sessions into an instructional sequence, leading to a *plan for instruction, lesson plan,* or *educational plan.*

Table 11-2 presents a way to organize and sequence these events of instruction—that is, how you will sequence the various activities you will carry out during sessions. It is based on Gagne's theory of instruction (Gagne 1965, 1985; Gagne et al. 2004), which has been widely used to design instruction using a variety of media (e.g., oral, written, computer-based, Web-based) for a variety of audiences (e.g., children, adults) and modified for health education design (Kinzie 2005) and on McGuire's step model of health communications (McGuire 1984). It also takes into account sequencing based on consideration of different learning styles, which is discussed in detail in Chapter 15.

This sequence is as follows:

- *Gain attention (A).* Devise activities to gain attention, pique interest, and increase awareness. Visuals, striking statistics, or personal stories that increase awareness of risk or of benefits to taking action or concrete experiences such as self-assessments are helpful here. In ongoing programs, review, reflection, and sharing are appropriate.
- *Present stimulus and new material (S).* Take into consideration the audience's prior knowledge, experience, and values. Here, focus

TABLE 11-2	**Sequencing Nutrition Education Strategies Within Session**
Sequence of Events of Instruction	**Theory-Based Nutrition Education Strategies**
Gain attention (A)	*Use attention-getter that is personally relevant for audience about behavioral goal, for example*
	• Risk information or self-assessment
	• Health benefits
	For ongoing sessions: Review and reflect
Present stimulus or new material (S)	*Tailor messages to audience's prior knowledge and values*
	Outcome expectations or perceived benefits: Demonstrate effectiveness of the desired behavior
	Affective attitudes: Increase reflection on affect/feelings about taking action
	Barriers/self-efficacy: Make desired action easy to understand and do
Provide guidance and practice (G)	*Provide food- and nutrition-related knowledge and cognitive skills to engage in actions*
	Use credible social models
Apply and close (C)	*Enhance application*
	Goal setting and action plans
	Provide social supports

on motivation by demonstrating the effectiveness of goal behaviors of the program for health outcomes or emphasize personal benefits. Make the desired action easy to understand and do. Use mini-lectures, learning activities, and visual presentations.

- *Provide guidance and practice (G).* Provide the knowledge and skills participants will need for the desired action. To take into account learning styles, use role models to demonstrate action, and hands-on activities to gain practice and mastery and hence increase self-efficacy.
- *Apply and close (C).* Help participants consider how they will apply what has been learned and write a personal action plan (or implementation intention). For ongoing sessions or a program, strengthen self-regulation skills and personal agency. Provide social support for participants' action plans. Summarize, wrap up, and bring the session to closure. Participants should be clear about the central messages of the session.

Motivational or promotional activities are usually conducted first, whether within a session, over a series of sessions, or in a multicomponent nutrition education intervention. The nutrition science information you present in this phase is of a *why-to* nature. However, motivational activities are still needed throughout the intervention to promote active deliberation and to reinforce motivation.

Strategies to facilitate the ability to take action usually follow motivational activities. The food and nutrition information you present and self-regulation skills participants practice in this phase are of a *how-to* nature.

This sequencing is useful for all types of sessions. This general sequence should be used for all sessions. If you do not have much time, you can select one or two strategies within each event of instruction to focus on but still address both motivational and skills objectives within the same session. If you have the opportunity to conduct several sessions, you may want to start with the motivational-phase activities and continue with action-phase activities in the second and later sessions. This has a downside—the same participants may not come to all sessions. Or you may be working with an already motivated group—mothers who want to know how to feed their children, for example, or those at risk of diabetes who want guidance on what to eat. Even in this instance it is helpful to start each session with an attention-getter, and then provide short motivational activities to strengthen the group's attitudes, reinvigorate their motivation, and renew their commitment to act before moving into skill building in the food and nutrition area and in self-regulation.

Sequencing by the Transtheoretical Model's Stages of Change

You can also sequence educational activities and learning by individuals' stage of readiness to make dietary changes. **Table 11-3** describes the 10 processes of change of the transtheoretical model. Educational activities that facilitate the movement through the stages of motivational readiness form a sequence rather similar to the events of instruction and steps of health communication just described. Although all the processes of change are used in all stages, in general experiential processes are used more often during the early stages of motivational readiness, and behavioral processes are used more often during the later stages of change. In the early stages, the experiential processes of change emphasized are consciousness-raising, dramatic relief, environmental reevaluation, and self-reevaluation.

In the later stages, the processes often used for behavior change are the relapse prevention strategies of counterconditioning, management of reinforcements, control of environmental stimuli, and social liberation

| TABLE 11-3 | Transtheoretical Model: Processes Associated with Stages of Change and Implications for Intervention Strategies |

Processes of Change	Stages When More Often Used	Brief Description of Change Process Within the Individual	Intervention Strategies
Consciousness-raising	PC to C	Increasing one's awareness about causes and consequences, seeking new information about healthy behavior	Increase awareness of individuals' eating patterns (e.g., F&V intake) through self-assessment and feedback, confrontations, media campaigns
Dramatic relief/ emotional arousal	PC to C	Emotional experience of threat followed by relief if action is taken	Personalizing risk, personal testimonies, role playing, trigger films, media campaigns to address feelings
Environmental reevaluation	PC to C	Assessing how one's behaviors affect others and the physical environment	Empathy training, documentaries
Self-reevaluation	C to Prep to A	Appraisal of one's image of oneself	Assisting individuals to clarify their values; imagining themselves as active and healthy; believing that behavior change is part of their identity
Self-liberation	C to Prep to A	Believing in ability to change; consciously making a firm commitment to act	Commitment-enhancing techniques such as contracting and public group decisions
Helping relationships	A to M	Enlisting social support for the healthy behavior change	Build rapport; create a supportive environment through groups, buddy systems, and calls
Counterconditioning	A to M	Substituting alternative thoughts and behaviors for less healthful eating behaviors	Teach new ways of thinking (self-talk) about behavior; new food- and nutrition-related skills
Reinforcement and rewards management	M	Increasing rewards for healthful eating and decreasing rewards for unhealthful eating practices	Overt rewards such as tee-shirts; incentives; verbal reinforcement; teaching individuals to reward themselves
Stimulus or environmental control	M	Removing cues to less healthful eating and adding cues for more healthful eating	Provide instruction on how to restructure environment; refrigerator magnets with reminders; tip sheets
Social liberation	All	Selecting and advocating for environments that support healthful food practices	Provide environmental supports such as more F&V in schools or worksites; advocacy; policy

Note: PC = precontemplation; C = contemplation; Prep = preparation; A = action; M = maintenance; F&V = fruits and vegetables.

(see Chapter 5 for details). Consequently, if you wish to design educational activities and learning experiences by stages of change, you can use intervention activities that are appropriate for each stage.

■ CASE STUDY

We now apply the information in this chapter specifically to the ongoing case study. Most educational plans should address both motivational mediators as well as facilitators of action. The sequence usually is for motivational activities to be conducted first, followed by skills building and application activities. Because there are so many mediators, strategies, and activities that could be used, for illustration purposes the case study presents the educational plan or lesson plan outlines for two hypothetical sessions—one in this chapter directed at motivational-phase strategies and one presented in Chapter 12 directed at action-phase strategies. However, for most situations, you would have both motivational and skills objectives and activities in the same session.

The Educational Plan: Features

The educational plan consists of the following features:

- The behavioral goal of the educational session or sessions from Step 1.
- The nutrition education program objectives from Step 4.
- Several general educational objectives for the session or series of sessions. These objectives convert theory variables into a format that the nutrition educator can use to create relevant educational activities. Thus, for each general objective the nutrition educator indicates the mediator that the objective seeks to address.
- Specific educational objectives and the practical activities or learning experiences that the nutrition educator creates to reach these objectives. These specific objectives and activities together will achieve the stated general objectives, the achievement of which will help the participants reach their behavioral goals.

The Educational Plan: Matrix Format for Designing the Session

The case study first presents an example of the design version of the educational plan in a matrix format.

- *In the first column* are listed each of the potential mediators of behavior change—which are also the theory constructs—from the theory model in Step 3 that the lesson will address.
- *The second column* states the specific educational objective(s) for each mediator.
- *In the third column*, we check whether the objectives cover all three domains of learning—head, heart, and hand—and include a range of complexity of objectives. These are usually arranged from most simple to most complex within a session or program.
- *The fourth column* first indicates the *theory-based strategies* (such as shown in Table 11-1) to operationalize the potential mediators, and then describes (briefly) all the practical educational activities, learning experiences, or messages that we plan to use to carry out the theory-based strategies.
- *In the final column*, we review each mediator, objective, and activity row and decide where in the sequence of instruction it would best belong (A, S, G, C). Is the activity an attention-getter (A), or is it providing new informational that is motivational (S), or is it how-to information with opportunity to practice (G), or

is it goal-setting or other closure activity (C)? This review helps the nutrition educator sequence activities during the session appropriately.

Back and Forth Between Objectives and Activities

In designing the educational plan for the case study, we went back and forth between objectives and activities. As we viewed the objectives, we thought of interesting and relevant activities that we could create to help the middle school students achieve the objectives. We then carefully reviewed the extent to which these activities would address the objectives set forth. The result of this back-and-forth approach is the lesson plan that is shown.

Re-Arrange Sequence

We then re-arranged the sequence of the items in the design matrix so that they are in the order that we will use to conduct the activities—A, S, G, C. The final re-arranged design matrix is shown in the case study.

The Educational Plan: Narrative or Teaching Format for Delivering the Session

For use in actually delivering the educational plan to the middle schoolers, the design matrix is converted into a narrative or teaching format. This teaching format for the session is also shown in the case study.

■ YOUR TURN: COMPLETING THE STEP 5 WORKSHEETS: STRATEGIES AND THE EDUCATIONAL OR LESSON PLAN

You can now apply the information in this chapter to state general and specific educational objectives for a session and design of educational strategies to address the mediators that you identified and the educational objectives that you have stated. These strategies should then be sequenced into an instructional plan for how to proceed, showing the events of instruction. The resulting plan goes by many names, such as the *lesson plan* or *education plan* for a single session, a *curriculum* for several sequenced sessions, a *media message plan*, or the *intervention guide* for an intervention with many components. Designing activities is a very fluid process in which you go back and forth between designing activities and sequencing them appropriately. After pilot testing, you may want to change or rearrange activities.

Sequencing Activities Is Important

How exactly you arrange your sequence of educational strategies depends on many factors that are specific to the needs of your audience and the theory guiding your intervention. In general, though, you want to begin each session with activities to gain the attention of the group, move to activities to enhance motivation and promote contemplation by presenting new material that builds on what they already know and can do, and then focus on activities to build skills and strengthen self-efficacy or collective efficacy. Some kind of closure or take-home message is important. Help the group to consider how to apply the message, perhaps through some kind of personal or group action plan. These events of instruction have been labeled in this chapter as: gain attention (A), present stimulus or new material (S), provide guidance and practice (G), and apply and close (C) (refer to Table 11-2). The same systematic process is needed for the design of all nutrition education messages and activities, such as brochures, newsletters, posters, media messages, or campaigns.

The Educational or Lesson Plan: Using a Matrix Format to Design the Education Plan

It is useful to first develop a lesson or educational plan outline using a matrix format as shown in the worksheet and case study. Here, you first state the behavioral goal of the session, and then write general educational objectives to achieve the behavioral goal. These objectives should be directed at the key mediators of change. You then write specific objectives for each of the mediators that your theory suggests that you address. Achievement of these specific objectives can help the group participants achieve the desired behavioral goals. You then create learning experiences, activities, and content that will achieve the specific objectives. The matrix format enables you to see whether you have addressed all the educational objectives that you set and whether the activities are appropriate in terms of domain of learning and level of complexity. The information in Chapters 15 and 17 about practical tips for working with a wide range of groups is very helpful here as you design your educational sessions.

The Educational or Lesson Plan: Developing a Teaching Format to Deliver the Plan

You then convert the matrix into a more detailed narrative lesson plan that you will actually use when you are with a group. The case study provides a sample lesson plan showing how the matrix format is used to design the session and how the narrative or teaching format is used for delivery. Use the worksheet at the end of this chapter to develop your educational plan for a real or hypothetical educational session.

- Think of a catchy title that will be meaningful to your audience. It should motivate people to come to your session or pique their interest if they are required to attend.
- Place an overview or outline of activities and a materials list at the beginning of the teaching plan. That way you will have the entire session in mind and all of the materials ready.
- For each educational activity, create a heading with a title and indicate the mediator(s) addressed.
- Convert each of the activities in the matrix into a fuller description or narrative. Include all the specific information you will need when you are with the group.
- Write the educational plan such that someone else could deliver it.

- Be prepared. If the session involves a food preparation activity, make sure you have tested the recipes and that you have prepped the foods so they are ready for the participants (such as fruits and vegetables washed, stems cut off, etc.).
- Sequence the activities based on an order of instruction. You can use the one described in this chapter based on the work of education instruction specialists (Gagne et al. 2004): gain attention, present stimulus or new material, provide guidance and practice, and apply and close. If the session involves hands-on activities, think through the flow—will it work with the size of group that you have?
- A sense of closure is especially important. This is a good time to provide an opportunity to apply what the audience has learned. A clear take-home message or simple action intention or plan will be very useful.

Pilot Testing the Educational Plan

If your program is more than a one-time event, all the learning experiences designed should be extensively pilot tested with the intended audience. If food is used, test the recipes and preparation procedures for taste acceptance and feasibility. Using focus groups, direct observation, and interviews, assess whether activities are acceptable and effective with the intended audience.

Educational Plans in Practice

The educational plan or lesson plan formats as presented here may seem quite specific, detailed, and almost rigid. It is important to have such a plan, but it is understood that you will apply the education lesson plans fluidly in the actual setting. You may find yourself needing to adapt the lessons to the situation on the ground. At the same time, even approaches that seem very informal with a strong focus on learner-centered education require that you develop strong, theory-based educational plans. Ideally these plans would be developed in collaboration with the intended audience. You will always interact with the group and adjust the content and activities as needed. Tips about how to deliver the educational plans in practice in a group setting and how to develop accompanying materials, such as handouts, posters, or newsletters are described in Part III of this book, which is about methods of implementing and delivering nutrition education.

Questions and Activities

1. In the context of this book, what does *learning* mean? Define and describe. How is learning related to education and behavior change?

2. Describe carefully the relationship between potential mediators, theory constructs, theory-based strategies, and diet-related action or behavior change.

3. Compare what *instruction*, *instructional framework*, and *instructional design* mean. How are these terms related to theory-based strategies and learning experiences?

4. What is a lesson plan or educational plan?

5. State the four events of instruction and a give a one- to two-sentence description of each in your own words. How do you see the sequence as useful for you? If not useful, explain why not.

6. For practice, state one educational strategy for each of the potential motivational mediators of the behavior of increasing intake of calcium-rich foods among teenage girls shown in the accompanying table. For each strategy, describe at least one educational activity or learning experience.

Potential Motivational Mediator	General Theory-Based Strategy	Specific Educational Activity or Learning Experience
Perceived risk		
Outcome expectations/ perceived benefits		
Perceived risk		
Affect/feelings		
Behavioral intention		

References

Ammerman, A. S., C. H. Lindquist, K. N. Lohr, and J. Hersey. 2002. The efficacy of behavioral interventions to modify dietary fat and fruit and vegetable intake: A review of the evidence. *Preventive Medicine* 35(1):25–41.

Armitage, C. J., and M. Conner. 2000. Social cognition models and health behavior: A structured review. *Psychology and Health* 15:173–189.

Baranowski, T., E. Cerin, and J. Baranowski. 2009. Steps in the design, development, and formative evaluation of obesity prevention-related behavior change trials. *International Journal of Behavioral Nutrition and Physical Activity* 6-6.

Baranowski, T., K. W. Cullen, T. Nicklas, D. Thompson, and J. Baranowski. 2003. Are current health behavioral change models helpful in guiding prevention of weight gain efforts? *Obesity Research* 11(Suppl.):23S–43S.

Buchanan, D. R. 2000. *An ethic for health promotion: Rethinking the sources of human well-being*. New York: Oxford University Press.

Carmody, T. P., J. Istvan, J. D. Matarazzo, S. L. Connor, and W. E. Connor. 1986. Applications of social learning theory in the promotion of heart-healthy diets: The Family Heart Study dietary intervention model. *Health Education Research* 1(1):13–27.

Contento, I., G. I. Balch, S. K. Maloney, et al. 1995. The effectiveness of nutrition education and implications for nutrition education policy, programs, and research: A review of research. *Journal of Nutrition Education* 27(6):277–422.

Dewey, J. 1929. *The sources of a science of education*. New York: Liveright.

Doak, C. M., T. L. Visscher, C. M. Renders, and J. C. Seidell. 2006. The prevention of overweight and obesity in children and adolescents: A review of interventions and programmes. *Obesity Review* 7(1):111–136.

Freiere, P. 1970. *Pedagogy of the oppressed*. New York: Continuum.

———. 1973. *Education for critical consciousness*. New York: Continuum.

Gagne, R. 1965. *The conditions of learning*. New York: Holt, Rinehart & Winston.

———. 1985. *The conditions of learning and theory of instruction*. 4th ed. New York: Holt, Rinehart & Winston.

Gagne, R., W. W. Wager, J. M. Keller, and K. Golas. 2004. *Principles of instructional design*. Boston: Cengage.

Halverson, R., and M. Pallack. 1978. Commitment, ego-involvement and resistance to attack. *Journal of Experimental Social Psychology* 14:1012.

Iowa Department of Public Health. 2005. Pick a better snack. http://www.idph.state .ia.us/pickabettersnack.

Johnson, D. W., and R. T. Johnson. 1987. Using cooperative learning strategies to teach nutrition. *Journal of the American Dietetic Association* 87(9 Suppl.): S55–S61.

Kinzie, M. B. 2005. Instructional design strategies for health behavior change. *Patient Education and Counseling* 56:3–15.

Levy, J., and G. Auld. 2004. Cooking classes outperform cooking demonstrations for college sophomores. *Journal of Nutrition Education and Behavior* 36:197–203.

Lewin, K. 1943. Forces behind food habits and methods of change. In *The problem of changing food habits. Bulletin of the National Research Council*. Washington, DC: National Research Council and National Academy of Sciences.

Liquori, T., P. D. Koch, I. R. Contento, and J. Castle. 1998. The Cookshop Program: Outcome evaluation of a nutrition education program linking lunchroom food experiences with classroom cooking experiences. *Journal of Nutrition Education* 30(5):302.

Lytle, L., and C. Achterberg. 1995. Changing the diet of America's children: What works and why? *Journal of Nutrition Education* 27(5):250–260.

Manoff, R. K. 1985. *Social marketing: New imperatives for public health*. New York: Praeger.

McGuire, W. J. 1984. Public communication as a strategy for inducing health-promoting behavioral changes. *Preventive Medicine* 13:299–313.

Petty, R. E., and J. T. Cacioppo. 1986. *Communication and persuasion: Central and peripheral routes to attitude change*. New York: Springer-Verlag.

Pomerleau, J., K. Lock, C. Knai, and M. McKee. 2005. Interventions designed to increase fruit and vegetable intake in adults can be effective: A systematic review of the literature. *Journal of Nutrition* 135:2486–2495.

Radke, M., and E. Caso. 1948. Lecture and discussion-decision as methods of influencing food habits. *Journal of the American Dietetic Association* 24:23–41.

Rokeach, M. 1973. *The nature of human values*. New York: Free Press.

Schwarzer, R. 1992. Self-efficacy in the adoption of maintenance of health behaviors: Theoretical approaches and a new model. In *Self-efficacy: Thought control of action*, edited by R. Schwarzer. Washington, DC: Hemisphere.

Shaya, F. T., D. Flores, C. M. Gbarayor, and J. Wang. 2008. School-based obesity interventions: A literature review. *Journal of School Health* 78(4):189–196.

Tyler, R. W. 1949. *Basic principles of curriculum and instruction*. Chicago: University of Chicago Press.

In Step 5, you use your theoretical model, philosophy of nutrition education, and nutrition education program objectives to create (1) educational plans for the individual-level components and (2) environmental support plans for environmental/policy components.

These pages of the Step 5 worksheets are devoted to designing educational plans for activities directed at individuals, referred to here as the individual-level components. Generally, the primary individual-level component consists of one or more group sessions. (You can also use these worksheets to design other individual-level components, such as newsletters and media-related activities.)

You should have **one** educational plan for **each** group session you design (or newsletter or other component directed at individuals).

At the end of the Step 5 worksheets for the individual-level components, you will have the following products:

Step 5A: General educational objectives for each session or series of sessions directed at the same behavioral goal

Step 5B: An overall design plan for the session in the form of a matrix that links mediators, objectives, and activities

Step 5C: A narrative educational plan that translates the matrix into a form ready for teaching or presenting

Use these worksheets as an organizational guide to help you design your educational plan and translate theory mediators into educational activities. Electronic versions of these worksheets are available at http://nutrition.jbpub.com/education/2e/. If you are unable to access the worksheets electronically, you can write onto this blank worksheet or create a text document that uses the same flow of information.

> **NOTE:** For the case study, we present educational plans that focus on only one of the program's goal behaviors: increasing fruit and vegetable intake. Generally, educational plans include activities based on both motivating and facilitating mediators. For illustrative purposes, we present two lessons and divide them into one educational plan that focuses primarily on motivational mediators (Chapter 11) and a second educational plan that focuses on facilitators of behavior change (Chapter 12). We have done this to highlight the numerous strategies and activities that are possible for addressing motivating and facilitating mediators.

Step 5A: General educational objectives

Educational plan title: The Whys of Colorful Eating (educational plan focusing on potential motivating mediators)

Program goal behaviors: Students will increase their fruit and vegetable intake (youth to aim for 2.5 or more cups per day).

Write the general educational objectives.

Mediator (from Step 3)	General educational objectives
Physical outcome expectations (perceived benefits)	Demonstrate understanding and appreciation of the importance of eating a variety of fruits and vegetables
Physical outcome expectations (perceived risk)	Evaluate their own intake of fruits and vegetables compared with recommendations
Physical outcome expectations (barriers)	Identify barriers to intake of fruits and vegetables and propose ways to overcome them
Physical outcome expectations (perceived benefits)	Express enjoyment of, and positive attitudes toward, eating a variety of fruits and vegetables
Goal intention	State intention to increase own fruit and vegetable intake

Step 5B: Designing the educational plan: matrix format

Design your educational (or lesson) plan in matrix format. Write specific objectives for the mediators in your theory model (Step 3). Identify the learning domain and level for each objective. Then write the theory-based strategy you will employ to address the mediator and create educational activities that will be meaningful, interesting, and appropriate for your audience and will operationalize strategy.

Sequence your educational activities based on the events of instruction. After you have completed creating activities for each of the mediators in your theory model, go back through the design matrix and carefully identify each of the strategies/activities as to where it should fall in a sequence suitable for implementing with your audience. Label each activity as to whether it will be used to (A) gain attention, (S) present stimulus or new material, (G) provide guidance and practice, or (C) apply and close the session. These are referred to as the "Events of Instruction" or "EoI."

Carefully re-order the matrix. If the mediators and the related activities you have created are not listed at first in your matrix in the properly sequenced order (i.e., gain attention to apply and close), then carefully re-order the matrix so all activities as well as mediators and objectives are in the proper sequenced order ready to use to create your educational plan or teaching plan.

Mediator (from Step 3)	Specific educational objectives	Learning domain / level*	Theory-based** strategy and educational activities, experiences, and/or content	EoI
Physical outcome expectations (perceived benefits)	State benefits of eating F&V: energy; hair and skin; build strong bones and muscles State the key reasons for eating a variety of F&V ("a rainbow of colors")	C: comprehension A: valuing	Health benefits/pros of behavior** •Create list of group's perceived benefits of F&V on newsprint. •Emphasize the need for variety of intake (a colorful plate). List the five colors: blue/purple, green, white, yellow/orange, red. •Provide scientific evidence that eating F&V makes for strong bodies; clear up misconceptions.	A/S
Physical outcome expectations (perceived risk)	Describe risks to health from eating too few F&V Evaluate personal risk of not eating enough F&V	C: comprehension A: valuing	Self-assessment; personalizing risk** •Checklist or recall of own intake of F&V and compare with recommendation for number and colors.	S
Barriers/self-efficacy	Identify barriers to eating F&V Propose ways to overcome barriers to eating F&V Describe ways in which F&V can be easy to eat	C: comprehension A: valuing	Overcoming barriers** •Group brainstorms barriers to eating F&V; list on newsprint. •Group brainstorms ways to overcome barriers. •Group discusses ways to make behavior easy to do.	G
Social norms	Describe the role of peers in influencing food choices Appreciate that vegetables are cool to eat	A: valuing	Exposing peer pressure; modeling** •Students express what peers say when they eat F&V. •Provide relevant models (media models, stories) eating F&V, showing it is cool.	G
Benefits	Appreciate that fruits and vegetables taste good	A: valuing	Direct experience with food** •Provide a fruit salad or vegetables/dips for tasting.	G
Goal intention	Evaluate the pros and cons of eating a variety of colors State an intention to add a fruit/vegetable a day to diet	C: evaluation A: valuing	Values clarification and decisional balance** •Group activity: present value statements and discuss in group. •Individual worksheet record pros and cons of eating more F&V. •Make individual decisions about actions to take.	C
*C = cognitive domain; A = affective domain; P = psychomotor domain.				

Step 5C: Educational plan

Write a narrative educational plan, based on your design matrix, that you will actually use to deliver your session. Think of a catchy title that will be meaningful to your audience. Make sure that activities are sequenced based on order of instruction. For each educational activity create a heading with a title and the mediator(s) addressed. Then write a detailed procedure for the activity. It is customary to place an overview or outline of activities and a materials list at the beginning of the teaching plan.

The Whys of Colorful Eating

Overview of Content (50 to 60 minutes)
1. Introduction: overview and gain attention
2. Brainstorm and record on newsprint the benefits of eating F&V
3. Emphasize importance of different colors
4. Fill out 24-hour recall checklist to assess colorfulness of F&V intake
5. Brainstorm and use newsprint to record barriers to eating F&V
6. Brainstorm ways to overcome barriers/discuss how to make eating all the colors of the rainbow easier
7. Discuss influence of peers and provide alternate models
8. Appreciate the rainbow of fruits and vegetables by tasting F&V
9. Group values discussion
10. Pros and cons worksheet of adding F&V to your diet
11. Goal-setting and wrap up

Materials
- Five to 10 different F&V, such as eggplant, blueberries, zucchini, kale, green grapes, jicama, potato, carrots, kumquat, tangerine, tomato, and strawberry
- Copies of the 24-hour recall checklist and pros/cons and goal-setting worksheets
- Fruit salad or vegetables and dip
- Newsprint
- Markers
- Pencils or pens

Procedure

1. **Introduction. Overview, gain attention (3 minutes)**
   Demonstrate the wide variety of colors that are found in F&V. Hold up F&V. Ask the following series of questions to facilitate conversation: What is the name of this food? Have you seen this food before? Have you eaten this food before? Are there other foods that are similar in color? Are there other foods that are similar in shape? Encourage participation from the whole group. Discuss why it is important to eat a rainbow of colors. (Address any behavior problems immediately and talk about the importance of creating a positive, supportive environment.)

2. **Benefits of F&V. Brainstorm and record on newsprint (6 minutes) (perceived benefits)**
   "Now that we are familiar with how a variety of different F&V look, we are going to continue to explore what we already know about F&V. Let's make a list of some of the benefits of eating a wide range of F&V." Discussion will follow; ensure that the following benefits of eating F&V are covered: provides essential vitamins, minerals, fiber, and other nutrients; can increase energy; helps make hair and skin healthy; builds strong bones and muscles; decreases risk for certain diseases.

3. **Benefits of F&V. Emphasis on importance of different colors (3 minutes) (perceived benefits)**
   List the following colors on newsprint: blue/purple, green, white, yellow/orange, and red. Emphasize a need for a variety of different colored F&V. Different colors reflect the presence of different phytonutrients. Explain that by eating all different colors, they are eating a wide range of different nutrients. Tell students that instead of needing to remember that orange colored vegetables are filled with carotenoids and dark blue/purple fruits, like blueberries, are filled with resveratrol, they should remember to eat the rainbow and they will eat all the different nutrients they need! Ask the group if there are any questions to clear up misconceptions.

4. **Self-assessment of intake. 24-hour recall checklist to assess colorfulness of F&V intake (9 minutes) (perceived risk)**
   Distribute checklist and ask participants to think about what F&V they ate yesterday (or during the past week). Each participant should write down the F&V they ate from each color group. Discussion starters: Is there a rainbow on your plate? What colors are you missing?

5. **Barriers to eating F&V. Brainstorm and record on newsprint (5 minutes) (barriers and self-efficacy)**
   Make a list of the reasons why it is sometimes hard to eat all the colors of the rainbow. Ask students what prevents them from eating all the different colors. Ensure that the following topics are mentioned: lack of time, not available, my parents don't buy/cook them, dislike taste.

6. **Brainstorm ways to overcome barriers. Discuss how to make eating all the colors of the rainbow easier (6 minutes) (self-efficacy)**

   Based on the list of barriers, ask for suggestions on ways to overcome each barrier. For example: lack of time: pre-cut vegetables; whole fruit for a snack; dislike taste: provide culturally appropriate suggestions on how to prepare. Record on newsprint. Ask for other suggestions about how to eat a variety of foods. If there is a color that most participants seem to be lacking, this is the time to focus on that particular color.

7. **Social influences. Discuss influence of peers and provide alternate models (5 minutes) (social norms)**

   What might your friends say when you choose to eat F&V or bring them as a snack? Allow for adequate discussion time. If the participants suggest that it might be seen as "uncool," provide alternate stories or media models that show F&V consumption as "cool." Make sure that the models are appropriate for the specific age, gender, and culture of the group.

8. **Tasting F&V. Appreciate the rainbow of fruits and vegetables by tasting F&V (10–20 minutes) (benefits)**

   Provide a rainbow fruit salad or a rainbow vegetable plate with dips for the participants to enjoy. Depending on time and facilities, allow participants to prepare the snack.

9. **Group values discussion (5 minutes) (values clarification)**

   Now that you have discussed the importance of eating a rainbow of F&V, and participants have eaten a great snack with a rainbow of colors in it, ask the participants for their thoughts now about F&V. Facilitate discussion by presenting value statements using a scale of 1–10, such as, How important is it to you to eat a rainbow of different F&V? How likely do you think it is that you will eat a rainbow of different F&V during the next week?

10. **Pros and cons of adding F&V to your diet (5 minutes) (benefits versus barriers)**

    Hand out pros and cons worksheet. Ask the participants to write at least three personal pros and three cons about eating a rainbow of different colored F&V.

11. **Goal setting and wrap up (8 minutes) (goal intention)**

    Review the reasons why and ways to increase the colorfulness and number of F&V in diet. Encourage participants to make a clear statement about what actions they will take in the next week. For some it might be adding one F&V a day to their diet, for others it might be adding a different colored F&V. Take a few minutes to fill out the worksheet. Ask participants, "Will some of you now share the goals you set for yourself?" After a participant reads his or her goal, ask if others have a similar goal. Encourage the members of the group to support each other in reaching their goals. Thank the group and include any reminders about future meetings or events.

In Step 5, you use your theoretical model, philosophy of nutrition education, and nutrition education program objectives to create (1) educational plans for the individual-level components and (2) environmental supports plans for environmental/policy components.

These pages of the Step 5 worksheets are devoted to designing educational plans for activities directed at individuals, referred to here as the individual-level components. Generally, the primary individual-level component consists of one or more group sessions. (You can also use these worksheets to design other individual-level components, such as newsletters and media-related activities.)

You should have **one** educational plan for **each** group session you design (or newsletter or other component directed at individuals).

At the end of the Step 5 worksheets for the individual-level components, you will have the following products:

Step 5A: General educational objectives for each session or series of sessions directed at the same behavioral goal

Step 5B: An overall design plan for the session in the form of a matrix that links mediators, objectives, and activities

Step 5C: A narrative educational plan that translates the matrix into a form ready for teaching or presenting

Use these worksheets as an organizational guide to help you design your educational plan and translate theory mediators into educational activities. Electronic versions of these worksheets are available at http://nutrition.jbpub.com/education/2e/. If you are unable to access the worksheets electronically, you can write onto this blank worksheet or create a text document that uses the same flow of information.

Step 5A: General educational objectives

Educational plan title: _____

Program goal behaviors: _____

Write the general educational objectives.

Mediator (from Step 3)	General educational objectives

Step 5B: Designing the educational plan: matrix format

Design your educational (or lesson) plan in matrix format. Write specific objectives for the mediators in your theory model (Step 3). Identify the learning domain and level for each objective. Then write the theory-based strategy you will employ to address the mediator and create educational activities that will be meaningful, interesting, and appropriate for your audience and will operationalize strategy.

Sequence your educational activities based on the events of instruction. After you have completed creating activities for each of the mediators in your theory model, go back through the design matrix and carefully identify each of the strategies/activities as to where it should fall in a sequence suitable for implementing with your audience. Label each activity as to whether it will be used to (A) gain attention, (S) present stimulus or new material, (G) provide guidance and practice, or (C) apply and close the session. These are referred to as the "Events of Instruction" or "EoI."

Carefully re-order the matrix. If the mediators and the related activities you have created are not at first listed in your matrix in the properly sequenced order (i.e., gain attention to apply and close), then carefully re-order the matrix so all activities as well as mediators and objectives are in the proper sequenced order ready to use to create your educational plan or teaching plan.

Mediator (from Step 3)	Specific educational objectives	Learning domain/level*	Theory-based strategy** and educational activities, experiences, and/or content	EoI

*C = cognitive domain; A = affective domain; P = psychomotor domain.

266

Step 5C: Educational plan

Write a narrative educational plan, based on your design matrix, that you will actually use to deliver your session. Think of a catchy title that will be meaningful to your audience. Make sure that activities are sequenced based on order of instruction. For each educational activity create a heading with a title and the mediator(s) addressed. Then write a detailed procedure for the activity. It is customary to place an overview or outline of activities and a materials list at the beginning of the teaching plan.

Overview of Content   **Materials**

Procedure

CHAPTER

12

Step 5: Translating Behavioral Theory Into Educational Strategies: A Focus on Facilitating the Ability to Take Action

OVERVIEW

Chapters 11 and 12 focus on selecting theory-based strategies and creating practical educational activities to achieve educational objectives and on sequencing the strategies into educational plans ready for implementation within groups or through other channels. The focus of *this* chapter is on designing practical educational activities or learning experiences to facilitate the ability of participants to take action. The information in Chapter 5 will help you with this step in the design process.

CHAPTER OUTLINE

- Introduction
- Selecting theory-based strategies to facilitate the ability to take action
- Action planning
- Skill building in food- and nutrition-related knowledge and skills
- Strengthening self-regulation processes and personal agency
- Case study
- Your turn: completing the Step 5 worksheets

LEARNING OBJECTIVES

At the end of the chapter, you will be able to:

- Describe the kinds of theory-based strategies to address potential mediators that are particularly important in facilitating the ability to take action
- Design specific educational activities or learning experiences to make practical the theory-based educational strategies designed to address potential mediators of target behaviors
- Sequence the educational objectives and strategies to create a lesson plan or educational plan
- Demonstrate skill in creating an educational plan or lesson plan

■ INTRODUCTION: FACILITATING THE ABILITY TO TAKE ACTION

Eating is very personal—and people like their eating patterns. Making changes in them is usually undertaken with some ambivalence: individuals want to eat for health, but they also gain psychological satisfaction, a sense of belonging to their culture, and enjoyment from their food.

And eating is not optional, unlike some other health-related behaviors such as smoking. Therefore, people's choices usually require trade-offs and difficult decisions. Not surprisingly, translating intentions into action is often fraught with difficulties. Even when people are motivated to make changes, they are not always able to act on their interests and motivation because of the press of other concerns and barriers. This intention–action gap is a common phenomenon to which all individuals can attest. How, then, can nutrition educators improve individuals' abilities to act on their motivations? What educational strategies can you design that facilitate the translation of intentions into action? (**Figure 12-1** and **Figure 12-2** highlight Step 5, as discussed in Chapters 11–13.)

Bridging the Motivation–Intention Gap

Theory proposes that progress toward engaging in an action or practice will not occur simply because individuals judge that the behavior or practice is highly desirable and feasible. Motivation alone is not sufficient to initiate health-promoting personal change. Evidence suggests that there are two major approaches to bridging this gap: nutrition educators can provide *relevant knowledge and skills* and assist individuals to strengthen their *self-regulation skills*, particularly the skill of setting goals, and they can foster supportive *environments* that make the action easier to do. This chapter focuses on the first approach. The next chapter focuses on the second. The environment presents many challenges to eating healthfully and being active, so individuals need knowledge and skills to navigate the environment successfully. At the

same time, health promotion efforts should seek to make the environment easier to navigate.

How Nutrition Educators Can Assist Individuals to Bridge the Gap

Consider the following example. A nutrition educator has been asked to make a presentation to a group of community women who are concerned about the high rate of diabetes in their community and who want to learn how to eat more healthfully. The nutrition educator decides that she will present a session where she provides them with a list of actions they can take, such as reading food labels, watching the fat and sugar in foods, and portion control. After about 20 minutes, she notices that the group is getting restless.

What is going on here? Certainly, nutrition information and skills are very important for those who are already motivated, which these women are. However, eating more healthfully is difficult and requires more than information. It requires, in addition, a set of skills called self-regulation skills. Here, individuals choose specific action goals and develop specific action plans to achieve these action goals. They learn how to make choices, to direct and take charge of their own behavior, and to pursue their action goals, even in the face of difficulties,

That is, in general, taking action and maintaining it for the long term require the food- and nutrition-related knowledge and skills necessary for taking action, but also enhanced self-regulation skills to use that knowledge and those skills in the service of taking action. This represents the action-phase component in the integrative conceptual framework for translating and implementing nutrition theory-based education presented in Chapter 9 (Figure 9-4). Consequently, this chapter describes theory-based strategies to:

- Build food- and nutrition-related skills
- Strengthen self-regulation skills

The strategies are summarized in **Table 12-1**. In designing your sessions or program, you will most likely go back and forth among these various strategies and between strategies in this chapter and those described in Chapter 11.

■ SELECTING THEORY-BASED STRATEGIES TO FACILITATE THE ABILITY TO TAKE ACTION

Your selection of educational strategies depends on the theory or model for the intervention that you created in Step 3 and your educational philosophy. Increasing evidence suggests, however, that for this phase, self-regulation models, social cognitive theory, integrated models, and grounded theory from extensive interviews are the most helpful (Pelican et al. 2005; Bisogni et al. 2005).

Remember, *theory-based strategies* are ways to operationalize each of the personal mediators of behavior change for educational and instructional purposes, and hence the mediators and strategies are often called by the same name. Table 12-1 shows the connections between theory constructs, potential mediators of change, and theory-based strategies, and practical educational strategies or learning experiences.

It is important to design educational activities that are engaging and fun, involve the affective as well as the cognitive domain, and include the psychomotor domain where appropriate. People generally remember 10% of what they read, 20% of what they hear, 30% of what they see, 50% of what they hear and see, 70% of what they say and write, and 90% of what they say as they do a thing (Wiman & Mierhenry 1969).

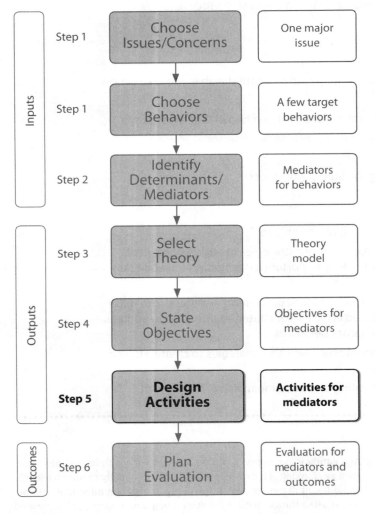

FIGURE 12-1 Flowchart for steps in designing theory-based nutrition education: Step 5.

Inputs: Collecting Assessment Data			Outputs: Designing the Theory-Based Intervention			Outcomes: Evaluation Plan
Step 1 ⟵⟶	Step 2 ⟵⟶	Step 3 ⟵⟶	Step 4 ⟵⟶	Step 5 ⟵⟶		Step 6
Analyze issues and audiences to state program behavioral goals	Identify potential mediators to achieve program behavioral goals	Select theory, philosophy, and components	State objectives for mediators	Design theory-based strategies and activities for mediators		Plan evaluation
Tasks • Analyze issues and select audience • Identify behaviors or patterns contributing to issue • Specify behavioral or action goals of the program	*Tasks* • Identify personal psychosocial mediators • Identify environmental support mediators	*Tasks* • Select theory or create appropriate model • Clarify philosophy (education and content) • Determine program components	*Tasks* • State educational objectives for psychosocial mediators • State change objectives for environmental support mediators	*Tasks* • Design activities to address psychosocial mediators • Design activities to address environmental support mediators • Implementation plan		*Tasks* • Design outcome evaluation plan • Determine tools to measure impact • Plan process evaluation
Product • *Description of issue of concern* • *Statement of action or behavioral goals for program*	*Product* • *List of potential mediators for action or behavior goals*	*Product* • *Theory/model for program, philosophy, and components*	*Product* • *Objectives for each mediator*	*Product* • *Educational plans for sessions linking mediators, objectives, and strategies* • *Environmental support plans*		*Product* • *Evaluation plan* • *List of indicators and measures for outcomes* • *Procedures and measures for process evaluation*

FIGURE 12-2 Stepwise Procedure for designing theory-based nutrition education: Step 5.

■ ACTION PLANNING: DEVELOPMENT OF IMPLEMENTATION INTENTIONS OR ACTION PLANS

How can you assist individuals to move from motivation to action, from intention to reality? Theory and evidence suggest that the following theory-based educational strategies are useful.

Action Plans

Translating behavioral intentions and goals into action is greatly facilitated by the formation of implementation intentions (Armitage 2004). These are also called action goals. Some audiences prefer the term *action plans* because the word *goals* seems too lofty. The term *contracting* is sometimes also used because it involves a contract between the person and himself or herself. These implementation intentions or action goals are volitional (conscious-choice) strategies that are designed to ensure that the behavioral goal or goal intentions are translated into action. Thus, whereas behavioral goals take the form of "I will eat more fruits and vegetables daily," action goals or implementation intentions take the following form: "In the next week, I will add orange juice at breakfast, eat a fruit for a snack midafternoon, and add one vegetable to my dinner in the evening."

Why Action Plans Are Effective

Implementation intentions are effective because they link the specific actions to a given situation so that when the situation arises, such as breakfast time, individuals do not have to think and make a new decision each time (Gollwitzer 1999). Such planning ahead means the behavior

will require less mental effort each time. This is especially important because healthful food- and nutrition-related behaviors are often perceived as difficult or even unpleasant to implement, even if they are desirable and feasible (e.g., switching from a high-fat to a low-fat diet, switching from eating takeout to cooking own food, starting to exercise daily, buying local foods). You should provide action goal or action plan worksheets for individuals to complete. Have someone else in the group sign as a witness to the action plan, and where appropriate and comfortable for the group to do so, have the group participants discuss with each other their action plans. Such verbalization can enhance a sense of commitment.

■ SKILL BUILDING IN FOOD- AND NUTRITION-RELATED KNOWLEDGE AND SKILLS

Although how-to knowledge or instrumental knowledge is not enough to motivate individuals to take health-related actions or to make changes in their diets—motivation is necessary, it *is* necessary for individuals to act on their motivations and achieve their behavioral goals and action plans. Thus, individuals need both motivation and ability to act, both why-to information and specific how-to knowledge and skills, to carry out the actions.

Knowledge and Cognitive Skills

After individuals have decided to take action on the behaviors or practices targeted by your program, they may still need specific knowledge and skills to carry out the actions. For example, individuals may not

TABLE 12-1	**Linking Theory, Strategies, and Educational Activities**	
Potential Mediator of Behavior Change (Theory Construct)	**Theory-Based Strategies for Potential Mediators of Behavior Change**	**Practical Educational Activities, Learning Experiences, Content, or Messages**
Goal setting	Goal setting and implementation or action plans	Teach goal-setting skills, provide contracts/pledges or action plan forms
Behavioral capability (knowledge and how-to information)	Food- and nutrition-related knowledge and cognitive, affective, and behavioral skills to engage in actions: • Teaching of how-to information • Food and nutrition skills building • Active methods • Discussion and facilitated dialogue • Guided practice	Presentations for passive learning and providing how-to information Active methods for higher-order learning: discussions, role plays, worksheets, games, and interactive learning experiences to teach needed food- and nutrition-related skills to engage in behavior; food preparation skills
Self-efficacy	Social modeling of behavior Guided practice to encourage mastery of behavioral skills Exhortations or persuasion so as to overcome doubt	Make the desired actions easy to understand and do: • Clear instructions • Demonstration of the behavior by respected social model • Direct experience (e.g., food preparation or cooking) with guidance and feedback • Give feedback on performance, emphasizing achievements and difficulties already overcome
Reinforcements	Provide reinforcements and rewards	Verbal praise, tee-shirts, drawing for prizes, or awards
Self-regulation	Strengthen self-regulation skills (self-influence or self-control) • Self-monitoring skills for progress toward goal • Goal maintenance • Coping self-efficacy • Managing cues from environment Developing personal policies, routines, and habits (TTM: Counterconditioning, rewards management, stimulus control)	Identify and prioritize competing goals; provide self-monitoring forms and tips; protect action goals from distractions: mindful eating, conscious attention (self-talk), and planning ahead; develop strategies for coping with difficulties Tip sheets on personal policies for purchasing foods, meal patterns (e.g., always eat breakfast, bring lunch to work), eating out
Social support	Social support (TTM: Helping relationships)	Create supportive group environment; encourage buddy system
Cues to action	Provide cues to action	Billboards, grocery bags, media messages, news articles, refrigerator magnets, and key chains with messages

Note: TTM = transtheoretical model.

know how to select foods for optimal health from the 50,000-item supermarket; evaluate the nutrition information that bombards them from magazines, newspapers, television news, advertising, and friends; or interpret medical information provided by their physicians. Food and nutrition education activities must therefore be directed at increasing basic knowledge and complex cognitive skills that will enhance people's power to take thoughtful action.

In discussing educational objectives in Step 4, you were reminded to write objectives that addressed several levels of thinking in the cognitive taxonomy, ranging from knowledge (recall of information) through comprehension, application, analysis, and synthesis to evaluation. Table

10-1 summarizes these levels of knowledge skills. Do not focus only on basic factual knowledge. All age groups are capable of all levels of learning; it is only the sophistication of the language and concepts that may differ. For example, do not assume that for young children or low-literacy audiences, educational activities should be set at low levels of cognitive learning such as recall of information or comprehension. Even second graders can evaluate. It is good practice to include information on the cognitive level of each activity in your educational plan to ensure that activities are well distributed across levels.

You can build on the current knowledge of your audience, which you learned about in Step 2. This will help you avoid providing information

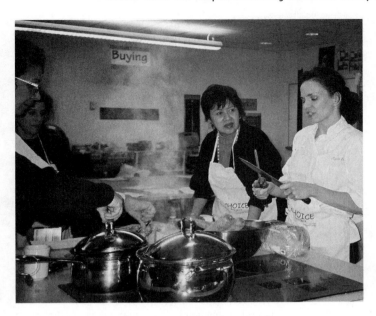

The skill of cooking fresh vegetables can boost confidence.

they already know, which can come across as condescending, or information that is too complex. In a group setting, encourage the audience to share information with each other.

Provide Factual Knowledge and Increase Comprehension

As you have seen, *knowledge* has been defined for the purposes of developing educational programs as "the recall of specifics and universals, the recall of methods and processes, or the recall of a pattern, structure, or setting" (Krathwahl, Bloom, & Masia 1964, p. 201). In the area of food and nutrition, knowledge might include the ability to recall such facts as the recommended guidelines for healthful diets appropriate for an individual's age, sex, and stage of life; which foods to select to meet the guidelines; serving sizes and how many servings one should eat of each food group in the food pyramid; and the ecological impact of different food processing techniques and packaging materials. *Comprehension* might involve understanding why fruits and vegetables are important in the diet or how to read a label.

- *Vivid information.* Such information can be provided through lectures, handouts, slides, discussions, and demonstrations. Just as nutrition messages are more likely to be motivating if they are vivid and personal, so also how-to nutrition information, especially for the general public, is more likely to be remembered if it is vivid and understandable in everyday terms. Graphs can be made using "foods" visually as units instead of abstract numbers (e.g., a stack of five teaspoons on top of each other instead of a plain bar graph to display the number of teaspoons of fat in foods).
- *Visuals and demonstrations.* Show photographs or models of foods to help the audience estimate portion sizes, or bring in boxes or containers of foods to show nutrient composition. (Tip: Containers should be empty so that audience members don't ask to take the foods home! This has the added advantage that you can use the containers again.) Demonstrations can be very effective, such as spooning out onto a plate the number of teaspoons of fat in a hamburger or burning a cracker to show that it has

"calories" in it. (Tip: Use a cracker that has a lot of fat and a loose weave for oxygen to get in.)
- *Other channels.* Other methods involve newsletters, flyers, and Web-based programs depending on the behavior or practice and the channel chosen (e.g., mass media, in-person). Correcting misconceptions at this time is very important if they constitute barriers to program participants' ability to take action.

Stimulate Higher-Order Thinking

Food and nutrition issues often are complex. To take action and maintain behavior change require not only knowledge of facts but also development of conceptual frameworks on which to hang isolated messages, called *knowledge structures* or *schemas*. Skills in analysis, synthesis, and evaluation are important here. Building such skills is more difficult than providing factual information.

- *Analysis* may involve comparing the sugar content of different beverages or the fat content of different fast foods.
- *Synthesis* may be planning a day's menu to incorporate four and a half or more fruits and vegetables (or just a plan as to when individuals will incorporate more fruits and vegetables in a day).
- *Evaluation* may involve rating several different food sources of calcium to select the best source based on some criterion such as price or impact on the body, or evaluating the amount of energy used to produce different types of food packaging.
- *Active methods* are usually more effective with most audiences: worksheets and hands-on, minds-on activities are appropriate to help people see connections between concepts and develop their conceptual frameworks for the given issue.

Skills in Critical Evaluation and Problem Solving

Depending on the behavior or practice that your program has targeted and the channel chosen (e.g., mass media, in-person), your nutrition education sessions may include activities directed at enhancement of critical reasoning skills to evaluate complex and controversial issues or to understand food and nutrition policies. Food choice criteria have become more complex, involving not only health concerns but also, for many people, concerns about the ecological consequences of consumption (e.g., conventional, organic, local), moral/ethical concerns (to eat meat or not), social justice concerns (e.g., who produced the food, under what working conditions), and food safety concerns. Thus, critical thinking skills are needed so that people can make informed trade-offs between criteria in making food choices.

Individuals also need such skills so that they can examine the arguments on both sides of an issue related to your target behaviors—for example, whether to reduce dietary fat or carbohydrates to lose weight, eat organic versus "regular" fruits and vegetables, or breast-feed or bottle-feed their infant. They need critical evaluation skills to analyze and resolve contradictions and develop personal policies that will guide their food-related activities on an ongoing basis. A cognitive understanding of the food system and its impacts provides a context for action. Food- and nutrition-related behaviors are also embedded in larger social, economic, and political contexts that need to be understood for the continued maintenance of change.

- *Trigger films or clips from the Web followed by discussion.* You can use trigger films and discussion to enhance critical thinking skills so participants can learn to evaluate controversial issues or develop complex understandings. The arguments for and against certain practices can be volunteered by the group and recorded on newsprint in a brainstorming format and then discussed and perhaps voted upon.

- *Debates.* Carefully designed activities such as written or oral critiques or debates can also be used to encourage analysis of issues. Here, participants should focus on the claims of the position, the evidence for and against the position and the strength of such evidence, and conclusions based on this evaluation of the evidence. When selecting opposing groups for a debate, to the extent possible assign group members to argue for the position that is contrary to their own personal position: this will greatly facilitate discussion and debate based on evidence rather than personal conviction. Use of these activities will depend on the learning style preferences of the audience as well as their comfort level with them. However, debates are interesting for all and should be considered. Low literacy does not preclude oral debates.

Affective Skills: The Importance of Feelings

Food is needed for survival, and changes in diets are often undertaken with some ambivalence. Survival and quality of life require that appetite and enthusiasm about eating be maintained. Yet people recognize that they may need to change some of their food practices for health reasons even if these current practices are psychologically or culturally beneficial. Or they may want to take action on food system issues to support broader goals and values (such as supporting local agriculture), even though doing so is personally inconvenient and more expensive.

In discussing educational goals and objectives in Step 4, you were reminded to write objectives that addressed several levels of engagement in the affective taxonomy, ranging from receiving (awareness and willingness to receive your message) through responding, valuing, organizing, and internalizing values. Table 10-2 summarizes these levels of affective engagement.

Designing Educational Activities at Different Levels of Affective Integration

Your activities should seek an appropriate level of affective engagement by your audience. Maybe you wish only for groups or audiences to become *aware* of an issue (mass media campaigns may seek this level). Or you may seek for your audience to actively *respond* during your sessions or program, participating instead of just observing, and beginning to respond with satisfaction to the educational activities and to form their own opinions. Most educational programs aim for the *valuing level* of engagement. Here, individuals make a commitment to the action recommended by the program, perhaps at first tentatively, but later with conviction. At that level of commitment, individuals are ready and willing to take action, moving from intention to action.

- *Review of activities.* Review your activities to see whether they encourage engagement and commitment. Depending on the issue and the audience, you may be able to design activities that assist individuals to build an internally consistent value system for guiding behavior by resolving conflicts and developing their own policies to guide action. See Chapter 10 for more details on the affective taxonomy.
- *Affective, cognitive, and behavioral skills complement each other.* Skills in the cognitive and affective domains accompany, and are usually integrated with, skills in the behavioral domain. For example, to be able to carry out a behavior, individuals need to be able to accurately observe and interpret a situation, to understand their own feelings in the situation, or to change how they think

about the situation from ways that are less accurate or productive to ones that are more productive (a process that is often called *cognitive restructuring*, or changing self-talk), to evaluate their own abilities to perform the behavior, to express themselves in ways appropriate to situations and persons, to express personal objectives, and to negotiate demands in an assertive and appropriate way. Check whether the education or lesson plans include the affective domain.

- *Facilitated discussion or dialogue.* In small groups, using facilitated discussion or dialogue is one way nutrition educators can deal with feelings and emotional issues. In facilitated discussion, group members share feelings and experiences; the process is described more fully in Chapter 15. Participants can also be divided into groups of three or four in which they can talk over questions such as the following: what is the hardest thing about trying to change the way we eat? What are some successful ways we have changed other habits that could be applied to this particular dietary behavior?

Skills Mastery and Enhanced Self-Efficacy

Self-efficacy is an important mediator of behavior change in the action phase of nutrition education. Self-efficacy may increase with increased level of skills, but self-efficacy is not the same thing as skills. Self-efficacy involves both skills and the confidence that individuals can consistently use their skills even in the face of impediments or barriers. Social cognitive theory argues that a person's feeling of self-efficacy or competence in being able to carry out a behavior is crucial to whether that person will perform the target behavior (Bandura 1986). Furthermore, an increased perception of control or feeling of success comes from becoming more skillful in performing the desired behavior. Skill acquisition is thus an essential step leading from intention to behavior.

Skills include behavioral skills such as food shopping, household food management skills, and time management skills. Shopping skills such as using a shopping list, stocking up on bargains, and using coupons have been shown to be related to nutrient intake in low-income households and are thus important. Physical skills include such skills as preparing foods, cooking, breastfeeding, growing a vegetable garden, and participating in sports.

Building Mastery and Self-Efficacy

Social cognitive theory (Bandura 1997) proposes a review of the many methods for facilitating mastery of skills and enhancing self-efficacy, yielding the following three specific instructional methods (Thoresen 1984) that can be applied to the acquisition of food preparation, cooking, breastfeeding, safe food handling, or other food- and nutrition-related skills as required for participants in your program to engage in the program's targeted behaviors or practices:

- *Clear instructions to individuals on how to perform the desired behavior.* You can enhance individuals' sense of confidence in their own abilities to carry out the goal behaviors or think analytically about issues when you provide them with clear and realistic instruction on how to perform the behavior or evaluate evidence critically. Examples include teaching participants how to make tasty low-fat meals, store fruits and vegetables correctly so that they do not spoil quickly, plant a vegetable garden, breast-feed, or handle foods safely in the home kitchen. Such teaching can be done by direct verbal instruction, using audiovisual media, role playing, or written instructions.

- *Social modeling, in which the skills are demonstrated.* Food demonstrations are a notable example. Such demonstrations can be live, on videotape, through visual mass media such as television, or in printed materials. Note the popularity of food shows and cooking demonstrations on television. Modeling is a powerful factor in motivating behaviors as well as an important instructional tool.

- *Guided practice with feedback.* This method is highly effective in both teaching skills and increasing self-efficacy. Cooking has been shown to improve cooking-related knowledge, attitudes, and behaviors more than food demonstrations (Levy & Auld 2004). Here, you create opportunities for individuals to practice the behavior (e.g., cooking a particular food) and provide them with specific feedback immediately after they have performed the desired behavior. Encouragement is useful because it can overcome participants' self-doubts. Early in the skills acquisition process, individuals should be encouraged to try out skills without evaluation by you or by themselves so that they can focus their attention on the skills to be acquired. This, of course, requires food preparation or cooking facilities to be available. However, many nutrition educators have developed ways to make cooking demonstrations, and even cooking by participants, possible by bringing with them all the needed food and equipment, including portable butane stoves or electric hot plates. Supermarket tours can enhance skills in shopping practices that are nutritionally healthy and ecologically sound.

Taken together, these three procedures result in a strategy referred to as *guided practice, behavioral rehearsal,* or *skills mastery.* You provide a demonstration of the desired behavior or skills, create opportunities for participants to practice what they observed with guidance on the performance of the task, make suggestions for improvement where necessary, and encourage them in their actions.

Complexity of Dietary Behavior Changes

Making dietary changes requires attention to a specific recurring array of behaviors and many specific actions that constitute the behavior, such as food shopping, eating out, or food preparation practices. It is the cumulative effects of these behaviors that have an impact on health. The environment in which dietary choices have to be made is quite challenging. One study found, for example, that to eat more fruits and vegetables, individuals said that they had to make more visits to stores, eating at friends' houses became more difficult, and buying takeout meals became more problematic (Anderson et al. 1998).

It is helpful to keep in mind that making changes in food intake involves different behavioral categories, such as the following:

- Decreasing or avoiding certain foods, food constituents, or beverages
- Adding foods to the diet
- Modifying foods

When you design sessions that involve behavioral skills, it is useful to keep these different behavioral categories in mind. The psychological, educational, and practical tasks may be very different for reducing and adding behaviors. Learning to avoid fat (or salt) means being able to recognize which types of foods it may be found in, learning to read food labels, and acquiring new food preparation techniques. Psychologically, it may mean giving up certain foods. Fruits and vegetables are easier to recognize, so this requires less education. In addition, psychologically,

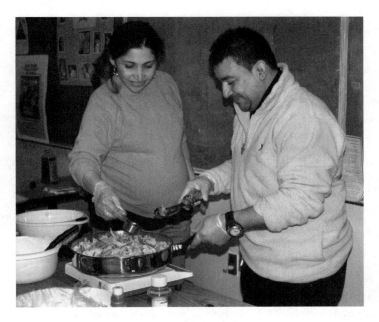

Learning to cook and eat healthful at the WIC clinic.

eating fruits and vegetables is about adding foods to one's diet and not having to give up certain favorite foods. Sometimes these behaviors are complementary, so they can be addressed together—for example, eating fruit rather than a high-fat snack between meals. Nutrition educators can help individuals think through these categories and which ones they would like to tackle first. For example, Kristal, Shattuck, and Henry (1990) found that excluding high-fat ingredients and preparation techniques and modifying high-fat foods were the most difficult to do but had the greatest impact on fat intake, whereas substituting specially manufactured low-fat foods for their higher-fat counterparts was the easiest to do but had the least impact on fat intake.

These behaviors are of course very culture bound and hence must be investigated for each intended audience. In addition, dietary behaviors are complex and the psychological motivations and skills needed are different depending on the food; you need to consider these factors when planning nutrition education.

■ STRENGTHENING SELF-REGULATION PROCESSES AND PERSONAL AGENCY

Self-directed change comes about when individuals are not only motivated but can exercise self-regulation. Self-regulation is the process through which individuals develop the ability to influence and direct their own actions or behaviors though their own efforts: this is often referred to as *self-control.* However, what is meant by the term is ability to take control or take charge of one's actions. Hence, the action phase of health behavior change is also referred to as the *volitional, conscious-choice,* or *action-control phase.* Several models describe the process (Bandura 1997; Gollwitzer 1999; Schwarzer & Renner 2000). Self-regulation is not achieved through willpower but through the development of self-regulation skills. Such skills are needed for both action initiation and action maintenance. Nutrition education interventions must therefore create opportunities for individuals to develop these skills and, through these, develop a sense of personal agency.

Nutrition Education in Action 12-1 describes the Squire's Quest program, which focuses on setting goals and providing skills. **Nutrition Education in Action 12-2** describes the Choice, Control, and Change program, where the development of a sense of personal agency is the central focus of the intervention.

Chief among the strategies to achieve self-regulation skills is the process known to professionals as goal setting, which was discussed in Chapter 5 (Locke & Latham 1990; Cullen, Baranowski, & Smith 2001; Shilts, Horowitz, & Townsend 2004). The term *goal setting* refers to a systematic behavioral change *process* that involves many of the educational or behavioral change strategies described earlier.

Note: The strategies described here use the language of nutrition education professionals. You would not necessarily use the same terms with the public. Examples are given of terms to use with the intended audience for each strategy.

Goal Setting

Goal setting works to motivate, bridge the intention–action gap, and maintain action in nutrition education program participants for a variety of reasons. It engenders a sense of commitment to the goal. By planning ahead, participants do not have to make a new decision every time a food choice situation arises, thus leading to less mental burden and to development of a routine. The statement of a goal sensitizes individuals so that they are more conscious or mindful as they make food choices. It gives them a sense of control over their own behavior. It builds their perceptions of self-efficacy and mastery. It creates self-satisfaction and a sense of fulfillment from having achieved their goals and contributes to the cultivation of intrinsic interest through active involvement in the process.

Goal setting is an example of taking charge of one's own behavior, or exercising agency, and is similar to the process of self-liberation in the transtheoretical model. Several reviews have shown that the goal-setting process can be very useful in the dietary arena (Cullen et al. 2001; Shilts et al. 2004).

Goals can refer to a variety of levels of states to be achieved:

- There are *end goals*, or *value goals*, which express long-range, deeply valued end states that serve as an orienting function in life, such as being healthy, being self-fulfilled, enjoying a high quality of life, contributing to the community, or living a life worth living.
- *Intermediate goals*, or *instrumental goals*, are behaviors or practices that people can engage in to achieve these end goals, such as eating a healthful diet or walking to get exercise (to support an end goal of a healthy life).

NUTRITION EDUCATION IN ACTION 12-1

Squire's Quest! A Multimedia Game

Increased consumption of fruits and vegetables by children has immediate benefits in terms of healthier growth and development and may reduce the risk of chronic disease later in life. Nutrition education can thus play an important role by addressing the mediators of eating more fruits and vegetables. Research evidence suggests that the most important mediators for children are increased availability and accessibility, preference, and skills in making fruit and vegetable recipes when they are responsible for making their own snacks. Squire's Quest was designed to increase consumption of fruits and vegetables in fourth-grade children by addressing these mediators.

Program

Squire's Quest was designed as a 10-session, computer-based, interactive multimedia game, with each session lasting about 25 minutes. The game was based on the following background story: the kingdom of 5A Lot was being invaded by the Slimes (snakes) and the Mogs (moles), who were desirous of destroying the kingdom by destroying its fruit and vegetable crops. The king (Cornwell) and the queen (Nutritia) were leading their knights to defeat the invaders. The knights had such names as Sir Sarah See-a-Solution and Sir Alex Try-to-Be-Right. The program invited children to commit to being a squire in the first session and to seek to become knights to help the king and queen.

The squire had to face many challenges in this quest. These involved acquiring skills and setting goals related to eating more fruits, juice, and vegetables. The squire prepared FJV (fruit, juice, and vegetable) recipes in a virtual kitchen and had the help of a wizard through the challenges. Many of the sessions were delivered by the castle robot. The children participated in decision-making activities, choosing between their favorite FJV and a more common snack. The decision criteria provided were based on the most important outcome expectancies reported by the child at baseline. Before the end of each session, the squire set goals to make a recipe during that session, eat a FJV serving as a meal or snack, or ask for FJV to be available at home. Through this game, children learned about serving sizes and finding and buying FJV, and acquired practice in decision making, goal setting, and using problem-solving skills as well as practical skills such as preparing recipes in the virtual kitchen. Computers were provided to the schools and the intervention was conducted in five weeks.

Evaluation

The program was evaluated with 1578 fourth-grade students in 26 schools. The schools were matched in pairs, and within matched pairs schools were randomly assigned to intervention or control conditions. The behavioral outcome was assessed immediately after the program based on four days of dietary intake data obtained through a multiple-pass, 24-hour dietary intake interview with the children. Results showed that children participating in Squire's Quest increased their FJV intake by 1.0 servings more than the children not receiving the program. This suggests that psychoeducational multimedia games can serve as an effective venue through which to provide nutrition education to children.

Source: Baranowski, T., J. Baranowski, K. W. Cullen, et al. 2003. Squire's Quest! Dietary outcome evaluation of a multimedia game. *American Journal of Preventive Medicine* 245:52–61.

NUTRITION EDUCATION IN ACTION 12-2

Choice, Control, and Change

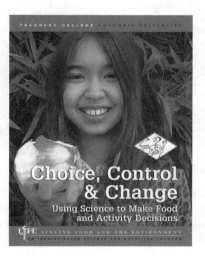

The Choice, Control, and Change (C3) program is an inquiry-based science education and health program for overweight prevention among middle school students. Given an environment that encourages overeating and sedentary behavior, the goal of C3 is for youth to become competent eaters who have a sense of personal agency and are able to navigate this environment. It is based on social cognitive and self-determination theories. The why-to information (outcome expectations) explores the interplay of biology, personal behavior, and the food system and meets various national standards for science education. Students collect scientific evidence to enable them to understand why healthful eating and ample physical activity are important. The how-to information focuses on teaching cognitive self-regulation skills and enhancing competence and personal agency. It is thus both a science education curriculum as well as a behavior-focused, theory-based nutrition education intervention. It addresses both why to and how to eat healthfully.

The program consists of 19 lessons, broken into five units. The lessons consist of exciting hands-on and minds-on nutrition and science activities:

- *Unit 1 Investigating Our Choices:* Students explore how the environment around us interacts with our biological predispositions to influence what we choose to eat and what activities we do.

- *Unit 2 Dynamic Equilibrium:* Students learn about energy balance in the human body and why and how the body functions better when it is in balance.
- *Unit 3 From Data to Health Goals:* Students collect and analyze their own food and activity data. They compare their data to the C3 goals, create action plans for change, and monitor their change process—through to the end of the curriculum. This gives students opportunities to discuss, debate, and defend the personal changes they are making, both with each other, and with significant others in their lives.
- *Unit 4 Effects of Our Choices:* As the students continue to work on their action plans for change they go deeper into why these changes are important to maintain long-term health and decrease risk for cardiovascular disease and type 2 diabetes.
- *Unit 5 Maintaining Competence:* Students integrate their understanding of science, connecting food and activity choices to health, and confirm their personal health commitments.

Evaluation

In a cluster-randomized control study, students in the program significantly reduced the reported frequency (days per week) and amount of sweetened beverages and packaged snacks as well as smaller sizes at fast food restaurants. There were no reported changes in fruit, vegetable, and water intakes. They also reported walking and taking the stairs more for exercise. Their outcome beliefs, self-efficacy, sense of competence, and autonomy became significantly more positive.

Sources: Contento, I. R., P. A. Koch, A. Calabrese-Barton, H. Lee, and W. Sauberli. 2007. Enhancing personal agency and competence in eating and moving: Formative evaluation of a middle school curriculum, Choice, Control, and Change. *Journal of Nutrition Education and Behavior* 39:S179–S186; and Contento I.R., P.A.Koch, H. Lee, A. Calabrese-Barton. Adolescents demonstrate improvement in obesity risk behaviors following completion of *Choice, Control, and Change*, a curriculum addressing personal agency and autonomous motivation. *J Am Diet Assoc* 2010;110: December.

Choice, Control, and Change is a curriculum module of the Linking Food and the Environment (LiFE) curriculum series from Teachers College Columbia University (http://www.tc.edu/life) and is available from the National Gardening Association. (http://www.gardeningwithkids.org/11-3320.html) The book cover is used with permission.

- *Specific action goals* refer to specific actions people can take to achieve these intermediate goals, such as "I will drink orange juice each morning for breakfast." In the goal-setting process, individuals generally focus on the intermediate or instrumental behavioral goals (or goal intentions) and on action goals to achieve them. These action goals are the same as implementation intentions. There are different ways to describe the goal-setting

process (Cullen et al. 2001; Shilts et al. 2004, 2009). One way is suggested in the following.

1. *Clarifying the behavioral goal.* For a behavior-focused intervention, behavioral goals are clearly specified by the intervention or program, such as eating a healthier diet, improving bone health through eating more calcium-rich foods and being more physically

active, eating more fruits and vegetables, and so forth. If the program's behavioral goal is quite broad, such as "participants will eat a healthier diet," then the individual will have some choices to make. The individual's behavioral goals might include, I will (or I intend to):

- Increase my intake of fruits and vegetables
- Increase my intake of calcium-rich foods
- Increase my intake of whole-grain foods
- Decrease my intake of high-fat, high-sugar foods

Depending on the duration and intensity that is possible for your program, you will usually want the participants to focus on only one or two goals to work on.

2. *Select or develop a self-assessment tool for participants.* Self-assessment involves identification of specific actions that participants are currently engaging in that relate to the behavioral goals of the intervention program.

For example, if the intervention or program's behavioral goal is to reduce fat in the diet, then participants need to identify the foods in their diet that contribute to their fat intake. Is it the amount of meat they are eating or the number of rich desserts? If the goal of the intervention is to increase fruit and vegetable consumption among audience members, how many servings are they now eating in a day? If the program's behavioral goal is to encourage eating locally produced foods, then how often do the participants visit farmers' markets or look for foods in the supermarket that are labeled as being local? This may further the recognition of the need for change. The self-assessment usually involves some kind of recording method, such as food records of one to three days, 24-hour dietary recalls, or checklists of the targeted foods or practices. **Figure 12-3** shows an example of a self-assessment tool for recording food intakes; it is for the EatFit program described in Chapter 5.

3. *Develop a system for scoring the self-assessment tool and generating appropriate specific action goals.* This system could be as simple as adding up the scores for different behaviors assessed in the self-assessment tool. In the EatFit example, the 24-hour recalls were analyzed for the programs' behaviors, which included increasing fruit and vegetable intake, decreasing fat intake, reducing added sugar intake, and increasing calcium intake. Physical activity behaviors included increasing strength and aerobic activities (Shilts et al. 2009).

4. *Provide instruction for setting effective action goals or action plans.* The general behavioral goals should be translated to specific action goals. Action goals should be clear and quantifiable, close in time, and attainable (Bandura 1986; Locke & Latham 1990; Shilts et al. 2004).

- *Clear and quantifiable (specificity).* The action goal should be specific. General behavioral goals have been shown to be ineffective for achieving changes in behavior. Specific action goals provide clear targets for action, indicating the type and amount of effort needed to achieve the goal. An example might be "I will drink orange juice for breakfast and add a vegetable to lunch" (to increase intake of fruits and vegetables from one to two cups daily).
- *Close in time (proximity).* Action goals to be accomplished in the immediate future are more likely to be effective than those set for a longer time frame because, in the latter case,

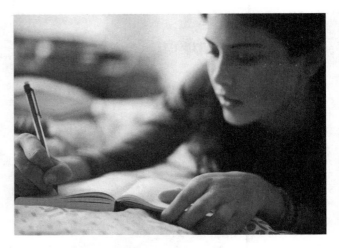

Self-assessment is a powerful tool.

it is easy to postpone action. For example, "I will eat 2 and a half cups of fruits and vegetables *today* by having orange juice at breakfast, eating a fruit for a mid-morning snack, adding a salad to lunch, and eating two vegetables for dinner" is likely to be more effective than stating, "I will eat more fruits and vegetables this month."

- *Reachable (difficulty).* The action goals should be difficult yet reachable. Those that are challenging but clearly attainable through extra effort are more likely to be motivating and satisfying. Difficult goals require more effort to achieve than easy ones do. It is the discrepancy between where individuals are and where they want to be that is motivating (Bandura 1986, 1997). Motivation can be sustained by setting progressively more difficult action goals, assuming that they are seen as reasonable and within reach. Very difficult or complex changes should be broken down into smaller units, and goals set for each of the units. The maxim is that the goal should be small enough to achieve but large enough to matter. For example, rather than set one action goal "to eat less fat and sugar and to eat more fruits and vegetables," individuals should set separate action goals and make them specific, such as "to add one dark green vegetable to my diet each day this week" or "to eat ice cream only twice this week."

5. *Create a contract, pledge, or action plan.* Commitment to an action goal is the personal resolve to pursue the goal. Personal commitment is strengthened by pledges that bind the individual to future action. The motivational effect of binding themselves to future action is largely the result of not wanting to renege on an agreement they have made. This is especially true if the goal is highly valued.

It is helpful to provide some kind of agreement form or worksheet on which group participants can state their commitment or pledge (**Figure 12-4**). The actual form is often called a *contract* because it involves a contract between the person and himself or herself. The word *contract* may not work with your audience. You should pilot test your form with the target group to find a term that is most appropriate for them. For example, it can be called an *action plan*. Each participant should sign one. Given that public commitment enhances the likelihood of following through on a pledge, it is best to have another member of the group, a friend, or

My Eating Record

1) Write down the foods you eat and drink as you go through the day.
2) Begin your record in the morning with the first thing you eat or drink and finish at bedtime with the last thing that you eat or drink.
3) Include those foods and drink consumed during breakfast, lunch, and dinner and do not forget to write down your snacks and munchies. A piece of gum, drink from the water fountain, a taste of cookie dough all count, so write them down.
4) Make sure to check out the hunger rating scale at the bottom of your food record: write down how hungry you were before you began to eat.

Help! How Much Did I Eat?

1 cup = a handful	1/2 cup = the size of an ice cream scoop
1 ounce of cheese = 4 dice	3 ounces of meat = a deck of cards
1 tsp = the tip of your thumb	1 medium-size fruit = 1 tennis ball
1 tablespoon = the size of your thumb	12 fluid ounces = 1 can of soda

Once you're done, log onto http://www.eatfit.net to see how your eating rates.

Name: _____

One Day Eating Record

Food/Beverage	Type/Description	Preparation	Amount Eaten	Where Did You Eat/Drink It?	Hunger Rating
Bread	Whole wheat	Toasted	1 slice	Kitchen	7

Hunger Rating Scale

1 —— 2 —— 3 —— 4 —— 5 —— 6 —— 7 —— 8 —— 9 —— 10

| Starving | | Pretty hungry | | A little hungry | Not hungry | | Pretty full | | Stuffed |

FIGURE 12-3 Example assessment tool from the EatFit program: Eating record.

Source: Shilts, M. K., M. Horowitz, and M. S. Townsend. 2004. An innovative approach to goal setting for adolescents: Guided goal setting. *Journal of Nutrition Education and Behavior* 36:155–156. Courtesy of M. K. Shilts, M. Horowitz, and M. S. Townsend, University of California–Davis.

family member also sign as a witness. **Table 12-2** contains some tips to go with the contract form, which can be made into a handout for the group. Some nutrition educators who work in classroom settings with younger children, who might lose contract forms, have students voluntarily sign a class book instead. The children then check off when they have attained the goal. This often is called a challenge sheet.

Other more informal formats also can be used. Children can be each asked to trace their hands on a large piece of newsprint and then to write in their action goal inside the hand. This collective contract can be hung up in the room as a reminder. Or, in a group setting with adults, particularly a low-literacy audience, a public verbal commitment may be appropriate.

6. *Build skills.* In many instances, program participants need to hone their existing skills or learn new ones to carry out the behaviors to which they have committed themselves. Becoming more skillful in performing the desired behavior also results in an increased perception of control or feeling of success. Possible activities to build skills are described in an earlier section of this chapter.

7. *Develop a tracking and feedback system (self-monitoring and self-evaluation).* The next step is for individuals and groups to track their progress to see how well they are doing compared with their action goals. Self-observation and self-evaluation are considered extremely important in the self-regulatory process. Such feedback can be provided through a tracking system that you develop for use by program participants. This may be quite easy for behaviors that are clearly visible or identifiable, such as eating fruits and vegetables. However, other behaviors may not be so easy, such as reducing fat in foods. In the latter case, you could come up with some clear definitions of higher-fat and lower-fat foods to make tracking possible. You can review the completed tracking forms and give individual feedback as well. Or the participants could give oral reports in group settings, if the action goals have been made public. In this case, individuals will get feedback from

the group also. Both individual and group feedback can be used, depending on the conditions under which the action goals were set. The focus should be on positive accomplishments rather than failures.

Figure 12-5 shows the tracking system used in the EatFit program for middle school students. The system consists of a graph in the form of a thermometer (one thermometer for tracking a student's eating goal and another for his or her fitness goal). Students shade in the thermometer starting at the bottom (cold) and move toward the hot end of the thermometer as they judge that they are reaching their goal.

8. *Create rewards and encouragement.* Achievement of the action goals can be rewarded by program staff, by collective action on the part of the participants, or by the individuals themselves, depending on the situation. Nutrition educators can provide reinforcement in many ways: verbal encouragement, smiles, and an approving, nonjudgmental tone of voice in all interactions with the group; or material rewards such as key chains, magnets, tee-shirts, or sweat shirts to those who participate or complete the program. For example, tee-shirts appear to be quite motivating to runners. A founder of the New York City Road Runners Club used to say, "Never underestimate the power of a tee-shirt!" Indeed, some runners are known to select races on the basis of the tee-shirts being given out. You can also give out raffle tickets to be drawn for prizes upon completion of the contract. The hidden messages in these reinforcements should be consistent and support the spoken, overt message. For example, rewarding children for being physically active with high-fat, high-sugar food products would not be supportive of the message. Present participants with certificates of achievement when they achieve their goals.

Individuals can also be encouraged to reinforce themselves in tangible ways, such as buying a new piece of clothing or a new piece of exercise equipment, or through their affective reactions, such as praising themselves when they meet their goals and problem solving when they fall short. Physiological and external reinforcements also influence goal achievement. Thus, knowledge that one's serum cholesterol level has declined can enhance an individual's commitment to eating a low-fat diet.

9. *Problem solving.* When participants do not attain their action goals, assist them to engage in problem solving and decision making to find more effective ways to attain the goals they set or to set new ones that are more attainable.

Goal Maintenance (Relapse Prevention)

In the area of food and dietary behavior, goal maintenance is a more appropriate concept than relapse prevention. Eating requires daily food choices and constant trade-offs among numerous alternative actions. Healthy food practices need to be maintained for the long term—indeed, permanently. Studies have found that no magic food changes are involved in making dietary changes. In interventions designed to lower fat intake, for example, people made changes in all high-fat food groups (Burrows et al. 1993). In interventions directed at fruits and vegetables, people made changes through conventional eating habit changes such as adding fruit juice as a snack or including a vegetable at lunch (Cox et al. 1998). Adding foods to the diet, such as fruits and vegetables, appears easier to do and maintain than removing a food or a food constituent such as fat.

An effective approach is to use a *general dietary framework*, not a prescriptive diet. This gives individuals control over their diets. You

TABLE 12-2	**What Works and Doesn't Work in Making Changes**
What Works	**What Doesn't**
Setting realistic goals and breaking your goal into small steps you can achieve	Setting unrealistic goals
Allowing for your food dislikes	Trying to include foods you don't like
Making small changes	Making drastic changes
Choosing foods you can get easily	Choosing foods you have to search for
Getting support from your family and friends	Trying to make changes all by yourself
Being flexible: compromising in some situations	**Being rigid:** trying to live up to your changes with absolutely no exceptions

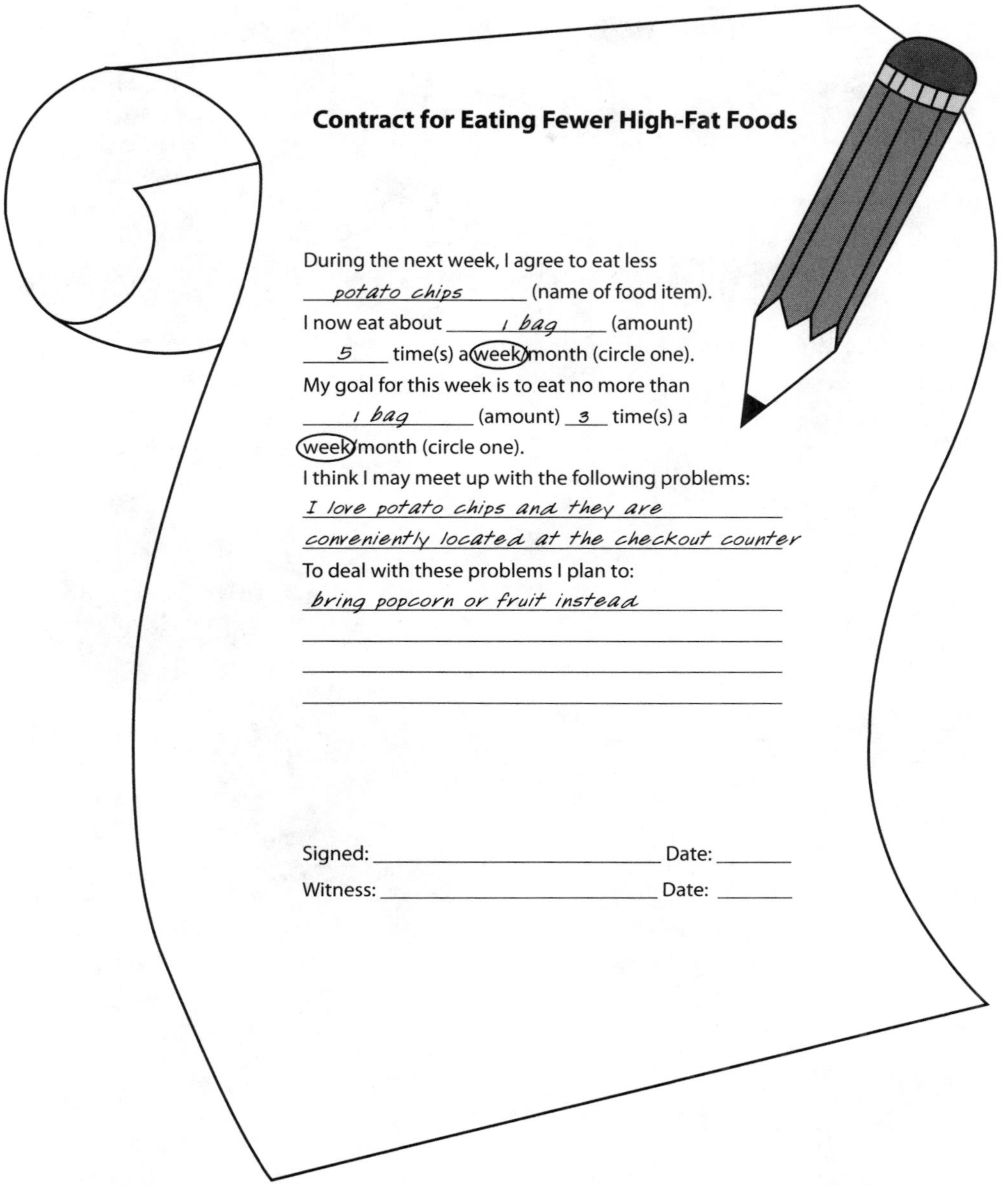

Contract for Eating Fewer High-Fat Foods

During the next week, I agree to eat less
_____potato chips_____ (name of food item).
I now eat about _____1 bag_____ (amount)
___5___ time(s) a (week)/month (circle one).
My goal for this week is to eat no more than
_____1 bag_____ (amount) _3_ time(s) a
(week)/month (circle one).
I think I may meet up with the following problems:
I love potato chips and they are
conveniently located at the checkout counter
To deal with these problems I plan to:
bring popcorn or fruit instead
_____
_____
_____

Signed: _____ Date: _____
Witness: _____ Date: _____

FIGURE 12-4 A sample completed contract for eating fewer high-fat foods.

can provide them with more than one way to change their diets and give alternative menu suggestions to enhance their ability to make their own trade-offs.

Another effective approach is to devise and provide to program participants some sort of *self-monitoring system* that is feasible and easy to use. For foods that are easily identifiable, such as fruits and vegetables, such a system is relatively simple—counting items and estimating the amounts in foods. In the dietary fat arena, visible fats are easily identified (such as butter and oils), and changes can be monitored. However, many nutrients are not visible, such as fat, salt, or fiber. Here, some kind of point system needs to be devised for self-monitoring purposes, and label reading skills become important.

In general, whereas the initial motivation for change is driven by *anticipated* positive consequences of making the change, maintenance of

change is motivated by *actual* positive experiences from the change, such as finding that eating healthful food is satisfying and pleasurable.

Prioritizing Competing Goals

Managing conflicting goals and competing priorities is at the heart of self-regulation for maintaining the behavior chosen. A major ongoing challenge in maintaining healthful practices is setting priorities between conflicting goals or desires, such as between the goal to eat more healthfully and a personal agenda that may involve work-related aspirations that do not leave much mental and physical time for planning and eating healthfully. At this time, the chosen behavioral goal, such as to eat healthful lunches at work, needs to be evaluated in relation to competing goals, such as the desire to be a productive worker and hence not to be gone too long from one's desk, and needs to be protected from these

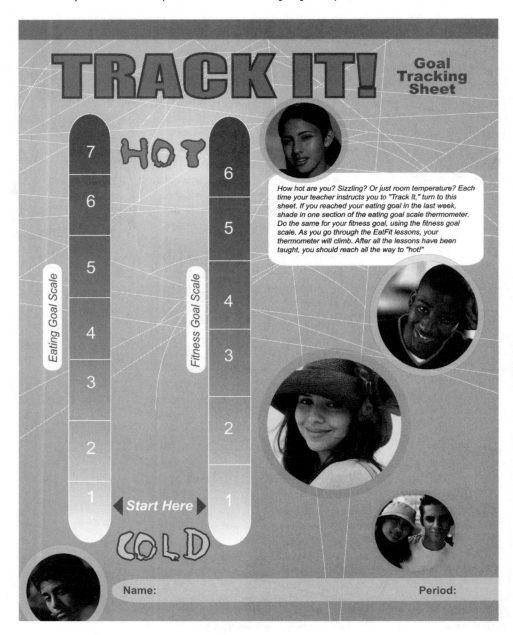

FIGURE 12-5 The EatFit program's goal tracking sheet.

Source: Shilts, M. K., M. Horowitz, and M. S. Townsend. 2004. An innovative approach to goal setting for adolescents: Guided goal setting. *Journal of Nutrition Education and Behavior* 36:155–156. Courtesy of M. K. Shilts, M. Horowitz, and M. S. Townsend, University of California–Davis.

competing goals if the chosen goal is determined to be more important. Nutrition educators should remember that implementing a new, more healthful behavior, such as adding fruit to the diet, does not automatically reduce less healthful habits such as eating high-fat, high-sugar snacks. Encourage participants to review each goal they are trying to achieve (e.g., eating fruits and vegetables, breastfeeding) in terms of its positive value to them, how important or desirable it is to them, how it relates to their larger life goals, how they will feel about achieving or not achieving the goal, and how much they have already invested, and then to reaffirm their commitment to their chosen goal. Your role is that of a collaborator and coach.

Protecting Action Goals from Distractions (Mindful Eating)

Goal maintenance relies on conscious control and attention. It is important to assist program participants to protect their goals from being interrupted and given up prematurely because of competing distractions. For example, a table that is full of tasty, high-fat foods presents a distraction to someone who has chosen the goal of eating lower-fat foods. The eating setting—ambiance, lighting, eating with others, or look of the menu—influences the amount of food eaten (Wansink 2006). Ask individuals to identify potential distracting situations and to make plans ahead of time to ignore these anticipated distractions. This can be done when participants verbally describe or imagine the situation and rehearse exactly what they will do and the positive outcomes they can expect from staying with their goals. You also can remind individuals just to be mindful about what they eat: think before they eat.

Attributions and Cognitive Restructuring (Self-Talk)

When individuals attempt to make changes in their eating patterns, they will likely experience both successes and failures. Their attributions of why they were successful or not will influence their sense of self-efficacy and future behavior. If they think their success (for example, in cooking) was because of a stable cause, such as their ability, they will have a higher expectation of success the next time compared with individuals who attribute their success to something unstable, such as luck. After failure, these effects are reversed. These attributions are sometimes called *self-talk*. You can assist individuals to develop more accurate attributions and new ways of thinking or self-talk. For example, encourage individuals to tell themselves they are not clumsy, but skillful, and to recognize that the great dish they have prepared results from the skills they have acquired, not luck, and to tell themselves they can do it again. This process is called *counterconditioning* in the transtheoretical model.

Focusing on Higher-Order Behavioral Goals in the Achievement of Action Goals

Higher-order behavioral goals can provide stability and facilitate choices among specific action goals in difficult situations. Encourage program participants to focus on the major goal when they are in difficult situations. For example, individuals may find themselves unable to eat the vegetables at lunch they had planned because of a birthday party for a coworker. They can fulfill their personal social goal at lunch and "reschedule" an extra vegetable serving at dinner to achieve their major health goal of eating more fruits and vegetables.

Linking Action Goals to Self-Identity

If the chosen goals can be seen as part of the identity of intervention participants, they are less likely to be devalued or postponed when competing goals emerge (such as deadlines at work). For example, if individuals come to think of themselves as health-conscious or ecologically responsible eaters, they will be more likely to stay with their action goals to eat more fruits and vegetables.

Coping Self-Efficacy

Goal maintenance also relies on emotion-coping strategies, such as the ability to ignore feelings of worry or of disappointment in not meeting the goals that were set. These strategies are important because many desirable food- and nutrition-related practices require effort—for example, seeking out farmers' markets to eat locally or learning to cook so as to gain control over what is eaten. Individuals' optimistic beliefs about their ability to deal with barriers, though a major hindrance in getting them motivated, may be helpful here because a new behavior may turn out to be much more difficult to adhere to than they had anticipated.

These beliefs are sometimes referred to as *coping self-efficacy*. Examples are "I can stick with a healthful diet even if I have to try several times until it works" or "I can stick with a healthful diet even if I need a long time to develop the necessary routines" (Schwarzer & Renner 2000). Or again, "I can stick with a healthful diet even when others in the family do not wish to do so." Thus, the nutrition educator should help program participants become aware that they have coping resources. Here again, having program participants practice positive, action-oriented self-talk (or cognitive restructuring) can be useful, reminding themselves that they are capable of taking action.

Managing Environmental Cues

Cue management is the process in which individuals remove cues to less healthful eating and add cues for more healthful eating. Provide instruction to program participants on how to restructure their personal environments. For example, they can reduce the number of less healthful foods in the household and keep them out of sight or make them less accessible and convenient. Such foods can be purchased and eaten occasionally or as treats. On the other hand, fruit can be washed, ready to eat, and left on the counter or in the refrigerator. Likewise, vegetables can be washed, cut up and ready to eat, and conveniently placed in the refrigerator. If a goal is to reduce the number of plastic bags used for groceries, then canvas bags can be placed on the front door knob or in the car, ready for use in the grocery store.

Help participants to be aware of environmental cues even in situations where they cannot control them and develop coping strategies. Two thirds of food purchases are unplanned and influenced by store displays and other marketing strategies. Participants should write out shopping lists.

Developing Routines and Habits

A major aim during the maintenance phase of dietary change is for the new behaviors to become automatic or habitual (Bargh & Barndollar 1996). When people repeatedly perform a behavior in a specific context (such as drinking orange juice at breakfast), the motivation (to eat more fruit) and its implementation instructions (drink orange juice at breakfast) become so integrated that as soon as they experience the situation (breakfast) the specific action is triggered in memory without the need for conscious decision making. Thus, repeated context-specific action leads to increasingly effortless enactment of the behavior.

Setting goals helps to initiate new habits. At first, achieving the goals requires conscious control, but repetition of the action leads to more unconscious control over behavior. Help program participants to develop routines. Assure them that even difficult behaviors will become easier when they become more routine (such as making a lunch to bring to school or to work each day).

Familiarity with Healthful Food

An important aim of nutrition education programs is for participants to enjoy eating the healthful foods that are the target of the programs. As you saw earlier in the book, there is considerable evidence that repeated experience with a food can increase liking and preference for it. Studies have found that those who decide to eat less salt eventually come to like foods with less salt. In the case of fat intake, when individuals use fat substitutes to reduce the fat content of their diet, they still like the taste of fat, but when they switch to naturally low-fat foods, they decrease their liking for the fatty taste (Mattes 1993; Grieve & Vander Weg 2003). One study of long-term maintenance of a low-fat diet found that using fat substitutes was easily adopted but did not contribute much to dietary fat reduction, whereas avoiding fat as a flavoring (such as sauces on vegetables or butter on bread) and eating less meat were difficult to adopt but contributed the most to reducing the overall fat content of the diet (Bowen et al. 1993). It should be noted that the former represents a substitution of one product for a similar one and is not a behavioral change, whereas the latter actions represent a change in behavior. Many of the study participants felt deprived, but those who successfully maintained the diet regimen found they no longer liked the taste of fat (Urban et al. 1992). It is clear that people eat what they like, but they also come to like what they eat. Hence, remind program participants to stay with their chosen dietary change long enough for them to come to like the new foods and, indeed, to find them pleasurable to eat.

Personal Food Policies

The ultimate goal in nutrition education is for individuals themselves to be able eventually to take charge of their food choices and practices by using self-regulatory processes such as those described in this chapter. These processes help them develop the skills necessary for influencing not only their own personal behavior but also the environments in which their food choices are made. Individuals can be encouraged to develop personal food policies to guide their dietary choices and food-related actions. They can decide, for example, that they will always eat breakfast, always have a vegetable at lunch, eat desserts only once a week, buy organic or local foods whenever there is a choice, shop at farmers' markets in season, eat at a fast food chain restaurant only once a week (or whatever frequency), and so forth. These food policies help guide decisions on an ongoing basis.

Management of Social Context

Most eating occurs in a social context, even if many meals are eaten alone. For example, food purchasing requires consideration of household needs. Thus, the mother of the household may decide to drink nonfat milk, but the rest of the family insists on whole milk. Should she then buy both kinds? Does she have space to store both kinds? If she decides to eat more plant-based, whole-grain meals, whereas the other family members want to eat hamburgers and french fries, will she make two meals? Or will she cook for herself and let the others fend for themselves? She will have to make trade-offs and negotiations between her desire for health for herself and her desire to maintain good family relationships. And of course mothers of young children also need encouragement and skills in feeding their children. Facilitated group discussions can be invaluable here as individuals meet with others like themselves to share ideas and challenges and how to overcome them. The nutrition educator can provide valuable assistance in the process. An example of such an intervention is discussed in **Nutrition Education in Action 12-3**.

Figure 12-6 depicts how mediators from theory can be translated into educational strategies and activities that are useful in action-phase sessions or program components.

■ CASE STUDY

We now apply the information in this chapter specifically to the ongoing case study to illustrate the process of selecting appropriate educational strategies for each of the mediators selected and of designing fun, enjoyable educational activities and needed content for group participants to achieve the educational objectives. This lesson is a follow-up to the one described in Chapter 11.

Educational Plan Design: Matrix Format

In the first column, we list each of the *potential mediators* of behavior change—which also are the theory constructs from our theory model. For each mediator, we now write *specific educational objectives*. In the next column, we indicate the theory-based *strategies* that we will use to address the potential mediators and briefly describe all of the *practical educational activities, learning experiences, or messages* that we plan to use to carry out the educational strategies. In the final column of the matrix, we list the "events of instruction" to help us *sequence* the activities during the session appropriately.

Educational Delivery Plan: Teaching Format

The teaching or narrative form for delivering the lesson is also shown for the case study. This is what we will take with us to implement the session.

■ YOUR TURN: COMPLETING THE STEP 5 WORKSHEETS: FOCUS ON TAKING ACTION

You can now apply the information in this chapter to the process of selecting appropriate educational strategies and designing learning experiences to achieve each of the behavioral goals of the program. As you saw in the last chapter, these strategies should be sequenced as events of instruction to provide a plan for how to proceed. The resulting plan is referred to as the *lesson plan* or *educational plan*, even though it will be used for in-person group activities with all ages and in all settings, particularly nonformal ones. By now you probably realize that designing learning experiences or activities is a very fluid process so that you will be going back and forth between designing activities, sequencing them, and writing educational objectives. In addition, after pilot testing, you may want to change or rearrange activities.

Sequencing Activities Is Important

How exactly you arrange your sequence of educational strategies depends on many factors that are specific to the needs of your audience and the theory guiding your intervention. In general, though, you want to begin each session or series of sessions with activities to gain the attention of the group, move to activities to enhance motivation and promote contemplation, and then focus on activities to build skills and strengthen self-efficacy or collective efficacy. Some kind of closure or take-home-message is important (Gagne et al. 2004). The same systematic process is needed for the design of all nutrition education messages and activities, such as brochures, newsletters, posters, media messages, or campaigns.

The Educational Plan: Using a Matrix Format to Design the Plan

It is useful to first develop a lesson or educational plan outline using a matrix format as shown in the worksheet and case study. Here, you first state the behavioral goal of the session, and then write general educational objectives to achieve the behavioral goal. These objectives should be directed at the key mediators of change. You then write specific objectives for each of the mediators that your theory suggests that you address. Achievement of these specific objectives helps the group participants achieve the desired behavioral goals. You then create learning experiences, activities, and content that will achieve the specific objectives. The matrix format enables you to see whether you have addressed all the educational objectives that you set and whether the activities are appropriate in terms of domain of learning and level of complexity. The

NUTRITION EDUCATION IN ACTION 12-3

Sisters in Health: An Experiential Program Emphasizing Social Interaction to Increase Fruit and Vegetable Intake Among Low-Income Adults

Sisters in Health was a community-based program to increase fruit and vegetable intake among low-income women that was designed to be implemented in small groups in real-life community settings, to be flexible, and to be easy to implement by community nutrition educators. It was based on facilitated group discussion and experiential learning, in which group members were interactively involved in discussing their knowledge, experiences, problems, and solutions with other group members.

Program

The program consisted of six 90-minute weekly meetings for groups of approximately 10 women, facilitated by community nutrition paraprofessionals trained through the Cooperative Extension Service. The program was based on extensive formative research or needs assessment.

Each session included the following:

- A welcome or warm-up activity, such as how the family liked the new dish tried at home
- A food preparation and tasting experience, such as creating and tasting a salad bar
- A group learning activity, such as adding or subtracting ingredients from a salad to boost nutrient density
- A take-home challenge, such as making at least one "enhanced salad" at home
- Feedback on the meeting and for planning the next one
- Low-cost incentives, such as cooking utensils and notebooks for recipes

All groups received the sessions "Getting Started," which focused on participants' familiarity with and preferences regarding fruits and vegetables, and "All About Me," which focused on recommendations and portion sizes. Four other sessions were chosen by the group (from eight), on topics such as "Scoring with Salads," "Kids and Vegetables," "Easier Than Pie: Fruit Anytime," and "Beat the Clock with Meals in Minutes." Such an approach combined flexibility and the needs and interests of the group with the need for prepprepared education plans for effective education.

Evaluation

The program's impact was evaluated in a nonrandom sample of 269 low-income adults in 32 intervention and 10 control groups using a quasi-experimental, pre- and postprogram evaluation design in which a control group received a budgeting or parenting program of the same duration and intensity. Intervention groups reported an increase in fruit and vegetable consumption, measured by a brief screener, of 1.6 times a day (compared with 0.8 in the control groups). Knowledge of the number of servings people should eat and self-efficacy did not increase (they may have already been high), but attitudes, knowledge of preparation methods, and satisfaction with how vegetables turned out did increase significantly. Group support, active learning experiences, food tastings, and food skill development were thus effective in increasing fruit and vegetable intake in these low-income adults.

Source: Devine, C. M., T. J. Farrell, and R. Hartman. 2005. Sisters in Health: Experiential program emphasizing social interaction increases fruit and vegetable intake among low-income adults. *Journal of Nutrition Education and Behavior* 37:265–270.

---

information in Chapter 15 about practical tips for working with groups is very helpful as you design your educational sessions.

The Educational Plan: Developing a Narrative Format to Deliver the Plan

You then convert the matrix into a more detailed narrative lesson plan or some other format that you will actually use when you are with a group. The case study provides a sample lesson plan showing how the matrix format is used to design the session and how the narrative format is used for delivery. The worksheet can be used to develop your educational plan for a real or hypothetical educational session.

- Think of a catchy title that will be meaningful to your audience. It should motivate people to come to your session or pique their interest if they are required to attend.
- Place an overview or outline of activities and a materials list at the beginning of the teaching plan. That way you will have the entire session in mind and all of the materials ready.
- Convert each of the activities in the matrix into a fuller description or narrative. Include all the specific information you will need. Don't count on remembering everything.

- For each educational activity, create a heading with a title and indicate the mediator(s) addressed.
- Write the educational plan with sufficient detail that someone else could deliver it.
- Be prepared. If the session involves a food preparation activity, make sure you have tested the recipes and that you have prepped the foods so they are ready for the participants (such as fruits and vegetables washed, stems cut off, etc,).
- Sequence the activities based on an order of instruction. You can use the one described in this chapter based on the work of educational instruction specialists (Gagne et al. 2004): gain attention, present stimulus or new material, provide guidance and practice, and apply and close. If the session involves hands-on activities, think through the flow: once the group starts to do food preparation, for example, it may be hard to get them back into a group listening mode. Can some of the instruction be provided concurrently with the activity?
- A sense of closure is especially important. This is a good time to provide an opportunity to apply what the audience has learned. A clear set of action steps or a goal-setting worksheet would be very useful.

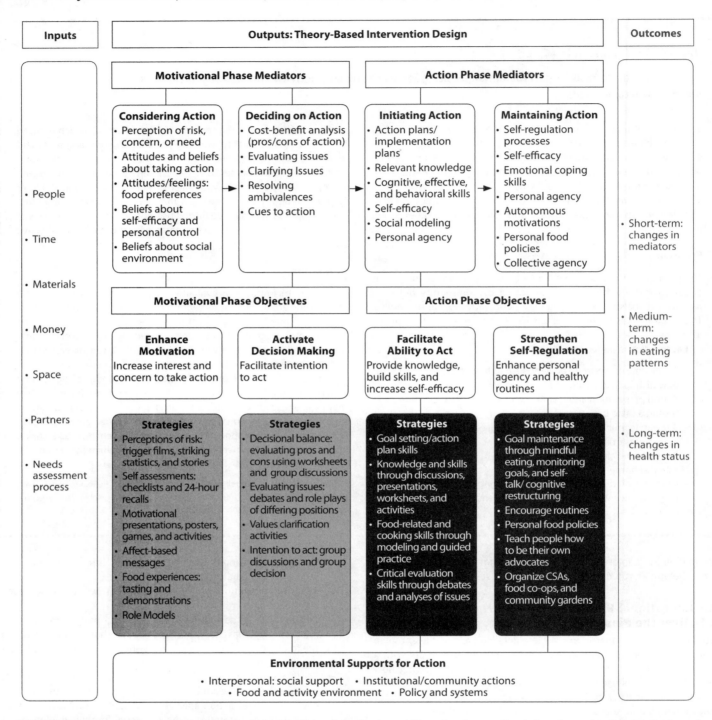

FIGURE 12-6 Integrative framework for translating behavioral theory into effective nutrition education practice: Action phase educational strategies and activities.

Pilot Testing the Educational Plan

If your program is more than a one-time event, all the learning experiences designed should be extensively pilot tested with the intended audience. If food is used, test the recipes and preparation procedures for taste acceptance and feasibility. Using focus groups, direct observation, and interviews, assess whether activities are acceptable and effective with the intended audience.

Educational Plans in Practice

The educational plans as presented may seem quite specific and detailed. However, it is very important to have such plans. Otherwise, you may not have a clear focus that serves the cause of helping program participants to achieve the behavioral goals that your program has set out. It is understood, however, that you may find yourself needing to adapt the education plans to the situation on the ground and to the backgrounds and interests of the *specific* group with whom you are working. Practical delivery methods are described in more detail in Part III of this book.

Questions and Activities

1. Why are goal setting and the development of action plans important for the effectiveness of nutrition education interventions? Discuss.
   a. What are three characteristics of effective action goals?
   b. Describe some practical ways that goal setting can be taught.
2. Describe three kinds of specific educational activities or learning experiences that you could conduct to strengthen self-regulation skills.
3. For practice, state one educational *strategy* for each of the following potential mediators that facilitate the ability to increase the intake of calcium-rich foods among teenage girls. For each strategy, describe at least one *educational activity or learning experience*.

Potential Mediator of the Ability to Take Action	Educational Strategy	Educational Activities or Learning Experiences
Perceived self-efficacy		
Social support		
Cues to action		

References

Achterberg, C. 1998. Factors that influence learner readiness. *Journal of the American Dietetic Association* 88:1426–1428.

Anderson, A. S., D. N. Cox, S. McKellar, J. Reynolds, M. E. Lean, and D. J. Mela. 1998. Take Five, a nutrition education intervention to increase fruit and vegetable intakes: Impact on attitudes towards dietary change. *British Journal of Nutrition* 80(2):133–140.

Armitage, C. 2004. Evidence that implementation intentions reduce dietary fat intake: A randomized trial. *Health Psychology* 23:319–323.

Bandura, A. 1986. *Foundations of thought and action: A social cognitive theory.* Englewood Cliffs, NJ: Prentice Hall.

———. 1997. *Self-efficacy: The exercise of control.* New York: WH Freeman.

Bargh, J. A., and K. Barndollar. 1996. Automaticity in action: The unconscious as repository of chronic goals and motives. In *The psychology of action: Linking cognition and motivation to behavior*, edited by P. M. Gollwitzer and J. A. Bargh. New York: Guildford Press.

Barnard, N. D., A. Akhtar, and A. Nicholson. 1995. Factors that facilitate compliance to a low fat intake. *Archives of Family Medicine* 4:153–158.

Bisogni, C. A., M. Jastran, L. Shen, and C. M. Devine. 2005. A biographical study of food choice capacity: Standards, circumstances, and food management skills. *Journal of Nutrition Education and Behavior* 37:284–291.

Bowen, D. J., H. Henry, E. Burrows, G. Anderson, and M. H. Henderson. 1993. Influences of eating patterns on change to a low-fat diet. *Journal of the American Dietetic Association* 93:1309–1311.

Brunner, E., I. White, M. Thorogood, A. Bristow, D. Curle, and M. Marmot. 1997. Can dietary interventions change diet and cardiovascular risk factors? A meta-analysis of randomized controlled trials. *American Journal of Public Health* 87:1415–1422.

Burrows, E. R., H. J. Henry, D. J. Bowen, and M. M. Henderson. 1993. Nutritional applications of a clinical low fat dietary intervention to public health change. *Journal of Nutrition Education* 25:167–175.

Cox, D. N., A. S. Anderson, J. Reynolds, S. McKellar, M. E. J. Lean, and D. J. Mela. 1998. Take Five, a nutrition education intervention to increase fruit and vegetable intakes: Impact on consumer choice and nutrient intakes. *British Journal of Nutrition* 80(2):123–131.

Cullen, K. W., T. Baranowski, and S. P. Smith. 2001. Using goal setting as a strategy for dietary behavior change. *Journal of the American Dietetic Association* 101:562–566.

Gollwitzer, P. M. 1999. Implementation intentions: Strong effects of simple plans. *American Psychologist* 54:493–503.

Grieve, F. G., and M. W. Vander Weg. 2003. Desire to eat high- and low-fat foods following a low-fat dietary intervention. *Journal of Nutrition Education and Behavior* 35:93–99.

Krathwohl, D., B. Bloom, and B. Masia. 1964. *Taxonomy of educational objectives: The classification of educational goals (affective domain).* New York: McKay.

Kristal, A. R., A. L. Shattuck, and H. J. Henry. 1990. Patterns of dietary behavior associated with selecting diets low in fat: Reliability and validity of a behavioral approach to dietary assessment. *Journal of the American Dietetic Association* 90:214–220.

Levy, J., and G. Auld. 2004. Cooking classes outperform cooking demonstrations for college sophomores. *Journal of Nutrition Education and Behavior* 36:197–203.

Locke, E. A., and G. P. Latham. 1990. *A theory of goal setting and performance.* Upper Saddle River, NJ: Prentice Hall.

Mattes, R. D. 1993. Fat preference and adherence to a reduced fat diet. *American Journal of Clinical Nutrition* 57:373–377.

Pelican, S., F. Vanden Heede, B. Holmes, et al. 2005. The power of others to shape our identity: Body image, physical abilities, and body weight. *Family and Consumer Sciences Research Journal* 34:57–80.

Satia, J. A., A. R. Kristal, R. E. Patterson, M. L. Neuhouser, and E. Trudeau. 2002. Psychological factors and dietary habits associated with vegetable consumption. *Nutrition* 18:247–254.

Schwarzer, R., and B. Renner. 2000. Social cognitive predictors of health behavior: Action self-efficacy and coping self-efficacy. *Health Psychology* 19:487–495.

Shannon, J., A. R. Kristal, S. J. Curry, and S. A. Beresford. 1997. Application of a behavioral approach to measuring dietary change: The fat and fiber-related diet behavior questionnaire. *Cancer Epidemiology, Biomarkers and Prevention* 6:355–361.

Shilts, M. K., M. Horowitz, and M. Townsend. 2004. An innovative approach to goal setting for adolescents: Guided goal setting. *Journal of Nutrition Education and Behavior* 36:155–156.

———. 2009. Guided goal setting: effectiveness in a dietary and physical activity intervention with low-income adolescents. *International Journal of Adolescent Medicine and Health* 21(1):111–122.

Thoresen, C. E. 1984. Strategies for health enhancement overview. In *Behavioral health: A handbook of health enhancement and disease prevention*, edited by J. D. Matarazzo, S. M. Weiss, J. A. Herd, and N. E. Miller. New York: Wiley.

Urban, N., E. White, G. Anderson, S. Curry, and A. Kristal. 1992. Correlates of maintenance of a low fat diet in the Women's Health Trial. *Preventive Medicine* 21:279–291.

Wansink, B. 2006. *Mindless eating: Why we eat more than we think.* New York: Bantam Dell.

Wiman, R. V., and W. C. Mierhenry. 1969. *Editors, educational media: Theory into practice.* Columbus, OH: Charles Merrill.

Zeitlin, M., and C. S. Formacion. 1981. *Nutrition in developing countries. Study II. Nutrition education.* Cambridge, MA: Oelgeschlager, Gunn, O'Hain.

In Step 5, you use your theoretical model, philosophy of nutrition education, and nutrition education program objectives to create (1) educational plans for the individual-level components and (2) environmental support plans for environmental/policy components.

These pages of the Step 5 worksheets are devoted to designing educational plans for activities directed at individuals, referred to here as the individual-level component. Generally, the primary individual-level component consists of one or more group sessions. (You can also use these worksheets to design other individual-level components, such as newsletters and media-related activites.)

You should have **one** educational plan for **each** group session you design (or newsletter or other component directed at individuals).

At the end of the Step 5 worksheets for the individual components, you will have the following products:

Step 5A: General educational objectives for each session or series of sessions directed at the same behavioral goal

Step 5B: An overall design plan for the session in the form of a matrix that links mediators, objectives, and activities

Step 5C: A narrative educational plan that translates the matrix into a form ready for teaching or presenting

Use these worksheets as an organizational guide to help you design your educational plan and translate theory mediators into educational activities. Electronic versions of these worksheets are available at http://nutrition.jbpub.com/education/2e/. If you are unable to access the worksheets electronically, you can write onto this blank worksheet or create a text document that uses the same flow of information.

> **NOTE:** For the case study, we present educational plans that focus on only one of the program's goal behaviors: increasing fruit and vegetable intake. Generally, educational plans include activities based on both motivating and facilitating mediators. For illustrative purposes, we describe two lessons and divide them into one educational plan that focuses primarily on motivational mediators (Chapter 11) and a second educational plan that focuses on facilitators of behavior change (Chapter 12). We have done this to highlight the numerous strategies and activities that are possible for addressing motivating and facilitating mediators.

Step 5A: General educational objectives

Educational plan title: The Whats of Colorful Eating (educational plan focusing on facilitating mediators)

Program goal behaviors: Students will increase their fruit and vegetable intake (youth to aim for 2.5 or more cups per day).

Write the general educational objectives.

Mediator (from Step 3)	General educational objectives
Self-efficacy	Demonstrate increased self-efficacy in eating a variety of fruits and vegetables (F&V) every day
Food and nutrition skills	Demonstrate increased knowledge and skills in incorporating fruits and vegetables into their daily food patterns
Goal-setting skills	Prepare action plans using goal-setting and decision-making skills to increase their consumption of F&V

Step 5B: Designing the educational plan: matrix format

Design your educational (or lesson) plan in matrix format. Write specific objectives for the mediators in your theory model (Step 3). Identify the learning domain and level for each objective. Then write the theory-based strategy you will employ to address the mediator and create educational activities that will be meaningful, interesting, and appropriate for your audience and will operationalize strategy.

Sequence your educational activities based on the events of instruction. After you have completed creating activities for each of the mediators in your theory model, go back through the design matrix and carefully identify each of the strategies/activities as to where it should fall in a sequence suitable for implementing with your audience. Label each activity as to whether it will be used to (A) gain attention, (S) present stimulus or new material, (G) provide guidance and practice, or (C) apply and close the session. These are referred to as the "Events of Instruction" or "EoI."

Carefully re-order the matrix. If the mediators and the related activities you have created are not listed in your matrix in the properly sequenced order (i.e., gain attention to apply and close), then carefully re-order the matrix so all activities as well as mediators and objectives are in the proper sequenced order ready to use to create your educational plan or teaching plan.

Mediator (from Step 3)	Specific educational objectives	Learning domain/level*	Theory-based** strategy and educational activities, experiences, and/or content	EoI
			Icebreaker: •In dyads, individuals discuss a time they felt good about their eating and another when they did not, and why.	G
Food- and nutrition-related knowledge	State the key reasons for eating a variety of F&V ("a rainbow of colors") Compare the nutrient content of F&V snacks with processed and packaged energy-dense snacks Estimate serving sizes of F&V	C: comprehension C: evaluation C: comprehension	How-to knowledge:** •Review reasons for eating a variety of F&V; key nutrients in them, health benefits, and need for variety of intake. •Show commonly eaten packaged energy-dense snacks; worksheet for students to calculate and compare fat and vitamin C content with F&V. •Show serving sizes; engaging group activity for estimating serving sizes (e.g., contest for answers).	S
Food- and nutrition-related skills	Describe how these F&V can be used in meals/snacks Prepare simple recipes using F&V State satisfaction in trying new F&V	C: application P: imitation A: valuing	Food skills:** •Present tips on how to use F&V in meals and snacks. •Provide exciting cooking experience if possible; or teens in groups make different snacks from new fruits and/or vegetables: salads, salsa. •Teens eat foods/snacks they prepared.	G
Goal setting	State clear personal action goals to eat more F&V Make action plan to eat all the colors during a given week	C: application A: valuing	Personal action goals:** •Teach skills in goal setting and in developing action plans to achieve personal action goals; provide contract forms. •Worksheet for action plan to eat all the colors during the following week.	G
Self-regulation skills	Appreciate the importance of recognizing hunger and satiety cues during a busy day Develop plan, incorporating F&V, to satisfy hunger when it occurs and to follow plan during a busy day	A: valuing C: synthesis A: organization	Goal setting and self-monitoring:** •Activity to teach students to identify hunger, mood, and cues for food intakes. •Provide action planning form for adolescents to plan F&V to eat during a busy day; make contract; develop way to monitor progress toward that goal; reward self when goal is achieved. •If more than one session, provide opportunities for feedback, rewards, and new goals.	G/C

*C = cognitive domain; A = affective domain; P = psychomotor domain.

Step 5C: Educational Plan

Write a narrative educational plan, based on your design matrix, that you will actually use to deliver your session. Think of a catchy title that will be meaningful to your audience. Make sure that activities are sequenced based on order of instruction. For each educational activity create a heading with a title and the mediator(s) addressed. Then write a detailed procedure for the activity. It is customary to place an overview or outline of activities and a materials list at the beginning of the teaching plan.

The Whats of Colorful Eating

Overview of Content (50 to 60 minutes)
1. Introduction and icebreaker
2. Review reasons for eating a variety of F&V
3. Worksheet comparing fat and vitamin C between various foods
4. Group serving size activity
5. F&V snack and meal tips
6. Prepare and eat a snack
7. Goal setting and action plans for eating a variety of different colored F&V
8. Hunger and mood discussion
9. Goal setting and action plans for eating F&V when hungry and wrap-up

Materials
- Worksheet to record fat and vitamin C content in food items
- Energy-dense snack labels (e.g., candy bars, chips, cookies, chocolates)
- Various F&V (e.g., lettuce, broccoli, different size apples, grapefruit, banana)
- Game prizes (e.g., stickers, temporary tattoos, pencils, small bounce balls)
- Bowls
- Blank paper and pencils
- F&V for snack
- Utensils necessary to prepare the snack (e.g., knives, cutting board)
- Action plan worksheets

Procedure
1. **Introduction and icebreaker (8 minutes)**
   Greet participants and introduce the lesson, the whats of colorful eating—what you can do to make sure you eat a rainbow of different colored F&V every day. Instruct participants to pair up with a partner they do not usually work with. The pairs will individually discuss a time they felt really good about their eating and another time when they did not, and why. Allow discussion for a few minutes and then ask pairs to switch speakers. Bring group back together. Ask if anyone wants to share his or her experience during the icebreaker. Remind the group that positive participation is encouraged.

2. **Review reasons for eating a variety of F&V (2 minutes) (benefits)**
   Begin by reviewing the reasons to eat a colorful range of F&V. Ensure the following are mentioned: provides essential vitamins, minerals, fiber, and other nutrients; can increase energy; helps make hair and skin healthy; builds strong bones and muscles for athletic performance; and decreases risk for certain diseases. F&V can be wonderful snacks.

3. **Worksheet comparing fat and vitamin C content between common snack foods (8 minutes) (behavioral capability)**
   Now that the reasons for eating F&V have been discussed, compare the fat and amount of vitamin C found in some common snack foods with the fat and vitamin C found in F&V. Provide nutrition labels of a few different energy-dense snack items, such as chips. Ask the participants to fill out the worksheets. Discussion: How did the energy-dense snacks compare with the F&V in terms of fat and vitamin C? How surprised are you at the difference?

4. **Estimating serving sizes. Group activity (10 minutes) (food-related skills)**
   Explain that knowing why we should eat F&V is as important as understanding how much we are eating when we have a portion of F&V. Divide into teams and play a game to guess the serving size, with the winner winning a prize. Take prepared bowls filled with a variety of different foods that have been previously measured for their portion size. Show each group the first bowl, for example one filled with lettuce, and ask each group to write down how many servings are in the bowl. If the bowl was filled with two cups, each group that guesses two servings will get a point. Continue the game with different F&V and portion sizes. Discussion: What do you think about the size of a serving? How often do you think about the serving size when you eat a food? Do you usually eat larger or smaller portions than the recommended serving size?

5. **F&V snack and meal tips (3 minutes) (food- and nutrition-related skills)**
   Ask participants to share one of their favorite F&V snacks, or ways to eat F&V at a meal. Ensure tips such as leaving fruit on the kitchen table to grab as a snack or cutting up a lot of veggies to make an easy grab-and-go snack are mentioned. Suggest having a piece of fruit at breakfast, F&V for snack, a salad during lunch or dinner, and discuss ways to cook vegetables.

6. **Snack time! Prepare and eat a snack (10–30 minutes) (food- and nutrition-related skills)**
Snack suggestions: veggies and dips, such as hummus, lemon yogurt, peanut butter, fruit salad, and green salad with dressing. Make sure all the participants are involved in the preparation. Encourage everyone to taste the food. Let the group know that positive feelings about the food should be shared, but negative ones should not. Remember to practice good food safety and clean up when you are done.

7. **Time to take action. Goal setting and action plans for eating a variety of different color F&V (5 minutes) (goal setting)**
Discuss the importance of practicing what has been learned every day. Encourage participants to set personal goals for eating more F&V by filling out the action plan worksheet. For example, set incremental goals of eating three different colors of F&V one week, four different colors the next week, and then all five the following week. Provide time for the students to fill in the worksheets. Ask if any of the students want to share what their goals are and how they hope to achieve them.

8. **Planning ahead (4 minutes) (goal setting)**
A sample lecture is as follows: The school day can be very busy, beginning from the moment you wake up. Many of you don't have time to eat breakfast before you leave the house, and then you rush from class to class. That means you can get quite hungry. Then you grab whatever is easiest to eat and whatever is at hand, so it is almost impossible to include F&V in your day. This happens to all of us. These ups and downs can affect our mood and our ability to learn. However, we can plan ahead, and carry some foods with us to eat when we get hungry and are not near food—such as bananas or apples.

 Instruct students to review their action plans and make them more specific: They can now write action plans that focus on bringing F&V with them and eating them when they are hungry. Participants can list three occasions when they anticipate they will be hungry during the day and write down specific actions they will take to incorporate F&V during these times.

9. **Self-monitoring (4 minutes) (self-regulation skills)**
Discuss ways to monitor progress. Encourage the members of the group to support each other and remember to reward themselves when they meet their goals! Thank the group and include any reminders about future meetings and events. If the group will continue to meet in the future, plan to follow up with the participants' successes and struggles working towards their goals.

In Step 5, you use your theoretical model, philosophy of nutrition education, and nutrition education program objectives to create (1) educational plans for the individual-level components and (2) environmental support plans for environmental/policy components.

These pages of the Step 5 worksheets are devoted to designing educational plans for activities directed at individuals, referred to here as the individual-level components. Generally, the primary individual-level component consists of one or more group sessions. (You can also use these worksheets to design other individual-level components, such as newsletters and media-related activities.)

You should have **one** educational plan for **each** group session you design (or newsletter or other component directed at individuals).

At the end of the Step 5 worksheets for the individual-level components, you will have the following products:

Step 5A: General educational objectives for each session or series of sessions directed at the same behavioral goal

Step 5B: An overall design plan for the session in the form of a matrix that links mediators, objectives, and activities

Step 5C: A narrative educational plan that translates the matrix into a form ready for teaching or presenting

Use these worksheets as an organizational guide to help you design your educational plan and translate theory mediators into educational activities. Electronic versions of these worksheets are available at http://nutrition.jbpub.com/education/2e/. If you are unable to access the worksheets electronically, you can write onto this blank worksheet or create a text document that uses the same flow of information.

Step 5A: General educational objectives

Educational plan title: _____

Program goal behaviors: _____

Write the general educational objectives.

Mediator (from Step 3)	General educational objectives

Step 5B: Designing the educational plan: matrix format

Design your educational (or lesson) plan in matrix format. Write specific objectives for the mediators in your theory model (Step 3). Identify the learning domain and level for each objective. Then, write the theory-based strategy you will employ to address the mediator and create educational activities that will be meaningful, interesting, and appropriate for your audience and will operationalize strategy.

Sequence your educational activities based on the events of instruction. After you have completed creating activities for each of the mediators in your theory model, go back through the design matrix and carefully identify each of the strategies/activities as to where it should fall in a sequence suitable for implementing with your audience. Label each activity as to whether it will be used to (A) gain attention, (S) present stimulus or new material, (G) provide guidance and practice, or (C) apply and close the session. These are referred to as the "Events of Instruction" or "EoI."

Carefully re-order the matrix. If the mediators and the related activities you have created are not at first listed in your matrix in the properly sequenced order (i.e., gain attention to apply and close), then carefully re-order the matrix so all activities as well as mediators and objectives are in the proper sequenced order ready to use to create your educational plan or teaching plan.

Mediator (from Step 3)	Specific educational objectives*	Learning domain/level	Theory-based strategy** and educational activities, experiences, and/or content	EoI
*C = cognitive domain; A = affective domain; P = psychomotor domain.				

Step 5C: Educational plan

Write a narrative educational plan, based on your design matrix, that you will actually use to deliver your session. Think of a catchy title that will be meaningful to your audience. Make sure that activities are sequenced based on order of instruction. For each educational activity create a heading with a title and the mediator(s) addressed. Then write a detailed procedure for the activity. It is customary to place an overview or outline of activities and a materials list at the beginning of the teaching plan.

Overview of Content

Materials

Procedure

CHAPTER 13

Step 5: Designing Strategies to Promote Environmental Supports for Action: Making Action Possible

OVERVIEW

This chapter describes how to design strategies to increase environmental supports for participants to take action on behaviors or practices targeted by the program. The information in Chapter 6 will be especially helpful to you with this step in the process.

CHAPTER OUTLINE

- Introduction
- Designing theory-based strategies to increase interpersonal social support and informational support
- Designing supportive environments through collaborations and partnerships
- Designing institutional-level food environment and policy activities
- Designing community-level food environment and policy activities
- Multiple-level community nutrition education
- Summary
- Case study
- Your turn: completing the Step 5 worksheets

LEARNING OBJECTIVES

At the end of the chapter, you will be able to:

- Describe general types of strategies that can be used to address potential environmental mediators of the actions, behaviors, or practices targeted by the intervention
- Recognize the importance of collaboration with decision makers and policy makers
- Select, from the potential environmental mediators of the goal behaviors identified in Step 1, those that are to be targeted in the intervention to increase environmental support
- Use theory, current nutrition education research, and existing evaluated programs to design specific strategies to address the relevant environmental support objectives written in Step 4
- Demonstrate skill in designing environmental supports for action

■ INTRODUCTION: PROMOTING ENVIRONMENTAL SUPPORTS FOR ACTION

In addition to motivation and skills, individuals need *environmental and policy support* to take action, the third component in our integrative conceptual framework for translating theory into practice and implementing nutrition theory–based education (refer to Figure 9-4). The aim here is for the healthful choice to be an easy choice.

We have seen that interventions are more likely to be effective when they are directed not only at personal psychosocial mediators of behavior change but also at factors in the interpersonal, organizational, community, and policy spheres of influence to make them supportive of healthful eating and active living (McLeroy et al. 1988; Gregson et al. 2001; Green & Kreuter 2005).

As a nutrition educator, you can create social and informational supports for the intended audience. These might include creating support groups for the program participants, working with peer educators, developing a family component to support school- or worksite-based programs, and creating informational environments that reinforce behavior and change social norms. (**Figure 13-1** and **Figure 13-2** highlight Step 5, as discussed in Chapters 11–13.)

Nutrition educators can also inform, educate, and form partnerships with others—food and service providers, decision makers with authority and power, and policy makers—to increase environmental supports for the behaviors or practices targeted by nutrition education programs. Nutrition educators work with institutions and communities to make healthful foods available and accessible and to develop policies that encourage and reinforce healthful eating and physical activity practices.

Nutrition Education That Addresses Multiple Levels

The logic model framework for nutrition education can be expanded to include activities at multiple levels of intervention. **Figure 13-3** shows a possible community nutrition education logic model, based on the Community Nutrition Education model for Supplemental Nutrition Assistance Program Education (SNAP-Ed), and summarizes the kinds of activities nutrition educators can conduct at various levels of influence on target behaviors. This chapter focuses on food environment and policy activities at the interpersonal, organizational, and community levels as they are relevant to the design of a specific program. In designing activities, choose from among the potential environmental support objectives that you wrote in Step 4 for your program goal behaviors, those that can be realistically targeted in the intervention, given your available time and resources.

■ DESIGNING THEORY-BASED STRATEGIES TO INCREASE INTERPERSONAL SOCIAL SUPPORT AND INFORMATIONAL SUPPORT

Nutrition educators can promote supportive environments by addressing social support, a potential environmental mediator of behavior change. Here, you seek to strengthen existing social networks to make them more supportive of the food- and nutrition-related behavioral goals of your program, such as increasing breastfeeding rates and duration (e.g., by involving the family in the intervention); developing new networks that are supportive of participants' desire to take action; and providing informational support as reinforcements and cues to action. These activities can be considered to be interpersonal-level support strategies.

Making Existing Networks More Supportive

You can design activities to encourage members of participants' current social networks to be more supportive of the behavioral goals of the programs. These networks might include parent associations in schools, employee associations at workplaces, or groups that meet regularly in communities and organizations.

Parental Support

For programs directed at preschool or school-aged children in school settings, parents are external to the students and are hence part of students' external environment. In this case, parents represent a new "audience" for whom general and specific educational objectives need to be written and educational activities designed in a process similar to that for the case study, as described in the last two chapters.

Educational Sessions

The most general approach is to design sessions with parents so that they can support their children's attempts to eat healthfully. These sessions will be based on your assessments in Steps 1 and 2 and the objectives that you stated in Step 4. A potential program for parents is shown at the end of this chapter for the ongoing case study with middle school youth.

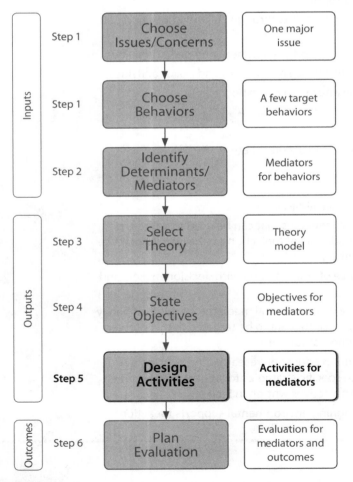

FIGURE 13-1 Flowchart of steps in designing theory-based nutrition education: Step 5.

Inputs: Collecting Assessment Data			Outputs: Designing the Theory-Based Intervention			Outcomes: Evaluation Plan
Step 1 ⟷	Step 2 ⟷	Step 3 ⟷	Step 4 ⟷	Step 5 ⟷		Step 6
Analyze issues and audiences to state program behavioral goals	**Identify potential mediators to achieve program behavioral goals**	**Select theory, philosophy, and components**	**State objectives for mediators**	**Design theory-based strategies and activities for mediators**		**Plan evaluation**
Tasks	*Tasks*	*Tasks*	*Tasks*	*Tasks*		*Tasks*
• Analyze issues and select audience • Identify behaviors or patterns contributing to issue • Specify behavioral or action goals of the program	• Identify personal psychosocial mediators • Identify environmental support mediators	• Select theory or create appropriate model • Clarify philosophy (education and content) • Determine program components	• State educational objectives for psychosocial mediators • State change objectives for environmental support mediators	• Design activities to address psychosocial mediators • Design activities to address environmental support mediators • Implementation plan		• Design outcome evaluation plan • Determine tools to measure impact • Plan process evaluation
Product	*Product*	*Product*	*Product*	*Product*		*Product*
• *Description of issue of concern* • *Statement of action or behavioral goals for program*	• *List of potential mediators for action or behavior goals*	• *Theory/model for program, philosophy, and components*	• *Objectives for each mediator*	• *Educational plans for sessions linking mediators, objectives, and strategies* • *Environmental support plans*		• *Evaluation plan* • *List of indicators and measures for outcomes* • *Procedures and measures for process evaluation*

FIGURE 13-2 Stepwise Procedure for designing theory-based nutrition education: Step 5.

Alternative Venues

In most communities, parents are very busy, and getting parents to attend nutrition education sessions may not be feasible. You will need to use alternate channels and design alternate educational activities that will fit into their busy schedules. Carefully determine the educational objectives of these alternate channels. In general, they are similar to the ones listed earlier: to stimulate awareness and interest, provide food- and nutrition-related knowledge and skills, and elicit parental support for your program, for example, by increasing the accessibility at home of the foods targeted by your program.

Home Activities

For programs in elementary schools, it is most effective to develop activities that children can do at home that require parental participation. Families can accumulate points for these activities, for which they can receive incentives and reinforcements. For programs with teens, colorful brochures featuring the targeted foods can be distributed to parents with school mailings; special program newsletters with activities, recipes, discount coupons, and information on the benefits of the targeted behaviors can be sent; and calendars with monthly eating tips can be distributed. You can provide taste tests, media displays, and activities at parent–teacher organization meetings and hand out colorful brochures. Again, the educational objectives of these materials should be clear. Carefully examine the mediated materials or food taste tests:

is their purpose to motivate, to provide knowledge and skills, or to do both? Which item or activity does which?

Family Support for Adults

In workplaces and outpatient clinics, it may be possible to provide educational activities for families to help them create a home environment that is supportive of participants' attempts to engage in needed or desired actions, such as a type 2 diabetes management diet or eating diets that are lower in saturated fat. Activities that have been found to be effective are written learn-at-home programs distributed through participants at the workplace, family newsletters, and family activities related to program goals that can be incorporated into workplace family holiday parties or picnics. For each of these activities, goals and objectives need to be developed so that the purposes of the activity are clear.

Peer Educators as Social Support

Peer educators have been used in a variety of settings, such as in schools, with low-income families through the Expanded Food and Nutrition Education Program (EFNEP), with older adults, and for breastfeeding promotion. The role of peer educators is not only to teach sessions and serve as models, but also to provide social support. You will need to provide professional development wherein you help peer educators understand the purposes and content of the program. They are a new audience to educate, and hence you will need to determine a set of goals

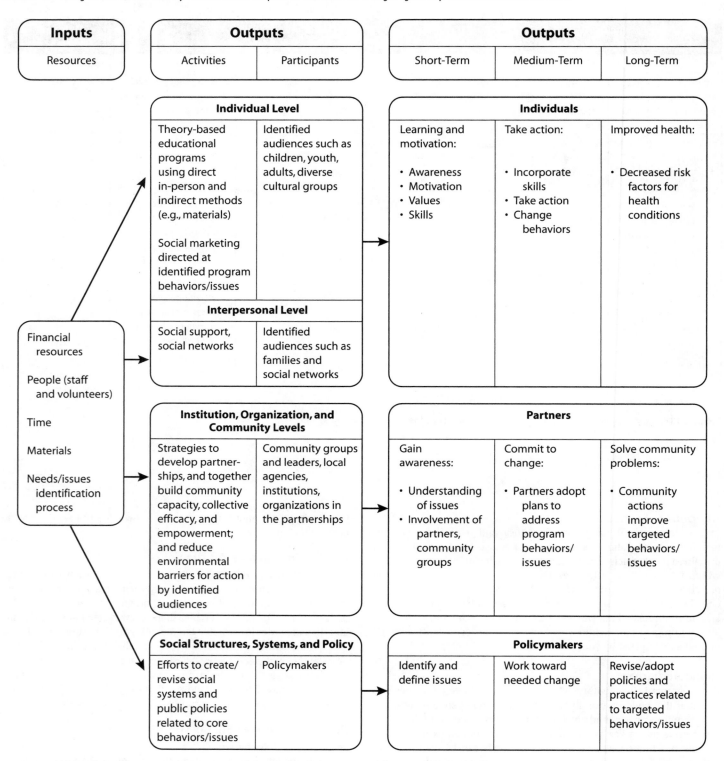

FIGURE 13-3 A nutrition education logic model framework addressing multiple levels of intervention.

Source: Based on Helen Chipman (national coordinator), Supplemental Nutrition Assistance program Education (SNAP-Ed), NIFA/USDA, and Land Grant University System Partnership. 2006, January. Community Nutrition Education (CNE) Logic Model, Version 2: Overview. http://www.nifa.usda.gov/nea/food/fsne/logic.html. Used with permission.

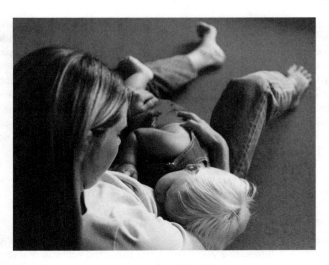

Breastfeeding mothers need peer and social support.

and objectives for their training and develop appropriate theory-based educational strategies.

Developing New Social Networks That Are Supportive of Change

Social support is incorporated into many health interventions through the development of new social groups, such as weight control groups at work, HIV support groups at a health center, cooking classes, or behavioral change sessions with participants in a program. Programs can also initiate new social networks in which individuals participating in the intervention can help each other (such as forming walking groups or buddy systems).

Support Groups

Nutrition programs frequently create social support by providing regular structured occasions for participants to meet and support each other. Such structured social support was identified in a review of nutrition education as one of the key elements that contributed to effectiveness (Ammerman et al. 2002). Weight loss interventions routinely incorporate social support groups, such as Weight Watchers. Interventions in schools, workplaces, and communities also have incorporated social support groups. Increasing social support through social networks means increasing one or more of the following kinds of support:

- *Emotional support:* Expressions of empathy, caring, love, and trust
- *Informational support:* Advice and suggestions
- *Appraisal support:* Information that is useful for self-evaluation
- *Instrumental support:* Tangible support and resources

Social Support Group Sessions

You must carefully design and facilitate social support group sessions: they are not just a matter of getting a group together and talking. Write educational objectives for the sessions that are directed at theory mediators and design activities for each objective. In other words, develop an educational plan. However, you implement it through facilitated dialogue and mutual support. The structure or agenda usually involves the following: individuals share how they did during the previous week or time interval in terms of successes and challenges (focus on suc-

cesses); group members assist each other from their own wealth of experience; you provide content where necessary and design learning tasks to promote active engagement and maintain support; you provide worksheets, handouts, food tasting, or cooking demonstrations when feasible; and time is set aside for the development of action plans or goal setting for the next session. If you are not the group leader, design a manual for the group leader that includes all this information and also a manual for participants. For participants, hand out session packets each time as you go along.

During the session, your role is to be a facilitator to guide the discussion. The participants are experts on their lives, even though you may be an expert on food and nutrition information. (Even here, participants can be very knowledgeable.) They come with prior experience and expertise. Invite them to share with each other and create dialogue. Build on the strengths of the group members and not their deficits.

Mutual Support

You can also foster social support by encouraging program participants to help each other through such strategies as forming buddy systems or walking clubs; creating an e-mail listserv to share ideas, experiences, and resources; and going out to eat together and practicing learned behavioral skills.

Creating Informational Supports for Program Behavioral Goals

To support the behavioral goals of the program, you can place information in public forums to serve as environmental supports by providing cues to action. For example, you can institute point-of-choice labeling of targeted foods such as fruits and vegetables or lower-fat foods in grocery stores or workplaces, distribute key chains that have program messages printed on them, hang posters on walls, and place flyers or brochures on tables in settings where program participants eat, such as cafeterias.

Information in public spaces can help establish social and community norms that are supportive of the behavioral goals of the program. For example, posters about breastfeeding in pediatricians' offices or posters on eating fruits and vegetables in restaurants, company cafeterias, health centers, and community centers can encourage people to see these behaviors as the social norm. Posters about taking the stairs can be placed in workplaces. Billboards in the community can also help to establish norms and serve as cues to action. Promotions through other

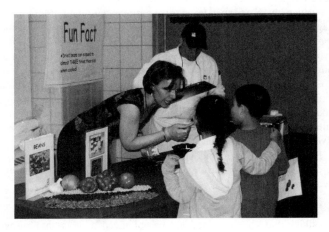

The school cafeteria can be a place for students to try new foods.

media, such as radio and magazines, can also be supportive of the behavior change that is targeted by the intervention.

■ DESIGNING SUPPORTIVE ENVIRONMENTS THROUGH COLLABORATIONS AND PARTNERSHIPS

It is increasingly clear that many of the food-, nutrition-, and physical activity–related issues of key concern cannot be addressed by nutrition educators working alone. You must work in collaboration with others to address issues such as preventing overweight, decreasing chronic disease risk, decreasing food insecurity, increasing intakes of fruits and vegetables, and increasing consumption of food from local farmers because changes in behavior require organizational- and community-level support as well as interpersonal support and individual action.

In the context of program design, changes in foods offered at nutrition education intervention sites, such as schools, workplaces, community centers, soup kitchens, food banks, or supermarkets, may require that nutrition educators work with partners to modify policy, social structures, and systems.

Collaboration and Partnership

Collaborations include a range of structural relationships, and different terms are often used to describe these, such as partnerships and coalitions (Rosenthal 1998; Gregson et al. 2001).

Clarifying Terms

Collaboration has been described as "a fluid process through which a group of diverse, autonomous actors (organizations or individuals) undertakes a joint initiative, addresses shared concerns, or otherwise achieves common goals. It is characterized by mutual benefit, interdependence, reciprocity, concerted action, and joint production" (Rosenthal 1998). In degree of involvement, collaboration ranges from loose networks through cooperation and coordination of effort to full collaboration. Collaboration has long been practiced in the field of nutrition. For example, nutrition educators have long collaborated with school food service personnel and with food assistance programs such as the Supplemental Nutrition Assistance Program, the Women, Infants and Children (WIC) program, and congregate meals programs for older adults to provide nutrition education in these contexts. Nutrition educators also can collaborate with public health departments in health promotion programs, with farmers in farm-to-school programs, or with community groups in gardening projects in schools and communities.

Partnerships are formed for reasons of organizational self-interest and pragmatism and can be for the long or short term. Partners have distinct resources and expertise that, if pooled, can expand possibilities for everyone: the whole becomes greater than the sum of its parts. Partners share responsibility and ownership of the effort or product.

Coalitions or *consortia* are another arrangement in which organizations, institutions, and sectors unite to develop a comprehensive approach. The focus is on social change, empowerment, and community building, and the activities include planning, community organizing, advocacy, and program development.

This book uses the general terms *collaboration* and *partnership* to describe the variety of arrangements in which nutrition education is involved.

Collaborations Are Important

It is likely that your program will be enhanced by collaborating with another group. Indeed, it may be that an environmental support com-

ponent to your program is made possible only by such partnership. For example, the environmental change objectives of your nutrition education curriculum in a school might require that you work in partnership with school food service personnel, school administrators, local wellness policy councils, and perhaps also school–parent associations. Similarly, changes in foods in many other settings, such as workplaces, might require your entering into collaborations with food vendors in those settings. In Chapter 10, you wrote several environmental support objectives for your program. This chapter describes examples of how they can be translated into action.

■ DESIGNING INSTITUTIONAL-LEVEL FOOD ENVIRONMENT AND POLICY ACTIVITIES

Food Environment and Policy Activities in Schools

Students in schools where à la carte foods and snack and beverage vending machines are available eat fewer fruits and vegetables at lunch (Cullen et al. 2000; Cullen & Zakeri 2004) and fewer fruits and vegetables and more saturated fat during the entire day (Kubik et al. 2003). Hence, changing the food environment means making changes in a variety of venues: school meals offerings, vending machines, à la carte offerings, food items in school stores, and foods used for fundraising programs and as rewards by teachers. These changes are all difficult to achieve, as discussed in Chapter 6, but change these you must if you are to support people's interest in healthful eating. Nutrition educators need different partners to bring about changes in these different venues because different people have decision-making power and authority over each venue, such as principals, food service personnel, teachers unions, and parent associations.

Local Wellness Policy

Legislation now requires every local district that participates in the federal school meals program to develop and implement a wellness policy. Such a policy must accomplish the following:

- Include nutrition guidelines for all foods available on the school campus during the school day
- Include goals for nutrition education, physical activity, and other school-based activities designed to promote student wellness
- Establish a plan for measuring the implementation of the policy
- Involve parents, students, and representatives of the school food authority, school board, administrators, and public in development of the policy

Although school *districts* have developed such policies, some plans may not be implemented fully in each *school* (Story et al. 2009). Policies also need to be evaluated and updated from time to time (Institute of Medicine 2007). Nutrition educators can serve as a valuable resource.

Depending on the scope and duration of your school intervention and the resources you have, you may incorporate the following strategies in assisting schools in implementing, revising, or updating the wellness policy to support healthy eating.

Activating Local Wellness Policy Councils

Legislation for the wellness policy requires that many stakeholders be involved. As a nutrition educator, you can contribute to the process by providing information to school administrators about the importance and benefits of conducting an assessment to describe the food environment of the school and by having an active wellness policy council.

Find out whether the school has an ongoing and active wellness council. Although school administrators are highly concerned about academic achievement issues, they are also interested in health. You may also work with teacher and parent associations to familiarize them with the purpose of such a council and member responsibilities. Potential student members can be solicited from the recommendations of the principal and teachers. Developing and maintaining such a council can be a challenge (Kubik, Lytle, & Story 2001). The team should consist of those who are willing to make a commitment to participate actively and to stay involved. Also ask:

- Does the school have a written food policy? Is nutrition addressed in it?
- Does the policy address soft drinks? Food for fundraising?
- Is there a policy about teachers/faculty using food as a reward or incentive?
- If the school already has a good nutrition wellness policy, is it being implemented? How is the school monitoring implementation?

Assessing the School Food Environment

An accurate description of current food-related practices and policies provides a framework for discussion and decision making, permits the school that you are working in to devise an appropriate action plan to implement its wellness policy, and provides a means by which to monitor progress. Several assessment tools are available to help with the process, such as the School Health Index (SHI) from the Centers for Disease Control and Prevention (CDC 2009a, 2009b; refer to https://apps.nccd .cdc.gov/SHI). These instruments are quite general, seeking information on broad policies such as the degree of commitment to nutrition and physical activity, quality meals, and a pleasant eating experience.

It is considered best that the school wellness council members conduct this assessment. You may help the group develop an assessment tool (or monitoring tool if a policy is already in place) and administer it. Or you may interview key informants, such as the school principal or assistant principal, the school food service director, or teachers. In addition to interviews, you will want to make direct observations of the foods and beverages available through various venues, such as school meals, vending machines, school stores, or competitive foods in the cafeteria (Kubik et al. 2001). This means that you will need to devise some kind of coding scheme that is fairly simple and directed only at the behaviors of interest to your program. For example, the TEENS intervention, which focused on increasing intake of fruits and vegetables and decreasing fat consumption, came up with a list of food items to promote, foods to neither promote or limit, and foods to limit (Kubik et al. 2001) and characterized foods in various venues according to this scheme.

Develop a Policy Implementation Plan

Whether implementing a policy or revising it, the group's task is now to analyze the school's food and nutrition assessment data that have been collected, come up with a shared vision, identify areas needing improvement, and develop action plans. The Institute of Medicine's nutrition standards are helpful here (Institute of Medicine 2007). Your role as the nutrition educator is to provide technical assistance in the form of relevant research data and to help the group think through issues and make choices.

Put the Plan into Action

The team may come up with very creative, manageable, and meaningful activities that are supportive of your program's behavioral goals.

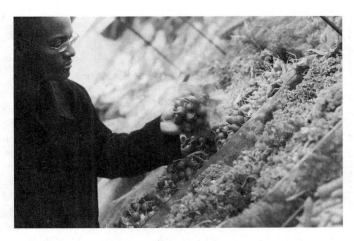

Incentives such as coupons can encourage more healthful eating.

For example, in the TEENS study, the nutrition advisory council set the policy that 50% of items offered in the school store should come from the "foods to promote" list; that instead of using high-fat, high-sugar foods as rewards for students, teachers would use "healthy food" coupons that students could redeem in the school cafeteria for baked chips, fruit, or low-fat desserts; and that they would produce and display posters advertising healthy choices (Kubik et al. 2001). Your role is to provide technical assistance and advice.

It should be noted that implementing food policies is fraught with barriers. Often opponents object to the policies for a variety of reasons and put enormous pressures on schools not to change, particularly when revenues are at stake. For policies to be actually implemented requires political will on the part of school administrators and parental support. In addition, it has been found that even though extra funding can initially enable schools to provide quality lunches, success cannot be sustained without changes in students' preferences for unhealthful foods and parental and community involvement in fostering healthy eating behavior. Coordination and communication among food service staff, teachers, and health educators have been found to be essential, as well as school-wide nutrition education (Cho & Nadow 2004), confirming that both individual-level and environmental-level strategies are needed so that individuals have both the willingness and skills as well as opportunity to take action.

Changes in School Meals

All schools are interested in offering quality meals that children will eat and a pleasant atmosphere in which to eat them (http://www .schoolnutrition.org). If you would like the school meals to be more supportive of your nutrition education program's behavioral goals, plan to meet with the school food service manager to discuss how you might collaborate. For example, if your program goal is to increase children's consumption of fruits and vegetables (or whole grains, or low-fat, high-calcium foods), you can discuss how the school meals program can be supportive, given the constraints of budget and staff. Clarify what your role will be. Perhaps the school food service staff is already providing the foods you are targeting but needs help with promotion. Maybe they could use some technical assistance with menu modification or with staff development. View the process as a collaboration of persons who have different but complementary knowledge and skills that are needed to enhance healthful eating in students.

NUTRITION EDUCATION IN ACTION 13-1

Making It Happen: School Nutrition Success Stories

The Team Nutrition program of the U.S. Department of Agriculture (USDA) is an example of nutrition education that is directed at both the individual and environmental levels. Team Nutrition focuses attention on the important role that nutritious school meals, nutrition education, and a health-promoting school environment all play in helping students learn to enjoy healthful eating and physical activity. In particular, it encourages collaboration among many partners, such as school food service personnel, teachers, school administrators, parents, and community organizations, to achieve these student outcomes. Such collaborations can help to establish wellness policies for schools.

Examples of what some school districts have done are described in a set of "success stories" collected by the Centers for Disease Control and Prevention (CDC) and Team Nutrition. These successful schools conducted the following policy and system change activities:

- *Made more healthful foods available.* Healthy foods were made available through various venues in the school, such as school meals, à la carte offerings, and vending machines, based on the fact that increasing the variety of nutritious choices makes it more likely that students will choose nutrient-dense foods and that they will see such foods as the norm.
- *Established nutrition standards.* The nutrition standards help schools select the foods to offer outside the national school meals program. Nutrition standards are the criteria that determine which foods and beverages can and cannot be

offered on a school campus. These standards resulted in most of the schools adding such healthful items as water, low-fat or nonfat milk, 100% juice, air-popped popcorn, fresh fruit, salads or salad bars, sandwiches, baked chips, and whole-grain breads.

- *Influenced food and beverage contracts.* These contracts gave vendors selling rights for up-front cash and noncash benefits to a school or district. Schools canceled them, did not renew them, or negotiated contracts that promoted more healthful eating.
- *Adopted marketing techniques to promote healthful choices.* Schools identified and offered healthful food products that were appealing and met the nutrition standards, placed these healthful products in sites that were easily accessible to students, promoted them so that students would be motivated to try the foods, and set the price at a level that encouraged students to purchase them.
- *Limited students' access to foods that were competitive to the national school meals program.* Most schools removed such less healthful items as sweetened beverages, candy, deep-fried foods, and snack cakes.

Source: Food and Nutrition Service, U.S. Department of Agriculture, Centers for Disease Control and Prevention, U.S. Department of Health and Human Services, and U.S. Department of Education. 2005, January. *Making it happen! School nutrition success stories* (FNS-374). Alexandria, VA: Authors.

Team Nutrition provides an example of collaborations between schools, parents, nutrition educators, community members, policy makers, and other stakeholders in improving the eating patterns of youth in schools. Some examples of successes are discussed in **Nutrition Education in Action 13-1**.

Use of Local Foods in Schools: Farm-to-School Programs

Many schools are introducing salad bars using fresh produce from local farmers' markets or local farms in farm-to-schools programs. Schools can buy many other farm-fresh foods, such as eggs, meat, beans, and honey. These programs are initiated locally. You may want to consider promoting these options if they are relevant to your program (French & Wechsler 2004). Farm-to-school programs usually also provide experiential learning opportunities through having farmers visit classrooms, sponsoring educational events at farmers' markets, and making field visits to farms. Children learn about local food and agriculture and are energized to try new foods when they see where their food comes from. Schools can fulfill their mission to provide wholesome, nutritious foods that children want to eat, and farmers have access to a new market. Information on the many activities in different states can be found at the National Farm to School Program website (http://www.farmtoschool .org) and in **Nutrition Education in Action 13-2**.

School Gardens

Schools are increasingly seeing the relevance and importance of having school gardens in which to grow vegetables. Children learn where food comes from and become more interested in nutrition. You may need to develop coalitions with knowledgeable individuals or groups to initiate and maintain such gardens if you do not have the expertise to do so within your own team but deem it an important supportive activity for your program. See http://www.edibleschoolyard.org for more information. **Nutrition Education in Action 13-3** describes an example of the use of school gardens to make changes in schools and in communities.

Food Environment and Policy Activities in Workplaces

Many of the strategies described previously also apply to environmental support activities in workplaces. However, they are usually more difficult to implement because food service operations are generally managed by external for-profit companies, which do not necessarily share the interest of the workplace in improved employee health.

If your program will be conducted in a workplace, you can include the following strategies in your plan.

- *Build collaboration and foster buy-in.* Make presentations, meet with, and educate key food service decision makers about the importance of your program's goals. You may need to work with

Farm-to-School Programs Connect Schools with Local Farms

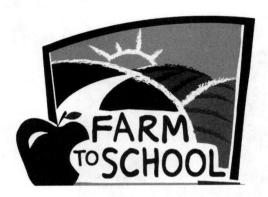

Farm-to-school programs are programs in which schools buy and feature farm-fresh foods such as fruits and vegetables, eggs, honey, meat, and beans in their menus; provide students experiential learning opportunities through class visits to farms, gardening, and recycling programs; and incorporate nutrition education into their activities. Farm-fresh salad bars are often offered as part of the National School Lunch Program, and local foods are often featured in the cafeteria or in fundraising events. Thus, farmers and schools develop partnerships so that local farmers have access to the school market and at the same time participate in programs designed to educate children about local farms and agriculture.

Legislation titled "Access to Local Food and School Gardens" as part of the Child Nutrition and WIC Reauthorization Act of 2004 permits schools to compete for grant funds to help school food service personnel develop procurement relationships with local farmers and equip their kitchen facilities to handle local foods. The program also supports agriculture-based nutrition education, such as school gardens, to teach students where their food comes from. There are an estimated 2000 farm-to-cafeteria programs in about 9,000 schools in 43 states that not only feed children fresh, local food, but get them excited about it.

Results of an evaluation showed positive impacts on many aspects of the school, among them:

- *Student impacts.* Improvements in student knowledge, attitudes, and behavior such as choosing healthier options in cafeteria, eating more fruits and vegetables at school and home, modifying daily exercise routines, and increasing social skills and self-esteem.
- *Teacher impacts.* Positive changes in their diets and lifestyles.
- *Food service operations.* Generally positive impacts on quality of foods offered, increased knowledge and interest of staff, increased participation rates, and higher labor costs but no clear indication whether overall costs increased.
- *Farmer impacts.* Increased income from schools, diversification of market, and increased collaboratives or cooperatives to supply schools.
- *Parent benefits.* Gains in interest and ability to improve family diets and help children make healthier choices as well as improved shopping for healthy and local foods.
- *Community benefits.* Increased interest in purchasing local foods and awareness of foods served in school cafeterias.

Sources: National Farm to School on the Web (http://www.farmtoschool.org) and A. Joshi and A. M. Azuma. 2008. Bearing Fruit: Farm to School Program Evaluation Resources and Recommendations. Occidental College, CA: National Farm to School Network, Center for Food & Justice.

---

a regional manager of the food service company as well as the site manager.

- *Use a phased approach: start with simple changes first.* With the manager, identify a short list of items currently served that meet your criteria for individual foods that support your program's behavioral goals (e.g., fruits and vegetables). Indicate these with signs and your logo. If these are well received, then using a computer analysis of nutrient content, identify entrées, soups, and other meal items that satisfy your criteria. When it is clear that these changes do not have a negative financial impact, the food service managers may be ready to make recipe modifications. Here, you can provide technical assistance for making changes.
- *Promote employee advisory committees.* Active participation of workplace employees is vital. Depending on the scope of your program, you may help to form a nutrition advisory committee made up of employees as well as management that will provide ongoing feedback and suggestions to food service personnel. Committee members can take over your functions for long-term institutionalization of food service changes.

■ COMMUNITY-LEVEL FOOD ENVIRONMENT AND POLICY ACTIVITIES

The extent to which you try to increase environmental supports at the community level for the behavioral targets of your intervention depends on the scope of your intervention and the resources available. Activities will most likely require collaboration with several to many other groups who have similar goals to those of your program.

Collective Efficacy and Community Action Plans

Collective efficacy is the belief of groups and community members that they have the capacity to take collective action to create change in their environment. Collaborations can lead to a sense of collective efficacy. Where you and your partners have similar goals, the group makes community action plans to address specific issues or achieve specific objectives (somewhat like goal setting for individuals). When the group is successful at bringing about change on one issue, the members feel self-efficacious and ready to take on other issues. Your role can be to work with others to develop a community plan that is also supportive

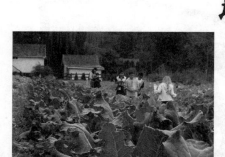

NUTRITION EDUCATION IN ACTION 13-3

Food $ense CHANGE: Cultivating Health and Nutrition Through Garden Education

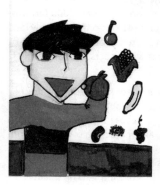

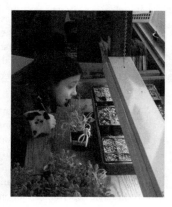

Learning about where food comes from: Indoor gardening.

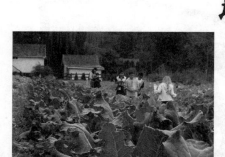

Learning about where food comes from: Visiting a farm

Food $ense CHANGE improves the nutrition of limited-income children and their families by teaching a nutrition curriculum enhanced by gardening, cooking, and other hands-on activities. In addition to teaching classroom lessons, primarily in elementary schools, CHANGE instructors act as a support system and resource for teachers as they incorporate nutrition education into their daily classroom work. CHANGE instructors also participate in school family nights and other family or adult outreach activities.

CHANGE teaches students how to make good food choices, how to grow food, and how to prepare healthy snacks and meals. Through outdoor garden education, students plant seeds, measure their growth, and harvest fruits and vegetables to eat. They learn where their food comes from and make the connection between what they eat, their health, and the environment.

The goals of CHANGE are as follows:

- Teach nutrition through gardening and cooking to limited-income youth and their families, resulting in the consumption of more fruits and vegetables and higher quality, nutrient-dense foods.
- Train teachers to integrate nutrition education into their existing curricula resulting in the delivery of consistent messages about healthy eating.
- Encourage behavior changes in Food $ense schools to create an environment of healthy eating.

The Food $ense CHANGE program in schools includes the following:

- The CHANGE curriculum that teaches nutrition experientially through gardening and cooking.
- The CHANGE curriculum of 40 lessons, taught in four 10-lesson units. There are two units for primary grades (1–3) and two units for intermediate grades (4–5).
- Enhancement of reading and comprehension skills, teamwork, math skills, science concepts, and creativity while students grow food plants in their classrooms and outdoor gardens and harvest produce for cooking and eating in class.
- Inquiry-based science and nutrition activities.

- Guidance and support for creating school gardens. Each garden meets the needs and environment of each school. Whether gardens are dug in the ground or grown in large containers, children learn about nutrition by experiencing the excitement of growing, harvesting, and cooking their own food.
- Field trips to local farms, where children have the opportunity to see where their food is grown, talk to the farmers, and learn valuable lessons about nutrition, fresh fruits and vegetables, and caring for the environment.

Results showed that about 75% to 85% of youth reported improved eating practices such as eating breakfasts that include three food groups and using food labels.

Healthy Food in Motion

After learning about food advertising in a CHANGE class, students asked why they don't see any ads for fruits and vegetables. As a result, Food $ense CHANGE decided to place fruits and vegetable advertisements drawn by children in metro buses. Children in 40 elementary school classrooms participated in a contest to draw the advertisements. One hundred twenty colorful expressions of health foods were chosen for the signs, which were accompanied by appropriate messages in multiple languages to reach all bus riders.

Adult Outreach

CHANGE educators use every opportunity to share information about healthy eating directly with parents. Parent newsletters, family nights, and other school and community events involving adults allow parents to meet and discuss the positive changes that nutrition education can make in the household. Educators provide parents with information to support the behavior changes being attempted by their children and to improve the household's eating habits.

Source: Washington State University King County Extension. 2006. Food $ense CHANGE. Funded by Supplemental Nutrition Assistance Program Education (SNAP-Ed). http://king.wsu.edu/nutrition/change.htm. Logo used with permission.

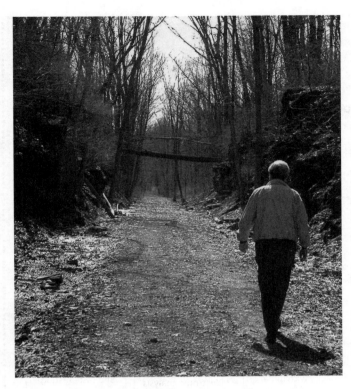

Converting old train tracks into walking and biking trails increases opportunities for people to be active.

of your program behavioral goals (e.g., such as increasing opportunities for participants to eat more fruits and vegetables or to walk more).

Designing Community-Level Activities

Active participation of community members in all activities is crucial—from planning to implementing to evaluating. Consequently, as described for institutional activities in schools and workplaces, your first activity is to locate decision makers in other organizations—whether these are grocery stores or community gardens—discuss your program with them, and seek strong collaborations. This collaborative group can decide on strategies. The following strategies can be considered, to the degree they are relevant for your program.

- *Provide point-of-purchase information.* You can collaborate with grocery stores relevant to your program and provide posters, brochures, and shelf labels for foods targeted by your intervention (Story, Kaphingst, et al. 2008). Shelf labels can enhance awareness of the foods and increase use of the information. The strategy of providing point-of-purchase information can also be used in restaurants and other places where food is served.
- *Provide coupons at stores and farmers' markets.* Your program may issue coupons for program participants to use in selected stores that are redeemable for foods relevant to your intervention, such as low-fat milk. Your program would need to pay for these. Government farmers' market coupon programs for various low-income populations have increased shoppers' attendance at farmers' markets and can be used as an environmental support to your program.

- *Work with community food assistance organizations.* Many community organizations are involved in providing food assistance to communities, such as food recovery or food gleaning programs, food banks, and community kitchens or soup kitchens. You may be able to link activities within your educational program to such programs in your community. If your nutrition education is being provided through these organizations, then the foods made available in these settings should be supportive of your program's behavioral goals. You may wish to develop policies as to which kinds of foods the organization is willing to accept for redistribution to those in need to ensure that they are wholesome and nutritious. America's Second Harvest (http://www.secondharvest.org) is a national food bank network of more than 200 regional member food banks and food rescue organizations.
- *Community-supported agriculture (CSA).* You may be able to link individuals in your educational program to community-supported agriculture. CSA helps to support family farms that are struggling to stay in business, while providing city people, particularly those in low-income neighborhoods, with access to high-quality, locally grown, affordable produce. During the winter and spring, the CSA farmer sells shares in his or her farm's upcoming harvest to individuals, families, or institutions. The share price goes toward the cost of growing and distributing a season's worth of produce and paying the farmer a living wage. Generally, each week from June through November, the CSA farmer delivers the week's share to a central neighborhood distribution site—usually a community center or house of worship. Members collect their food at their neighborhood sites. Organizations in your community may be able to link your program participants with local CSA farmers.

■ MULTIPLE-LEVEL COMMUNITY NUTRITION EDUCATION

The local- and state-level nutrition education networks and collaborations found in most states, and described in Chapter 6, provide an example of activities at many levels to improve the diets of youth and adults. Many networks are partnerships among a variety of groups, usually with funding from the USDA Supplemental Nutrition Assistance Program (SNAP)–Education and from state and other sources. These networks provide nutrition education to SNAP recipients and eligible individuals in a variety of settings. The primary partners, with contractual arrangements, are generally the state SNAP agencies and other agencies such as the state Cooperative Extension Service or department of health, whose task is to organize the networks in their state. The networks range from informal collaborations to formal funded entities. The average network has several dozen public- and private-sector member organizations as partners, such as the Cooperative Extension Service, WIC, welfare agencies, university nutrition or medical departments, professional and voluntary associations (such as the local American Cancer Society and American Diabetes Association affiliates), food banks and other food-related organizations, and for-profit organizations (such as supermarkets). Your program may want to become part of a local or regional nutrition network, make members aware of your program goals and become available to work collaboratively with others in the network to further your program goals.

An example of the kinds of multilevel activities conducted within a community is provided in **Nutrition Education in Action 13-4**. Rock on Café was a grassroots effort community program to achieve sustainable systems changes in school lunch programs through partnerships.

NUTRITION EDUCATION IN ACTION **13-4**

Rock on Café

Rock on Café was a grassroots community program to achieve sustainable systems changes in school lunch programs through partnerships. It was part of a larger program called Steps to a Healthier New York and involved four counties and 15 school districts, with the educational cooperative Board of Cooperative Educational Services (BOCES) as the lead organization.

Assessment Information

- The three leading *health issues of concern* for Steps to a Healthier New York were diabetes, obesity, and asthma.
- The *behaviors or practices* that contributed to these conditions were identified as poor nutrition, physical inactivity, and tobacco use.

The Intervention

- The *intervention theoretical model* was the social-ecological model, along with social marketing principles.
- The *nutrition education program objectives* were based on theory:

    1. *Individual level:* Educating students, parents, and food service directors (FSDs).
    2. *School level:* Repackaging healthy options, including content, preparation and presentation, and restriction of foods low in nutrition value occurred at the school level.
    3. *School and community social norms:* Involving school and community role models in the advertisements to be made so as to make healthy food choices the acceptable norm.
    4. *Regional policy to change food environment:* Food procurement, menu planning, and branding.

Evaluation Results

School-level impacts:

- Purchases of fresh fruit and vegetables increased by 14%.
- School meals consistently met the 30% fat guidelines and better.
- School lunch participation went up 3%.

Parent impact:

- Parents that thought the school lunch was a healthy option increased approximately 7% from 38% to 45%.

School food service:

- All FSDs rated the program as good to excellent.
- Use of a registered dietitian and consolidated food procurement were rated as most valuable.

Overall:

- Team building, organizational learning, community partnerships, and social marketing all contributed to the success and likelihood of long-term sustainability of the changes.

- *The intervention components and processes* were as follows:

Timeline and major activity	Intervention components	Intervention processes
Year 1: Program planning and team building	• Regional planning team • Regional food procurement initiative • Dietitian services contracted	• Secure support of FSDs, school superintendents • Conduct needs assessment • Establish short- and long-term goals
Year 2: Creating capacity with initial participation and training	• Education for FSDs • Electronic analysis of school foods served • Standardize lunch menus	• Student surveys and taste testing • Creating new recipes • Staff development and training
Year 3: Main intervention	• Social marketing/ branding • Key stakeholders' involvement • Education for children and parents	• Acquire support of community partners • Launch public relations campaign to spread message • Social marketing (stickers, posters, aprons, menu boards) • Data monitoring

Source: Johnson Y., R. Denniston, M. Morgan, and M. Bordeau. 2009. Steps to a Healthier New York: Achieving sustainable systems changes in school lunch programs. *Health Promotion Practice* 10:100S–108S.

■ SUMMARY

Nutrition education programs can work with partners to promote policy, food environment, and community interventions that increase supports for program participants to engage in the nutrition- and food-related behaviors targeted by the program. Thus, the food environments of intervention sites such as schools, Head Start programs, workplaces, and congregate meals sites for older adults can make healthful foods available and accessible as well as encourage and reinforce the behaviors or practices targeted by the program you are designing.

In *schools*, school-wide food-related policies can be developed addressing food and beverage availability, vending machines, and school stores as well as school cafeteria offerings to provide students the opportunity to have easy access to the healthful food choices being promoted by your program and to see healthful food practices modeled.

In *workplaces*, healthful alternatives can be made available in the cafeteria and in vending machines and can be promoted.

In *all settings*, the nutrition educator can work with decision makers to make healthful choices the easy choices. The active participation of community members and worksite employees as well as leaders through community organization and community building must be incorporated into any intervention. Indeed, community empowerment and collective efficacy are high priorities. Adopting these comprehensive approaches enhances the likelihood of improving the effectiveness of nutrition education interventions.

■ CASE STUDY

The ongoing case study is with middle school youth, addressing the behavioral goal of increasing their intake of fruits and vegetables. In Step 3 (refer to Chapter 9), two environmental components were selected for the intervention program in addition to a curriculum for youth in order to increase the opportunities of youth to enact program behavioral goals: one for changing the school environment and one for parents, family members, or other responsible adults. The case study in this chapter presents a program of activities to address the school environment and a potential program for parents.

Changing the food environment means working with decision makers and policy makers in the school setting to create a healthy food environment for the middle school youth. The case study states some potential general environmental and policy support objectives and then describes activities that can be conducted to achieve these objectives, involving changes in school meals, school-wide food policy, social support, and school information environment.

The family component focuses on providing motivation and skills to parents to help them to be more supportive of the behavioral goals targeted for their children. We do so by designing theory-based strategies to address potential mediators of change in the *parents'* behaviors. These strategies build on the educational objectives developed in Step 4 (Chapter 10). Although it is an educational program, it is considered an environmental support component because it is external to the primary audience (youth) and is designed to create an environment that is supportive of youth's motivation and skills in making healthy choices. Because family members are busy, the family component consists of only two group educational sessions—one directed at supporting youth's fruit and vegetable consumption and another at supporting them in reducing intakes of sweetened beverages—and two newsletters—one on packaged, processed, and high-calorie snacks and one on physical activity.

For illustrative purposes, the case study in this chapter presents one group session for family members on fruits and vegetables. Only the design matrix format is shown. The narrative educational plan can easily be derived from it and is not shown. The case study also shows you an example of a newsletter for family members on processed, packaged snacks. The theory mediators addressed by the text are shown in italics.

■ YOUR TURN: COMPLETING THE STEP 5 WORKSHEETS: A FOCUS ON ENVIRONMENTAL SUPPORTS

Intervention activities directed at increasing the opportunities for taking action can take so many different forms. A worksheet is provided to help you design these environmental supports.

Questions and Activities

1. Describe how you might make existing social networks more supportive for (a) children and (b) adults.
2. Describe several key features for designing a social support group for your intended audience so that it will likely be effective.
3. Describe three reasons why collaborations and partnerships are important in nutrition education and three reasons why they may be challenging. How might you overcome these challenges?
4. Describe the key steps in developing an effective school or work-site nutrition-related wellness policy. What is the role of the nutrition educator in this process?

References

Ammerman, A. S., C. H. Lindquist, K. N. Lohr, and J. Hersey. 2002. The efficacy of behavioral interventions to modify dietary fat and fruit and vegetable intake: A review of the evidence. *Preventive Medicine* 35(1):25–41.

Bogden, J. F. 2000. *Fit, healthy and ready to learn, a school health policy guide. Part I: Physical activity, healthy eating, and tobacco-use prevention*. Alexandria, VA: National Association of State Boards of Education.

Brener, N. D., L. Kann, T. McManus, B. Stevenson, and S. F. Wooley. 2004. The relationship between school health councils and school health policies and programs in U.S. schools. *Journal of School Health* 74:130–135.

Centers for Disease Control and Prevention. 1996. Guidelines for school health programs to promote lifelong healthy eating. *Morbidity and Mortality Weekly Report* 45(RR-9):1–33.

———. 2009a. *School Health Index: A self-assessment and planning guide. Elementary school version*. Atlanta, GA: Author. https://apps.nccd.cdc.gov/SHI.

———. 2009b. *School Health Index: A self-assessment and planning guide. Middle school/high school version*. Atlanta, GA: Author. https://apps.nccd.cdc.gov/SHI.

Cho, H., and M. Z. Nadow. 2004. Understanding barriers to implementing quality lunch and nutrition education. *Journal of Community Health* 29:421–435.

Cullen, K. W., J. Eagan, T. Baranowski, E. Owens, and C. deMoor. 2000. Effect of à la carte and snack bar foods at school on children's lunchtime intake of fruits and vegetables. *Journal of the American Dietetic Association* 100:1482–1486.

Cullen, K. W., and I. Zakeri. 2004. Fruits, vegetables, milk, and sweetened beverages consumption and access to à la carte/snack bar meals at school. *American Journal of Public Health* 94:463–467.

French, S. A., and H. Wechsler. 2004. School-based research and initiatives: Fruit and vegetable environment, policy, and pricing workshop. *Preventive Medicine* 39(Suppl. 2):S101–S107.

Glanz, K., and A. L. Yaroch. 2004. Strategies for increasing fruit and vegetable intake in grocery stores and communities: Policy, pricing, and environmental change. *Preventive Medicine* 39(Suppl. 2):S75–S80.

Green, L. W., and M. M. Kreuter. 2005. *Health promotion planning: An educational and ecological approach*. 4th ed. Mountain View, CA: Mayfield Publishing.

Gregson, J., S. B. Foerster, R. Orr, et al. 2001. System, environmental, and policy changes: Using the social-ecological model as a framework for evaluating nutrition education and social marketing programs with low-income audiences. *Journal of Nutrition Education* 33:S4–S15.

Institute of Medicine. (2007). *Nutrition standards for foods in schools: Leading the way towards healthier youth*. Washington, D.C.: National Academies Press.

Kramer-Atwood, J. L., J. Dwyer, D. M. Hoelscher, T. A. Nicklas, R. K. Johnson, and G. K. Schulz. 2002. Fostering healthy food consumption in schools: Focusing on the challenges of competitive foods. *Journal of the American Dietetic Association* 102:1228–1233.

Kremers, S. P. J., G. deBruijn, T. L. S. Visscher, W. van Mechelen, N. K. de Vries, and J. Brug. 2006. Environmental influences on energy balance-related behaviors: A dual-process view. *International Journal of Behavioral Nutrition and Physical Activity* 3:9.

Kubik, M. Y., L. A. Lytle, P. J. Hannan, C. L. Perry, and M. Story. 2003. The association of the school environment with dietary behaviors of young adolescents. *American Journal of Public Health* 93:1168–1173.

Kubik, M. Y., L. A. Lytle, and M. Story. 2001. A practical, theory-based approach to establishing school nutrition advisory councils. *Journal of the American Dietetic Association* 101:223–228.

McLeroy, K. R., D. Bibeau, A. Steckler, and K. Glanz. 1988. An ecological perspective on health promotion programs. *Health Education Quarterly* 15:351–377.

Medeiros, L. C., S. N. Butkus, H. Chipman, R. H. Cox, L. Jones, and D. Little. 2005. A logic model framework for community nutrition education. *Journal of Nutrition Education and Behavior* 37:197–202.

Michigan Department of Community Health. 2005. *The Healthy School Action Tool (HSAT)*. Lansing, MI: Author. http://mihealthtools.org/schools.

Rosenthal, B. B. 1998. Collaboration for the nutrition field: Synthesis of selected literature. *Journal of Nutrition Education* 30(5):246–267.

Story, M., K. M. Kaphingst, et al. 2008. Creating healthy food and eating environments: Policy and environmental approaches. *Annual Review of Public Health* 29:253–272.

Story, M., M. S. Nanney, et al. 2009. Schools and obesity prevention: Creating school environments and policies to promote healthy eating and physical activity. *Milbank Quarterly* 87(1):71–100.

U.S. Department of Agriculture. 2000. *Changing the scene: Improving the school nutrition environment*. Alexandria, VA: Author.

Wechsler, H., N. D. Brener, S. Kuester, and C. Miller. 2001. Food service and foods and beverages available at school: Results from the School Health Policies and Programs Study 2000. *Journal of School Health* 71:313–324.

In Step 5, use your theoretical model, philosophy of nutrition education, and nutrition education program objectives to create (1) educational plans for the individual-level components and (2) environmental supports plans for environmental/policy components.

These pages of the Step 5 worksheets are devoted to designing the environmental supports plan for the environmental/policy components. Generally, the environmental/policy components consist of activities directed at changes that impact one or more facets of the environment or policy as these relate to your program's behavioral goals.

You should have **one** support plan for **each** environmental/policy component you stated in Step 3.

At the end of the Step 5 worksheets for the environmental/policy components, you will have the following products:

> **Step 5D:** General support objectives for each environmental or policy component.

> **Step 5E:** A matrix that links mediators, objectives, and activities to help you design your support plan.

Use these worksheets as an organizational guide to help you design your environmental support plan and translate theory mediators into environmental and policy change activities. Electronic versions of these worksheets are available at http://nutrition.jbpub.com/education/2e/. If you are unable to access the worksheets electronically, you can write onto this blank worksheet or create a text document that uses the same flow of information.

NOTE: This case study presents two types of environmental/policy support components: one involving educational activities directed at the family to help students make changes, and one involving creating school environment and policy changes. For illustrative purposes, we describe the support plan that focuses on only one of the program's goal behaviors: increasing fruit and vegetable intake. This completed case study worksheet focuses on the school component.

Step 5D: General support objectives

Support plan title: The Whys and Whats of Colorful Eating (School Environment Component)

Program goal behaviors: Students will increase their intake of fruits and vegetables (youth to aim for 2.5 or more cups a day)

Write the general educational objectives.

Mediator (from Step 3)	General support objectives
Decision-makers' awareness and motivation	The nutrition education program will enhance motivation of school administrators to create healthy environment.
Food environment	The nutrition education program will provide many opportunities for youth to taste F&V.
Organizational food policy	The school will activate school wellness policy council to develop guidelines for foods available in school.
Information environment	The school will make cafeteria information environment supportive of eating fruits and vegetables.

Step 5E: Designing the support plan: matrix format

Design your support plan in matrix format. Write specific objectives for the mediators in your theory model (Step 3). Then, write the theory-based strategy you will employ to address the mediator and create support activities that will be meaningful, interesting, and appropriate for your audience and will operationalize strategy.

Mediator (from Step 3)	Specific support objectives*	Strategies to achieve environmental/policy support objectives
Decision-makers' awareness and motivation	Increase school administrators' beliefs in importance of healthful school environment (outcome expectations)	Individual meetings or presentations to staff about importance of healthful eating for learning; discussion of financial impacts, success stories.
Social support	Increase social modeling by valued celebrities	Bring in local celebrities for school assembly to talk about why they choose healthy eating patterns.
Food environment	School will provide many opportunities for students to taste F&V	Nutrition educators and food service staff will provide taste tests for F&V in the cafeteria.
	School food service personnel will increase fruits and vegetables in meals; obtained from local farmers in a farm-to-school program	Provide professional development and manuals for food service personnel; provide information on potential vendors for local produce.
Organizational food policy	Activate school food policy council to develop guidelines for foods available in school	Presentations to or conversations with school administrators, teachers, parent associations about need for school policies.
	School nutrition advisory council will develop food policies	Recruitment to council: administrators, food service staff, teachers, students, parents, and others.
	Develop guidelines of items in vending machines and school store	Provide technical assistance to develop guidelines for vending machine and school store items.
	Vending machines will carry healthful F&V items	Vendors will supply healthful items in vending machines; develop system for monitoring compliance.
	School stores will carry healthful F&V food items	Develop guidelines of items in school store (e.g., 50% will be healthful items); develop.
Information environment	Make eating F&V normative; develop posters for cafeteria; newsletter to family	Focus group with teens; design posters with teens about eating F&V; post them.

* Use your findings about the changes that could be made in your audience's environment (Step 2D) for each category to guide your writing of the specific objectives.

In Step 5, use your theoretical model, philosophy of nutrition education, and nutrition education program objectives to create (1) educational plans for the individual-level components and (2) environmental supports plans for environmental/policy components.

The pages of the Step 5 worksheets are devoted to designing the environmental supports plan for the environmental/policy component. Generally, the environmental/policy component consists of activities directed at changes that impact one or more facets of the environment or policy but can take other forms, such as media campaigns and activities directed at parents or families.

> **NOTE:** This case study presents two types of environmental/policy support components: one involving educational activities directed at the family to help students make changes, and one involving creating school environment and policy changes. For illustrative purposes, we describe the support plan that focuses on only one of the program's goal behaviors: increasing fruit and vegetable intake.
>
> These completed case study worksheets focus on the family component, which consists of one group session on fruits and vegetables conducted with parents or other primary adult caregivers. Because this component is directed at family behaviors, it involves developing an educational plan but this time directed at how parents or families might help their children eat more fruits and vegetables. Hence we use the same design matrix used when developing educational plans for the youth themselves (Steps 5A and 5B). The design matrix then can be converted to a narrative educational plan for delivering the family group session (not shown).

Step 5 (Modified): General educational objectives

Support plan title: The Whys and Whats of Colorful Eating (Family Component)

Family goal behaviors: Parents/family members will make a variety of fruits and vegetables available/accessible to their children

Write the general educational objectives.

Mediator (from Step 3)	General educational objectives
Physical outcome expectations (benefits)	Demonstrate understanding and valuing of the importance for their children of eating a variety of fruits and vegetables
Social support	Develop skills for providing social support to each other
Food- and nutrition-related skills	Develop skills in preparing and making fruits and vegetables accessible for their children
Goal intention	Demonstrate commitment to providing fruits and vegetables for their children

Step 5: Designing the educational plan: matrix format

Design your educational (or lesson) plan in matrix format. Write specific objectives for the mediators in your theory model (Step 3). Then, create educational activities that will be meaningful, interesting, and appropriate for your audience and will operationalize the mediators.

Event of instruction	Mediator (from Step 3)	Specific support objectives	Theory-based strategy and educational activities, experiences, and/or content
Gain attention (A)	Physical outcome expectations (benefits)	State benefits: energy, important for healthy growth, build strong bones and muscles for athletic performance	Use colorful visuals, striking statistics, or short trigger films to emphasize the importance of F&V for their children's health. Bring in a variety of differently colored F&V.
Present stimulus or new material (S)	Physical outcome expectations (benefits)	State the importance of eating a "rainbow of colors"	Provide colorful visuals of nutrients in differently colored F&V.
		Value importance of providing many opportunities for children to become familiar with different F&V	Learning task: to show that children need help to eat more F&V; parents can help.
	Social norms/ social models	State ways that other parents have made changes at home to support their children; recognize that media personalities support F&V intake	Have parents share their successes in providing F&V to children. Show pictures or film clips; tell stories of media personalities advocating F&V. Discuss parents as role models and the importance of talking about nutrition with their child; explain intent of TV advertisements.
Provide guidance and practice (G)	Physical outcome expectations (barriers)	Describe ways to select F&V to lower cost	Talk about and show data that buying in season and storing correctly can reduce costs.
	Self-efficacy	Describe how F&V can be used in meals and as snacks	Provide tip sheets and simple recipes.
	Social support	Appreciate that other parents share their challenges and successes	Provide family fun nights to meet other parents; share information; newsletters with parents' stories.
	Behavioral capability (food- and nutrition-related knowledge and skills)	Demonstrate skills in quick and easy preparation methods and recipes using F&V	Provide food demonstrations or food preparation tasks for parents to learn new recipes.
		Demonstrate skills to make F&V readily accessible and available to children	Describe ways to cut up vegetables and place in accessible shelf in refrigerator for children to eat; fruit washed and on the counter.
Apply and close (C)	Behavioral goal intention/action planning	State a commitment, in writing, to make F&V readily accessible and available to children	Parents will make an action plan for exactly when, how, and where they will make F&V available to their children.
	Reinforcement	Maintain their commitment to support children	Newsletters sent home on a regular schedule to reinforce healthful eating; tips and recipes.

Taking Control:
Eating Well and Being Fit

Small-sizing processed, packaged makes a big difference

Why Care About Your Child's Snack Choices

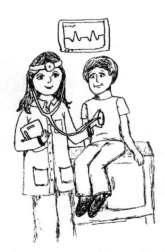

Snacks typically play a big role in the life of middle school students. They have active, busy lives and are often on the run from morning until night. Additionally, if they are growing they may be hungry much of the time. However, the snacks that are typically easily available in our food environment can be putting adolescents' health at risk. More and more adolescents are being diagonsed with conditions such as high levels of bood fat, high levels blood sugar and high blood pressure. *(Outcome expectations: Perceived risk)*

Did you know...

- A snack of three chocolate peanut butter cups has over 4 teaspoons of fat. The recommendation is to not exceed 13 teaspoons a day. They also have 8 teaspoons of sugar and the recommendation is to not exceed 12 ½ teaspoons a day.

You can see how snacks can easily add on extra fat and sugar in the diet. Having smaller portions of processed packaged snacks can help adolescents do what they want to be able to do today, and keep them healthy into the future. *(Perceived benefits)*

Great ways to small-size processed, packaged snacks and add snacks that pack in the nutrition adolscents need

Look over the tips below and model these practices with your child so that she or he will take on the same behaviors when making snack choices. *(Social modeling)*

- When given the choice between several sizes of a snack, such as chips or cookies, your child can choose the small size or split with a friend. (We suggest no more than one small snack each day)

- When buying snacks at a convenience store, your child can try snacks such as granola bars that usually have less sugar and fat than other snacks.

- Help your child to cut up fruit or vegetable in the morning and place in a sealed container. Also have fruits and vegetables easily available at home. This way your child will have snacks with lots of good nutrients that is naturally low in fat and sugar.

- Have your child eat balanced meals so that he or she gets filled up with healthful foods at mealtime and thus will be less likely to be grabbing for snacks.

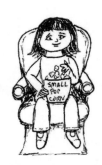

(Knowledge and skills)

For more information about Taking Control: Eating Well and Being Fit, stop by the parent room anytime!

In Step 5, use your theoretical model, philosophy of nutrition education, and nutrition education program objectives to create (1) educational plans for the individual-level components and (2) environmental supports plans for environmental/policy components.

These pages of the Step 5 worksheets are devoted to designing the environmental supports plan for the environmental/policy components. Generally, the environmental/policy components consist of activities directed at changes that impact one or more facets of the environment or policy as these relate to your program's behavioral goals.

You should have **one** support plan for **each** environmental/policy component you stated in Step 3.

At the end of the Step 5 worksheets for the environmental/policy components, you will have the following products:

    Step 5D: General support objectives for each environmental or policy component.

    Step 5E: A matrix that links mediators, objectives, and activities to help you design your support plan.

Use these worksheets as an organizational guide to help you design your environmental support plan and translate theory mediators into environmental and policy change activities. Electronic versions of these worksheets are available at http://nutrition.jbpub.com/education/2e/. If you are unable to access the worksheets electronically, you can write onto this blank worksheet or create a text document that uses the same flow of information.

Step 5D: General support objectives

Support plan title: _____

Program goal behaviors: _____

Write the general educational objectives.

Mediator (from Step 3)	General support objectives

Step 5E: Designing the support plan: matrix format

Design your support plan in matrix format. Write specific objectives for the mediators in your theory model (Step 3). Then, write the theory-based strategy you will employ to address the mediator and create support activities that will be meaningful, interesting, and appropriate for your audience and will operationalize strategy.

Mediator (from Step 3)	Specific support objectives*	Strategies to achieve environmental/policy support objectives

* Use your findings about the changes that could be made in your audience's environment (Step 2D) for each category to guide your writing of the specific objectives.

Step 6: Planning the Evaluation for Theory-Based Nutrition Education

OVERVIEW

This chapter describes key issues in designing and conducting evaluations and how they may be applied to planning the evaluation of theory-based nutrition education programs.

CHAPTER OUTLINE

- Introduction
- Evaluation
- What should be evaluated?
- Planning the process evaluation
- Planning the outcome evaluation
- Case study
- Your turn: completing the Step 6 worksheets

LEARNING OBJECTIVES

At the end of the chapter, you will be able to:

- State reasons for conducting evaluations of nutrition education interventions
- Distinguish between the major types of evaluation
- Explain the relationships among educational objectives, mediating variables, and measures of outcome
- Describe types of measures for evaluating mediators and behaviors
- Describe key features to consider in creating evaluation measures
- Judge the appropriateness of different evaluation designs for the given intervention and audience
- Demonstrate skills in designing an evaluation for a nutrition education intervention

■ INTRODUCTION: WHY EVALUATE?

You have designed your program activities carefully, basing them on theory and evidence, so that the program will be effective. Why then do you need to evaluate it?

Consider this example: An American Peace Corps volunteer went to Malawi to work in an under-five's clinic. There he saw many malnourished children and started trying to convince mothers to enrich their babies' food. He finally wrote and recorded a song with the following message: put pounded peanut flour in your baby's maize porridge and feed it to him or her three times a day if you want your child to weigh a lot. The song was a success; it became number one on the national radio hit parade. Did this very original and apparently successful approach to nutrition education change the mothers' behavior and improve the nutritional status of children in Malawi? Unfortunately, no one will ever know. Large amounts of dedication, creativity, and resources have often been invested in programs and no one knows their impact because the programs were not evaluated. As we can see in **Figure 14-1**, evaluation is an important component of nutrition education.

The Stepwise Procedure (**Figure 14-2**) serves as a way to translate theory into intervention practice and to provide ways to implement theory. In general, with the word *value* embedded in the term *evaluation*, it is not surprising that a simple definition of the term is that evaluation is the process of determining the value or worth of an enterprise. Consequently, evaluation serves research purposes, program evaluation purposes, or both.

For research purposes, nutrition educators investigate whether and how interventions influence potential mediators and how mediating variables influence nutrition behavior so that they can learn exactly how and why interventions do or do not work. Such understandings can be incorporated into evidence-based theory to enhance the effectiveness of nutrition education.

In practice settings, practitioners are held accountable for the programs they conduct. In these settings, evaluation can serve many functions, examples of which are given in the following list. These functions vary in their relative importance depending on the nature of the program and the context in which it occurs:

- Determining whether the goals and objectives of the nutrition education intervention have been met
- Judging whether the program has had impacts on the targeted behaviors or on the mediating variables of the behaviors
- Determining whether the message or content was suitable for the target group
- Providing information on whether the educational strategies and activities (such as format, duration, and frequency) were appropriate for the given group and contributed to the achievement of the behavioral goals and educational objectives
- Determining whether the program was implemented as planned, and if not, why not
- Providing for participation of, and feedback to, the intended audience
- Providing evidence to funding sources that their funding was well spent and achieved their goals or the larger goals of society (such as chronic disease reduction, overweight prevention, or healthy living among those with HIV)

Nutrition educators can use information such as this to improve the planning and implementation of the nutrition education program the next time around, as well as to judge its overall worth.

Evaluation also can serve sociopolitical functions. For example, evaluation may be used to improve public relations by demonstrating to the public how good the program is and how worthy it is of further public- or private-sector funding. An evaluation report released to the various media may also be used to increase the visibility of an organization's work or to apply political pressure for legislative action in the area of nutrition education.

Finally, evaluation may serve psychological functions. Learning that they have been effective can be very motivating for all involved in the nutrition education program, but especially to those actually delivering the programs to the intended audience—whether they are teachers, workplace employees, or community nutrition educators.

■ EVALUATION: FOR WHOM AND BY WHOM?

As you can see, then, evaluation serves many purposes. Who exactly is served by evaluation? And, who should conduct it?

Evaluation: For Whom?

Who should be served by an evaluation? Clearly, many people are interested in the information generated by an evaluation. The term *stakeholder* is usually used to refer to all those who have some stake in the outcome of an evaluation. Policy makers and nutrition education practitioners often have different opinions regarding what should be indicators of effectiveness, and a fair evaluation must take into account the different needs of the various groups involved. It is best to include all stakeholders early in the evaluation design process so that all needs are articulated and considered.

Food and Nutrition Educators

For most food and nutrition educators, whether they conduct sessions, create materials, develop curricula, or design mass media campaigns, the most important function of evaluation is to provide information about whether the intervention was effective, that is, whether it achieved the stated goals and objectives. It also is important to know what worked, what did not, and why. Other aspects of interest are as follows: were the learning activities and message content suitable? Was the educational

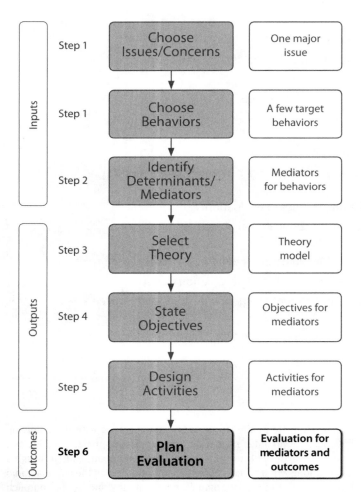

FIGURE 14-1 Flowchart of steps in designing theory-based nutrition education: Step 6.

Inputs: Collecting Assessment Data			Outputs: Designing the Theory-Based Intervention			Outcomes: Evaluation Plan
Step 1 ⟵⟶ **Analyze issues and audiences to state program behavioral goals**	Step 2 ⟵⟶ **Identify potential mediators to achieve program behavioral goals**	Step 3 ⟵⟶ **Select theory, philosophy, and components**	Step 4 ⟵⟶ **State objectives for mediators**	Step 5 ⟵⟶ **Design theory-based strategies and activities for mediators**		Step 6 **Plan evaluation**
Tasks • Analyze issues and select audience • Identify behaviors or patterns contributing to issue • Specify behavioral or action goals of the program	*Tasks* • Identify personal psychosocial mediators • Identify environmental support mediators	*Tasks* • Select theory or create appropriate model • Clarify philosophy (education and content) • Determine program components	*Tasks* • State educational objectives for psychosocial mediators • State change objectives for environmental support mediators	*Tasks* • Design activities to address psychosocial mediators • Design activities to address environmental support mediators • Implementation plan		*Tasks* • Design outcome evaluation plan • Determine tools to measure impact • Plan process evaluation
Product • *Description of issue of concern* • *Statement of action or behavioral goals for program*	*Product* • *List of potential mediators for action or behavior goals*	*Product* • *Theory/model for program, philosophy, and components*	*Product* • *Objectives for each mediator*	*Product* • *Educational plans for sessions linking mediators, objectives, and strategies* • *Environmental support plans*		*Product* • *Evaluation plan* • *List of indicators and measures for outcomes* • *Procedures and measures for process evaluation*

FIGURE 14-2 Stepwise Procedure for designing theory-based nutrition education: Step 6.

style or approach used appropriate? Were the print, audio, or video materials effective as used? Was it easy to implement the program as designed? What facilitated and what hindered implementation? If you are conducting one-shot educational events, this may be the only function of a brief evaluation carried out at the end of a given session. Such information can guide future activities with the same group or similar groups, or provide feedback that is helpful for the future.

The Sponsoring Organization or Funding Agency

The organization sponsoring your nutrition education sessions or program, whether it is a national or community governmental or private voluntary agency, school system, nonprofit organization, corporate worksite, or fitness center, needs evaluative information to determine whether the goals and objectives of the program are being met and whether the program is being well managed. Information may also be needed to satisfy funding agencies (if other than the sponsoring organization itself) demanding evidence for program effects. Evaluation results are important for decision making about future courses of action.

Participants

Those participating in the program, such as community members, workplace employees, or school students, have the greatest stake in its outcome or impact. For them, evaluation may provide a sense of accomplishment and self-worth or objective information on whether their eating patterns and health have improved. It also provides information to those participants who are paying directly for the nutrition education service (e.g., a cardiovascular risk reduction group) by which they can judge whether the effect was worth the money they spent. For school students, evaluation provides feedback on whether they have adequately acquired needed health knowledge and skills. For them, the evaluation activities may actually be interesting to do.

Evaluation: By Whom?

Who should conduct the evaluation depends on the scope of the nutrition education program. If you are providing only one or several in-person group sessions, you will probably be the one conducting the evaluation. If the nutrition education is more extensive, who should be involved depends primarily on two factors: the resources available and the need for objectivity.

Resources Available

Resources include not just time and money but also the technical skills needed to conduct the evaluation. Simple evaluations do not require many resources. Pencils, paper, a duplicating machine of some sort (optional), and knowledge of how to construct and analyze a simple questionnaire are probably all that is needed for a simple but formal quantitative postsession evaluation for a one-time educational event. An informal or qualitative evaluation requires even less in the way of physical resources but probably more technical skills: making verbal inquiries of participants about what they learned. However, evaluating a curriculum in nationwide field tests or evaluating a mass media campaign requires more resources. Such an evaluation requires people with the technical expertise for planning and implementing an evaluation design and analyzing the results. It also requires considerable time and money. Most nutrition education program evaluations are somewhere in between in scope.

Objectivity

For evaluation results to be credible, they need to be obtained in such a way that those reading the results believe that the results are objective. Should the evaluation, then, be conducted by some outside person or group? Although the advantage of this approach is that the results will be considered more credible, the outside evaluators may be less familiar with the program and may be culturally or socially different from those implementing or participating in the program. In-house evaluations, on the other hand, have the advantage that those conducting them are more familiar with the program, have access to more information, and are better able to identify problem areas as well as solutions to them. In many situations, it is possible to use both in-house and outside evaluations, with some aspects (e.g., pilot testing) primarily done by in-house personnel and others (e.g., outcome evaluations or those involving staff members' jobs) done by an outside person or group.

■ WHAT SHOULD BE EVALUATED? TYPES OF EVALUATION

There are three major types of evaluation that you can use to evaluate your program, depending on your needs: formative, outcome, and process. Formative evaluation involves pilot testing near the beginning of your program. Outcome evaluations are carried out at the end of the program to provide information on the overall effects of the program or intervention, and they are sometimes called *effect evaluations*. In process evaluation, you want to know whether the program was delivered to the persons for whom it was intended and whether it was implemented as designed or planned in order to help shed light on why your intervention worked well or did not.

Formative Evaluation or Pilot Testing

The function of formative evaluation or pilot testing is to develop or improve an ongoing activity such as programs or educational sessions. It is usually used during the early developmental or formative stages of program development. The information collected in this type of evaluation is intended to serve decision making about the sessions or program.

Formative research can determine whether the intended audience understands the messages. Also, pilot testing and revising each of the program components ensures that the program as a whole will be stronger. For example, you may now want to deliver the session/program activities with an audience similar to your intended audience to find out

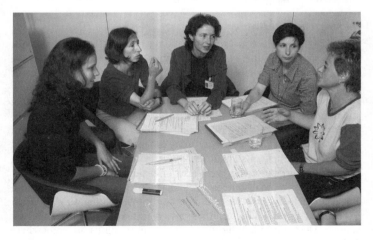

Among the considerations for practitioners as they design programs are goals, objectives, target audience, and appropriate activities.

whether the objectives are appropriate and the activities are interesting to the audience, sequenced logically, and can be delivered within the allotted time. You can now use such information to revise the objectives and educational activities of the curriculum. You also will want to test the food-related activities and recipes that are included. Formative evaluation also includes more systematic field tests carried out on the new curriculum or program materials before the final product is published. Here, you send this curriculum draft or manual of activities to a sample of teachers or community nutrition educators and ask them to implement the educational plans with a similar group to find out if (1) the objectives are clear, (2) the issues included are considered relevant, (3) the educational activities are appropriate, interesting, and feasible to carry out, and (4) the evaluation procedures are useful.

Outcome Evaluation: Outcomes and Impacts

Clarifying Terms

The terms *impact evaluations* and *outcome evaluations* refer to evaluations conducted at the end of the program and are statements of the results of the program (Medeiros et al. 2005). That is, did the nutrition education program actually accomplish what it was designed to accomplish? This type of evaluation carries the connotation of accountability.

Outcome evaluations address the question of whether anticipated group changes or differences occur in connection with the intervention. By itself, however, measuring outcomes may not provide definitive evidence that the observed outcomes are the result of the intervention. To definitively conclude that the observed outcomes are a result of the intervention, an *impact evaluation* has to be conducted (U.S. Department of Agriculture [USDA] 2005).

Impact evaluation involves use of a systematic research design or evaluation plan to eliminate alternative explanations for the observed differences. Such a design is called the *impact evaluation design* and is described later in this chapter.

Efficacy and Effectiveness Evaluations

In the research literature, a distinction is made between effectiveness and efficacy evaluations. An *efficacy evaluation* is one conducted under optimal conditions (such as when the researchers or program designers themselves deliver the program with outside funding and supports), whereas an *effectiveness evaluation* is evaluation of a program under real-world circumstances (such as conducted by teachers or by practitioner staff as part of their jobs).

Appropriate Outcomes: Short, Medium, and Long Term

Outcome evaluations are based on the goals and objectives of the nutrition education sessions or program.

Behavioral Outcomes

In behavior-focused, theory-based nutrition education interventions or communications, the primary outcomes to be assessed are usually the behaviors that are targeted by the program; that is, the assessment is of whether the *behavioral goals* of the program have been achieved, such as an increase in consumption of fruits and vegetables, breastfeeding, or use of electronic benefit transfer cards to shop at a farmers' market. These behavioral outcomes are considered *medium-term outcomes* in the community nutrition education logic model described in Chapters 6 and 13 (Medeiros et al. 2005).

Impacts on Mediators

You also want to measure whether the mediators of targeted behaviors, such as perceived threat, perceived benefits and barriers of taking action, preferences for healthful foods, self-efficacy, and intentions, as well as food- and nutrition-related knowledge and skills or goal-setting and self-influence skills have improved. In some cases, movement of participants through the stages of readiness to change may be measured. These are called *short-term outcomes* in the logic model. As discussed at some length in this book, these mediators are the targets of the general educational objectives of a program. Although demonstration of achievement of specific actions or behaviors is often sought for many nutrition education programs, achievement of these short-term outcomes may be all that can be expected given the duration, intensity, and scope of the program. If the research evidence indicates that there is a strong relationship between these mediating variables and the behavior itself, then changes in these mediators can serve as good indications that the impacts may be translated into action under suitable conditions. For example, in many studies the relationship between self-efficacy and behavior is strong so that an increase in self-efficacy in program participants may be meaningful. Information about changes in these mediators of behavior can also help to explain how and why the intervention or its component activities worked, or did not.

Physiological or Health Outcomes

In some educational interventions, physiological parameters are the desired primary end points, such as changes in serum cholesterol levels or weight. These are *long-term outcomes*, requiring educational interventions of considerable intensity and duration.

Choice of Outcomes

Choice of outcome may be influenced by the function of the evaluation and funding sources. At the time of designing the educational intervention, it is best to design ways to evaluate each *behavioral goal* (behavior) and each *general educational objective* (mediator of behavior). You must

decide whether to evaluate all the *specific* educational objectives and all the environmental support objectives, or only a sample of them. This will depend on the purposes of the evaluation and how detailed or comprehensive the evaluation needs to be.

Process Evaluation

In a process or program evaluation, you want to know answers to the following questions: Did the program reach the intended audience? How many attended? Was the program implemented as designed or planned? If so, what worked and what did not? If it did not work, why not? Were all the activities implemented? To what degree? How did participants judge the intervention activities or component? In terms of environmental support activities, process evaluation questions might include the following: How many coalition partners were involved? How effective was communication among partners? How did the partners feel about the program?

It is just as important to probe failures as successes. Failures may bring to light flaws in the original design and identify breakdowns in the internal operations of the program. Failures also help you understand the limitations of what the program can accomplish.

Linking the Evaluation Plan to Program Design

You should select evaluation procedures when you are planning the educational intervention so that the procedures can be incorporated into activities of the program. Even before you have implemented the program, you need to plan for the kinds of information you will need as you go along and at the end of the program, and design appropriate measurement tools. The logic model (**Figure 14-3**) can serve as the framework for evaluation. This figure is based on the integrative framework for translating theory into nutrition education practice described in Step 3, which is discussed in Chapter 9 (refer to Figure 9-4).

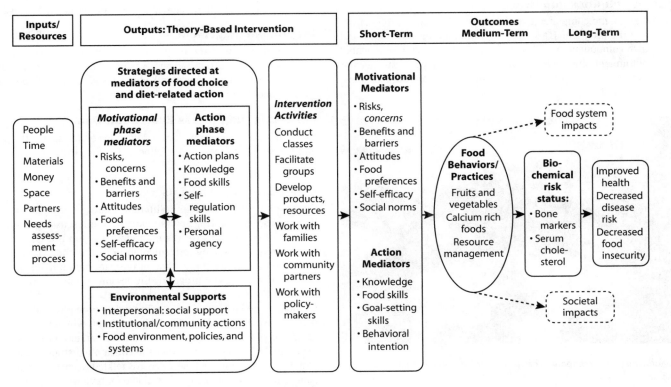

FIGURE 14-3 Designing the evaluation for theory-based nutrition education.

Because evaluation involves judgment of worth, it requires the development of some way to assess or measure worth. An analogy might clarify the difference between measurement and evaluation. In everyday terms, *measurement* is saying that the temperature in a room is 68°F; *evaluation* is saying, "I feel cold at this temperature." The measurement instrument (a thermometer, in this instance) has to be accurate and reliable, and your judgment has to be based on ruling out competing explanations for why you might feel cold (you might be sick that day and hence feeling cold). When you say, "It's cold today," you are mixing measurement and evaluation. *It* is not cold: *it* is 68°F (measurement); *you* feel cold (evaluation).

■ PLANNING THE PROCESS EVALUATION

This chapter describes process evaluation first because it is most familiar, tends to be done routinely, and is easier to design and carry out. You are participating in a process evaluation when, as a student, you complete an end-of-semester evaluation of the course and the instructor, or when, as a professional, you complete an evaluation instrument at the end of a conference or professional meeting asking for your opinions of the learning experience. Banks do it; airlines do it. This section describes the kinds of questions you might want to ask about the program you are designing.

Clarifying the Process Evaluation Questions

In general, process evaluation focuses on evaluating the input and output components of the logic model. Process evaluation questions might be related to program activities and reach, program implementation and fidelity, program design, and program management in some cases. During program implementation and at the end you may want to know the following.

Program Activities and Reach

- What are the components of the program? What are the materials of the program? (Descriptive information on how many and which components you designed, such as classroom plus school environment plus parent component, or groups plus media campaign; how often the sessions are held; what are the handouts, and so forth.)

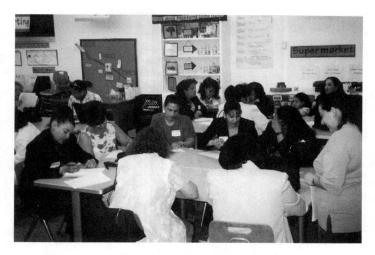

Evaluating the parent component can provide important information for a program.

- Did the program reach the intended target audience? To what extent? (What proportion of the intended audience participated or is participating?) How many participated or are participating?
- What were participants' and practitioners' degree of satisfaction with both the content of materials, learning activities, or media messages and the form in which it was delivered?
- If a coalition component was or is involved, how many partners or coalition members were or are there? What were or are their roles?
- What activities did coalition partners conduct separately or together?
- What degree of satisfaction did or do the coalition partners express about their participation?

Program Implementation and Fidelity

- How many of the activities designed for the program were actually delivered?
- Was the program implemented, or is it being implemented, as designed? How extensively (part or all)? How frequently?
- If the program was or is not being implemented as designed, why not? What are the obstacles?
- How well did the coalition function or is it functioning? Did coalition partners conduct the activities they committed themselves to do? If not, why not?

Program Design Review

- Are the program behavioral goals and educational objectives that you designed directed at, or consistent with, the issues identification and needs analysis data you collected in Step 1?
- Are educational strategies and learning experiences appropriately designed to achieve stated goals and objectives?
- Are educational strategies and learning experiences appropriately based on nutrition behavior theory and research findings?

Program Management

- How well was the program managed or is it being managed? Did it stay within budget? Was or is the flow of information to those needing it timely and adequate? Was the coalition managed satisfactorily?

Collecting the Process Evaluation Data

How you collect the evaluative data depends on the size of the program and the extent of the resources allocated to the evaluation phase of the program.

Using Existing Materials

Collection can involve many different strategies: examining existing documents, interviewing key individuals, and discussing matters with a group of participants (or the entire target group if it is a small one) as the program is being implemented or at the end. Making process evaluation possible requires that all program design materials such as the description of the program, the lesson or education plans used by the nutrition educator or given to participants, and handouts be maintained and easily accessible (in binders or in physical or computer files). These materials provide information on whether the behavioral goals and educational objectives are directed at, or consistent with, the needs analysis data and whether the educational strategies are consistent with theory and evidence. Records related to coalition partnerships should also be maintained and available for review—for example, meeting agendas, announcements of accomplishments, program plans, or products developed.

Developing Instruments

Gathering the evaluative data may also involve the development of appropriate instruments or forms for recording the data. These might include attendance sheets to provide information on number of participants, and instruments to assess fidelity to the program—such as a checklist of activities for each session for the nutrition educator to check off how much of the session content was delivered and note whether other material was added. If ongoing records are to be obtained from the participants, such as three-day food records, you need to design some way to keep track of whether these records were turned in. You will also want to develop an evaluation form for participants to complete, asking them to rate the usefulness of the nutrition education experience—whether it was one session or a program of several months. More important, it should ask them to state which parts of the program were most useful and which least useful, what topics should have been covered in greater depth or less, and what other topics or activities should have been included.

You can use the data collected in a formative way to decide how to improve participation rates and degree of satisfaction with the program; how to improve the process of delivery, such as better training for personnel, better materials, or more clarity about intervention strategies; or how to improve management. The data collected in an evaluation at the end of the program can be used to identify specifically why the program was or was not effective in bringing about desired nutritional goals. In other words, information obtained about program functioning can help to interpret the results obtained from the outcome evaluation about the effectiveness of the program (or lack of it).

■ PLANNING THE OUTCOME EVALUATION

Figure 14-3 provides the framework for designing the outcome evaluation. As you can see, you can measure short-, medium-, and long-term outcomes. Planning the outcome evaluation generally involves the following steps:

1. Clarifying the outcomes that will be evaluated
2. Specifying indicators and measures of outcome effectiveness and data collection methods
3. Designing and testing the instruments or tools for measuring program effectiveness
4. Constructing an appropriate evaluation plan to measure impacts

Clarifying the Outcomes That Will Be Evaluated

Outcome evaluations are based on the goals and objectives of the nutrition education sessions or program. Hence, at the time of designing the educational intervention, it is best to design ways to evaluate each behavioral goal, general educational objective, and environmental support objective. So, in a major way, your evaluation outcomes have already been determined by your statement of objectives. Outcomes of a nutrition education program can thus be evaluated in terms of mediating variables, behaviors or practices, or health outcomes, as shown in Figure 14-3.

Criterion of Effectiveness

At the outset, you need to clarify what you will use as the criterion of effectiveness for a given program. Selection of outcomes should be based on the purpose, duration, and power of the intervention.

Behaviors or Practices

What exactly is meant by "behavior" in this intervention? For example, will achievement of the actual behavior change (such as increased intakes of fruits and vegetables) or engagement in the targeted actions by the intended audience (such as buying at farmers' markets) be used as the criterion of outcome effectiveness? On the other hand, for an intervention of short duration, the behavior change expected can be quite small, such as trying new vegetables when offered. Changes in behaviors, food intakes, or practices are considered to be medium-term outcomes in the logic model shown in Figure 14-3.

Physiological or Health Outcomes

Will outcome effectiveness be judged not just on whether participants engaged in the target behaviors but also on whether there were changes in the physiological parameters or risk factors for health problems that result from engagement in the targeted actions, such as change in weight or biochemical markers? These are referred to as long-term outcomes.

Mediating Variables

On the other hand, is behavior change an appropriate criterion for the particular audience or for the power, duration, or intensity of the intervention? Will behavioral intentions be sufficient? Will improvement in the stages of motivational readiness to change be sufficient? Are changes in mediators of behavior an appropriate measure of the outcome of the given intervention? If you are conducting only one or two sessions, changes in awareness and motivation and in relevant knowledge and skills may be appropriate outcomes. These are referred to as short-term outcomes in the model.

Participant Choice

Perhaps the philosophical approach of the program is that participants will choose which changes to make or whether even to make any. What criteria will you use to evaluate effectiveness? How will you report to stakeholders the effect of the program?

Specifying Indicators and Measures of Outcome Effectiveness and Data Collection Methods

To evaluate outcomes of your program, you need to develop some indicators of effectiveness.

Indicators are the ways to operationalize theoretical constructs, activities, and behaviors to identify that change has occurred or that an action has been taken with respect to the desired outcome.

Measures are the specific tools or instruments that you use to evaluate the change that has occurred. You need to select the indicators and measures that are appropriate for your program.

Linking Outcomes, Indicators, and Measures

To evaluate outcomes you will develop tables that have the following columns: "Outcomes," "Indicators for Achievement of Outcomes," and "Measures for the Indicators" as shown here:

Outcomes	Indicators of Achievement of Outcomes	Measures/Instruments for the Indicators
Mediator Outcomes Outcome expectations (benefits)	Learner demonstrates understanding of benefits of eating fruits and vegetables.	List of statements why fruits and vegetables are important for health; learner checks agreement or disagreement with statements

Outcomes	Indicators of Achievement of Outcomes	Measures/Instruments for the Indicators
Behavioral Outcomes Increased intake of fruits and vegetables	Self-report of increased intake of specified fruits and vegetables.	Food frequency questionnaire for 15 fruits and vegetables
Health Outcomes Heart disease risk	Improved serum cholesterol levels.	Finger prick or blood draw and lab analysis for serum cholesterol level
Environmental Supports School food service personnel provide meals high in fruits and vegetables, prepared in a healthy way	Staff follows recommended food purchasing procedures and preparation methods.	Food purchasing procedures: review of purchasing records Food preparation methods: review of recipes and observation, using checklists

The following subsections discuss some potential indicators and measures in four categories: (1) short-term outcomes: mediators of goal behaviors, (2) medium-term outcomes: goal behaviors, (3) long-term outcomes: physiological parameters, and (4) environmental supports for goal behaviors. For each, the methods for colleting the data are described along with the measures. Tables 14-1 through 14-4 provide detailed versions of the tables for all four categories of outcomes.

Evaluating Impacts on Mediators: Short-Term Outcomes

As stated earlier, general educational objectives are written to address potential mediators of action or behavior change. Thus, impacts on mediators—short-term outcomes—are evaluated on the degree to which these general educational objectives have been achieved. Excerpts from the ongoing case study are shown in **Table 14-1** to illustrate. The full set of outcomes, indicators, and measures are shown in the case study at the end of the chapter.

Mediators as Core of Translating Theory to Nutrition Education Intervention

You used mediators as the basis of your educational objectives, and you used them as the basis for designing educational strategies to address the educational objectives. Now they will be the basis of your evaluation—which is another reason why you design the evaluation at the same time as goals, objectives, and strategies.

You may not want to measure impacts on all of the potential mediators (or mediating variables)—some may be more important than others for judging the effectiveness of the intervention. Now is the time to specify which mediating variables you will actually measure, and then state what will indicate that the program has been effective in changing a given potential mediating variable.

Indicators

The *indicators* can include the following (depending on your theory or model):

- Increased awareness of risks or issues of concern
- Increased outcome expectancies or beliefs in the perceived benefits or pros of action
- Decreased sense of the barriers or cons of change
- Increased preferences for or enjoyment of targeted foods or behaviors
- Improved attitudes or feelings toward the targeted behaviors, such as healthy eating
- Increased understanding of the participant's own social norms and skills

TABLE 14-1	Evaluating Impacts on Potential Individual-Level Psychosocial Mediators of Goal Behaviors: Examples	
Outcomes for Mediators	**Indicators of Achievement of Outcomes (Based on General Educational Objectives)**	**Measures/Instruments for the Indicators**
Outcome expectations	Increased understanding of benefits of eating more F&V; knowledge of scientific basis for eating F&V *Specific indicators:* List of specific benefits and understandings	Scale on benefits with responses of 1 to 5, from strongly disagree to strongly agree; instrument on benefits: multiple-choice questions on impact of F&V on health and disease risk reduction
Barriers	Decreased perception of barriers to eating fruits and vegetables *Specific indicators:* List of specific potential barriers	Scale with responses of 1 to 5, from strongly disagree to strongly agree on items listing barriers
Attitudes	Improved attitudes toward F&V and toward self eating specific fruits and vegetables *Specific indicators:* List of specific attitudes	Scale with responses of 1 to 5, from strongly disagree to strongly agree, on attitudes about specific F&V; and on self eating more F&V (e.g., "I feel I am taking care of myself when I eat F&V")
Self-efficacy	Increased confidence in being able to eat more F&V *Specific indicators:* Confidence in various situations, including difficult ones	Scale with responses of 1 to 5 on how confident participant feels about eating F&V (e.g., "If I wanted to, I am sure I would be able to eat more vegetables at lunch")
Behavioral capability	Increased food- and nutrition-related knowledge and improved skills in incorporating F&V into their daily food patterns *Specific indicators:* List of specific knowledge and skills	Knowledge and skills instrument: Multiple-choice questions and some open-ended questions related to importance of variety and serving sizes; ways to add F&V to daily diet

Note: F&V = fruits and vegetables.

- Increased self-efficacy
- Increased understanding of moral or ethical responsibility issues
- Increased food and nutrition knowledge related to the behavioral goals of the program
- Improved skill in selection of targeted/healthful diets
- Increased skill in preparation of targeted/healthful foods
- Improved stage of readiness to take action or to change
- A stated intention to engage in the action or to change
- Improved ability to engage in a goal-setting process for the program goal behaviors

For social marketing or communications campaigns, the following are important indicators:

- Recall of advertisements or other messages
- Level of exposure to various other interventions within the campaign—such as classes, workshops, health fairs or festivals, food demonstrations attended, or materials brought home from school or workplace

Measures/Instruments and Data Collection Procedures

- *Survey instruments.* You can measure changes in indicators in various ways, although the most usual way is through the use of survey instruments. Theory constructs or mediating variables are operationalized as a series of questions that participants answer or a series of statements to which the participants respond. Many formats can be used. For most mediators, participants are given a series of statements and asked to indicate their opinion on a 5-point agreement scale such as whether they strongly disagree (given a score of 1), disagree (given a score of 2), are neutral (given a score of 3), agree (given a score of 4), or strongly agree (given a score of 5). Statements might include "I feel that I am helping my body by eating more fruits and vegetables" (perceived benefits), "I feel that fruit is too expensive" (perceived barriers), or "People in my family think that I should eat more fruits and vegetables" (perceived social norms).

  A scale might also be stated in terms of amount or frequency. For example, "In your household, how much control do you have in buying/preparing the food you eat?" with a scale ranging from "very little control" to "complete control." Self-efficacy is often measured in terms of how confident individuals are in being able to carry out a given action, such as "How sure are you that you can eat two or more vegetables at dinner?" or "How sure are you that you can add more vegetables to casseroles and stews?" The range of responses might be from "not at all sure" (score of 1) to "very sure" (score of 5). Individuals' readiness to take action can be measured using a series of statements that place them in one of the stages of change: "I am not thinking about eating more fruit" (precontemplation), "I am thinking about eating more fruit" (contemplation), "I am planning to start eating more fruit within 6 months" (contemplation), "I am definitely planning to eat more fruit in the next month" (preparation), "I am trying to eat more fruit now" (action), and "I have been eating two or more servings of fruits a day for at least six months" (maintenance).

- *Data collection methods.* Some examples of instruments to measure mediators are shown in Tables 8-2 and 8-3. These instruments can be given using a pencil-and-paper format (most common). Participants usually complete the instruments on their own. Questions are usually read aloud to young school-aged children or low-literacy audiences, who then complete the questionnaire. The

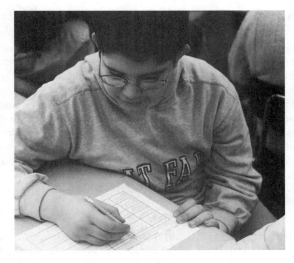

Children like questionnaires if the questions are interesting.

questionnaires should look inviting and be motivational to complete, using pictures, drawings, or other visuals to add interest. Various interactive approaches can also be used. One interactive approach used with school-aged children is to alternate team games to answer some questions with individual responses to questionnaires tapping mediating variables and behavior (Eck, Struempler, & Raby 2005). Instruments can be read aloud to individuals in an interview setting where literacy is low. They can also be administered through computer or Web-based technologies.

- *Scoring the data.* To evaluate whether there have been improvements in the selected mediators of behavior, you calculate changes in scores in these variables. You average the score of all participants for each of the questions in the pretest given at the beginning of the program, and you average the score of all participants on the same instrument given as a post-test at the end of the program. You then examine whether there has been an improvement in scores and whether this improvement is statistically significant. (You will generally also compare this improvement to that of a group that did not participate in the program to see whether the improvement is a result of the program.)

  In many programs, the changes in indicators are expressed in terms of percentage of individuals who demonstrate ability to engage in skills that are relevant to the behavioral target of the program, such as the percentage who can adjust menus or prepare foods to achieve the goal behaviors (e.g., reduce fat, increase fruit and vegetable content of menus) or who can set goals, develop action plans, and practice self-regulation skills.

- *Qualitative data.* Information on impacts on mediating variables can also be obtained through in-depth interviews, focus groups, and other qualitative methods (Straus & Corbin 1990). In this case, the interviews are first transcribed and then analyzed for categories and emerging themes. The analysis involves an iterative or repeated process, in which cases are first reviewed and the data grouped into categories or codes that may be based on prior research or program goals. As new cases are reviewed and added to the coding scheme, the categories and themes may change. This is repeated until there is consensus that the codes have captured all the information. The findings may also be shared with the recipients as validation.

Evaluating Impacts on the Program Goal Behaviors or Practices: Medium-Term Outcomes

In behavior-focused and evidence-based nutrition education, increased engagement in the program goal behaviors is usually the major outcome of interest in an evaluation. This outcome is usually sought by various stakeholders, including participants themselves. Individuals usually give of their time and effort to participate in nutrition education programs because they desire to lose weight, eat more healthfully, or in a way that fosters sustainability of the food system, or for other reasons. You will need to select the indicators and measures that are appropriate for your program. The following are some potential indicators and measures for you to consider.

Indicators

Indicators of behavioral outcomes can include the following:

- Improvement in behavior(s) targeted by the program. This could include increased intake of certain foods (such as fruits and vegetables or calcium-rich foods), decreased intake of targeted foods (such as sodas or high-fat, high-sugar foods), eating a healthy diet (as defined by the program), or increased physical activity.
- Improved intake of nutrients derived from specific foods, such as a decreased percentage of fat in the diet or an increased amount of carotene or calcium.
- Engagement in behaviors or practices targeted by the program. These are visible food-related actions that individuals take. The behaviors can be very specific, such as eating one or more servings of vegetables at lunch and dinner; drinking sweetened beverages; eating breakfast; or eating at a fast food restaurant. Behaviors can also involve practices such as shopping at local farmers' markets or buying organic foods.

Measures and Data Collection Methods

Tools for measuring behaviors depend on the exact indicators of effectiveness chosen, the level of accuracy desired, the purpose of the evaluation, the size of the group, and the resources available. A detailed discussion of these methods is outside the scope of this book: they are usually described in nutritional assessment books. Many of the ones commonly used in nutrition education interventions have been reviewed (Kristal & Beresford 1994; Willett 1998; McPherson et al. 2000; Hersey et al. 2001; Keenan et al. 2001; McClelland et al. 2001; Medeiros et al. 2001; Contento, Randell, & Basch 2002). In brief, they may include the following:

Food Intake

- *Observations of intake.* This usually involves observing how much of meals that were served is eaten or thrown away; thus, the method is often called measurement of estimated plate waste. This can be done by preweighing the average serving size of each item served. Individuals or groups, such as students sitting together, are observed, or asked to leave their trays, and the amount left on each plate is recorded on a predesigned recording sheet or is videotaped and analyzed. This is a very labor-intensive method and requires trained personnel. It is also time-consuming for the participant (called *respondent burden*).
- *Recalls of foods consumed, usually over the previous 24 hours (24-hour dietary recall).* Here, program participants are asked to recall all the foods and beverages that they consumed during the previous 24-hour period. This is usually done individually but can also be done as a group, such as a class. The recalled foods can be manually scored for the quantity of intakes of the foods targeted by the program, such as fruits and vegetables or calcium-rich foods, or they can be converted into nutrients of interest to the program, such as percentage of fat in the diet, using a computer diet-analysis program. This is a very labor-intensive method and requires trained personnel; respondent burden is moderate.
- *Food records.* In this instance, participants keep a record of their intakes of foods and drinks over a one-, three-, or seven-day period. The records can be analyzed for foods targeted by the program or for nutrients, as for the 24-hour recalls. This too is a very labor-intensive method, requiring trained personnel, and respondent burden is very high.
- *Food frequency questionnaires.* There are standard food frequency questionnaires that you can use that contain fairly long food lists. Individuals indicate how frequently they have eaten foods on this list during the past year or some other time period. The foods on this list can again be scored for the individual foods of interest or can be converted to nutrients, again using a computer program. These standardized questionnaires usually use forms that can be optically scanned. These can be self-administered in a group setting. The respondent burden for participants is moderate, and lower than for the methods listed previously (Willett et al. 1987; Block et al. 1992).
- *Food intake checklists or short food frequency questionnaires.* These are food frequency questionnaires that are usually shorter than the ones described in the last item and may include behaviors as well as intakes of specific foods (e.g., Kristal et al. 1990; Yaroch, Resnicow, & Khan 2000; Townsend et al. 2003). An example of a validated short food frequency instrument is shown in Table 7-1.
- *Brief food intake checklists or screeners.* These are even shorter food frequency questionnaires, involving only a short list of the foods of interest, such as fat intake screeners or fruit and vegetable screeners. Some examples are the Centers for Disease Control and Prevention's Behavioral Risk Factor Surveillance System (BRFSS) (Serdula et al. 1993), the National Cancer Institute's 5 A Day fruit and vegetable screener (NCI 2000), or the Rapid Screener for Fat and Fruit and Vegetable Intake (Block et al. 2000).
- *A note about food frequency questionnaires.* The food list must use an appropriate inventory of foods commonly eaten by the audience you are working with, and the names of the foods should be clearly understood by the audience (these often differ by ethnic group). Food frequency questionnaires tend to overestimate intakes and so are best used to compare intakes before and after the nutrition education program rather than to provide estimates of actual intakes. They also ask about intake over a time span of a month to a year, and hence may not be suitable for short-term school or community programs.

Eating Behaviors or Patterns

- *Food behavior checklists or questionnaires.* These instruments or tools measure specific observable food-related *behaviors*, such as behaviors related to high-fat diets, eating fruits and vegetables, buying local or organic foods, shopping practices, food safety behaviors, or food insecurity. In one such instrument (Shannon et al. 1997), the *behaviors* related to reducing fat in the diet are categorized as modifying foods to make them lower in fat, avoiding fat as a seasoning or condiment or in cooking, using lower-fat substitutions, or replacing high-fat foods with fruits and vegetables and other lower-fat foods. Those related to fiber are categorized as eating cereals and grains, eating fruits and vegetables, and substituting high-fiber for low-fiber foods.

- *Eating patterns.* These tools provide information on specific eating patterns, such as whether the participants are eating breakfast.

Diet Quality

- *Dietary quality indices or questions.* Sometimes a single question can be used, such as "How would you describe the quality of your diet?" Other instruments provide an assessment of the overall quality of the diet. A prime example is the USDA's Healthy Eating Index. The index is available online for use by individuals (http://www.mypyramidtracker.gov).

Evaluating Impacts on Physiological Parameters: Long-Term Outcomes

In some nutrition education programs, the expected outcomes are reduced risk for chronic disease or improved health. Indicators are improvements in nutritional status (iron deficiency, bone health) or in physiological disease-risk status.

Measures include the following:

- *Biochemical or physiological measures.* A variety of measures is used. For example, for those with diabetes, maintenance of appropriate blood glucose levels may be the appropriate measure; for weight gain prevention programs, body mass index (BMI) may be the primary outcome measure. For heart disease prevention programs, serum cholesterols may be used as the outcome measure.

Evaluating Changes in Environmental Supports

Tools to measure environmental and policy changes are emerging, such as tools to evaluate the quality of school wellness policies (Schwartz et al. 2009) or community-level changes (Glanz, Sallis, et al. 2005, 2007; Sallis, Orleans, et al. 2009).

However, indicators and measures of program effectiveness in terms of changes made in the environment to make it more supportive of nutrition education program goals are usually very specific to each program. Some examples are shown here, but you will need to develop specific indicators and measures for your program.

Table 14-2 describes some examples of possible indicators and measures that can be used to evaluate the impact of a program on interpersonal-level social support provided by parents to their children and by coworkers and administrators in workplaces. These measures can be administered

TABLE 14-2	Interpersonal-Level Support of Healthful Behaviors: Examples	
Outcomes	**Indicators of Achievement of Outcomes**	**Measures (Surveys) for Indicators**
Parents/Households		
Behaviors	Parents/family members state that they have increased availability and accessibility of targeted healthful foods for their children Parents develop and implement polices about child eating behaviors	Parents indicate from a list whether healthful foods targeted by the program are present in the home and offered at meals (e.g., Marsh, Cullen, & Baranowski 2003). Parents indicate from a list their policies with respect to children's tasting new foods and choosing how much to eat; rewarding eating (e.g., Ventura & Birch 2008).
Outcome expectations *(perceived benefits)*	Increased understanding of the impact of F&V on health.	Knowledge instrument (written or oral) on role of various nutrients in F&V in health and disease (multiple choice).
Social modeling	Parents/adults in household are serving as role models for their children by increased consumption of healthy foods targeted by the program	Parents report quantity and frequency of personally eating a list of fruits and vegetables (e.g., Reynolds et al. 2002).
Worksites		
Social support	Increased coworker and/or family support for targeted healthful behaviors	Individuals complete surveys; for example, on whether coworkers, family, or social support group members never, seldom, sometimes, or often: • Compliment their attempt to eat healthfully • Bring in healthful foods or fruits or vegetables for them to try • Encourage them to eat more healthful foods (Sorensen, Stoddard, & Macario 1998)
Social networks	Increased number of social support groups and high degree of functioning within groups	Observations of support group functioning and checklists Qualitative interviews of group participants and group facilitators

before and after the program; changes in scores on these measures are indicative of the impact of the program on these outcomes.

Multiple Levels

Many changes in environments to make them more supportive of healthful eating require the collaboration and partnership of nutrition educators with various individuals and groups that provide food or services or have decision-making power in that environment, such as school administrators, workplace and institutional managers, community organizations, and food providers, as described in Chapter 13. **Figure 14-4** shows a framework for evaluating the multiple levels of intervention that may be addressed by an intervention.

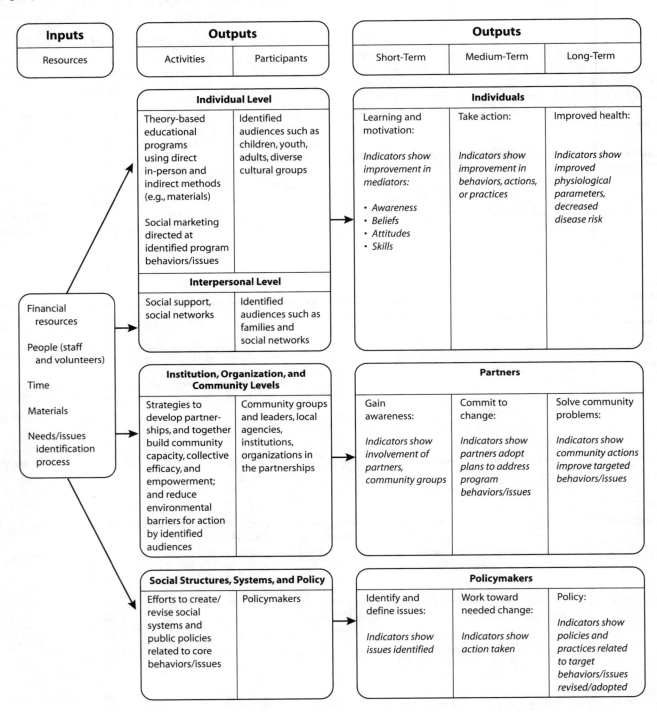

FIGURE 14-4 A logic model for evaluating nutrition education that addresses multiple levels of intervention.

Source: Based on Helen Chipman (national coordinator), Supplemental Nutrition Assistance program Education (SNAP-Ed), NIFA/USDA, and Land Grant University System Partnership. 2006, January. Community Nutrition Education (CNE) Logic Model, Version 2: Overview. http://www.nifa.usda.gov/nea/food/fsne/logic.html. Used with permission.

In schools, the food environment is more controlled than it is in workplaces. The intervention, and hence the evaluation, can be more formal and systematic. In workplaces, the changes usually involve adding food options to existing menus and making some changes rather than implementing systematic changes. It is possible to change informational environments and hence social norms, for example, by placing walking prompts in stairwells. The number of people taking the stairs in a given time can provide an estimate of impact. **Table 14-3** describes possible

<table>
<tr><td colspan="3">**TABLE 14-3**   **Institutional-Level Food Environment and Policy Supports: Examples**</td></tr>
<tr><td>**Outcomes (Based on Objectives)**</td><td>**Indicators of Achievement of Outcomes**</td><td>**Measures or Instruments for the Indicators**</td></tr>
<tr><td colspan="3">*Food Environment*</td></tr>
<tr><td>School food service personnel or workplace food vendors will provide healthful meals.</td><td>Behaviors: Staff follows recommended food purchasing and preparation methods

Food quality reflects changes recommended by program</td><td>Interviews and observations using checklists to identify how many, which, and how often recommended practices are carried out

Review of purchase records

Analysis of planned and actual menus (computer nutrient/food composition programs); observation of food services on-site</td></tr>
<tr><td>Workplace food service personnel or vendors will conduct food-related activities in the cafeteria.</td><td>Increased promotional activities in cafeteria</td><td>Checklist completed by staff on number of activities per month

Review of quality of foods promoted: checklist or observation</td></tr>
<tr><td>School or workplace stores will carry healthful food items.</td><td>Guidelines for school stores developed and implemented

Increased number/proportion of healthful items in stores</td><td>Review of guidelines (process)

Count of number and/or proportion of healthful items available in stores</td></tr>
<tr><td>School, workplace, or health care setting catering will use foods from local farms or local processors.</td><td>Increased number or proportion of selected foods from local sources</td><td>Count of number and/or proportion of foods from local sources being served in cafeteria meals during appropriate season</td></tr>
<tr><td colspan="3">*Information Environment*</td></tr>
<tr><td>The information environment will be supportive of:

• Healthful eating
• Walking stairs</td><td>Posters: Positive and consistent messages about healthful eating provided throughout the school

Informational materials

Posters promoting stair walking in area organizations</td><td>Number of posters designed and posted; content consistent with program goals

Number of brochures, newsletters distributed

Survey of students/employees: number read, degree of satisfaction, what learned

Number of posters displayed; impact on number taking the stairs</td></tr>
<tr><td colspan="3">*Policy Environment or Organizational Climate*</td></tr>
<tr><td>Food policies are supportive of healthful eating.</td><td>Schools: Active wellness policy council

Participation on council of a variety of stakeholders

Policies for foods available in schools or workplaces encourage healthful eating

Worksites: Existence of employee advisory boards; active participation on board; number of activities conducted</td><td>Review of documents; interviews

Review of minutes of meetings; lists of participants; agendas

Mission statements; annual reports with a description of policies (existing and newly adopted) that have been implemented (number and degree of implementation)

Minutes of meetings; lists of participants; agendas

Survey instrument of participatory strategies (e.g., Linnan et al. 1999; Ribisl & Reischl 1993)</td></tr>
<tr><td>Organizational climate is supportive of healthful eating.</td><td>Assessment of organizational climate</td><td>Schools: Changes in scores on a school health index or score card

Worksites: Changes in scores on checklist of workplace policies and environment (e.g., Heart Check; Golaszewski & Fisher 2002)</td></tr>
</table>

indicators and measures of change for institutional environmental supports. **Table 14-4** lists possible indicators and measures for community food environment and policy supports.

Role of the Nutrition Educator

The role of the nutrition educator is to provide technical assistance to the program team on food and nutrition issues in order to design evaluation instruments where measures are carefully linked to theory and program objectives.

Criteria of Effectiveness

For each of the measures you choose to evaluate the program, you also need to decide the level of change that you will consider as necessary to judge effectiveness. Will a statistically significant change be the demonstration of effectiveness (such as a significant increase in intake of fruits and vegetables or rate of breastfeeding)? Or will the change have to reach some criterion level (such as 4 or more cups of fruits and vegetables per day or exclusive breastfeeding for six months)? For stages of readiness to change, will any movement be considered acceptable or does the movement have to be from motivation to action (e.g., from precontemplation or contemplation to preparation or action)?

In terms of change objectives directed at environmental supports for the targeted behaviors, what will serve as criteria of effectiveness? All changes made at the 100% level (e.g., all school meals are to be 20% to 35% fat), or an average for the week? Is the criterion whether fresh fruits and vegetables are available every day, or just some days? Should the criterion be the availability of low-fat options in all worksite cafeteria meals or some? By what percentage should Supplemental Nutrition Assistance Program Electronic Benefits Transfer cards used at farmers' markets increase?

A community could state the following as their environmental support objectives and include specific criteria of effectiveness as follows:

For schools in the community:

- Support Wellness Policy Council Activities so that 70% of schools will conduct a school assessment using the School Health Index or similar tool
- Close streets adjacent to 50% of schools that lack adequate gyms or playgrounds between 3 and 7 pm
- Facilitate enforcement of existing regulations about low-nutrient, high-calorie vending machine food in 50% of schools

For community activities:

- Create four new walking paths in the community
- Double the number of sites where the city-financed exercise classes will be held
- Add one supermarket in the community, which currently has small stores only
- Display walking prompts in stairwells of 70% of area organizations

Designing and Testing the Instruments or Tools for Measuring Program Effectiveness

There is no handbook of evaluation tools or instruments for nutrition education from which you can select one that is right for you. There are many reasons for this: nutrition education interventions need to be

TABLE 14-4	**Community-Level Food Environment and Policy Supports: Examples**	
Outcomes	**Indicators of Achievement of Outcomes**	**Measures or Instruments for the Indicators**
Community capacity: Increased capacity to support healthful actions Increased collective efficacy	Coalitions, collaboratives, or partnerships: number, type, depth, and strength of partnerships	Number of organizations in the coalition or partnership Scales to describe the extent and depth of the partnerships; contributions of each partner, effective functioning (Gregson et al. 2001)
	Commitment to address targeted behaviors/practices Collaboratives or partnerships work together to initiate and implement specific actions to support agreed upon health behavior goals	Number of meetings held on program issue (minutes of meetings, documentation); evidence of concrete written plans (short-term impact), evidence of implementation of plans (medium-term), evidence of increased community access to affordable and healthful food and opportunities for being active (long-term impact)
Information environment	Nature and frequency of media coverage; community events (to enhance social norms for action)	Print media: Number of news articles, inches of column space times circulation Electronic media: Minutes/seconds of airtime and monetary value of that time Pubic relations events: Amount of materials disseminated
Community food environment Grocery stores will highlight items supportive of program's targeted behaviors	Number of grocery stores that now carry or highlight targeted foods Degree to which labels are in place; signage in place Number of farmers at farmers' markets; number who accept Supplemental Nutrition Assistance stamps	Data from grocery store association or organization; interviews Observations at the sites using checklists Data from green market association or government agency

specific to the behavior that has been selected as the focus and to the intended audience. Rarely are two interventions identical. Tools need to be appropriate to the specific intervention, so it is not easy to find one that is exactly appropriate for the intervention you are designing. However, research on instrument development is ongoing, and many usable tools are being constantly generated and tested. These can be identified through a search of the literature or government sources. The *Journal of Nutrition Education and Behavior, Journal of the American Dietetic Association*, and *International Journal of Behavioral Nutrition and Physical Activity* are rich sources of potentially useful instruments. There are many other journals as well. For example, some instruments have been validated with low-resource adult audiences in the domain of reducing fat in the diet or increasing fruit and vegetable intake; some have been validated for upper elementary school-aged children, and so forth. When selecting, adapting, or developing a new instrument, you need to consider the topics discussed in the following subsections.

Appropriateness

In some types of educational interventions, the educational activities that participants will complete can also serve as evaluations. For example, in school food and nutrition education, activities in community nutrition education, or WIC clinics, many of the evaluations work best as activities that participants will complete as part of the learning units. In this case, some system must be set up to record the results of these evaluation activities.

In most cases, nutrition educators use specific instruments administered separately from the educational activities. These should measure achievement of the behavioral goals and general education objectives directed at mediators. These measures need to be appropriate for the intended audience. If you need to design your own instruments, remember that designing such instruments is not easy, even for a one-time session or for short interventions. How much time and effort you should spend on such instruments depends on the purpose of evaluation and the degree of measurement accuracy needed or desired.

The most commonly used procedure is to identify those instruments that are close to your intervention in terms of behavioral focus and mediators addressed and to modify or adapt them for use with your specific audience. If you are working with adolescents or a low-income audience, for example, check whether the instrument you have identified as potentially useful has been developed and validated for that group. Whether you modify or develop your own, you will need to consider the issues related to nutrition education tools or instruments described in these subsections.

Validity

Validity is a generic term that refers to different kinds of accuracy—the degree to which the instrument adequately or correctly measures the variable or concept under study, whether that variable is in the domain of knowledge or of mediating variables, or is a behavior. The following list provides a brief description of the different types of validity. Check for these when you are reading nutrition education intervention articles, selecting your instrument, or developing your own:

- *Content validity.* Are the items on the test, questionnaire, or inventory reasonably representative of the larger domain or content covered? For dietary intake, are the items on the food frequency questionnaire truly representative of what is typical for this audience? If you are interested in knowledge about fruits and vegetables, are the items representative of that domain?

- *Face validity.* Face validity is an aspect of content validity in which a panel of experts reviews the instrument to ensure that it measures what it is intended to measure. In addition, from pilot testing with the intended audience, are the language, formats, and procedures of the instrument understandable and reasonable from the program participants' point of view?

- *Criterion validity.* Does the score generated by the instrument correlate well with data obtained with a criterion measure? For example, does the fruit and vegetable questionnaire correlate well with seven-day food records or serum carotenoid levels (which are considered as standards)?

- *Construct validity.* Does the instrument clearly measure the construct it is supposed to be measuring, such as outcome expectations or self-efficacy?

Reliability

Reliability is a measure of the consistency and dependability of the instrument. There are several kinds of reliability:

- *Reproducibility, or test-retest reliability.* Consistency or stability over time. It is the degree to which the instrument, used at different times with the same people, will give the same result.

- *Internal consistency.* Consistency within a set of items. Is the instrument internally reliable or consistent? For example, if you have four self-efficacy items, is there consistency among them? For knowledge items, split-half reliability or KR-20 coefficient is usually calculated, whereas for mediating variables, item-total correlations or Cronbach's alpha coefficient (Cronbach et al. 1980) are calculated.

- *Interrater reliability.* Consistency among data collectors. If two or more people will be collecting the information or coding it, has interrater reliability been established? For example, do two nutritionists code the fruit and vegetable intake data from 24-hour recalls in the same way?

Sensitivity to Change

Sensitivity is the degree to which an instrument can detect changes resulting from an intervention.

Cognitive Testing: Readability and Understandability

- *Readability* is the ease of comprehension of the evaluation tool by the intended audience given its vocabulary, sentence length, writing style, or other factors. Reading-level formulas can help make that determination.

- *Understandability* goes beyond readability to assess whether the instrument content is understood by the audience the way you intend. This can be judged by having participants tell you what they think each question means or is asking about, a process called *cognitive testing*. Even if you choose to use an existing instrument, you should still test it for understandability with your particular audience.

Qualitative Data

Qualitative data, such as information from observations, in-depth interviews, focus groups, or open-ended surveys, also are subject to reliability and validity considerations. In this case, the criteria are dependability, credibility, and trustworthiness.

- *Dependability* is somewhat like reliability in that other people need to be able to follow the procedures and decision trail of the original investigator to understand how the findings were obtained; documentation of all steps is thus crucial.

- The *credibility or trustworthiness* of the findings is indicative of validity. Credibility is increased through engagement with the individuals over a sufficiently long time to understand the phenomenon being studied, through persistent observation, and through the use of several sources and methods to study the same phenomenon, yielding consistent information. This process is called *triangulation*. Often, the findings are shared with the participants for verification, called *peer debriefing*. In addition, the findings need to ring true to readers in that they can recognize an aspect of human experience is being described, even though they have only read the study.

Validating and Pilot Testing Instruments

Extensive pilot testing of instruments and data collection procedures is absolutely essential. This cannot be emphasized enough. Whether borrowed or developed anew, instruments must be tested with your particular audience. When you are conducting a one-time or two-session program, you may not have the opportunity to pilot test extensively. But even here, if at all possible, check for content validity by asking colleagues to review your instrument, and have a few members of the intended audience complete it: check for readability and understanding and ask them when they think of it. Revise accordingly before using.

Examples of Validation Studies of Instruments

The general procedure is to compare your instrument to a criterion. One study compared a short calcium food frequency (taking about 5 minutes to complete), in an online version and printed version, with three-day food records as the criterion and found it to have a good correlation (Hacker-Thompson, Robertson, & Sellmeyer 2009).

The food behavior checklist shown in Table 7-1 and the tool for assessing indicators of psychosocial mediators of fruit and vegetable intakes shown in Table 8-2 were validated for low-income audiences as follows: items related to fruits and vegetables were compared to serum carotenoid levels. Other items were compared to nutrient intakes derived from three 1-day dietary recalls (Murphy et al. 2001; Townsend et al. 2003; Townsend & Kaiser 2005). A similar process was used to validate a brief fruit and vegetable tool (Townsend & Kaiser 2007). Readability of the instrument is very important in enhancing validity and reliability. The behavior instrument shown in Table 7-1 was extensively tested, at which time it was found that low-literacy audiences preferred photographs of food items over words or line drawings, color over black and white, and specific recognizable brands of items over generic ones (Townsend et al. 2008). A sample of questions from the new version, which includes photographs, is shown in **Figure 14-5**.

Constructing an Appropriate Evaluation Plan to Measure Impacts

The purpose of an evaluation plan or design is to ensure that evaluation results are caused by the nutrition education program and not by some other confounding factors. Thus, evaluation plans are designed to rule out competing explanations for the results that you get. This allows you to measure the true impact of the program. The nature of the design depends largely on which plan is most feasible given the type of power, duration, or intensity of the educational intervention and the context in which it is occurring and the financial and time resources and expertise available to you.

Experimental Designs

The *true experimental design* or *randomized control trial* (RCT) is considered ideal for research purposes. It is routinely used in clinical research studies. In this design, individuals, WIC clinics, schools, or worksites are randomly assigned to two groups, one receiving the nutrition education program (intervention condition) and the other receiving the usual education or another unrelated intervention (the control condition) of equal duration and intensity. Both groups are given test instruments before and after the intervention. One major advantage of this design is that the randomization process ensures that significant differences in outcomes are attributable to the program. A disadvantage is that randomization is very difficult to do in practice settings.

Quasi-Experimental Designs

Quasi-experimental designs are traditionally viewed as more realistic models for field evaluation studies. The most common design within this category is the *comparison-group design with pretest and post-test* in which one group receives the program and is compared with a second matched comparison group that does not receive the program and is selected from a similar population and matched on various characteristics, such as age, gender, ethnicity, or socioeconomic status. Both groups are given pre- and post-tests. Gain scores are compared between the two groups. In school settings, this means that entire classes may be matched with similar classes in the same school, or entire schools matched with other schools. WIC clinic groups receiving an intervention may be matched with groups from WIC clinics with similar characteristics. Although these designs do not guard against all competing explanations for the results, they do control for various important sources of error while remaining a fairly workable method for most programs in practice settings.

Nonexperimental Designs

Nonexperimental designs use two common approaches. In the *one-group pretest and post-test design*, scores are compared before and after the program in the same group. There is no comparison group. In the *post-test-only design with nonequivalent comparison groups*, the scores of those who have received the program are compared with a similar group that did not receive the program. These designs make it difficult to rule out other explanations. However, such designs are often the only ones feasible in practice settings and can provide important insights.

Time Series Designs

In *interrupted time series designs*, a number of observations are made over a period of time as a baseline, and then the program is introduced. A series of observations is then made after the program. If the scores remain constant for a time before the program and then increase after the program and remain constant at that higher level for some time after the program, the increase may be attributable to the program. This conclusion is strengthened if the observations are accompanied by time series observations of a no-treatment comparison group. Again, although many sources of error remain, this design can provide some insight into the effectiveness of the program.

Surveillance Studies

Surveillance studies monitor the status of a population or group on outcomes of interest such as dietary intakes or attitudes toward healthful eating. Such studies can document how a group is doing over time but cannot explain what causes the observed status.

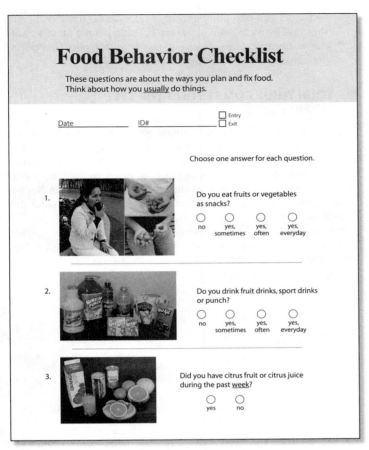

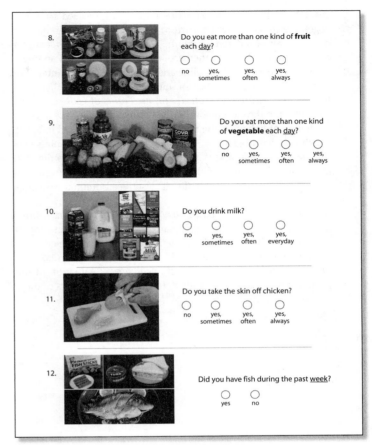

FIGURE 14-5 Food Behavior Checklist.

Source: Sylva, K., Townsend, M. S., Martin, A., and Metz, D. 2007. *Fruit and Vegetable Checklist*. University of California Cooperative Extension; University of California, Davis. http://townsendlab.ucdavis.edu. Reprinted with permission.

Qualitative Evaluation Methods

Qualitative evaluation methods can be used as an alternative to quantitative designs or as a complement to them. These methods are generally inductive in nature and rely on such strategies as observations, structured and semistructured individual and group interviews, focus groups, historical records, and questionnaires. Qualitative methods can boost the power of quantitative methods by focusing on the dynamics and contexts of change because the latter tend to focus on the outcomes of the interventions. Qualitative methods also enlarge the observational field to capture actual, and often unintended, changes. Qualitative methods can help to develop and delineate program elements, such as current practices, values, and attitudes of participants, leadership styles, staffing patterns, and relationships among program activities.

Conducting Evaluations Ethically: Informed Consent

Evaluations should be conducted ethically. This means that you should obtain informed consent from program participants to participate in the evaluation. Participants should not be coerced into completing evaluation activities. Their responses should be anonymous or confidential and should not jeopardize them in any way. Participants should not be denied essential services on the basis of their responses or lack thereof.

■ CASE STUDY

The ongoing case study with middle school youth addresses the goal of increasing their intake of fruits and vegetables. The conceptual framework for evaluating the intervention described in the case study uses a logic model as shown in the case study figure. The inputs of the program are the resources invested. The outputs include the activities conducted within the three major components of the program—students, parents, and school environment—and the specific theory-based strategies that are used to address the specific mediators of behavior change: motivational mediators, action mediators, and environmental mediators. As you can see from the model, student outcomes can be short, medium, or long term. Given the resources available, the case study intervention will measure short-term and medium-term student outcomes. Long-term outcomes are shown and can be measured later in time.

The evaluation in the case study shows the potential methods for evaluating the impact of the intervention on the behavioral goal, the general educational objectives directed at the potential mediators of the behavioral goal. For each of these impacts, indicators of achievement of impacts are shown as well as the measures used as follows:

- *Impact of program on goal behaviors.* The behavioral goal is for adolescents to increase their intake of a variety of fruits and vegetables. The indicator for this impact is increased fruit and vegetable intake. The measure to be used is a food frequency questionnaire validated for youth. The *criterion of effectiveness* is a statistically significant increase in the intake of fruits and vegetables compared with baseline and compared with the intakes in a matched comparison class of middle school students.

- *Impacts of educational strategies on mediators of goal behaviors.* Recall that to develop theory-based strategies to address specific mediators of behavior, the mediators are first expressed in terms of educational objectives. The case study evaluation plan lists the mediators first, and then the educational objectives directed at the mediators, along with indicators of achievement of each of the mediator outcomes. Finally, it describes potential measures to use.
- *Impacts of the program on the school in the environment component.* The case study evaluation plan lists the environment support outcomes, indicators of achievement of outcomes expressed in the form of objectives, and potential measures or instruments.
- *Impacts of the program on family behaviors.* Evaluation of impacts of the program on family behaviors and mediators of these

behaviors as a result of the family component is not shown, but these behaviors and mediators are evaluated in the same way as the youth curriculum component, using similar types of indicators and measures now focusing on family behaviors.

■ YOUR TURN: COMPLETING THE STEP 6 WORKSHEETS

As noted previously, designing nutrition education programs is an iterative process in which you go back and forth between various tasks. The design of evaluation methods goes hand in hand with the design of educational strategies. Thus, at the time when you are designing each of the educational objectives and educational strategies in Steps 4 and 5, consider an evaluation method. This is the time to finalize the evaluation methods.

Instructions and examples have been given throughout the chapter for how to design evaluations for your program. Evaluations are very varied and the possibilities are numerous, so the worksheets provide overall guidance for the evaluation process.

Questions and Activities

1. Give three reasons why it is important to evaluate nutrition education, no matter how briefly.
2. Distinguish between outcome and process evaluation.
3. In terms of evaluation, describe each of the following terms, indicating the relationships among them and to educational objectives:
   a. Outcomes
   b. Indicators
   c. Measures
   d. Instruments
   e. Evaluation plan
   f. Data collection methods
4. Describe four ways for measuring each of the following:
   a. Behavioral outcomes
   b. Potential mediators of behavioral outcomes
   c. Policy change
   d. Changes in school or community food environment
5. Distinguish between a true experimental design or randomized control trial (RCT) and quasi-experimental designs.
6. Distinguish between validity and reliability in terms of evaluation instruments. What is the relationship between these two features?
7. Think of a practice setting in which you will provide six nutrition sessions to low-income women. What would be a good evaluation design to measure the impact of your program? Describe the design and the kinds of outcomes you think would be practical to measure.

References

Block, G., C. Gillespie, E. H. Rosenbaum, and C. Jenson. 2000. A rapid screener to assess fat and fruit and vegetable intake. *American Journal of Preventive Medicine* 18:284–288.

Block, G., F. E. Thompson, A. M. Hartman, F. A. Larkin, and K. E. Guire. 1992. Comparison of two dietary questionnaires validated against multiple dietary records collected during a 1-year period. *Journal of the American Dietetic Association* 92:686–693.

Centers for Disease Control and Prevention. 2004a. *School Health Index: A self-assessment and planning guide. Elementary school version.* Atlanta, GA: Author.

———. 2004b. *School Health Index: A self-assessment and planning guide. Middle school/high school version.* Atlanta, GA: Author.

Chang, M. W., S. Nitzke, R. L. Brown, L. C. Bauman, and L. Oakley. 2003. Development and validation of a self-efficacy measure for fat intake behaviors of low-income women. *Journal of Nutrition Education and Behavior* 35:302–307.

Contento, I. R., J. S. Randell, and C. E. Basch. 2002. Review and analysis of evaluation measures used in nutrition education intervention research. *Journal of Nutrition Education and Behavior* 34:2–25.

Cronbach, L. J., et al. 1980. *Toward reform of program evaluation: Aims, methods, and institutional arrangements.* San Francisco: Jossey-Bass.

Eck, S. M., B. J. Struempler, and A. A. Raby. 2005. Once upon a time in America: Interactive nutrition evaluation. *Journal of Nutrition Education and Behavior* 37:46–47.

Freedman, D. S., and G. Perry. 2000. Body composition and health status among children and adolescents. *Preventive Medicine* 31:S34–S53.

Glanz, K., J. F. Sallis, et al. 2005. Healthy nutrition environments: Concepts and measures. *American Journal of Health Promotion* 19(5): 330–333, ii.

———. 2007. Nutrition Environment Measures Survey in stores (NEMS-S): Development and evaluation. *American Journal of Preventive Medicine* 32(4): 282–289.

Golaszewski, T., and B. Fisher. 2002. Heart Check: The development and evolution of an organizational heart health assessment. *American Journal of Health Promotion* 17:132–153.

Gregson, J., S. B. Foerster, R. Orr, et al. 2001. System, environmental, and policy changes: Using the social-ecological model as a framework for evaluating nutrition education and social marketing programs with low-income audiences. *Journal of Nutrition Education* 33:S4–S15.

Hacker-Thompson, A., T. P. Robertson, and D. E. Sellmeyer. 2009. Validation of two food frequency questionnaires for dietary calcium assessment. *Journal of the American Dietetic Association* 109(7):1237–1240.

Hersey, J., J. Anliker, C. Miller, et al. 2001. Food shopping practices are associated with dietary quality in low-income households. *Journal of Nutrition Education and Behavior* 33:S16–S26.

Keenan, D. P., C. Olson, J. C. Hersey, and S. M. Parmer. 2001. Measures of food insecurity/security. *Journal of Nutrition Education* 33(Suppl. 1):S49–S58.

Kohl, H. W., J. E. Fulton, and C. J. Casperson. 2000. Assessment of physical activity among children and adolescents: A review and synthesis. *Preventive Medicine* 31:S54–S76.

Kristal, A. R., B. F. Abrams, M. D. Thornquist, et al. 1990. Development and validation of a food use checklist for evaluation of community nutrition interventions. *American Journal of Public Health* 80:1318–1322.

Kristal, A. R., and S. A. Beresford. 1994. Assessing change in diet-intervention research. *American Journal of Clinical Nutrition* 59(Suppl.):185S–189S.

Linnan, L. A., J. L. Fava, B. Thompson, et al. 1999. Measuring participatory strategies: Instrument development for worksite populations. *Health Education Research* 14:371–386.

Marsh, T., K. W. Cullen, and T. Baranowski. 2003. Validation of a fruit, juice, and vegetable availability questionnaire. *Journal of Nutrition Education and Behavior* 35: 93–97.

McClelland, J. W., D. P. Keenan, J. Lewis, et al. 2001. Review of evaluation tools used to assess the impact of nutrition education on dietary intake and quality, weight management practices, and physical activity of low-income audiences. *Journal of Nutrition Education* 33:S35–S48.

McPherson, R. C., D. M. Hoelscher, M. Alexander, K. S. Scanlon, and M. K. Serdula. 2000. Dietary assessment methods among school-aged children. *Preventive Medicine* 31:S11–S33.

Medeiros, L. C., S. N. Butkus, H. Chipman, R. H. Cox, L. Jones, and D. Little. 2005. A logic model framework for community nutrition education. *Journal of Nutrition Education and Behavior* 37:197–202.

Medeiros, L., V. Hillers, P. Kendall, and A. Mason. 2001. Evaluation of food safety education for consumers. *Journal of Nutrition Education* 33:S27–S34.

National Cancer Institute. 2000. *Eating at America's Table Study: Quick food scan.* Bethesda, MD: National Cancer Institute, National Institutes of Health. http://riskfactor.cancer.gov/diet/screeners/fruitveg/allday.pdf.

Reynolds, K. D., A. L. Yaroch, F. A. Franklin, and J. Maloy. 2002. Testing mediating variables in a school-based nutrition intervention program. *Health Psychology* 21:51–60.

Ribisl, K. M., and T. M. Reischl. 1993. Measuring the climate for health at organizations. Development of the worksite health climate scales. *Journal of Occupational Medicine* 35:812–824.

Sallis, J. F., C. T. Orleans, and D. M. Buchner. 2009. Active living research: A six-year report. *American Journal of Preventive Medicine* 36(2S):S1–S72.

Schwartz M., A. Lund, H. Grow, et al. 2009. A comprehensive coding system to measure the quality of school wellness policies. *Journal of the American Dietetic Association* 109(7):1256–1262.

Serdula, M., R. Coates, T. Byers, et al. 1993. Evaluation of a brief telephone questionnaire to estimate fruit and vegetable consumption in diverse study populations. *Epidemiology* 4:455–463.

Shannon, J., A. R. Kristal, S. J. Currry, and S. A. Beresford. 1997. Application of a behavioral approach to measuring dietary change: The fat and fiber-related diet behavior questionnaire. *Cancer Epidemiology, Biomarkers and Prevention* 6:355–361.

Sorensen, G., A. Stoddard, and E. Macario. 1998. Social support and readiness to make dietary changes. *Health Education Behavior* 25:586–598.

Straus, A. L., and J. Corbin. 1990. *Basics of qualitative research: Grounded theory procedures and research*. Newbury Park, CA: Sage.

Thompson, F. E., and T. Byers. 1994. Dietary assessment resource manual. *Journal of Nutrition* 124(11 Suppl.):2245s–2317s.

Townsend, M. S., and L. L. Kaiser. 2005. Development of a tool to assess psychosocial indicators of fruit and vegetables intake for 2 federal programs. *Journal of Nutrition Education and Behavior* 37:170–184.

———. 2007. Brief psychosocial fruit and vegetable tool is sensitive for the U.S. Department of Agriculture's Nutrition Education Programs. *Journal of the American Dietetic Association* 107(12):2120–2124.

Townsend, M. S., L. L. Kaiser, L. H. Allen, A. Block Joy, and S. P. Murphy. 2003. Selecting items for a food behavior checklist for a limited-resources audience. *Journal of Nutrition Education and Behavior* 35:69–82.

Townsend, M. S., K. Sylva, A. Martin, D. Metz, and P. Wooten-Swanson. 2008. Improving readability of an evaluation tool for low-income clients using visual information processing theories. *Journal of Nutrition Education and Behavior* 40(3):181–186.

U.S. Department of Agriculture. 2000. *Changing the scene: Improving the school nutrition environment*. Alexandria, VA: U.S. Department of Agriculture, Food and Nutrition Service. http://www.fns.usda.gov/tn/Healthy/index.

———. 2005, September. Nutrition education: Principles of sound impact evaluation. *Office of Analysis, Nutrition, and Evaluation Newsletter*. Alexandria, VA: U.S. Department of Agriculture, Food and Nutrition Service. http://www.fns.usda .gov/ora/menu/FSNE/FSNE.htm.

Ventura, A. K., and L. L. Birch. 2008. Does parenting affect children's eating and weight status? *International Journal of Behavioral Nutrition and Physical Activity* 5:15.

Willett, W. C. 1998. *Nutritional epidemiology*. New York: Oxford University Press.

Willett, W. C., R. D. Reynolds, S. Cottrell-Hoehner, L. Sampson, and M. L. Browne. 1987. Validation of a semi-quantitative food frequency questionnaire: Comparison with a 1-year diet record. *Journal of the American Dietetic Association* 87(1):43–47.

Yaroch, A. L., K. Resnicow, and L. K. Khan. 2000. Validity and reliability of qualitative dietary fat index questionnaires: A review. *Journal of the American Dietetic Association* 100(2):240–244.

In Step 6, you plan the evaluation for your program. The outcomes are the personal mediators from your theory model, the program goal behaviors, and the selected health issues. You will also evaluate changes in food environment–policy supports.

At the conclusion of the Step 6 worksheets, you will have the following products:

Step 6A: Diagram of conceptual framework for program evaluation.

Step 6B: Indicators of and measures for evaluating individual level changes (e.g., mediators, behaviors, health outcomes).

Step 6C: Indicators of and measures for evaluating environment-policy supports.

Use the provided worksheets as a guide to plan your evaluation. Electronic versions of these worksheets are available at http://nutrition.jbpub.com/education/2e/. If you are unable to access the worksheets electronically, you can write onto this blank worksheet or create a text document that uses the same flow of information.

> **NOTE:** This part of the case study focuses on only one of the program's goal behaviors: increasing intake of fruits and vegetables. If you create a program with multiple goal behaviors, you will need to complete the worksheets for each of the behaviors.

Step 6A: Program evaluation conceptual framework

Diagram the conceptual framework that will guide your program evaluation.

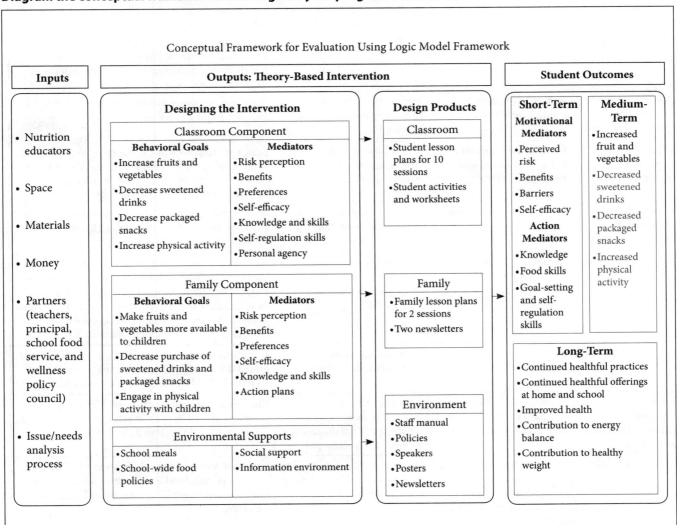

Conceptual Framework for Evaluation Using Logic Model Framework

Inputs	Outputs: Theory-Based Intervention		Student Outcomes

Inputs
- Nutrition educators
- Space
- Materials
- Money
- Partners (teachers, principal, school food service, and wellness policy council)
- Issue/needs analysis process

Outputs: Theory-Based Intervention

Designing the Intervention

Classroom Component

Behavioral Goals	Mediators
• Increase fruits and vegetables	• Risk perception
• Decrease sweetened drinks	• Benefits
• Decrease packaged snacks	• Preferences
• Increase physical activity	• Self-efficacy
	• Knowledge and skills
	• Self-regulation skills
	• Personal agency

Family Component

Behavioral Goals	Mediators
• Make fruits and vegetables more available to children	• Risk perception
• Decrease purchase of sweetened drinks and packaged snacks	• Benefits
• Engage in physical activity with children	• Preferences
	• Self-efficacy
	• Knowledge and skills
	• Action plans

Environmental Supports

• School meals	• Social support
• School-wide food policies	• Information environment

Design Products

Classroom
- Student lesson plans for 10 sessions
- Student activities and worksheets

Family
- Family lesson plans for 2 sessions
- Two newsletters

Environment
- Staff manual
- Policies
- Speakers
- Posters
- Newsletters

Student Outcomes

Short-Term

Motivational Mediators
- Perceived risk
- Benefits
- Barriers
- Self-efficacy

Action Mediators
- Knowledge
- Food skills
- Goal-setting and self-regulation skills

Medium-Term
- Increased fruit and vegetables
- Decreased sweetened drinks
- Decreased packaged snacks
- Increased physical activity

Long-Term
- Continued healthful practices
- Continued healthful offerings at home and school
- Improved health
- Contribution to energy balance
- Contribution to healthy weight

Step 6B: Evaluation plan for individual change component

Identify indicators of achievement for the selected goal behaviors, mediators, and health issues as well as potential measures/instruments to assess the achievement.

Behavioral outcome	Indicator of achievement	Measures/instruments
Increase students' intake of fruits and vegetables (youth to aim for 2.5 cups or more per day)	A statistically significant increase in intake of fruits and vegetables compared with baseline and compared with the intakes of students in a matched comparison middle school	A food frequency questionnaire validated for youth

Mediator outcomes	General educational objective	Indicator of achievement	Measures/instruments
Physical outcome expectations (perceived benefits)	Demonstrate understanding of the importance of eating a variety of F&V	Improved scores on instrument measuring understanding of the impact of F&V on health and disease	Benefits: Scale with responses of 1 to 5 (strongly disagree to strongly agree). Outcomes may include: have more energy, make stronger, help me do well in school, help maintain weight. Knowledge instrument: Multiple choice questions on scientific evidence linking F&V and skin health, bone development, disease risk reduction; importance of variety.
Physical outcome expectations (perceived benefits)	Express enjoyment of eating a variety of F&V	Improved scores on tool measuring preference for specific F&V	Scale with responses of 1 to 5 (dislike a lot to like a lot) for a list of 15 F&V.
Physical outcome expectations (perceived risk)	Evaluate their own intake of F&V compared with recommendations	Increased scores on instrument measuring perceived risk	Scale with responses of 1 to 5 on perceptions of risk about (not) eating enough F&V (e.g., "I eat enough F&V to keep me healthy"; "I am at risk for some diseases because I do not eat enough F&V").
Physical outcome expectations (perceived barriers)	Identify barriers to intake of F&V and propose ways to overcome them	Decreased scores on instrument measuring perceived barriers	Scale with responses of 1 to 5 on perceived barriers to eating more F&V (e.g., "Cost is a barrier when I eat F&V").
Self-efficacy	Demonstrate increased self-efficacy in eating more F&V each day	Improved scores on an instrument measuring self-efficacy about increasing F&V intake	Scale with responses of 1 to 5 on how confident learner feels about eating F&V (e.g., "If I wanted to, it would be easy to eat more vegetables"). Questions would also ask about difficult situations: "If I decided to eat fruit every day, I would do so even when I did not feel like eating fruit/when there are sweets."
Goal intention	State intention to increase own F&V intake	Increased scores on instrument measuring goal intentions	Items with responses from 1 to 5 on "I intend to add more F&V each day at lunch/dinner/as snack" and "It is likely I will add more F&V each day to my diet."
Behavioral capability (relevant knowledge and skills)	Demonstrate knowledge and skills in incorporating F&V into their daily diet	Increased scores on instrument measuring knowledge and skills about adding F&V to daily diet	Knowledge and skills instrument: Multiple choice questions and some open-ended questions, scenarios about ways to add F&V to daily diet.
Goal-setting skills	Prepare action plans using goal-setting and decision-making skills to increase their consumption of fruits and vegetables	Demonstrate increased ability to use specific skills in setting goals, making plans	Scenarios with questions about setting goals, planning ahead, and developing strategies to overcome roadblocks; multiple choice questions based on scenarios.

Health outcome	Indicator of achievement	Measures/instruments
Decrease in reported rates of obesity	A statistically significant decrease in student BMI compared with baseline and the BMI of students in a matched comparison middle school	Calculation of individual BMI using self-reported height and weight data for entire population

Step 6C: Evaluation plan for environmental/policy supports component

Identify indicators of achievement for the selected environmental/policy supports targeted by your program.

Environment support outcomes	Indicator of achievement (general support objectives)	Measures/instruments
Decision-makers' awareness and motivation	The nutrition education program will enhance motivation of school administrators to create healthy environment.	• Records of administrator attendance at school food policy council • Documentation of support for school food policy council, food service changes, and cafeteria-based social marketing messages
Food environment	The nutrition education program will provide many opportunities for youth to taste F&V through taste tests in cafeteria and greater incorporation into meals.	• Document number of events, taste testings • Interviews and observations using checklists to identify how many, which, and how often recommended practices are carried out • Review of purchase records • Analysis of planned and actual menus (computer nutrient/food composition programs)
Organizational food policy	The school will activate school food policy council to develop guidelines for foods available in school.	• Membership list • Review of meeting minutes • Copy of guidelines • Change in number of healthful items available in vending machines and in stores from start of guidelines to end of school year
Information environment	School will make cafeteria information environment supportive of eating fruits and vegetables.	• Number of posters and other signage supportive of eating fruits and vegetables

In Step 6, you plan the evaluation for your program. The outcomes are the personal mediators from your theory model, the program goal behaviors, and the selected health issues. You will also evaluate changes in food environment–policy supports.

At the conclusion of the Step 6 worksheets, you will have the following products:

Step 6A: Diagram of conceptual framework for program evaluation

Step 6B: Indicators of, and measures for, evaluating individual level changes (mediators, behaviors, health outcomes)

Step 6C: Indicators of, and measures for, evaluating environment-policy supports

Use the provided worksheets as a guide to plan your evaluation. Electronic versions of these worksheets are available at http://nutrition.jbpub.com/education/2e/. If you are unable to access the worksheets electronically, you can write onto this blank worksheet or create a text document that uses the same flow of information.

Step 6A: Program evaluation conceptual framework

Diagram the conceptual framework that will guide your program evaluation.

Step 6B: Evaluation plan for individual level component

Identify indicators of achievement for the selected goal behaviors, mediators, and health issues as well as potential measures/instruments to assess the achievement of outcomes.

Behavioral outcome	Indicator of achievement	Measures/instruments

Mediator outcomes	General educational objective	Indicator of achievement	Measures/instruments

Health outcome	Indicator of achievement	Measures/instruments

Step 6C: Evaluation plan for environmental/policy supports component

Identify indicators of achievement for the selected environmental/policy supports targeted by your program.

Environment support outcomes	Indicator of achievement (general support objectives)	Measures/instruments

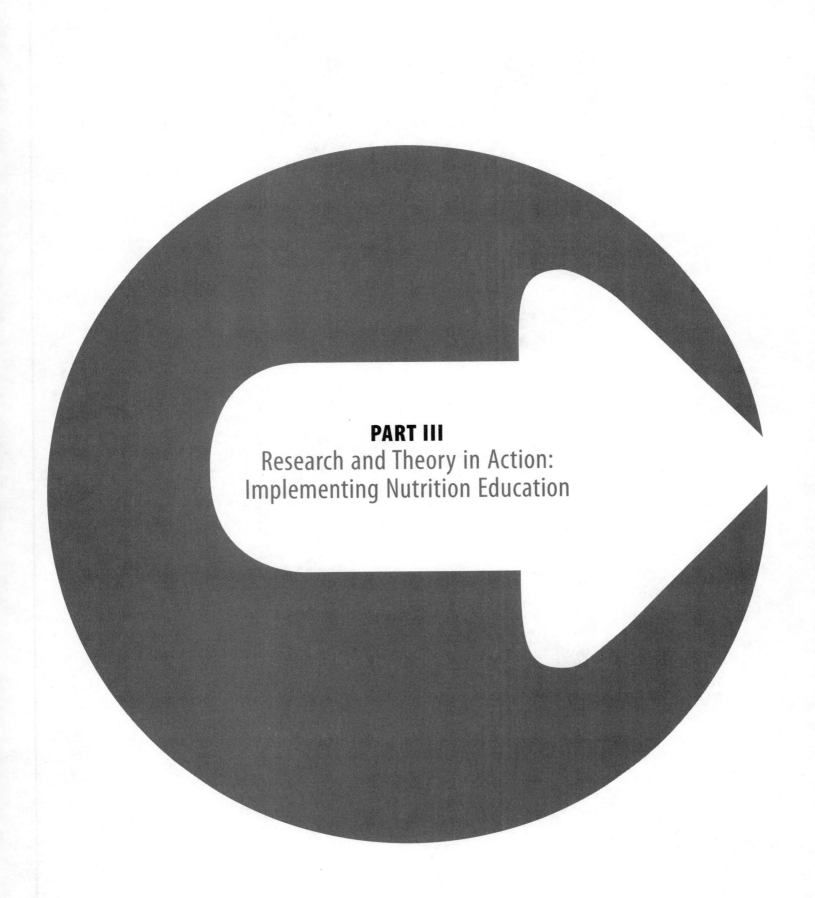

PART III
Research and Theory in Action:
Implementing Nutrition Education

CHAPTER 15

Communicating Effectively in Group Settings

OVERVIEW This chapter provides an overview of communication principles, learning styles, and group dynamics and how they can inform practical methods for implementing nutrition education with groups.

CHAPTER OUTLINE
- Introduction
- Basic communication model
- Understanding learning styles
- Implementing learning in groups
- Oral presentations and workshops
- Summary

LEARNING OBJECTIVES At the end of the chapter, you will be able to:
- Describe basic principles of communication and a communication model for nutrition education
- Apply learning style research in delivering nutrition education
- Use information on group dynamics to more effectively deliver nutrition education
- Describe key features in conducting facilitated group discussions and dialogues
- Apply public speaking principles to making presentations and leading workshops

■ INTRODUCTION: UNDERSTANDING COMMUNICATION

You have attended a comedy show and laughed all the way through. You want to share the jokes with your friends, so you decide to memorize one of the routines word for word. You present the jokes to your friends and do not get the same laughs. Why not? Because you were not able to *deliver* the jokes in the same way the comedian did. He was effective because of his manner of presentation, his facial expressions, the inflections of his voice, his gestures, and most important, his perfect sense of timing. Likewise, a wonderfully designed nutrition education session can be ruined by poor delivery. This does not mean that wonderful delivery

will turn a poorly designed session into an effective one. The issue you want to address must be important and relevant to the group. But having something to say or planning an interesting session is not enough. You must also know how to deliver it.

You have designed the nutrition education program, including its goals and objectives and theory-based education strategies, and have laid out your evaluation plan. You are ready to do what you like to do most—conduct nutrition education. Now what? How exactly should you proceed in the designated setting? Part III describes exactly how to deliver the intervention in practice through a variety of channels, including group sessions, printed materials, and other media. Conducting group activities and developing other supportive activities require numerous skills even after the intervention content and activities have been carefully planned. This chapter focuses on working with groups, and the next chapter focuses on implementing nutrition education through a variety of other channels that might accompany group sessions, such as supporting visual media, written materials, grocery tours, health fairs, mass media communication campaigns, social marketing activities, and other venues.

Although the design and delivery of nutrition education are described in different sections of the book, you will probably go back and forth between these two activities. For example, as you think about how exactly you will deliver what you have designed, you may find that you need to go back to Step 5 of the Stepwise Procedure to make changes in your educational plans to make them more in line with your delivery strategies. Because all interactions among people involve communication, communication is at the heart of nutrition education with groups. This chapter begins with a brief description of communication.

Communication is one of those terms we use frequently and yet would have a hard time defining. The word comes from the Latin *communis*, meaning "common." In general it refers to all methods of conveying thought and feeling between individuals. Most definitions have in common the notions that communication is the process of sending and receiving messages and that for a transmission of messages to be successful, a mutual understanding between the communicator and the recipient must occur. Communication refers to what is expressed verbally or nonverbally; it applies to articulated words and to unvocalized feelings. In a broad sense, then, communication includes all methods that can convey thought or feelings and describes interactions between individuals and groups as well as between various media and people.

The term *interpersonal communication* is often used to describe the communication context that involves direct, face-to-face interaction among persons, whether one on one or in small groups. The term *mediated communications* is often used to describe the communication that occurs through some nonpersonal channel such as television or radio, printed materials, telephone, and advertising.

■ BASIC COMMUNICATION MODEL

How much time do you spend each day talking with other people? If you are like other adults, you spend about 30% of your waking hours talking with or communicating with others. Thus, people are all very familiar with the notion of communication. Communication consists of very complicated processes that are described in numerous books and articles. This chapter briefly describes only its chief features. First, it describes a model that captures the basic elements of communication, and then it expands on this model for the nutrition education context.

This model states that communication involves the following components arranged in the following sequence:

1. Communication source, or sender
2. Message (sent through one or more channels)
3. Channels
4. Receivers (audience)

In the case of nutrition education, the communication source or sender is the nutrition educator, who sends a message (which can be as simple as "Eat more fruits and vegetables" or much more complex, such as how to get children to eat healthfully) through channels such as lecturing, making a presentation, leading a group discussion, newsletters, interactive media, or mass media campaigns to receivers, who are

groups or individuals, such as mothers of young children, who *attend* to the message, *comprehend* it and *process* it cognitively and affectively, and *act on it*, either by accepting it or rejecting it.

This basic model is clearly unidirectional, with a message being sent by a source to receivers, who receive the message somewhat passively. It does not capture the richness and complexities of interactions *among* individuals in groups that influence message processing. For example, in group discussion, all individuals take turns being the sender and the receiver through the channel of speaking. However, this model can be used to implement some mediated communications through nonpersonal media and in interpersonal settings such as presentations and lectures, where there is very little interaction among group members. After exploring the basic components of this model, the chapter then describes how the communication process is modified by complex interactions in social settings, where much of deliberate nutrition education occurs.

Communication Source Characteristics

First, recognize that just as individuals cannot *not* behave, so too in any situation involving social interaction they cannot *not* communicate. This means that you, as the nutrition educator, are communicating at all times, regardless of whether you are conscious of it or whether the communication is intentional or successful. Communication of the message is more likely to be effective if nutrition educators have the following characteristics.

High Credibility

Nutrition educators are more likely to have high credibility if they are perceived by the audience as having competence and trustworthiness. Competence refers to having the skill, knowledge, and judgment relevant to the issue. Credibility can be *extrinsic*, which refers to the audience's perception of the source before the message is delivered (e.g., by virtue of the nutrition educator's position or reputation), or *intrinsic*, which refers to the image of authoritativeness that the nutrition communicator, such as a speaker to a group, creates as a direct result of how the message is delivered.

To increase credibility, then, when you introduce yourself or are introduced you need to let the audience know your professional qualifications and experience. This needs to be done with sensitivity: you cannot be boastful or self-serving, but you should not be overly modest either. The audience needs to know that you are qualified to lead the group. It will help them relax and feel that they are in good hands. How you come across during the session also influences your credibility and trustworthiness. For instance, if your tone is authoritative and you are organized, the audience will be much more convinced than if you sound tentative.

Trustworthiness refers to nutrition educators coming across as having no ulterior motives for the opinions they offer or the actions they advocate. That is, they have "good motives." To ensure an audience's trust, you need to make clear to audience members that you are not using the occasion to sell something to them. If you do represent your own business or practice or a given group, corporation, or industry, you need to indicate this clearly to the audience.

Attractiveness or Dynamism

Sources are more effective when they are likable or attractive in the sense of having an attractive and dynamic personality and being seen as healthy. This is especially true when the audience is not initially motivated. Your enthusiasm will go a long way.

Similarity or Common Ground with the Audience

Effectiveness is enhanced if the audience perceives that the nutrition educator has some common ground with the audience or at least a sense of affinity with them. Communication specialists point out that because emotion always influences decisions, the audience must sense that the communicator understands their problems and cares. Empathy, or affinity with the audience, is called for, not sympathy, which can be patronizing. Audiences need to feel that they are respected.

Thus, you are more effective if you establish some common ground by initially expressing some views that are also held by the audience and by demonstrating understanding of the opinions and lives of group members. For example, while discussing the topic of food labels, you may want to acknowledge how confusing and time-consuming reading food labels can be (a personal story can be very powerful here). Then, go on to provide the necessary label-reading skills. In discussing parenting practices, you can express understanding and respect for what the (parent) audience members face on a day-to-day basis. Again, a personal story about your own children, or children you have worked with, can be very helpful. It is important to be authentic, however. Using the latest hip language with a group of teenagers, for example, when it is obvious that this is not congruous with who you are and how you would normally speak, will only make the teenagers think you are phony.

Message Characteristics

Every communication has a content aspect, which is the manifest or overt information being conveyed. These are the words you speak, the message you are trying to convey, or the illustrations and pictures you present. Every communication also has an implied or metacommunication aspect, which is information about the information, or a set of rules for interpreting the manifest information, whether this is conveyed consciously or not. In verbal communications it could be your tone of voice or facial expressions. In the case of printed messages, metacommunication could be conveyed through the pictures you use, the layout, and the ordering of content. This meta-level information provides the audience with rules for interpreting the content: it helps the audience judge whether the nutrition educator thinks the information being presented is really important or whether the nutrition educator is being humorous or serious.

Message Characteristics to Increase Processing by Audience

Message characteristics have been the focus of this book and are at the heart of Step 5 of the Stepwise Procedure, described in Chapters 11 to 13. A health message or nutrition communication is really a set of arguments for a particular behavior or practice or information on how to take action, or both. These arguments are based on the perceived benefits or outcome expectations for the given practice for the intended audience that have been discussed throughout the book. These arguments are referred to as "why-to" or motivational information. These arguments form the basis of much of your nutrition education content. Such information can be based on the scientific evidence for the desirability of the behavior or practice, such as breastfeeding or eating calcium-rich foods. It can also be based on benefits of a personal nature or can address some emotion related to the practice. An example given before is the Pick a Better Snack campaign: here the message about eating fruits and vegetables focuses on overcoming barriers to taking action by showing how easy it is to do. This message thus also addresses an attitudinal or emotional aspect—that is, it is not a bother to eat fruits and vegetables.

Messages can also convey information and skills of a "how-to" nature, such as how to read a food label or how to prepare a given food.

Elaboration Likelihood Model (ELM)

The elaboration likelihood model of communication proposes that individuals differ in their ability and motivation to process educational messages, or arguments, thoughtfully (Petty & Cacioppo 1986). (See Chapters 4 and 11 for more details.) To increase the *ability* of the audience to process messages, make your messages straightforward and clear, repeat or reinforce them, and present them with a minimum of distractions. To increase the *motivation* of the audience to process messages, make the messages unexpected or novel, memorable, culturally appropriate, and, most important, personally relevant. You can express the messages in terms of what participants will gain from taking action, as well as what they will lose by not taking action. Messages can involve humor, warmth, or other attributes as found to be appropriate for a given audience. The use of emotion-based messages through materials and activities has been shown to be especially effective (McCarthy 2005). Use these principles whether you deliver the messages through the mass media, brochures, newsletters, or in a group setting.

Nonverbal Communication Accompanying the Message

When you deliver nutrition education in person, nonverbal communication always accompanies the verbal message and is often more influential than the verbal. Receivers learn to trust their interpretations of the nonverbal messages because they know that these cannot be consciously selected or controlled by the sender. Indeed, communication experts believe that the image the nutrition educator projects may account for more than half of the total message conveyed to a group at first meeting. Nonverbal communication includes facial expressions, tone of voice, eye contact, gestures, and touch. Nonverbal cues, particularly facial expressions and tone of voice, can express acceptance and support for group members or judgment and disapproval.

Nonverbal cues can indicate whether you are working *with* the group to state barriers and identify ways to overcome them or manipulating them to come up with the solutions you think are best. Educators are often judgmental and do not know it; however, the audience is very quick to pick up on it. For example, a nonjudgmental tone is straightforward and sounds provisional instead of dogmatic or defensive. Tone of voice and mannerisms can also express whether you respect the group and consider yourself a member or whether you feel superior. Compare expressions such as "You may not be able to grasp this, but believe me, I have been doing this for 10 years and it works," with "That sounds like a good idea. I have worked with others who found it did not work for them, but you are the one who must be satisfied with the eating pattern. So, you can experiment and find whether it works for you. Let us know how it goes." As you work with groups or make a presentation, be very aware of the nonverbal messages that you are transmitting.

Nonverbal communication also accompanies verbal communication through nonpersonal channels, such as videos, media campaigns, websites, posters, and newsletters. The graphics, colors, visual images, and music or sounds used all convey information. Thus, you must select all these features carefully to support the message.

Receiver or Audience Characteristics

Identifying the characteristics of the audience is extremely important in any health communication model. This is done through a process of assessment of audience interests, needs, and characteristics, sometimes called *formative research* or *marketing research*. In the Stepwise Procedure for designing theory-based nutrition education, the predisposition and interests of receivers are carefully identified in Steps 1 and 2, where you analyze the behaviors and practices of the audience and the potential mediators of these behaviors and practices, such as their stage of emotional readiness to change and which social psychological factors influence their food-related practices. This information forms the basis of your educational design in Step 5 and therefore will not be repeated. The following are a few characteristics that are likely to affect how audience members may attend, comprehend, and react to the message.

Personal Motivation to Process the Message

Audience members are predisposed to react to messages in a particular way by their own experiences, beliefs, attitudes, and habits. Successful communication takes into account these predispositions and the reasons behind them. That is, the message must be personalized or tailored to the predispositions, outcome expectations, attitudes, and needs of the audience, as has been emphasized throughout the book, to increase motivation to process the message. As noted earlier, these personalized messages should be meaningful and memorable.

Message-Processing Skills

Audience members' skills in processing the message also influence the effectiveness of the communication. Receivers must understand, process, and elaborate on a message before it can have an effect on their attitudes or behaviors. Thus, receivers' abilities to listen, read, think about, or understand the nutrition concepts you wish to communicate are important considerations when designing and delivering the message. Make the message clear and straightforward for the given audience, but never condescending.

Life Situation

Sometimes other things are going on inside receivers that may interfere with their willingness and ability to process messages. As researchers have noted, cognitive information is filtered through affective states (Achterberg 1988). Audience members who are sick or in pain or who are anxious and worried cannot attend to messages as well as those who are calm and well. This means that the messages or session content and methods you use must gain the attention and affect the comprehension of the audience taking into account such interference.

Learning Styles

Participants' preferred learning styles influence how much attention they pay to a message. For example, in the context of group sessions, listening to you lecture may be the last thing a group of adolescents will want to do, whereas a cadre of executives may be perfectly comfortable listening to your message; they may indeed prefer this mode of communication. These learning styles are explored in greater detail later in this chapter.

Social Roles

The social status roles of the audience also influence response to the message. These roles are behaviors expected of people because of their position in society—for example, the role of "mother," "busy executive," and so forth. Audience members must feel that the message is appropriate for their role in society.

Communications in Social Context

The complexity of food- and nutrition-related behaviors and the social nature of communication has led to a more complex understanding of nutrition communications (Gillespie & Yarbrough 1984). The social context of communications also affects their reception in various ways.

The receivers' reference groups may influence response to the message. People are socially organized, with formal or informal group memberships or reference groups. These can be peers, family, and others whose opinions are valued by audience members. Research indicates that the response to messages is a social phenomenon that involves not only what the audience members think of the messages but also what trusted others, such as family members, close friends, or coworkers, think of the message. That is, individuals' responses are influenced by what they think others will think of their new opinions or actions. For example, teenagers will be more likely to change beverage choices if they think the change would be acceptable to their peers.

Communication Is a Two-Way Street

The nutrition educator and receivers both provide inputs into the communication process. Communication is a two-way, not a one-way, street. The nutrition educator designs the sessions, but the audience provides inputs, more formally through the needs analysis process (as in Steps 1 and 2 of the design process) and *always* during the sessions themselves. This is often called *feedback*. As you saw earlier, people cannot *not* communicate. This means the audience in a group setting cannot not communicate to the nutrition educator as well. Even in a very structured situation such as a lecture class, it has been found that when students in one half of the class look bored, pass notes, and start having side conversations and those in the other half are fully alert and interested and asking questions, the instructor will soon direct all of his or her attention to the latter half of the class. The audience has thus shaped the behavior of the communicator.

Communication Is Interactive

Complex interactions among individuals influence outcome. This interaction may be of two types: between the audience and the communicator, and between audience members and their reference groups or peers. These complex interactions influence acceptance or rejection of the communication. The nutrition educator and the audience communicate with each other verbally or nonverbally, consciously or unconsciously, and these interactions influence outcome, as just noted. Others also influence audience members in the group. For example, if the reference group norm for teens is that answering the nutrition educator's questions during question-and-answer periods is not cool, then you will need to find other ways to engage students, such as small group discussions or projects.

Consequently, messages and group sessions are more likely to be effective if interactions between the communicator and the audience and between the audience members and their peers are built into the communication process. For example, women are more likely to adopt breastfeeding if they think this practice will be acceptable in the eyes of their peers. Here a group process whereby women can share their perceptions and feelings with others in the audience would enhance communication. Successes and challenges can be shared, and mutual learning can take place. Indeed, Freire's dialogical method of critical consciousness-raising (Freire & Shor 1987) or Vella's method of facilitated dialogue (Vella 2002) may be very suitable in certain circumstances. In this process, educators or communicators pose questions and engage in dialogue with the group to facilitate understanding of the causes, consequences, and possible solutions of problems identified by the group. These issues are discussed in greater detail later in this chapter.

Implementing nutrition education as designed requires attention to the considerations regarding the characteristics of the communicator, audience, and message just discussed. Next, explore in greater detail two characteristics of receivers that influence how they will process nutrition messages: their styles of learning and their social interactions in group settings.

■ UNDERSTANDING LEARNING STYLES

One of the receiver characteristics that you need to keep in mind is that individuals have different learning styles. A given audience may have one predominant learning style, but more likely, the group will include people with different learning styles. Thus, different types of learning activities are needed within each session to accommodate these differences. The various design features emphasized in Step 5 took learning style into consideration, although it was not stated at the time. Here, the different learning styles are first described and then related to the design features in Step 5.

Kolb's Model of Learning Styles and Experiential Learning

Based on his research of the experience of learning, Kolb proposes that individuals differ in the way they understand their experience of, and adapt to, the world, and that these variances can be placed on a continuum of perception (Kolb 1984). At one end of the continuum are the sensing/feeling individuals who project themselves onto the current reality of each experience by sensing and feeling their way around. Conversely, people on the thinking end of the continuum tend to analyze experiences logically through their intellect. People do move back and forth on the continuum, but most have a comfortable "hovering place." Each of these two kinds of perception has strengths and weaknesses. Both are valuable. Learners need both perspectives.

The second way in which people learn differently is in how they process experiences and information. When confronted with learning new things, some people watch and reflect first to filter the experience through their own value system. Other people jump in and act immediately, saving the reflection for later, if at all. Watchers need to internalize; doers need to act. Neither way is better, but rich learning involves both.

When these two kinds of perceiving and processing are looked at together, a four-quadrant learning style model is formed (**Figure 15-1**).

- *Imaginative learners* process information reflectively and process it by intuiting and feeling. They want the world to be a meaningful place for them and therefore strive to connect personally to the content they are learning. They believe in their own experience and are interested in people and culture.
- *Analytic learners* perceive information abstractly and process it reflectively. They learn by thinking through concepts and pay attention to expert opinions. They are industrious and thrive in traditional classrooms and nutrition education lecture settings. Verbally skilled and avid readers, analytic learners sometimes see ideas as being more fascinating than people.
- *Commonsense learners* perceive information abstractly and process it actively. They learn by applying theories to practice and are avid problem solvers. They need to know how things work and wonder how (and if) what they learn in a nutrition education session can be of immediate use to them.
- *Dynamic learners* perceive information concretely and process it actively. They learn by trial and error and are enthusiastic about new things. They are at ease with people and enjoy taking risks and wrangling with change. Dynamic learners pursue inter-

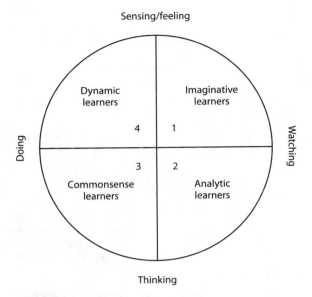

FIGURE 15-1 The four major learning styles.
Source: Kolb, D.A. 1984. *Experiential learning.* Englewood Cliffs, NJ: Prentice Hall.

ests through a variety of avenues, and therefore the structure of formal nutrition education sessions seems limiting to them.

Kolb (1984) suggests that each session or series of sessions include learning activities that address each of these learning styles in the following sequence: concrete experiences, observations and reflections, formation of abstract concepts and generalizations, and testing the implications of concepts in new situations (**Table 15-1**).

1. The sessions can begin with asking participants to investigate their own prior knowledge, attitudes, or behaviors through an activity. This is called self-assessment in earlier chapters. There may be other concrete ways to make the session personal and relevant to the participants.
2. The second part of the session or program can address why-to knowledge for the audience to observe and reflect on, such as the latest scientific information about the benefits of taking action. This could be a mini-lecture, incorporating graphs and visuals where appropriate. Together these two sections of the sessions will increase interest and motivation.
3. The next part can focus on activities for the individuals to begin to form their own understandings of the issues related to taking action, such as through needed how-to knowledge and skills.
4. Finally, the group can take steps to apply the knowledge gained by setting goals for specific actions they will take (Beffa-Negrini & Cohen 1990).

As you can see, these steps reflect the instructional sequence advocated by Gagne (1985) and modified by Kinzie (2005) that was used as the basis of the educational plan or design sequence in Step 5. That sequence of the events of instruction, as you recall, is as follows:

1. Gain attention.
2. Present stimulus or new material based on the prior knowledge and experience of the audience.
3. Provide guidance and practice.
4. Apply and close.

TABLE 15-1

Learning Activities to Address Each Learning Style

What does using the learning style approach look like in terms of instructional activities? Use activities to address all the learning styles by "teaching around the cycle."

Quadrant and Learner Type	Focus	Educational Activities
Quadrant 1: Imaginative learners		
Creating a concrete experience	Focus on sensing and feeling. Activate knowledge by making learning meaningful. The focus is on the learners and how they can connect to themselves what is being learned. The aim is motivation of learners.	Trigger films, demonstrations, hook questions, brainstorming, word webbing, puzzles, observations, games
Quadrant 2: Analytic learners		
Observing, reflecting, and analyzing experience; integrating reflective analysis into concepts	Focus on watching/reflecting. Assist learners to gain knowledge by introducing needed content. Learners reflect on prior experience from quadrant 1 and develop concepts and skills. The aim is to facilitate ability to take action.	Discussions, mini-debates, journals or logs, thinking questions, analyses of pros and cons, mini-lectures (graphs and charts, pictures or overheads, summaries), readings
Quadrant 3: Commonsense learners		
Developing abstract concepts and/or skills; practicing skills	Focus on thinking. Assist learners to examine how they can apply what they have learned. The aim is to provide opportunities for practice.	Making or completing graphs/charts, drawings, conclusions; case studies; writing activities; "minds-on" worksheets
Quadrant 4: Dynamic learners		
Practicing and adding something of oneself; analyzing application for relevance or usefulness	Focus on doing. Encourage creativity and self-expression by asking group members to take what they have learned and practiced and expand on it in their own way. The aim is to challenge the group to incorporate new motivations, learning, and skills in an ongoing way into their lives.	"Hands-on" activities; contracts, commitments, or action plans; developing products or videos, puzzles and/or skits, and simulations; field study; field visits

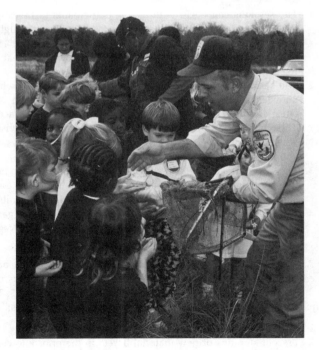

For younger children, a trip to a farm to see how vegetables and fruit are produced may be a great way to create a more hands-on learning experience.

Learning style research tells you *how* to design activities in each of the events of instruction so as to incorporate different learning styles. Such an approach integrates behavioral nutrition theory, learning styles research, and instructional design principles.

Note that as nutrition educators, we tend to teach according to our own learning style preferences, so we should be aware of our preferences and follow this sequence to ensure that you deliver nutrition education in ways that will reach individuals with different learning styles and enrich their repertoire of ways of learning (and perhaps your own at the same time!). With this information about learning styles in mind, you may need to go back and revise your educational plan or lesson plan and educational strategies to be appropriate for these considerations.

■ IMPLEMENTING LEARNING IN GROUPS

You have already designed learning experiences for nutrition education group sessions in Step 5. The following discussion concerns how to deliver the educational experiences that you have planned.

Methods for Implementing Learning Experiences

The sessions that you have designed may be delivered through many different instructional formats, such as lectures, demonstrations, hands-on learning tasks, and group discussions. These various formats are described in the following subsections.

Lecture

Lecture is still the predominant educational delivery method used today. It is how most people were taught, and many educators tend to teach as they were taught. During lecturing, group participants play a passive role as learners while the leader assumes the role of expert. As noted earlier, people remember only 10% of what they hear, so lecturing is not considered the most desirable method for reaching the public. A survey found that a group of mothers in the Women, Infants, and Children (WIC) program, struggling with complex issues regarding getting their children to develop healthful eating patterns, gave lectures a very low rating.

The lecture method should not be ruled out entirely, however. It can be useful in classroom settings when presenting new information that students will be required to master later on or at professional meetings when new information is presented to participants. In addition, lecture may be the preferred style of some types of learners. For example, one study examined the usefulness of social cognitive theory–based strategies such as taste testing, role playing, brainstorming, and goal setting to improve business executives' away-from-home eating behaviors (Olson & Kelly 1989). The study found that these busy business executives hated the use of hands-on behaviorally based activities. They were already interested in making changes in their eating practices and wanted the necessary how-to information delivered quickly and compactly. Activities just took too long. This affirms the importance of finding out audience learning style preferences in the needs analysis in Step 2.

Generally, lecture works best when it is delivered in short, palatable bites. The average person can listen for no longer than 10 minutes before needing to stop to process the information being taken in. Visuals such as charts, graphs, and pictures enhance the presentation of vital information while helping to accommodate learners who are not keen on the lecture as a viable mode of delivery. Analytic learners may be amenable to a longer lecture, whereas dynamic learners will begin to squirm after the first 5 minutes. Of course, listening to an engaging nutrition educator on an issue of interest will make any lecture seem shorter.

Short mini-lectures can be embedded in an otherwise activity-based session. For example, a mini-lecture is very useful during the part of the session in which scientific evidence of perceived outcomes of behavior, both positive and negative, is presented. Likewise, a mini-lecture may be useful for providing evidence-based information about effective actions for reducing risk or improving health, whether personal, community, or environmental.

Brainstorming

Brainstorming is an effective method for getting groups of participants to generate lists in a creative way. Everyone has a creative streak in them, and educators need to get rid of the blocks that keep good ideas pent up. Establishing rules for brainstorming helps participants keep on track and feel safe enough to contribute. Dynamic and imaginative learners prefer brainstorming over passive learning strategies. Brainstorming can be divided into two phases, for which the rules are as follows.

Phase One

- All critical judgment is ruled out; all ideas count.
- Wild ideas are expected; spontaneity, which comes when judgment is suspended, will flourish. Practical consideration is not important in this phase.
- Quantity, not quality, counts.
- Pool ideas and build on the ideas of others.

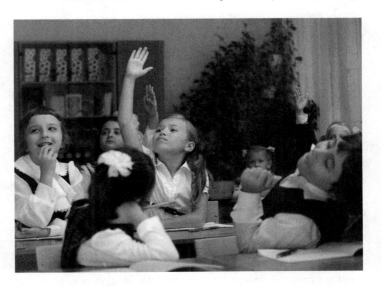

Brainstorming provides an effective, interactive way to involve everyone in a nutrition education lesson.

Phase Two

- Apply critical judgment—evaluate proposed ideas for feasibility.
- As a group, decide on the one or two best options if the group is interested in taking action.

Brainstorming can be useful in nutrition education for such purposes as generating a list of barriers to eating healthfully among teenagers, ways to get children to eat more healthfully, or easy meals for working moms to prepare.

Demonstrations, Including Cooking Demonstrations

Demonstrations can serve many functions. They can be used to show how something is done. They can also serve a motivational role and help the group explore ideas and attitudes. Often they serve both functions. For example, cooking demonstrations can teach skills. At the same time, they reduce the barriers to action in the participants watching and thus enhance their motivation and likelihood to take action. Other demonstrations do not specifically teach skills but are designed to enhance motivation. For example, you can spoon out the amount of fat or sugar in some popular fast foods and sweetened beverages. This will mean bringing to the sessions the target foods. Consider bringing empty wrappers of the demonstration foods because the audience may want to know what you plan to do with the food after you are done. Saying you will throw it away gives the message that you are comfortable with wasting food (not an appropriate message for any audience, and especially inappropriate for a low-income audience). Or they may ask if they can take it home, which of course undermines your latent message.

Conducting demonstrations means that you must have all the materials you need at the site or must bring them with you. It has often been said that a major qualification for a nutrition educator is the willingness to take materials with you to sites, including food or food ingredients. Those with cars often find that their trunks are full. Those in inner cities using public transportation find other means. For example, one nutrition educator uses a suitcase on wheels to bring needed materials to sites: one that is large enough to include a portable butane stove plus a few needed pots and pans, utensils, paper towels, and so forth. She takes it in taxicabs and buses. A second major qualification of a nutrition educator is the willingness to be flexible, that is, to use whatever is available to make the demonstration work. For example, if you want to show how blood vessels can get clogged during a lifetime of eating high-saturated-fat foods, you may not be able to purchase the demonstration materials. But you can buy some clear tubing in a hardware store (to serve as the blood vessel), solid cooking fat, some food coloring, a funnel, and a large bowl. You can place some of the fat in the tubing to block it partially (you do not want to block all of it), dissolve red food dye in water, and pour it through the funnel into the tube, with the large bowl ready to catch the colored water.

It is important to practice demonstrations ahead of time to know that they will work under the circumstances of your session. This is especially important for demonstrating food preparation skills.

Activities and Learning Tasks

Activities and experiences can heighten learning in a way that no passive learning can. Indeed, as noted before: "I hear—and forget; I see—and remember; I do—and understand." In addition, you know from earlier in this chapter that active learning not only increases awareness but also enhances motivation. The doers—dynamic and commonsense learners—prefer hands-on learning. This includes the many activities and learning tasks that you might design for your participants, such as calculating fat or sugar content in foods, completing checklists, sorting items into categories, completing worksheets comparing foods in terms of cost and nutritional content, or analyzing local restaurant menus for the most healthful meals. If it is feasible, other learning experiences might be taste testing, cooking or simple food preparation, grocery store tours, and visits to farms or farmers' markets. Refer to Table 15-1 for a summary of kinds of activities that can be done, particularly with youth.

Debates

Debates offer a lively vehicle for highlighting the two sides of an issue. There is much controversy in the area of foods and nutrition, as you are aware. Instead of lecturing about the pros and cons of a given matter, have participants research each side and then go at it in the session. All learners will enjoy a good debate, but the doers—dynamic and com-

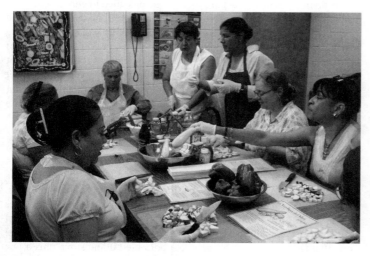

Group tasks can build empowerment and group cohesion.

monsense learners—will probably prefer to do the debating, whereas the watchers will be content to sit and absorb the show. Good issues for debate might include whether to take dietary supplements, whether children should drink low-fat milk, and how to introduce healthy foods into the home.

The instructional strategies mentioned here are effective, diverse methods that promote learning across the styles spectrum. Most of them involve active participation in which group participants step beyond the role of passive sponges. Important in each of these approaches is for the nutrition educator to evaluate whether the task involves purely hands-on work or whether there is indeed a thinking, minds-on dimension serving the learning objectives that you have stated in your educational plans.

Discussions

Discussions are one of the most constructive strategies for learning. In traditional schooling, a quiet classroom was considered a productive one. However, higher-order thinking skills require complex cognition, which is facilitated by individuals verbalizing what they know, do not know, or want to know (Johnson & Johnson 1991).

As a nutrition educator, you can encourage group participants to talk to each other. For example, use the enthusiasm that participants have for each other to promote learning. Passive learning, such as listening to the nutrition educator talk, does not employ the richer cognitive processes that promote memory, elaboration, or attitudinal changes. Imaginative learners enjoy discussions regarding "what if" questions, analytic learners "why" questions, and commonsense learners "how" questions; dynamic learners appreciate all three perspectives.

Interesting discussion questions in each category for nutrition education might include the following.

What if . . .

- You could only eat three foods for a whole week—what would they be?
- You lost the ability to taste—would you still enjoy eating?
- We could get all the nutrition we needed from one food—would everyone eat that food and only that food?

Why . . .

- Can't we just eat ice cream for all our nourishment?
- Do people gain weight?
- Is there not enough food in the world to feed everyone?

How . . .

- Does the food you eat turn into you?
- Come there isn't one perfect food?
- Did the first loaf of bread get baked?

Next is a discussion of the nature of groups and group dynamics, followed by a description of how to use facilitated group discussions in nutrition education.

Creating Environments for Learning

Kurt Lewin, who is considered a leading developer of the field of social psychology and who made profound contributions to the understanding of motivation of behavior, as noted earlier in the book, is also generally considered to be the founder of modern group dynamics. His work on field dynamics or field theory has had enormous influence on the understanding of human behavior in the context of others.

Lewin on Group Dynamics

He emphasizes that individuals' beliefs, attitudes, and habits are intimately related to those of the groups to which they belong. Humans, who always live in groups, are constantly involved in dynamic interactions with others. These interactions can be symbolic or can be affective and emotional in nature. In his view, the group is not the sum of its members. It is a structure that emerges from the interaction of behaving individuals who constantly and dynamically adjust to each other to form a "field" (Lewin 1951). The result of this mutual adaptation is a set of ever more complex patterns of behavior within the group. Neither the individual nor the group structure has an independent existence—they are mutually and dynamically dependent on each other, resulting in a set of group dynamics (Lewin 1935, 1947).

Since then, investigators have conducted considerable research to try to understand the dynamics of human behavior in groups, including such concerns as the roles of group members, settings and purpose, cohesive and disruptive forces in group behavior, group learning, collective problem solving, and group leadership styles. Such understandings have led to applications in psychotherapy, education, the management of organizations, and other settings. Because most learning about food and nutrition is social in nature, these understandings are especially important to nutrition educators. There are many kinds of groups, from groups convened to accomplish specific tasks (e.g., committees, teams at work) to those involving formal and nonformal classes. Most of this chapter is devoted to understanding the kinds of dynamics that exist in the nutrition education groups with which you work and the skills required of the group leader.

Social Climate and Learning

Lewin always liked to put his ideas to the test and to work out their practical implications. He therefore conducted many studies on "social climates." In one, Lewin and his collaborators set out to investigate the effects on their members of small groups organized along "democratic," "authoritarian," and "laissez-faire" patterns. The study involved task groups of 10-year-old youths in boys' clubs (Lewin, Lippitt, & White 1939). The studies were experimental in nature and carefully controlled. The setups and results are shown in **Table 15-2**.

The results suggest that the authoritarian atmosphere impairs initiative and independence and breeds hostility and aggression. In some groups the children were apathetic and bodily tensions increased. In the laissez-faire group, there was low morale, poor quality of work, and much frustration. The democratic climate permitted the children to thrive. The same kinds of results were obtained from a controlled experiment with workers in various kinds of work climates (Lewin 1947, 1948). Workers' resentment toward authoritarian management was found to reduce productivity. When workers could air their views and participate in the decision-making process, their motivation improved and their productivity exceeded previous levels.

Group Decision Method for Changing Food Habits

These findings led Lewin to a series of experiments on changing people's food beliefs and attitudes (or *values*, as he called them) and food habits. During World War II when meat was scarce, he and his collaborators conducted several studies to compare "the relative effectiveness of a lecture method and a method of group decision for changing food habits"

TABLE 15-2	**Group Dynamics: Leadership Patterns and Social Climate in Groups**		
	Authoritarian	**Democratic**	**Laissez-Faire**
Setup of social climate			
	All policies determined by the leader	All policies a matter of group discussion and decision, assisted by the leader	Complete freedom for group or individual decision, with no participation by leader
	Leader dictates the work task and work companions of each person	Work tasks decided by group, and members chose with whom to work	Complete nonparticipation by leader
	Leader was "personal" in his praise and criticism; impersonal and aloof, but friendly and nonhostile	Leader was "objective" in his praise and criticism; participated as a group member	No comments unless specifically asked; no participation or interference with course of events
Result			
	Greater quantity of work	Slower, but more motivated	Less and poorer quality of work
	Greater hostility and competition	Increasingly productive	Greater amount of time on horseplay
	Greater aggressiveness (30 times greater than in the democratic climate)	Greater friendliness and teamwork	Talked more about what they should be doing
	Greater dependence	Greater satisfaction	More aggressive than democratic and less than authoritarian
	Less originality on tasks	Praised more frequently	Expressed preference for democratic (after experiencing all three)

Sources: Lewin, K., R. Lippitt, and R. K. White. 1939. Patterns of aggressive behavior in experimentally created "social climates." *Journal of Social Psychology* 10:271–299; Lewin, K. 1947. Frontiers in group dynamics. Concept, method, reality in social science: Social equilibria and social change. *Human Relations* 1:5–41; and Lewin, K. 1948. *Resolving social conflicts: Selected papers on group dynamics.* New York: Harper.

(Lewin 1943). These studies were experimental in nature and carefully controlled for leader effect and socioeconomic and ethnic differences. In one study with housewives, Lewin compared these two ways of encouraging people to eat organ meats (kidneys, sweetbreads/brains, and beef hearts), purposely chosen because they are normally rejected. The lecture used health, status, and patriotic appeals, followed by handouts with recipes. The second method involved a short presentation by the leader, also linking the problem of nutrition to health, status, and the war effort. Then there was ample opportunity for the women to discuss why they rejected these meats and to share experiences with each other. They then identified ways to overcome barriers (with ideas from the leader if needed). Next, the group members were ready to make a decision whether to try one of these meats the following week using the recipes provided. They verbalized their decision to the others. Of the women in the lecture-only setting, only 10% served one of the recommended foods, whereas of those who had an opportunity to discuss and make a group decision, 52% served the recommended foods.

Lewin conducted a similar study with a different audience—college students—emphasizing whole-grain bread. In this case he compared a "request" to the students to eat more whole-grain bread instead of white bread with group decision and obtained similar results (Lewin 1943). His work suggests, therefore, that group dynamics are important and that a democratic social climate, in which group members have the opportunity to be involved in making decisions for themselves, is more conducive to social change than other social climates. He emphasized that the method was one of *group decision* rather than just group discussion because closure in terms of decision making was considered important to the approach, along with public commitment. Such commitment made in the context of supportive peers was a motivating factor to make good on one's commitment to oneself. As Lewin noted, no pressure tactics were used; instead, "the group setting gives the incentive for the decision and facilitates and reinforces it" (Lewin 1943).

Since then, there has been considerable research on group structure and development, group behavior, leadership issues, group learning, and group development in a variety of settings, such as education, worksites, and communities. There have also been numerous professional conversations about the appropriate roles of educators and group members, particularly in work with adults (Rogers 1969; Brookfield 1986; Vella 2002). All, however, agree that creating an emotionally safe learning environment is crucial.

Creating Safe Learning Environments Conducive to Change

Many of the individuals nutrition educators work with want to make changes in their lives but are also afraid to do so. Food- and nutrition-related behaviors are embedded in so many other aspects of their lives that making a change in this one aspect may involve drastic changes in other aspects. Educators and psychologists (Rogers 1969; Freire & Shor 1987; Knowles 1990; Vella 2002) note that learning environments must be challenging enough to stimulate growth but also safe enough to allow people to grow and change in perspectives, knowledge, attitudes, motivation, and action. Cooperative learning is more effective than competitive learning in this context (Johnson & Johnson 1991). This means respecting that individuals come with a set of fears and defenses. It also means that the design of the sessions, the atmosphere in the room, and your approach to the situation should all signal that this is a safe space and time to learn and change. This feeling is especially important for adult learners in nonformal settings. Group leaders, such as nutrition educators, are often referred to as *facilitators* of such learning groups, rather than teachers or instructors.

Participants in any group bring with them a set of fears. The following list describes a few of them. **Box 15-1**, based on work by Sappington (1984), discusses how you can address these fears to make the learning environment safe for participants.

- *Outcome fears.* These include participants' fear that they will not get what they want, that the information and activities may not be relevant to their personal needs, that there will not be enough time, and that the session will go over time.
- *Interpersonal fears or social concerns.* These are often the greatest barrier to significant learning and change. They include fear of embarrassment, looking stupid or incompetent to peers or to the nutrition educator, criticism by others in the group, being called on when one is not ready, judgment of one's beliefs or positions, feeling vulnerable, unfamiliarity with others in a new group, or competition with others.
- *Evaluation fears.* These include fear of failure at the tasks that have been chosen and fear that one's verbal responses are not correct.
- *Internal fears.* The deepest fears that group participants often bring are those that challenge their self-concept. Fear of incompetence or inadequacy arises from a genuine fear of not being able to do what is suggested. Changing would suggest that previous beliefs, attitudes, or actions were inferior or bad.

In general, safe environments are created when people feel respected; when their feelings are honored, their self-worth is assured, and their fears are overcome; and when the "delights of growth outweigh the anxieties of growth." Building safe learning environments is a crucial part of facilitated group discussion and dialogue, which is described next.

Facilitated Group Discussion as an Educational Tool: Focus on Adults

The importance of facilitating learning and change through emotionally safe group learning environments has recently been brought to the attention of nutrition educators, or brought *back* to their attention, considering that Lewin conducted the first group discussion and group decision work in the food habits area and Rogers focused on this issue in the 1970s. Although an emotionally safe learning environment is important for all age groups, discussions tend to be most useful for adults.

Guided discussions can range considerably in the degree to which the nutrition educator exerts leadership. You may make presentations with added activities; these would not be considered facilitated discussions. Or you may design sessions with open-ended questions and discussion but following a specific lesson plan. Or you may provide mini-lectures interspersed with guided discussion. These approaches are the most widely used and are appropriate for many group settings. There are group learning situations in which the entire session is devoted to a facilitated discussion. These adult group learning settings are described variously as facilitated group discussions, facilitated dialogue, or learner-based education (Abusabha, Peacock, & Achterberg 1999; Sigman-Grant 2004; Husing & Elfant 2005), which vary somewhat in the degree of leadership provided by the nutrition educator. This approach is described in Chapter 17.

No matter whether the entire session is a facilitated group discussion or consists of mini-lectures interspersed with guided discussion, the role of the facilitator is to guide the group unobtrusively and to encourage interaction among members. You can do this by addressing questions posed to you to other group members, by saying things such as, "Do you have any reactions to that or suggestions, Maria?" You can also look away from the speaker in the group as he or she attempts to

---

Box 15-1 Creating a Safe Learning Environment

The following lists present ways to reduce audience fears and create a safe learning environment.

Outcome Fears

- *Provide a welcoming start.* Make sure the room is comfortable in terms of light, heating, and ventilation. Arrange the setting or seating to be appropriate to the learning situation. Conscious decisions need to be made about whether to arrange seating in a circle or half circle (more intimate than rows), around tables, and so forth. Have coffee out if appropriate, and name tags.
- *Greet the group and introduce yourself.* If appropriate to the setting and size of the group, have the group members introduce themselves as well.
- *Set the time frame.* Let the audience know approximately how long the session will last.
- *Make your competence and experience clear, either through prior material you hand out or through your introduction.* This will make the group feel confident in your being able to provide a valuable experience for them.
- *State the objectives of the session clearly and provide a brief overview of the agenda or activities.* This will make the participants feel assured that the material will be relevant to their needs and that the activities are well organized.

Interpersonal Fears

- *State ground rules about how individuals will relate to each other.* Ask the group to contribute so that all are comfortable with the rules. Key ground rules are to respect each other and the facilitator and to listen to each other.
- *Design activities to be done first in dyads and then in small groups.* Do this before having a large group discussion.
- *As the facilitator of the group, provide nonjudgmental responses to individual contributions.* By listening carefully to the feelings behind the questions and comments, you can gauge the fear or safety level in the individual and the group. Model the desired behavior and use warm, accepting humor where appropriate.

Evaluation Fears

- *Validate each response either verbally or by writing responses on newsprint.*
- *Provide nonjudgmental responses.* For example, rather than saying that what a group member said was "not quite accurate," thank the person for bringing up that point because it is something that many others also think, and then say, "The latest information on that point is . . . "
- *Provide constructive feedback.*

Internal Fears

- *Be respectful of each individual.*
- *Validate individuals' past experiences.*
- *Use genuine dialogue as the approach.* Ask open-ended questions and listen to responses so as to allow for the free-flowing exchange of ideas so that all group members can learn from each other.

---

make eye contact with you. The speaker will soon get the idea that he or she should look to others for responses. A good way to increase group interaction, especially at first, is the following technique: tell the group that after a given person speaks, he or she will pick the next person who wishes to speak, who will then pick the next person, and so forth.

The facilitator also needs to know when and how to take control. This depends on the degree of leadership you have decided is appropriate for the given group. Although an authoritarian approach can stifle group discussion, being too uncertain, timid, or laissez-faire can make the group feel unsure of itself and undermine your authority in the group. You can retain your authority while setting up an open, safe, and democratic social climate. When the group goes off track, you can gently bring it back by saying something such as, "Those are important issues, but the issue we are addressing today is *x.*"

Understanding Group Dynamics in Nutrition Education Sessions

Even if you have designed engaging activities and wish to incorporate group discussion, you can confront situations that consistently plague instructors and group discussion leaders. If you are not ready to face spontaneous aspects of group dynamics, you may find yourself distracted, frustrated, or even becoming hostile. Defuse the anxiety by considering ahead of time how you will respond in some situations you might face, such as those shown in **Box 15-2**. These situations can be issues of authority (yours) and power (the audience's). The following list presents some ways you might handle these situations. In facilitated discussions or dialogues of groups that have met for some time, members of the group may take on many of the following roles.

- *Quiet members.* It is important to respect all individuals in the group in terms of whether they wish to participate in discussions or not. They may be shy, or their quietness may be cultural. However, silence may also be a reflection of boredom, indifference, or a person's sense of superiority, timidity, or insecurity. Thus, it is important for you to figure out why group members are silent. If they are shy or insecure, it is helpful to provide activities such as icebreakers, brainstorming, or working in dyads or small groups. You can also reinforce and praise each attempt they make to speak up in the group. Sometimes quiet members really wish to speak up and will do so if you give them some encouragement, using smiles, nods, and perhaps asking them to respond. If they have blank expressions, it would be unwise to invite them to participate.
- *Dominant or talkative members.* The most common problem facilitators have is what to say to those who are overly dominant and talkative. It is important to handle the situation carefully

$\mathcal{B}ox$ **15-2   Give Your Session a Fair Trial: Be Aware of the Effects of Group Dynamics**

You know your content. You have designed activities that are based on theory and research and are engaging, interactive, and fun. But you confront situations that have plagued instructors and discussion leaders forever. If you are not ready to face spontaneous aspects of group dynamics, you may find yourself distracted, frustrated, or even hostile. Defuse the anxiety ahead of time. These can be issues of authority (yours) and power (the audience's).

Consider how you would handle each of these chronic instructional problems:

1. Only a few people are on time. When should you begin?
2. People arrive late (missing critical content or instructions).
3. One person dominates the session.
4. People do other work while you are presenting.
5. Some refuse to join the activity.
6. Many tangents are raised.
7. Someone wants to link every issue to a long personal story.
8. A heated argument erupts over a content issue.
9. People leave early or exit the room frequently.
10. Someone thinks he or she should be teaching the session rather than you.
11. Someone nods off.
12. Two people chat continuously at the back of the room or within the circle.
13. Some people are much more informed on the topic than you.
14. You are asked a string of questions you cannot answer.
15. Some people let it be known that the only reason they are there is because they are required to be.

Source: Morin, K. 1998. Presentation at Teachers College, Columbia University, New York.

understood. Others are talkative because they enjoy talking or they believe that they can raise their status within the group by sharing information. They will not stop talking even when you or others in the group have paraphrased what they said or reflected their feelings. In this case, you might want to acknowledge their contributions and then say that short comments are easier for others to follow and that lengthy comments tend to lose people. If the pattern persists, you may need to talk with the participant privately. Talkative group members are often unaware of the fact that others may not appreciate their lengthy comments. You can emphasize that you have noticed that others want to talk but cannot because time is always limited in group learning settings.

- *Distractors or disrupters.* These individuals may carry out side conversations or make side comments to the group or frequently get up and leave the room, disrupting the group, whether the nutrition educator is presenting or leading the discussion or others are talking. Generally, you need not embarrass members who are engaged in side conversations if these are brief and intermittent. If the conversations are disrupting, you might stop talking and ask the individuals involved an easy question or ask them to share their thoughts with the group. If the disruptions persist, you should speak with them in private and point out that their behavior distracts and disrupts learning and is disrespectful of others.

- *Complainers.* Some participants are always complaining about some aspect of the group or about the physical surroundings. Acknowledge them and thank them for their concern. Ask them for suggestions for alternate approaches. Indicate that you will explore their suggestions and then be firm about staying on track. If the complaining persists, again take the individuals aside and talk with them privately.

- *Digressors.* These group members constantly digress from the main issues of the discussion or activities by talking about matters unrelated to the issues. You can respond by saying, "What you say is interesting, but let's get back to . . ." Or you can ask, "How does this relate to what we are talking about?" Or again, "This is interesting, but given our time constraints, we can discuss these issues later if we have time."

- *Resistors.* These individuals say that whatever is being proposed by you or the others can't be done, or they just can't do it. This response may stem from fear or insecurity. Acknowledge their feelings and indicate that all change is difficult and that they can take one step at a time. If possible, partner them with someone else in the group who can provide support.

- *Know-it-alls.* Some group members may indicate that they know more than you and keep correcting you. Acknowledge that they seem to know a lot. You might ask them about their sources of information. Even if you believe the source is very questionable, ask them what makes them believe the source. Remain questioning and probing. You might also ask the others in the group to respond. It may be effective for you to place such persons in some leadership role.

- *Wisecrackers.* Some degree of humor may be helpful in the group. However, you will need to determine when the humor stops being helpful in relieving tension and starts interfering with group learning. This usually occurs when more attention is focused on the person who is making the wisecracks than on what is being said. You can say to the person, with a smile and in a tone that suggests that you appreciate what he or she has said, that it is

because what you do will have an impact on all the others in the group. It is crucial to treat individuals with respect and not to humiliate or embarrass them. Being disrespectful is not only hurtful for the individual but also makes others in the group feel unsafe and uncomfortable.

Several techniques may be effective in dealing with dominant or overly talkative participants. Some people are overly talkative because they are insecure and repeat themselves because they are not sure that the points they are making have been understood. If this is the case, you might interrupt them gently but firmly by thanking them for their response, paraphrase concisely what they have said or reflect their feelings so that they feel they have been understood, and then turn to others for responses. Usually these participants will stop talking because they feel they have been time to get back to the issues. If the wisecracks continue, you may have to say it again, but with a firm tone.

- *Latecomers.* If one or two individuals are late for an ongoing group or learning situation, you may ignore it. However, if they are consistently late, you may need to say something such as, "I know it is not always easy to get here on time, given the traffic and your situation, but I do want to remind us all that learning works best when we are all here from the beginning of the group session. It is also respectful of the others who may have made considerable effort to be here on time." If lateness persists for some individuals, you may want to talk with them privately to find out what the issues are for them. If the entire group consistently arrives late, you will need to carefully examine your own hidden messages to the group. Perhaps you do not start or end on time. This may convey the message that the group is not that important and thus not worth being on time for. This will arouse considerable resentment, particularly from those who make an effort to be on time. It may be interpreted as disrespect for group members' time.

ORAL PRESENTATIONS AND WORKSHOPS

Leading group discussions is not the only way to implement nutrition education with groups. The session or sessions that you have designed may be delivered as a presentation, a series of presentations, or as workshops. Or you may make a mini-presentation followed by group discussion. The principles of communication described at the beginning of the chapter are particularly useful here.

Preparing and Organizing Oral Presentations

The key to holding the attention of the group in delivering your designed session as an oral presentation is to be well organized, focused, concise, and coherent. Use of theory and the Stepwise Procedure is important here, even if the steps are abbreviated.

When you first begin making presentations, you might have the impulse to tell the audience everything you know about food and nutrition. Yet listening requires concentration on the part of the audience. By covering too much, you overload our audience. In the procedural model for designing theory-based nutrition education described earlier in the book, it is very important to write clear goals and objectives for educational plans or session guides. This is even more important if you are delivering the session through the channel of an oral presentation.

Whatever the presentation's length may be, you have a limited time and you should be very clear about what you want to accomplish in that time. These are your objectives. What kinds of changes do you wish to take place in the audience—greater awareness of an issue, more motivation to consider action, or readiness to take a specific action? The audience should leave the presentation with the ability to state the main goal of the presentation and several supporting arguments or pieces of evidence, or *why-to* information, and a clear understanding of the conclusion or of what they should now do and *how to* do it. Thus, being organized is extremely important.

In addition, being organized throughout enhances your credibility. The audience gets only one chance to grasp your ideas and will become impatient if you ramble from one idea to another. The introduction to the session topic, discussion of the objectives of the session, explanations of learning activities, and transitions between activities should flow into each other in an organized fashion. Handouts, flip charts, PowerPoint slides, videos, and other ancillary materials should be ready for use and organized.

The Introduction

Presentations are generally described as having three parts: an introduction, body, and conclusion. Each serves a specific purpose. The functions of the introduction are to establish the speaker's credibility and goodwill, gain the attention and interest of the audience by providing an overview of what the *audience* will gain from the presentation, develop rapport with audience, and preview what the *presenter* intends to cover. The order of the first two functions may differ depending on the situation. If you have been adequately introduced, you may go directly to a way to gain the interest of the audience.

In terms of the first purpose of an introduction, credibility is established if you appear to be competent and trustworthy, as noted at the beginning of the chapter. Thus, when you introduce yourself or are introduced, let the audience know about your credentials and experience—with sensitivity and without bragging, of course—so as to indicate that you are qualified. For example, you can say, "In an article I wrote . . ." or "From my work with . . ." Your credibility does not necessarily depend only on your own accomplishments. You can say, "I have been interested in this issue for some time and have read widely on it." As discussed earlier, your being qualified helps the audience relax and feel reassured that they will get something out of the presentation. Your effectiveness is also enhanced if you can establish some common ground and connections with your particular audience. For example, you can say something like, "As those of us who live in this community can attest . . . ," "As a mother of three children myself, I know how difficult it is . . . ," or "I know how hard it is to find out where the food in our grocery stores comes from."

A major function of the introduction is to get the attention and interest of the audience. This is done by focusing on what the audience will gain from the presentation. The design section of this book emphasizes the importance of designing activities at the beginning of a session to be motivational, focusing on "what's in it for me." Here are a few ways to do this in the format of a presentation. They must all be relevant to your topic.

- *Relate the topic or issue to the audience in a way that is personal.* For example, if you are talking to a group of teenagers about world hunger, you might begin with the following: "How many of you barely got to school for your first class today? You jumped out of bed, showered, dressed, and were out the door without breakfast. By ten o'clock you are more aware of your growling stomach than of what the teacher is saying. You say to your classmate, 'I'm starving.' Imagine feeling like that all day, not just for an hour or two before lunch. And day after day. This is what it is like for millions of teenagers around the world."
- *Emphasize the importance of your topic or the issue.* On the issue of eating locally, you might begin with, "Every hour of every day, America is losing x acres of farmland, land that produces the food we all need to survive and grow. We want for there to be farmland for our children and our children's children, to produce the food they will need."
- *Make an intriguing statement.* For example, a presentation to teenagers about the importance of bone health and osteoporosis prevention could begin as follows: "Every day our bones are broken down and dissolved, and every day they are rebuilt. We do not see it happening or feel it happening, but it is happening nonetheless. We can't stop the breaking-down process. But what we eat can make a big difference in how well and how much bone is rebuilt."

- *Ask a stimulating question.* The question can be rhetorical or a way to get the audience to think about the topic in a new way. "What is the first word that comes to mind when I use the word *elderly*? The word *adult*? *Older adult*?" This can then lead into a speech about the experience and needs of older adults.
- *Tell a story.* Any story you tell should be clearly relevant to the main goal of the speech. "It happened about a week ago. I was early to a meeting at work, and several of us were chatting. One of my colleagues asked, 'How's your AIDS going?' The room fell silent as the others all looked at me. I then said, 'You mean my speech on AIDS and nutrition. It's going well.' There was palpable relief in the room, but for a moment I understood what it is like for someone to have AIDS in our society."

After gaining the audience's attention, you should devote the final section of the introduction to a clear statement of the main topic of the presentation and a listing of the points you will cover or issues you will address. Preferably your presentation should consist of only three or four main points, which are the three or four objectives of your session. By demonstrating that you are clear and organized, you also increase your credibility. Your credibility is also enhanced when the supporting materials you use are professional looking and clear. Chapter 16 discusses this issue in depth.

The Body

The body of the presentation consists of the objectives and content that you designed earlier using the procedural model for designing theory-based nutrition education. In translating these objectives and content into the format of an oral presentation, your first task is to identify the main points you want to make. These main points are usually the information on why to consider a food- or nutrition-related action and how to take action. This should be your "educational plan" from Step 5 of the design model. Because these main points are the central focus of your presentation, choose them carefully, phrase them precisely, and arrange them into some kind of strategic order.

From your educational plan, you can develop a speaking outline for use on the day of the presentation. Its aim is to help you remember what you want to say. Label the introduction, body, and conclusion. Make sure your outline is clear and easy to read. It is helpful to use large enough type so that you can see the main points just by glancing down. Some people like to put their notes on index cards, large enough so that the notes are clearly readable. You may be using slides throughout. These will contain only key ideas; thus, it is important, even in this instance, to have a speaking outline with key information on it. The PowerPoint program provides space to make notes on each slide. Those pages can serve as your speaking outline, with crucial supporting information on them.

It is also useful to write out the first few sentences for the beginning of the presentation—especially the dramatic opening you have planned—and the beginning of each new section so that the transitions are smooth. Make other notations as needed, such as "pause." Be sure to include important technical information so that you do not forget. You will probably also want to write out your conclusion. Rehearse from this speaking outline. Here are some factors to consider as you plan the body of your presentation.

- *Message vividness versus data summaries.* People tend to give greater weight to vivid and personalized information. Case studies, personal examples, and visual images such as slides are more vivid than recitations of facts, and people can remember and recall

them more easily even though they may be less representative of the issues you are presenting. Statistical data and impersonal information, on the other hand, are less vivid and thus will have less of an impact on attitudes and behavior, even though they may be more accurate. The challenge is to use personal and vivid—but accurate—information if you wish to be effective in increasing awareness, concern, or active contemplation. Statistics can be presented in a vivid way.

- *A single message versus many ideas.* A message or session should provide enough information to be convincing, enhance decision making, or provide new skills, yet it must be manageable in length and complexity. You do not need to tell the audience everything you know about an issue! Too many ideas, especially if they are thrown together haphazardly, create clutter in the receiver's mind so that no single message comes through clearly or sticks. Remember that the audience has only one chance to hear each idea. It is better to have a single message or theme in a given session, supported by a few clearly developed ideas or arguments, than to have too many different ideas. These supporting ideas are the "main points" in your outline. Plan to have only two to five main points because the audience can't keep track of too many more of them. Each main point should have one single idea, which should be worded clearly and later spoken with emphasis so that the audience will know it is one of your main points. "Less" is definitely better than "more" in this context.

    Being focused on your message does not mean that you should be simplistic. You should not underestimate the amount and depth of information that many people want. Indeed, oversimplistic messages may frustrate the audience because they do not provide the information the audience needs and may even lead to misunderstandings. Knowledge of the audience helps you judge the correct level of complexity. You can obtain this knowledge from a needs analysis or from the individuals or organization that invited you to make a presentation.

- *One side versus two sides.* Should you present only one side of a controversial issue or both sides? It is often more effective, and enhances your credibility, to present both sides. It shows that you know and understand more than one viewpoint and have taken a stand in light of these differing viewpoints. It can be quite powerful to present objections or counterarguments to your own message (that breastfeeding is best, for example) and then show how these objections are invalid or do not negate your message.

- *Order of presentation of main points or arguments.* The order of the main points depends on the purpose of the presentation; this book consistently suggests that focusing on motivational information first followed by how-to information is a good way to organize nutrition education presentations. But other orders are appropriate depending on the audience, issue, and setting.

- *Emotional appeals.* As you have seen, the audience is more likely to consider your message seriously if they believe you are credible and the evidence you present for taking action is strong and persuasive. However, you can deliver the why-to information in a fashion that has a greater impact if the words you use appeal to people's feelings as well as their reason. These issues are discussed earlier in the book in regard to most learning objectives having an affective as well as a cognitive aspect. This is just to remind you to use language vividly and clearly to help the audience effectively process your message emotionally as well as cognitively. For example, one way to say to mothers of young children that they should make sure their children get enough calcium for good teeth is to say, "You have the opportunity to give your child a smile for a lifetime" and show a photo of a child with a great smile (McCarthy 2005). Vivid examples can also convey feeling (e.g., what it is like to be hungry or to have AIDS and not be able to cook or shop for oneself), as noted earlier. Most important, it is your sincerity and conviction that the audience will feel and respond to.

The Conclusion

The conclusion of the presentation is extremely important. Its main purpose is to reinforce the audience's understanding of the central idea or their commitment to the main goal of the presentation. The conclusion is what you want the audience to remember, to make a commitment to, or to take action on. You may want to summarize your speech briefly. You have heard the old advice that in a speech one should "tell the audience what you will tell them, tell them, and then tell them what you told them." Your communication will be more effective if the conclusions are explicitly stated than if the conclusions are implied. You might refer back to the introduction to show your progression of ideas and how they led to the conclusion. You might also conclude with some kind of dramatic statement.

Delivering the Oral Presentation

As the presenter, you will be sized up by the audience from the moment you enter the room, so it is important that their impressions of you from the very first are positive. You should arrive early, meet the audience, smile, chat, and look confident whether you feel that way or not. This relaxes the audience or group and makes them want to listen to what you have to say. It also helps establish that you have an attractive personality. Appropriate attire and grooming also contribute to your credibility. After you have been introduced, walk confidently and with poise to where you will speak from, such as the front of the room, behind a podium, or onto a stage. Take a moment to look at the audience, smile, and make eye contact here and there with audience members. This establishes that you are interested in the audience, not just in what you want to say.

It is important to create a safe learning environment by continuing to develop rapport with the audience through looking at them and being comfortable with them. This gives permission for the audience to ask questions and make comments, if appropriate given the size and setting. You will need to decide whether you want audience members to ask questions throughout or at the end.

Room Arrangements

Another reason to arrive early is to check out the physical arrangement and technology in the room. Depending on the size of the group and the physical setup of the room, you may have the opportunity to arrange the seating to encourage effective learning in that setting. Decide whether you want to rearrange the seating to be in a circle, around tables, or some other arrangement. If you will be using audiovisual materials, be sure you know how to operate the equipment you will be using. Check out the temperature settings. If you will be using flip charts or newsprint to record group responses, make sure you have the markers you need. Make sure your handouts are ready to distribute.

Some speakers like podiums or lecterns. However, these present a barrier between you and the audience, and it is important to create an arrangement that allows you to connect with the audience. Instead, you could use a table on which to place your materials. What, then, to do

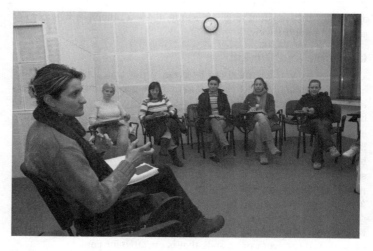

If you arrive early, you can rearrange your teaching area so it encourages communication and learning.

with your notes? You may be able to see them from the table, or keep them in your hand. You may find it useful to place your notes on cards that you can hold in your hand.

Nervousness and Anxiety

You should never share your internal feelings of nervousness or anxiety. Others cannot see or feel your anxiety unless you bring it to their attention by saying such things as how nervous you are, how intimidating the audience seems, or that you did not have a chance to prepare. Even if asked, do not acknowledge your fright. The group wants to learn and enjoy, and a safe learning environment is established when you seem relaxed and comfortable. When audience members are aware of the leader's fragility or stage fright, they become nervous in sympathy and start worrying for you instead of focusing on your message or the activities you have planned. The best way to reduce nervousness and anxiety is to be well prepared and to rehearse your presentation ahead of time.

Reading the Presentation or Speaking from an Outline

How you write and how you speak are usually very different in terms of language use and sentence structure. When speaking, people tend to use simpler words, shorter sentences, and more informal language. Some nutrition educators are able to write speeches in a way that sounds conversational, much as speechwriters do for politicians. Most people are not good at this kind of speechwriting, however, so that reading from a written text can be extremely dull. A memorized speech can also be dull. In both cases, the presentation becomes a monologue, spontaneity is lost, and the tone can become monotonous. Generally, therefore, you should not read or memorize the presentation. Instead, you should rehearse and deliver the speech from the speaking outline you have developed.

Time Management

Paying attention to how you are doing in terms of your outline and the time available for your presentation is crucial. However, you should find a way to monitor the time without your audience being aware of it. Looking constantly at your watch can give many unintended messages, such as that you can't wait for the presentation to be over or that you are afraid you are going to go over time. Place a timepiece where you can see it unobtrusively.

Language and Diction

The language you use needs to be clear, vivid, and appropriate. The audience members cannot go back to figure out something you said, as they could if they were reading a book. Therefore, what you say has to be clear and understandable the first time around. Use familiar words and the active voice instead of passive voice to the extent possible. The language you use should also be appropriate to the occasion (formal or informal) and to the audience. To be effective, the words, idioms, and style of the presentation must be suitable to the group, culturally appropriate, and nonsexist. The language you use should also be appropriate for you. As noted earlier, you have to be authentic to who you are; you can't be someone else—telling jokes or using hip language when these can be seen as forced and inconsistent with your personality and background. You can work out a style that is effective for you.

However, your diction is also important. Your credibility with the audience is influenced by your diction. When you misarticulate words, such as saying "wanna" for "want to" or "wilya" for "will you," and mispronounce words, such as "revelant" for "relevant" or "nucular" for "nuclear," the audience may develop negative impressions of you. Likewise, the use of *ums*, *ahs*, and "you knows" between words can grate on the audience. Listen to yourself speak when you rehearse, and train yourself to speak with clear diction in settings such as these.

Voice, Volume, Pitch, and Rate of Speaking

No matter what kind of voice you were born with, you can learn to make good use of what you have to make effective presentations. Whether you use a microphone or not, adjust your volume to the acoustics of the room. You want the individuals in the last row to hear you, but you do not want to shout. Your natural pitch could be high or low, but your speaking will be livelier when you vary your pitch by going up and down as you emphasize a point or ask a question. By varying your pitch (these variations are called *inflections*), you convey a variety of emotions and come across as dynamic, as opposed to when you speak in a monotone. Your inflections reveal whether you are being sincere or sarcastic, angry or anxious, and interested or bored. Enthusiasm about what you are saying goes a long way.

Pacing the rate (or speed) at which you speak is also important. If you speak too slowly, you may bore your audience. But if you speak too fast, the audience may not be able to keep up with your ideas. They may also get anxious because they suspect you are anxious. Indeed, people do tend to speed up when they are nervous. So pay attention to your pacing and practice a speed that seems appropriate for the audience. Pause from time to time at the end of a section for a point to sink in or for the audience to catch up with you. Because your mind can go much faster than your speaking, scan the group for "feedback" as you speak. Do they appear bored or puzzled? You might adjust what you are saying to fit your feedback.

Provide Signposts and Summarize Periodically

Provide signposts as to where you are in the speech, saying, for example, "first . . . ," "second . . . ," and so on. Use signposts to emphasize important points you want to make as well. You can say things such as, "The most important thing to remember about X is . . ." or "Above all, you need to know . . ." Summarizing periodically is also very helpful. As you begin the second main point, you could summarize in one sentence the key idea of the first point before proceeding.

Nonverbal Communication

As noted previously, nonverbal communication can be as powerful as the verbal communication it accompanies. Your personal appearance, facial expressions, gestures, bodily movement, and eye contact all convey information to the audience, and you want this information to be favorable so that the audience will focus on your message and not on you.

Listeners always see speakers before they hear them. There is evidence that how a speaker dresses and is groomed affects a speaker's credibility and reception considerably. The Madonnas and Einsteins of the world can get away with looking or wearing whatever they wish; the rest of us cannot. The main point is that you want the audience to focus on the message and activities you have designed, not on your personal appearance and grooming. So, check out the setting before you go to judge what will be appropriate to the audience and setting and to who you are. Remember that you will also be seen as a representative of the nutrition education profession.

When and how much to move can present a challenge. You can look for opportunities to break the invisible barrier between presenter and audience, so moving toward the audience or moving around a little can be helpful. However, pacing back and forth, fidgeting with your notes or with coins in your pocket, or playing with your hair are signs of nervousness and can be distracting. At the other end of the spectrum, standing rigidly in the same place signals nervousness. Pay attention to what you do, and practice coming across as confident. Saying to yourself, "I like the audience and the audience likes me" can be helpful.

What to do with your hands can be problematic. Clasp them behind your back? Put them in your pockets? Let them hang at your side? How much should you gesture? There are no rules about this, and people are all comfortable with different ways of holding their bodies and with when and how to gesture. The best way to think about this issue is that whatever you choose to do should appear natural and should not distract from your message.

Eye contact with the group helps you to establish a bond with the group. Look at individuals, not at some space between people, and move your eye contact from person to person around the entire room. Don't focus only on one side of the room or only on those who look most interested. How you look at the audience is also important—pleasantly, personally, and with sincerity. You want to convey that you are pleased to be there, that you have something important to say, and that you want them to believe that the message is important.

Delivering the Conclusion

The audience may be keeping track of your three or more points and may thus know that you are almost finished. However, you should still signal that you are coming to a conclusion by using such phrases as "in conclusion" or "in summary." The conclusion should be quite short; once you say "in summary," do not go on and on, and certainly do not say "in summary" multiple times! Come rapidly to the end.

Co-presenting or Co-leading Group Sessions

Often two people will be involved in making the presentation. This has many advantages: you can prepare together, and each brings special strengths. This is likely to increase the quality of the presentation. When you are co-presenting, you can draw energy from each other. By interacting with each other, you are likely to be more lively and enthusiastic. In addition, many of the tasks described earlier can be shared. Thus, while one person is speaking, the other can be monitoring the audience and keeping track of time and how the content is being covered. Co-presenters can also help each other out if necessary. If one gets off track or goes blank, the other can jump in. Experienced co-presenters have suggested the following formats for how two presenters can work together (Garmston & Bailey 1988):

- *Tag team.* In the tag-team format, one person presents and then the other does. This method is especially useful for those who do not regularly co-present together or when there is considerable material to cover and it is easier for each person to become an expert for each segment.
- *Speak and add.* In the speak-and-add format, one person is the lead presenter and the other is the support person. The lead is in charge of the content and decides when and how to proceed. The support person adds information when it seems useful or appropriate.
- *Speak and chart.* In the speak-and-chart format, the lead person presents content and elicits responses from the audience, and the support person records the information on newsprint or on an overhead transparency. Both presenters must be clear about their roles, and the support person must be able to record the ideas of the lead or the audience quickly and without comment.
- *Duet.* In the duet format, both presenters are on stage together and each presents content in small chunks of about two minutes each. The presentation thus goes back and forth. The presenters stand five to seven feet apart, but look at the audience and each other to cue each other in. They may move toward each other when they speak and move back when they are not speaking. This works best when the two people are experienced presenters or have rehearsed carefully.

Delivering Nutrition Education Workshops

The term *workshop* is used to describe many different kinds of group sessions. Usually, the term refers to some kind of professional development activity, but this is not always the case. Generally, workshops run longer than presentations do, but not always. They also usually involve more than one leader—but again, not always. What they *do* have in common is that they involve active participation of the group members. Workshops usually consist of a number of the activities described earlier in this chapter: presentations, group discussions, and group activities, which will not be repeated here.

The workshop can be structured somewhat like a presentation in the sense of having an introduction, a body, and a conclusion. The workshop usually begins with a group introductory activity or icebreaker to establish a safe environment and sense of cohesiveness. If the group is small enough, you can ask participants to state what they most want from the experience. This is then followed by an overview of the objectives of the workshop, the main issues to be covered, and expectations.

You can deliver the main body of the workshop using a variety of formats to address all the learning styles discussed earlier. This involves a sequence proposed in the design system described earlier. Thus, there should be concrete hands-on experiences or self-assessments to investigate the audience's own prior knowledge, attitudes, or behaviors; mini-presentations of needed information; time for work in groups to develop skills; and opportunity to apply the skills in their professional or personal lives.

The conclusion should be carefully planned to bring a sense of closure to the workshop, to summarize what has been accomplished, and to provide an opportunity for the group members to state how they plan to use the information and skills in the future.

■ SUMMARY

Working with groups is at the heart of nutrition education. This chapter describes many ways for nutrition educators to work with groups. Different methods work for different audiences, different situations, and different purposes. The aim in all cases, however, is for the method used to be effective in communicating the objectives of the messages you designed in such a way that the group becomes motivated to actively contemplate your message and to take action when appropriate. Effective communication involves understanding the communication process and the factors that influence it. Working with groups requires understanding different learning styles and how best to create a safe and challenging learning environment for all. It also requires understanding group dynamics and being able to manage difficult situations. Working with groups is challenging and hard work, in both planning and delivery. However, working with groups can be very rewarding for you, the nutrition educator, and a great experience for participants when the environment is safe and the learning experience is carefully planned and effectively delivered.

Questions and Activities

1. Think back to an occasion in a professional setting when you presented an idea for a group to consider and act on. Analyze your interaction in terms of the purpose of your communication and the effect on your listeners. Were you successful in your communication? Why or why not?

2. On a sheet of paper, create a table with two columns. Label one "Characteristics that make nutrition educators *effective* communicators in a group setting." Label the other one "Characteristics that make nutrition educators *ineffective* communicators in a group setting." In each column, list and briefly describe what you think are the five most important characteristics for that category. Candidly review your current strengths and weaknesses in terms of these characteristics. Pick three you would most like to improve.

3. Describe four learning styles that have been identified by some educators. Which kind of learning style best describes you? What can you do to make a group learning experience effective for different kinds of learners?

4. Compare and contrast the following methods for delivering nutrition education to groups: lectures, demonstrations, debates, and facilitated group discussions.

5. Describe authoritarian, democratic, and laissez-faire social climates in terms of the impact of each on the amount of learning that takes place, work accomplished or productivity, and feelings of the group. Have you experienced each of these kinds of social climate? How did you respond in each case? Which did you prefer? Why?

6. List four things you could do to create a safe learning environment for a group of adults. Would you plan the same way if the group was an after-school program made up of upper elementary school children? Explain.

7. If you were the leader of a group, how would you handle the following kinds of group members? Quiet members, complainers, those who dominate the conversation, digressors, those engaged in side conversations, and those who are consistently late.

8. What are some key features for holding the attention of a group when you are making an oral presentation?

9. Why is the introduction to a presentation or talk so important? What are its key components?

10. Why is it important to have a speaking outline?

11. Compare how you usually deliver oral presentations with five of the recommendations in this chapter. Candidly evaluate how many of these recommendations you have been using. Which of the recommendations do you think you will adopt in the future and why? What would you add to the list of recommendations in this chapter, based on your own experience?

12. Rehearse in front of the mirror a presentation you are planning to give. What do you think you are conveying nonverbally?

13. List all the ways you can enhance your credibility as a nutrition educator when you lead a group or make a presentation.

References

Abusabha, R., J. Peacock, and C. Achterberg. 1999. How to make nutrition education more meaningful through facilitated group discussions. *Journal of the American Dietetic Association* 99:72–76.

Achterberg, C. 1988. Factors that influence learner readiness. *Journal of the American Dietetic Association* 88:1426–1428.

Beffa-Negrini, P., and N. L. Cohen. 1990. Use of learning style theory in the development of a nutrition education program to reduce cancer risk. *Journal of Nutrition Education* 22:106A–B.

Brookfield, S. 1986. *Understanding and facilitating adult learning: A comprehensive analysis of principles and effective practices*. San Francisco: Jossey-Bass.

Freire, P., and I. Shor. 1987. *A pedagogy for liberation: Dialogues on transforming education*. New York: Bergin & Garvey.

Gagne, R. 1985. *The conditions of learning and theory of instruction*. 4th ed. New York: Holt, Rinehart, & Winston.

Garmston, R., and S. Bailey. 1988, January. Paddling together: A co-presenting primer. *Training and Development Journal* 52–56.

Gillespie, A.H., and P. Yarbrough. 1984. A conceptual model for communicating nutrition. *Journal of Nutrition Education* 17:168–172.

Husing, C., and M. Elfant. 2005. Finding the teacher within: A story of learner-centered education in California WIC. *Journal of Nutrition Education and Behavior* 37(Suppl. 1):S22.

Johnson, D., and F. Johnson. 1991. *Joining together: Group theory and group skills*. Englewood Cliffs, NJ: Prentice Hall.

Kinzie, M. B. 2005. Instructional design strategies for health behavior change. *Patient Education and Counseling* 56:3–15.

Knowles, M. S. 1990. *The adult learner: A neglected species*. 4th ed. Houston, TX: Gulf.

Kolb, D. A. 1984. *Experiential learning*. Englewood Cliffs, NJ: Prentice Hall.

Lewin, K. 1935. *A dynamic theory of personality*. New York: McGraw-Hill.

———. 1943. Forces behind food habits and methods of change. In *The problem of changing food habits* (National Research Council Bulletin 108). Washington, DC: National Academy of Sciences.

———. 1947. Frontiers in group dynamics. I. Concept, method, reality in social science: Social equilibria and social change. *Human Relations* 1:5–41.

———. 1948. *Resolving social conflicts: Selected papers on group dynamics*. New York: Harper.

———. 1951. Field theory in social science. *Selected Theoretical Papers*. New York: Harper.

———. 1958. Group decision and social change. In *Readings in social psychology*, edited by T. M. Newcomb and E. L. Hartley. New York: Holt, Rinehart, & Winston.

Lewin, K., R. Lippitt, and R. K. White. 1939. Patterns of aggressive behavior in experimentally created "social climates." *Journal of Social Psychology* 10:271–299.

McCarthy, P. 2005. Touching hearts to impact lives: Harnessing the power of emotion to change behaviors. *Journal of Nutrition Education and Behavior* 37(Suppl. 1):S19.

Olson, C. M., and G. L. Kelly. 1989. The challenge of implementing theory-based intervention research in nutrition education. *Journal of Nutrition Education* 22:280–284.

Petty, R. E., and J. T. Cacioppo. 1986. *Communication and persuasion: Central and peripheral routes to attitude change*. New York: Springer-Verlag.

Rogers, C. 1969. *Freedom to learn*. Columbus, OH: Merrill.

Sappington, T. E. 1984. Creating learning environments conducive to change: The role of fear/safety in the adult learning process. In *Innovative higher education*. New York: Human Services Press.

Sigman-Grant, M. 2004. *Facilitated dialogue basics: A self-study guide for nutrition educators—Let's dance*. University of Nevada, Cooperative Extension, NV.

Vella, J. 2002. *Learning to listen, learning to teach: The power of dialogue in educating adults*. Hoboken, NJ: Jossey-Bass.

CHAPTER 16

Beyond Groups:
Other Channels for Nutrition Education

OVERVIEW   This chapter provides an overview of how nutrition education can be delivered through various other channels, such as the use of visuals, printed materials, mass media strategies, and social marketing activities.

CHAPTER OUTLINE

- Introduction
- Using supporting visuals in group sessions and oral presentations
- Developing and using written materials
- Educational activities using other channels
- Mass media and social marketing activities
- Using new technologies
- Summary

LEARNING OBJECTIVES   At the end of the chapter, you will be able to:

- Apply design principles for developing supporting visuals for group sessions and oral presentations and state guidelines for their use
- Develop written materials for use in nutrition education
- Describe how to deliver nutrition education through activities such as cooking, supermarket tours, and health fairs
- Understand key principles of health communications and social marketing
- Implement nutrition education social marketing activities
- Recognize that there are many other channels and venues for nutrition education

▪ INTRODUCTION

A nutrition educator has been asked to speak to a class of teenagers about healthy eating. She begins the session by showing the group a number of food items familiar to this audience: a regular hamburger and a supersized one, and a variety of highly processed packaged snacks. She then shows them a can of solid shortening (fat used in baking) and asks them how many teaspoons of fat are present in each food. She does this as follows. Using a teaspoon, she begins to spoon out the shortening onto a plate until the audience tells her to stop. There are gasps in the group when they see how much fat is present in their favorite foods and snacks.

An old saying tells that one picture is worth a thousand words. People understand what speakers say, find it more interesting, and remember more when visual and other media are used in addition to the verbal message. As noted in an earlier chapter, people remember 20% of what they hear but 50% of what they both see and hear and 90% when they are actively involved in talking about it as they do something. Today's audiences grew up in the television and computer ages and are used to obtaining information visually as well as orally. About 99%

of households have television and adults spend an average of 15 to 17 hours weekly watching. Some two thirds of households have computers and spend several hours each day on them, particularly young people. People watch videos and see advertising billboards. They are used to being bombarded with information and persuasion from a variety of high-quality media sources. These media affect all age groups.

Using visual aids and written supporting materials with presentations or group discussions is thus important for nutrition education. These supporting media might include slides, overhead transparencies, models, food packages, handouts, or other materials. When the supporting materials are of high quality, they will enhance your credibility, make you seem more prepared, and enhance the effectiveness of your message. Supporting visual media are especially important for low-income groups who have limited reading ability and for those whose first language is not English. When real foods are used and tasted, the addition of other senses, such as sight and touch, as well as smell and taste, enhances the message.

Channels other than group sessions and oral presentations can also be important for delivering nutrition education messages, such as health fairs, church newsletters, billboards, social marketing media campaigns, or Web-based interventions. These channels are becoming increasingly important as people have less and less time to attend group sessions.

This chapter describes the use of visual and written media as supporting aids for group sessions as well as the use of other channels to deliver supporting nutrition education for the group intervention.

■ USING SUPPORTING VISUALS IN GROUP SESSIONS AND ORAL PRESENTATIONS

Humans are visual creatures. When news stories on television about events such as tsunamis, hurricanes, or earthquakes are accompanied by visual images, particularly those showing the suffering of individuals, the impact is dramatic. Often before the news program is over, relief organizations are deluged by calls from viewers wanting to make a donation.

Using supporting visuals or visual aids in nutrition education has many advantages, chief among them being that they make your message clearer and more lively. You can outline the main points and thus help the audience or group follow the key messages you wish to convey. Or you can show real objects or pictures, or present a graph of the statistics that you are quoting. These will make the message more vivid. Using supporting visuals also stimulates interest. And, of course, your audience will be more likely to remember your message. In the scenario at the beginning of the chapter, the teens will be more likely to remember how much fat is in some common foods because of the demonstration, and this may help them in their food choices. The next subsection discusses various visual media that you can use. Consider the following questions as you choose which to use:

- Who is the audience? What kinds of visual media are most appropriate for this audience? For example, a low-literacy audience may need different kinds of visuals from a highly educated audience.
- What will the audience prefer?
- What is the setting? Will you be in the front of a long room in which people in the back will be able to see slides but not real objects such as foods?
- What is the size of the audience? Ten, 25, 50, or 100 or more? Some visuals, such as food models, work well only with a small audience, whereas others, such as slides, can work with larger audiences.

- What equipment is available in the room?
- What length of time do you have? What kinds of visuals will fit into that time? For example, a videotape may take too long, but you could use excerpts.
- How much time do you have to prepare the visuals?
- What skills do you have to develop the visuals that you need? Can someone else assist you?

Types of Supporting Visuals

You can use a variety of visuals to support and reinforce your message, ranging from real foods to slides.

Real Objects: Foods and Packages

Showing real foods or packages can have a dramatic impact and make your objectives clearer. For example, a session on the importance of eating a variety of fruits and vegetables can begin with you bringing in an array of differently colored fruits and vegetables and asking the audience if they can identify them or have tasted them. You can bring in and show low-fat food products for a session on reducing fat in the diet. You can also bring in a variety of packaged food products for a session on label reading or as examples of low-fat snacks. Real objects are especially useful for showing portion sizes of different items, such as sodas or small, medium, and large sizes of movie-theater popcorn.

It is best to bring in *empty* packages and containers (such as empty soda cans and popcorn buckets), particularly for the less healthful items: they are easier to carry, you do not have to worry about the foods perishing, and you do not have to decide what to do when individuals want to take the items home! To avoid distraction for the audience, it is best to keep these kinds of visuals out of sight until you are ready to show them. It is also useful to bring in cups and measuring spoons if you want to show serving sizes of foods.

- *Advantages:* Realistic; dramatic; enhances motivation; improves understanding of the message and increases retention. Objects and packages are portable.
- *Disadvantages:* Some foods are perishable; not suitable for groups larger than 15 to 20 members.

Models of Foods and Other Nutrition-Related Objects

Models of foods are actual-sized, realistic, three-dimensional models made of plastic or rubber. They are especially useful for showing the sizes of servings of foods recommended by dietary guidelines and for foods that are perishable, such as meats (e.g., hamburger, chicken). Other kinds of models can also be used, such as models of the heart or of clogged arteries.

- *Advantages:* Food models are realistic, portable, and can show actual portion sizes of foods. Other models can be selected to illustrate complex organs or processes.
- *Disadvantages:* Cannot be seen in groups larger than 15 to 20 members.

Poster Boards

For many settings, poster boards prepared ahead of time can be very effective. Pictures from magazines or empty packages of various kinds of food items can be mounted onto poster boards for display. You may also be able to glue on pockets in which you place various pictures or cards of items that you can pull out to show as you need. You can also display pie charts, bar graphs, and line graphs. You may develop a collection of these poster boards to use for sessions focusing on different behaviors.

How exactly to keep poster boards standing presents a challenge that must be resolved before the occasion. A sturdy grade of poster board or foamcore and a method to keep it standing must be devised.

- *Advantages:* Inexpensive; portable; very helpful when there is not much equipment in the room.
- *Disadvantages:* Fragile when carried; limited amount of information; cannot be used with large groups; can get worn with repeated use.

Flip Charts

A flip chart with a display easel is very useful in a setting without much equipment. Flip charts consist of large pads of newsprint sheets that are fastened or glued together at the top. Write on the newsprint with crayon or felt-tip pens that do not bleed through the paper. Use a dark-colored pen, and write large enough for everyone in the group to read. You can prepare the sheets ahead of time to contain graphs, pie charts, written outlines, clip art, and so forth. Each sheet is flipped over at the top when you have finished showing the information. Flip charts are particularly useful for group brainstorming activities. The ideas can be recorded and then the sheets torn off and attached to a wall or blackboard for all to see. The sheets can also be taken away after the meeting. Use of different-colored pens can be very helpful.

- *Advantages:* Inexpensive; prepared flip charts can be reused from group to group; appropriate in informal settings such as senior centers or community programs; audience friendly, particularly when information is being collected from the group; information collected during the session can be preserved.
- *Disadvantages:* Cannot be seen in groups larger than 20 to 25 members; inconvenient to carry; requires someone to write clearly and quickly if it is being used to capture ideas of a group; prepared flip charts can get worn with repeated use.

Chalkboard

The chalkboard, too, can serve as a visual aid. It can be very useful if you write legibly and large enough for all to see and can spell well.

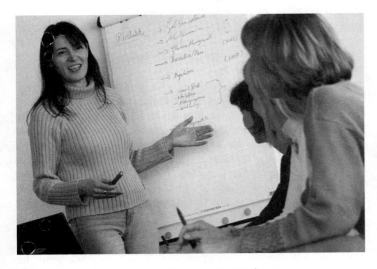

Flip charts are an inexpensive way to engage your audience.

However, it is important not to turn your back to the audience and talk to the board. It also takes time to write on the board, so you need to practice talking and writing at the same time, while facing the audience as much as possible during the process.

- *Advantages:* Inexpensive; easy to use.
- *Disadvantages:* Presenter often talks to the board; takes time to write material; poor handwriting reduces effectiveness.

Slides (PowerPoint, Freelance, Persuasion, Presentation)

Increasingly, those making presentations or working with groups use computer software programs such as Microsoft PowerPoint, Lotus Freelance, Adobe Persuasion, or Corel Presentation to create images involving just about everything from text to graphs, charts, and tables (**Figure 16-1**). Photographs can also be scanned in with high fidelity. There are ways to include animation, sound, and video clips, allowing for multimedia presentations. The images are sharp and multicolored and can be made any size you need. The presentation can be printed out on paper and used as a handout at the beginning of the session for the audience to follow along or at the end as reinforcement.

It is best to use colors and graphics on the slides that can be seen without turning off the lights. This helps you maintain contact with the audience. Make the slides visually compelling (**Figure 16-2**)—use of high technology does not automatically make a presentation interesting. There are now many designs to choose from, and you should exploit these options.

It takes considerable time to learn how to use the software; design the text, graphs, and charts; import images from other sources; and organize all these in a way that is appropriate. So, give yourself plenty of time to create the visuals. Arrive early and run through your presentation before the audience or group arrives. In addition, always carry a backup disk or flashdrive. If you have printed out your slides as handouts, you can use the handouts as the basis of your talk if the equipment fails. Finally, be prepared to give your presentation or conduct the group session without the slides if you have to!

- *Advantages:* PowerPoint-type slides provide high-quality lettering, charts, and graphics. Careful use of color and animation can enhance motivation. Your presentation can be saved to a CD or a flashdrive or mini-drive and easily transported from your home or office to the place of presentation. Slides are relatively easy to create once you have learned the program.
- *Disadvantages:* The necessary equipment is expensive and not always available in field settings for nutrition education such as senior centers, after-school settings, or community group education. Use of slides can distance you from the audience, especially when the room is dark and you cannot see the audience. It is easy to put too much information on a slide.

Design Principles for Preparing Supporting Visuals

You have probably experienced the presenter who begins a presentation by saying, "I know that you can't read this, but . . ." You wonder why the presenter even bothered with the supporting visual! Whatever the form of the supporting visuals you are preparing, following certain guidelines will help you make them effective (Smith & Alford 1989; Knight & Probart 1992; Raines & Williamson 1995). Public speaking expert Lucas (2004) provides useful guidelines that have been adapted here for use in nutrition education.

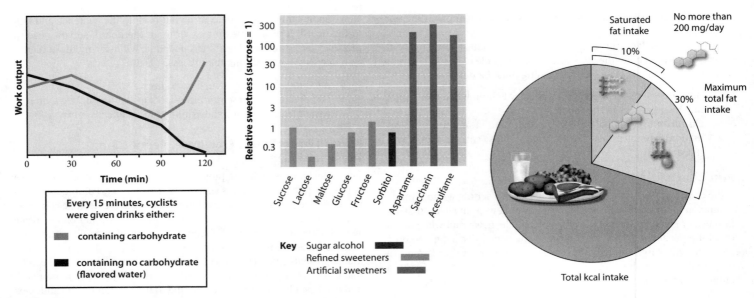

FIGURE 16-1 Example of effective line chart, bar graph, and pie chart presentations.

Source: Insel, P., R.E. Turner, and D. Ross. 2004. *Nutrition.* 2nd ed. Sudbury, MA: Jones and Bartlett Publishers.

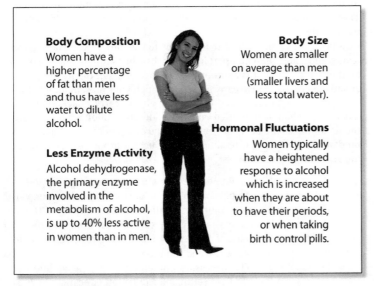

FIGURE 16-2 Example of effective slide presentation.

Source: Insel, P., D. Ross, K. McMahon, and M. Bernstein. 2010. *Nutrition.* 4th ed. Sudbury, MA: Jones and Bartlett Publishers.

Clear and Simple Supporting Visuals

Supporting visuals should be simple, clear, and directly relevant to your message. They are aids, not the centerpiece. Use only as many real objects and models as are necessary to help visualize what you are talking about. Make slides, flip charts, and overhead transparencies concise; use the fewest words possible, to which you will add as you speak. Thus, the visual will contain much less information than you will actually present: it should not be something that you will read word for word and say nothing else. Each slide or overhead should present only one idea or one set of ideas. It is suggested that the number of words

be limited to between 20 and 36. Some have recommended "the rule of six," which is to use no more than six lines of text and no more than six words per line (Raines & Williamson 1995). This may be overly restrictive, but the principle is not to load the slide with information from margin to margin.

Reproductions of tables and graphs from journal articles or books are rarely effective. Such tables are meant to be studied at the reader's leisure while being held about a foot or so away. They cannot be processed and understood in the few seconds available during a presentation. Unless you are presenting to a professional audience, simplify the tables and graphs and render them boldly so that they can be understood quickly (**Figures 16-3** and **16-4**). In addition, carefully consider the background you will use. Computer software programs provide numerous different background formats from which to select. However, use simple designs. When you make supporting visuals too busy or complicated or you put too much information on them, you are more likely to confuse your group than enlighten them.

Supporting Visuals Large Enough for the Audience to See

Presenters often have the urge to put a lot of information on the supporting visuals and hence to make the information too small. Remember, though, that if no one can see it, it is not only useless but also may provoke annoyance of the audience. Think about the size of the audience and their distance from you as you select or make your visuals.

For computer-generated slides, use font sizes that can be read from the back of the room when projected. It is recommended that for titles you use font sizes of 36 points; for subtitles, 24 points; and for the text, 18 points. Making fonts bold may increase readability. Capital letters are suitable for short titles of five to six words or fewer, but a combination of capital and lowercase letters is preferable for longer titles. All caps are more difficult to read, especially for those of lower literacy (Smith & Alford 1989). Number lists or use bullets, and underline words for emphasis. Keep paragraphs short.

Older students' (4th - 6th grade) pre-test and post-test scores. Analysis of Variance (ANOVA) comparing the four study conditions on the pre-test and post-test, and post hoc analysis to calculate significant differences between specific groups; unit of analysis is students

	Older students, 4th-6th grade									
	Pre-test					Post-test				
	CS + FEL 4 classes	CS only 5 classes	FEL only 4 classes	Com. 3 classes		CS + FEL 4 classes	CS only 5 classes	FEL only 4 classes	Com. 3 classes	
	M±SD (n)	M±SD (n)	M±SD (n)	M±SD (n)	F p**	M±SD (n)	M±SD (n)	M±SD (n)	M±SD (n)	F p
Preferences for plant foods (range 1-5)	2.96±.61 (68)	3.14±.61 (86)	3.20±.64 (65)	3.26±.71 (42)	2.56 NS	3.30±.58[ab] (68)	3.49±.59[a] (84)	3.11±.59[b] (61)	3.29±.62[ab] (43)	5.06 .002
Attitudes (range 1-4)	2.63±.44[a] (68)	2.83±.41[b] (83)	3.01±.42[c] (63)	2.73±.34[ab] (42)	10.16 <.001	2.78±.43 (67)	2.83±.46 (82)	2.91±.46 (65)	2.76±.42 (39)	1.32 NS
Knowledge (range 0-12)	9.68±3.19[a] (68)	11.67±3.13[b] (86)	11.48±3.42[b] (66)	10.26±2.84[ab] (43)	6.40 <.001	16.96±3.72[a] (68)	16.19±3.31[ab] (86)	14.48±3.73[b] (66)	11.05±2.81[c] (43)	29.77 <.001
Self-efficacy in cooking (range 1-4)	3.22±.52 (68)	3.31±.47 (86)	3.26±.41 (66)	3.18±.53 (42)	.85 NS	3.31±.43[a] (68)	3.50±.33[b] (86)	3.28±.49[a] (66)	3.27±.54[a] (43)	4.51 .004
Behavioral Intentions										
Food Intentions Subscale (range 1-4)	2.23±.60 (68)	2.33±.62 (84)	2.38±.49 (65)	2.25±.48 (41)	1.03 NS	2.30±.60 (67)	2.40±.60 (85)	2.33±.55 (64)	2.67±.52 (43)	.38 NS
Paired Food Choice Subscale (range 0-7)	2.34±1.38 (68)	2.67±1.57 (84)	2.58±1.37 (65)	2.37±1.13 (43)	.89 NS	2.92±1.38 (66)	2.95±1.70 (82)	2.95±1.43 (62)	2.59±1.38 (41)	.65 NS

CS = Cookshops
FEL = Food & Environment Lessons
Com. = Comparison
Com. = Comparison
higher scores are always "better"

[abc] different superscripts signify significant differences between those study groups
* n reported for each group was the number of students who took both the pre and post test; actual number of students in the classes was much larger
** ANOVA calculated significant differences among the four groups; to calculate significant differences between specific pairs of groups, Tukey Homogeneous Group Subsets Tests were used

FIGURE 16-3 Example of ineffective presentation of data for general audiences.

Cookshop Results for Older Children (Grades 4–6)

	Cookshop + lessons	Cookshop only	Lessons only	Control	Pre-post Cookshop (Lessons)
Preferences for plant foods (1-5)	3.2	3.4	3.1	2.8	<.001 (ns)
Attitudes (1-4)	2.8	2.8	2.9	3.2	ns (ns)
Knowledge (0-25)	16.1	16.1	14.1	11.3	<.001 (<.05)
Self-efficacy in cooking (1-4)	3.2	3.3	3.0	3.0	<.05 (ns)
Plate waste (%)	74	78	91	97	<.10 (ns)

FIGURE 16-4 Example of good presentation of data for general audiences.

Choice of Colors

Use of color increases attention. However, it is possible to have too many colors in a supporting visual. Use color sparingly and design it carefully. Use one to three colors at the most, and use them consistently. It is best to decide on the major focus of the visual and select that color first. An effective practice is to select dark lettering or print on a light background. Some argue for using a dark background, particularly dark blue. In this case the graphics and lettering should be larger and white, or some strongly contrasting, bright color such as yellow. Do not use black on blue. The biggest danger in using a dark background is that the lettering and graphics may not be bright enough to see. In addition, a dark background usually requires that the room lights be dimmed, which means you lose touch with your audience.

Appropriate Fonts

Most computers come with dozens if not hundreds of different fonts or typefaces that you can use. It is best to choose those that are simple and easy to read. Also, limit the number of different fonts you use in any given presentation. For example, use a squarer font in capitals for the title and a rounder font for the text. The rounder fonts are usually called *serif* because they have little feet. The squarer typefaces are called *sans* (from the French meaning "without") *serif*, or without feet. A third style is called *decorative* and includes all those that do not belong in the other two categories.

The following list presents some common fonts and their appropriateness.

More Effective	Less Effective
Courier (serif)	Apple Chancery
Times or Times New Roman (serif)	Lucinda Handwriting
Arial (sans serif)	Harrington
Helvetica (sans serif)	**Textile**

Guidelines for Using Supporting Visuals

Having selected or designed your supporting visuals with care, you need to give careful consideration to how you will use them when you are with your group. You will want to ensure that you use them effectively to get your message across.

Ensure That Your Audience Will Be Able to See Your Visuals

When you plan on using visuals such as poster boards, be sure to arrive early so that you can identify where you will place them so that all can see. Will you have access to easels? If not, where can you place them so that they will not fall over? If you are using objects, where will you place them so that all those in the audience can see? If you are using slides or overheads, do not stand in front of them and block the vision of the audience.

Show Your Supporting Visuals at the Appropriate Time

If you are using real objects such as food, food models, or food packages, do not show them to the audience until you are talking about them with the group. Leave them in cardboard boxes or bags until you are ready, or cover them up if you need to place them on a table in front of the audience. The same is true of poster boards or flip charts. Ensure that a blank sheet or a sheet with the title of the session is facing the audience as they come in. Likewise, for slides and transparencies, use a title slide as the audience or group enters, and introduce a blank (for slides) or cover up a transparency when you are not using the visuals. When you are finished, cover them up or put them away so as not to distract the audience.

Maintain Contact with Your Audience at All Times

When you use overhead transparencies, slides, or poster boards, you might often find yourself facing the visuals and not your audience. Be sure you only glance at the visuals and continue talking to your audience so that you maintain eye contact with them.

Use Handouts and Materials Appropriately

You may have only one visual, such as a photo or object, that you want to pass around while you speak. However, doing so will cause you to lose the attention of those who currently have it in hand and are looking at it and distract all the others who are wondering about it. At professional meetings you may hand out copies of your PowerPoint presentation for the audience to follow along and take notes. Do so at the beginning or place them on the chairs before the audience comes in. But in most other settings, it is best to pass out materials such as handouts at the end. If you make handouts for everyone and wish to hand them out at various times, do so at strategic points and allow time for all individuals to receive them before proceeding. Recognize, however, that these actions may be distracting.

■ DEVELOPING AND USING WRITTEN MATERIALS

Written materials in this context refers to short printed pieces such as handouts, flyers, brochures, tip sheets, booklets, and recipes that will be used with some intended nutrition education audience. Printed materials have many advantages compared with the other media described so far. Printed materials can be kept. Whereas messages in the visual media fly by, people can read and digest printed information at their own pace and refer to it over time. Printed media can provide information that can be read in private. Many individuals may be reluctant to ask questions in a group setting or to discuss issues they have. But they may be eager to receive information provided in handouts or brochures that they can take home. And, of course, printed materials can reinforce information discussed in a group setting or provided in a presentation.

The design of written materials should involve similar considerations to that of the six-step model used to design the group intervention itself. Many of the guidelines described earlier for designing supporting visuals apply to supporting printed pieces as well. This section highlights guidelines that may be useful for nutrition educators who are developing simple supportive materials. The advent of desktop publishing makes it possible for most people to develop and design a variety of materials that is pleasing to the eye and of good quality. However, the services of a graphic designer, professional writer, or editor may be necessary to ensure high quality in the design and readability of written materials.

Planning the Printed Piece

The effectiveness of printed materials is improved if you have clear answers for the following questions for each printed piece:

- *What is the primary purpose for each printed piece?* If you could accomplish just one goal, what would it be? Is this a promotional piece designed to generate interest in the group program or is it an information piece that will be used in conjunction with the program? You should be able to say, "The primary purpose of this flyer is to get people to come to the group nutrition education session" or "The purpose of this poster is to make eating a variety of colors of fruits and vegetables seem cool to teens." In other words, is the purpose to enhance motivation to take action and activate decision making (why-to information), or is the material to be used to reinforce the session by providing food and nutrition information that facilitates skills acquisition (how-to information), or some combination of both? What theoretical framework is being used? Which personal mediators of behavior change are addressed? In the example just given with teens, the purpose is to enhance motivation by addressing social norms (why to take action)—a primary theory construct in both social cognitive theory and theory of planned behavior.
- *What are the secondary purposes?* A printed piece usually has more than one goal. However, when you try to accomplish several goals, you risk not accomplishing any of them very well. So, think carefully about which goal is your primary purpose and which goals are secondary. Perhaps the primary goal of your poster is to increase motivation, but you also want the poster to have information about eating five to nine servings of fruit and vegetables a day (how-to information). If this is your secondary purpose, you will want to consider a format that makes this clear—perhaps by using smaller lettering or positioning it lower on the page. Remember that there are also unstated purposes, which are the impressions people get from reading your printed piece. In the previously mentioned case of posters for teens, if the posters are hung up or placed in the cafeteria, the unstated purpose may be that the school is concerned about teens' health and welfare. A common unstated purpose is for the reader to see you as professional and credible, or to see your organization or agency as a leader in the field.
- *What actions or behaviors do you want the audience to take?* What do you want individuals to do as a result of reading your piece? Individuals are more likely to take action if you lay out specific suggestions for what actions they can take. For example,

in a brochure on cancer risk prevention, what specific actions are you aiming for? Do you want the individuals to go to a medical facility to get screened? Then spell out how to do so. Do you want them to eat more fruits and vegetables? Then say so and tell them how to do so. Is it a policy document about actions a school can take to ensure a healthy school food environment? Then spell out what a school can do. What would you like the audience to do with the printed piece itself? Pass it on? Then say so. Put on the refrigerator door or on a bulletin board? Say so.

- *How will the printed piece be used?* Will the piece be used only in conjunction with the group intervention? Will it be used during the session and/or taken home? Or should it be able to stand alone?
- *Who is the intended audience?* What is their background in terms of cultural or religious traditions? What are their attitudes and values in relation to the issue or behavior you wish to address? What is most likely to get their attention? Here you should go back to Step 2 of the Stepwise Procedure model for designing nutrition education (Chapter 8) for details on conducting an audience analysis.

  What are the characteristics of the audience, such as age, sex, cultural group, or educational level, that might influence the nature and design of the piece? For example, individuals with low literacy skills will require different approaches than those with high levels of education. What does the intended audience prefer in terms of types of content and layout? A good needs analysis is extremely important here.
- *What length do you need?* A common urge is to want to tell the audience everything in one printed piece. But it is important to be selective. Do you have enough to say to require a booklet, or will a brochure do? Will a flyer do instead of a poster? If you have too much information for one printed piece, consider breaking up the information into several different handouts, flyers, or brochures.
- *What resources are available for this project?* The most frequently required resources are time, energy, and money. Needing a piece of printed material by a certain date will influence the nature of what you will be able to generate and produce. Likewise, your energy is limited. So, think through carefully what you are able to do given your time. Perhaps someone else can work on it or at least help you with it. Finally, most nutrition educators work with limited budgets. This calls for creativity and careful thinking. Perhaps instead of a poster, a flyer will do. Or a lighter paper will do. Or printing with several shades of one color will work as well as several colors.
- *How will you evaluate the effectiveness of these materials?* It is important to obtain feedback on the materials, if not from written evaluation forms then from asking the recipients of the materials. You may also discuss with other members of your team such questions as the following: Did the printed pieces fulfill their purpose? What did the readers learn from them? How much time, effort, and money did it take to produce them? Was it worth it? How can they be improved?

Making Your Printed Materials Motivating and Effective

You want your printed pieces to be effective with your audience. Some suggestions follow.

Tailor the Piece to Your Audience

Your audience will be more interested in your printed materials if they can immediately see that the information is relevant to them. This means that you need to know your audience well. A careful analysis as outlined in Steps 1 and 2 of the Stepwise Procedure model for designing nutrition education (described in Chapters 7 and 8) can provide you the information you need. In particular, you need to know the audience's food- and nutrition-related knowledge, their attitudes and values in relation to the issue in your printed material, their living situation, what magazines they read and what visual media they watch, and what their tastes are in terms of written materials.

Make the Writing Motivational and Reader-Friendly

Start with an Attention Grabber

It is important to gain and hold the attention of your readers just as you plan to do when designing lesson plans or presentations for an audience. Several ways to do this are by beginning your printed piece with one of the following:

- *An interesting anecdote or personal story, preferably of someone similar to the audience and involving a situation familiar to them.* "As a group of teens entered the school cafeteria last week, they were surprised to discover it had had a complete makeover and looked very cool."
- *A surprising fact or startling statistic.* "The rate of obesity is increasing. At current rates, all individuals in the United States will be overweight by the year *x*."
- *An intriguing question.* "Did you know that it has been estimated that one in three children today will develop diabetes during their lifetime?"
- *A checklist.* Create a checklist of foods or food-related behaviors addressed by the printed piece, such as a list of high-fat foods and fruits and vegetables, and ask readers to check off whether they eat them on most days. Come up with a score and tell them to read the rest of the printed material to learn how to eat a healthier diet.
- *A quiz.* Beginning with "Can you name five vegetables that are red or purple in color?" is likely to engage your readers.

Motivate the Reader

You are very interested in food, nutrition, and health, but you can't assume that the reader shares your enthusiasm! Describe the importance of the issue you are addressing, such as eating school meals. List the benefits of the actions you are writing about, such as eating breakfast or calcium-rich foods. Make clear to readers what is in this for them. Again, your needs analysis information from Step 2 is important here.

Put Important Information First

Assume that the reader will read just the first sentence, the first paragraph, or the first page. So place the most important information first rather than bury it in the middle of the document. Avoid lengthy introductions and long explanations at the beginning.

Be Simple and Direct

You are not writing a novel or poem. You are trying to communicate with the reader about important food- and nutrition-related information. So write simply and directly. To do this, consider the following tips:

- *Keep the words simple.* The field of nutrition is full of technical terms, and nutrition educators often use them when simple ones will do. Often the simplest words have the fewest syllables. Thus, use *better* instead of *more advantageous*, and *use* instead of *utilize*.

- *Use the active voice rather than passive voice.* Active voice makes the writing more personal and lively. For example, instead of "The program participants will be provided with handouts," say "The nutrition educator will provide program participants with handouts."
- *Write strong sentences.* Vary the length of sentences, but generally keep them short. Varying the length of sentences changes the pace for readers and makes the writing more interesting. But express only one idea per sentence. Long and complex sentences are difficult to understand and may discourage people, particularly those with low literacy, from reading. Aim for about 9 to 10 sentences per 100 words.
- *Keep paragraphs focused.* Begin sentences with the main topic. For example, say, "Watching your weight is very important when you have diabetes," rather than "When you learn that you have diabetes, it is important for you to watch your weight." Begin each paragraph with the topic sentence and keep the paragraph to one key idea or theme.
- *Aim for the right reading level.* Determine the appropriate reading level for your audience. It is often said that the eighth-grade reading level is best for most general printed pieces, and the fifth-grade level for low-literacy audiences. Computer programs will now give you information on the reading level or readability scores for the document you are writing. You can also calculate the SMOG (simple measure of gobbledygook) score as follows: take 10 sentences each from the beginning, middle, and last paragraphs of the document. Count how many words in these 30 sentences have three or more syllables (polysyllabic words) and look up the approximate grade level in **Table 16-1**. Readability is also influenced by concept density, so keep each paragraph to only one concept or message.
- *Be professional and accurate.* Writing can take on many different styles, from humorous to chatty to serious. Regardless of style, use a professional tone in your writing. Being concise, clear, and readable will increase your credibility. Make sure your information is accurate.
- *Use a positive tone.* This does not mean you should be a Pollyanna. You know only too well that the news in the area of foods and nutrition is often dire. It means speaking to your readers in a respectful and positive manner. Being negative or condescending does not help you communicate your message.
- *Be consistent in your vocabulary, particularly for technical information.* For example, use *hypertension* or *high blood pressure*, but not both interchangeably.

Design Considerations

Make the written material look easy to read. The following tips can help:

- *Keep the document as short as you can.* You might try to say too much in your printed materials. The piece ends up looking crowded and difficult to read—and so it is not read.
- *Use more headings and keep them simple.* Break up the piece with more headlines and make them vivid and informative. This way, the reader who only skims the piece will get something out of it. Rather than "Introduction," use "An Overview of the Senior Program." Instead of "Picky Eaters," use "Ways to Handle Picky Eaters."
- *Use more paragraphs and make them shorter.* Short paragraphs make for easier reading, especially in brochures and flyers. Long paragraphs make the page look dense and may discourage readers.
- *Include adequate white (empty) space.* Many educators think of empty or white space between paragraphs or in large margins as wasted space, waiting to be filled. However, it has been found that having adequate white space makes a piece easier to read. It is better to sacrifice some text than to have no white space.
- *Divide wide columns of text into two narrower columns for easier reading.* Lines that are too long strain the eye and make readers lose track of the content, whereas lines that are too short cause the eye to jump back and forth. A line length of 50 to 70 characters is best because it is less tiring to the eye.
- *Make text left justified with a ragged right margin.* Left-justified text with a ragged right margin is easier to read because the ragged right profile helps the eye distinguish one line from the next. Full justification (lines that go to the same left and right margins) is difficult to read because it is hard to distinguish the lines and the eye has to adjust to different spacing between letters. Indenting the paragraphs is also important.
- *Use a simple font, especially with low-literacy audiences.* As emphasized earlier for designing visuals, using simple fonts and adequate font sizes can help the reader, particularly low-literacy audiences. Remember also that all caps are more difficult to read.
- *Use bullets where appropriate.* Bullets are useful when the information lends itself to a list. Tips, procedures, and things to do can all be listed with bullets. Bulleted lists break up the text and make brochures, handouts, and tip sheets easier to read.

Examples of print materials from the Pick a Better Snack campaign are shown in **Figures 16-5** and **16-6**. Figure 16-5 shows an article about eating apples to be printed in a newspaper, and Figure 16-6 shows text that can be used for a flyer, poster, or print ad in a magazine or newspaper. You can see that these materials exemplify all the tips described earlier.

TABLE 16-1	Calculating Reading Levels: SMOG Conversion Table	

Total Polysyllabic Word Counts	Approximate Grade Level (± 1.5 grades)
0–2	4
3–6	5
7–12	6
13–20	7
21–30	8
31–42	9
43–56	10
57–72	11
73–90	12
91–110	13
111–132	14
133–156	15
157–182	16
183–210	17
211–240	18

Source: McLaughlin, G. H. 1969. SMOG grading: A new readability formula. *Journal of Reading* 12:639–646.

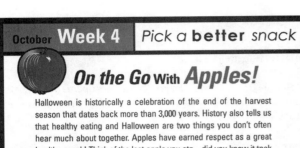

On the Go With *Apples!*

Halloween is historically a celebration of the end of the harvest season that dates back more than 3,000 years. History also tells us that healthy eating and Halloween are two things you don't often hear much about together. Apples have earned respect as a great healthy snack! Think of the last apple you ate – did you know it took the energy from 50 leaves to produce that one apple, which was most likely picked by hand just for you? No tricks involved – apples are a great treat, whether they're fresh, baked, microwaved, sauced or pressed for juice!

There are thousands of varieties of apples that come in all shades of reds, greens and yellows. Each has its own unique taste. Whichever type strikes your fancy, choose apples that are firm, without soft or bruised spots or wrinkled skin, and have a pleasant smell. Always wash apples with cold water before eating. Some apples are waxed to preserve freshness and increase storage time.

Wash. Eat. (how easy is that?)

Take Apples *With You!*

- Fill kids' bellies with apples and other healthy foods before they go out trick-or-treating. Chances are they won't overindulge as much on candy.

- Rent a Halloween movie. Munch on apple slices during the thriller.

- Try a new, food safety-friendly version of bobbing for apples. Cut an apple into slices. Tie one end of a piece of dental floss around each apple slice. Tie the free end of the floss to a broom handle. Have each person, holding his/her hands behind their back, take a bite of the apple slice as it swings through the air. Use a fresh piece of floss and apple slice with each person.

- Sliced apples smeared with cream cheese or peanut butter or dipped in yogurt are a great snack when you're in a rush or on a road trip.

Quick Nibble:
Every single McIntosh apple tree has a "family tree" that goes back to the very first McIntosh, discovered by John McIntosh growing wild on his farm in Dundas County, Ontario. That tree lived for 90 years.

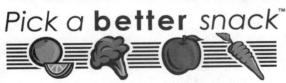

Pick a **better** snack™ was developed in partnership with the Iowa Nutrition Network and the USDA's Food Stamp Program and Team Nutrition – equal opportunity providers and employers. For more information about the Iowa Nutrition Network, call the **Iowa Department of Public Health** at **(800) 532-1579**.

Cut. Eat.

(how easy is that?)

Pick a **better** *snack*™

Serving Suggestions

Spread cabbage leaf with low-fat cream cheese. Roll it up and eat.

Dip cabbage wedges in a low-fat dressing. Use green or red cabbage.

Shred cabbage and mix with low-fat lemon yogurt. Add canned pineapple and mandarin oranges for a more interesting flavor.

Iowa Nutrition Network
PROMOTING HEALTHY LIFESTYLES

Provided by Iowa Nutrition Network, Iowa Dept. of Public Health, with funding from USDA's Food Stamp and TEAM Nutrition Programs.

FIGURE 16-5 (Left) Example of good printed material: Printed newspaper story using a template.
Source: Iowa Pick a Better Snack Social Marketing Campaign. http://www.idph .state.ia.us/pickabettersnack/default.asp. Used with permission of Iowa Nutrition Network, Iowa Department of Public Health and Iowa Department of Education.

FIGURE 16-6 (Above) Text that can be used for a flyer, poster, or print ad in a magazine or newspaper.
Source: Iowa Pick a Better Snack Social Marketing Campaign. http://www.idph .state.ia.us/pickabettersnack/default.asp. Used with permission of Iowa Nutrition Network, Iowa Department of Public Health and Iowa Department of Education.

A Caution

You may think that anything that is hands-on and innovative will be appreciated by your audiences. However, that may not always be the case. A survey of mothers in Head Start and Expanded Food and Nutrition Education Programs found that participants did not judge all program activities to be equally enjoyable or effective. Their evaluations led to the tips found in **Box 16-1**.

Box 16-1 Helping Low-Income Consumers Achieve the 5-a-Day Goal: Tips for Nutrition Educators

Focus group interviews and surveys with low-income women found that the following were effective and enjoyable ways to promote fruit and vegetable consumption.

Taste Testing

- Provide tasters with the recipe and demonstrate the preparation steps
- Offer ways to prepare "old favorites" (e.g., broccoli, carrots, apples)
- Offer the opportunity to taste new and unusual fruits and vegetables

Recipe Booklets

- Limit number of ingredients (no more than five)
- Ingredients should be low cost and on hand
- Limit number of steps; they should be quick and easy to do
- Do not include steps that use lots of dishes
- Do not use terms that people might not understand
- Include nutrition information about fat and calories
- Include a picture of how it should turn out
- Include tips for how to get the best buys when shopping for fruits and vegetables

Take-Home Items (Freebies) with Useful Information or Reminders

- Calendars (with reminders to eat fruits and vegetables; recipes; health information)
- Refrigerator magnets
- Magnetized shopping lists
- Tote bags
- Coffee mugs, or juice cups for kids
- Coloring books with recipes for kids
- Fruits and veggies (to make at home the recipes they tasted)

The following methods were least popular. Participants made the following suggestions for incorporating these elements if you decide to use them.

Videos

- Show videos for no more than 10 to 15 minutes at a time
- Select only videos that have "good actors" and "good music"
- Use food demonstrations and taste testing, or other hands-on activities, in conjunction with the video

Handouts or Brochures

- Discuss them with the group (don't just give to clients to take home)
- Make them colorful/appealing
- Keep them simple, to the point, and useful to the clients

Lecture-Style Presentation

- Be an enthusiastic speaker with a positive attitude
- Have personal experience with the topic
- Avoid use of technical terms (but also do not talk down to the group)

Source: Based on focus group interviews conducted in March 1996, with Expanded Food and Nutrition Education Program groups and Head Start and WIC moms (*n* = 61). Participants graded each of 20 methods using a scale ranging from A+ (12) to E (0). These methods included videos, group discussions, presentations, posters, refrigerator magnets, handouts, storybooks, coloring books and songs for children, recipes, mugs, and tote bags. The tips were generated from these scores. (Michigan Public Health Institute and Michigan Department of Community Health, presentation at the annual meeting of the Society for Nutrition Education, 1997.)

■ EDUCATIONAL ACTIVITIES USING OTHER CHANNELS

Nutrition educators engage in many activities in addition to conducting discussion groups, making presentations, and developing supporting written and visual materials. These include such activities as organizing health fairs and grocery store tours and conducting cooking classes. For all of these activities, plan ahead using the six-step Stepwise Procedure model for designing nutrition education described in Part II of this book.

Planning the Activity

The effectiveness of your activity is improved if you are clear about the following:

- *What is the specific purpose of the activity?* The objectives of the activity should be clear. You should be able to say, "The primary purpose of this activity is to get people to come to the group nutrition education session" or "The purpose of this activity is to teach skills in food selection (or in cooking) so that the audience

is able to follow the recommendations of the program." In other words, is the purpose to enhance motivation to take action and activate decision making (why-to information) or is it to provide food and nutrition information and facilitate skills acquisition for those already motivated (how-to information), or some combination of both? What theoretical framework is being used? Which personal mediators of behavior change will be addressed?

- *What actions or behaviors do you want the audience to take?* Do you want the behavioral outcome of the activity, such as a health fair, to be that participants will become aware of and attend the full program you are offering? Is it a freestanding activity with specific behavioral goals? For example, you may organize a health fair at which participants can be screened physiologically for a condition, such as blood pressure, or screened using a behavioral checklist, such as for their intake of fruits and vegetables. This may be followed by handouts about what to do. Thus, spell ut clearly what you wish the action outcomes to be for the activity.

Guidelines for Nutrition Education Through Other Channels

Channels such as cooking experiences, health fairs, or grocery store tours are useful for conveying food- and nutrition-related information. The following guidelines can help.

Cooking or Food Preparation as Nutrition Education

Just about everyone is interested in food, and participating in preparing it can be motivating. There is also evidence that cooking can be effective as a means of nutrition education beyond other hands-on activity-based nutrition education (Liquori et al. 1998; Brown & Hermann 2005). Consequently, nutrition education programs often include a session, or part of a session, in which the participants cook or prepare some items that they then all eat together. Following are some tips for conducting such activities.

Getting Started
Consider the following:

- *What are your objectives?* Be clear about the purpose or objectives of the food preparation activities. Do you wish to enhance motivation through the activity? For example, do you want to encourage the group members to try new foods? Is it an application of other material learned? Or is it primarily a skills-building activity for those already motivated? Do you want to assist participants to learn new ways of making familiar recipes more healthful?
- *What is the time frame?* What is the time frame that you have available for this activity? Is this a one-time session? How long? Or will this be a series of cooking sessions with a consistent group? These differences will influence your selection of objectives, recipes, and activities.
- *Who is your audience?* Do they come from a variety of ethnic groups with different cultural backgrounds, or are they somewhat homogeneous? Are they low income? These considerations will influence your recipe development.
- *What is the group's cooking skills level?* For example, are you working with teens with few skills or experienced older women with many skills? In all cases, make clear to the group the relationship of this activity to the rest of the nutrition education session or set of sessions.
- *What are the facilities?* Is there a stove in the setting or will you have to bring a butane stove or hot plate? Are there any utensils? Thus, you must check out the facilities ahead of time. If there are no cooking facilities and it is not possible for you to bring a heat source, you can still develop recipes that involve active food preparation such as making a salad. These factors will all influence the recipes you choose.
- *How large will the group be?* Will all the group members participate in the same food preparation or will you have several cooking stations preparing different recipes?
- *What ingredients and materials will you need?* Materials include all the utensils you will need as well as all the food items you will need. When bringing perishable foods, you need to consider issues of food safety, such as travel time in terms of keeping items cold and leaving food out at room temperature for any length of time. You may need to consider a cooler or ice packs. If you will have several stations, you may need several sets of utensils. If you have a lot of food materials, you will need sturdy boxes or suitcases on wheels.

Making the Cooking Experience Motivating and Effective
The following guidelines can help.

- *Tailor the experience to your audience.* Your audience will be more interested in food preparation if they can immediately see that the items being prepared are relevant to them, such as healthy and convenient snacks for teens or modifications of recipes for older adults. This means you need to know your audience well.
- *Make the cooking experience culturally appropriate.* One of the most visible and interesting ways in which people express their cultural and ethnic identity is through the food they will or will not eat. Hence, it is very important that the recipes you choose and the practices you recommend and teach take into consideration cultural differences between groups.
- *Test the recipes carefully ahead of time so that you know that they will work—no matter how simple they seem to be.* Test that they can be prepared in the setting in which the group will prepare them.
- *Always show respect for all participants.* Some may not like the recipes or have different levels of cooking skills, willingness to engage, and adventuresomeness in trying new foods. After all, preferences in food and eating are very personal. All participants bring valuable insights and past experiences to the table, and these should be honored.
- *Divide tasks into small group "assignments."* Each group may make a separate recipe or components of the same recipe.
- *Assemble all ingredients, materials, and utensils needed for each group ahead of time.* Place the ingredients for each group at a designated station or in a bag or box until you are ready to use them.
- *Review the recipes with the entire group.* Write the recipes on flip charts. If the group speaks English as a second language, record the recipe in their language of origin as well as in English. You may need to read the recipe, depending on the literacy level of the group.
- *Select the appropriate time within the session to do the food preparation activity.* You may lead a group discussion plus mini-lecture session first and conclude with the food activity as a skills development activity. Or you may have planned a series of cooking sessions for a group using food preparation as a primary form of nutrition education. In this case, interweave discussion of nutrition content with cooking, and provide motivational, why-to information as well as how-to food- and nutrition-related information. It is best not to talk too long before getting the group members started on the food preparation; provide information as you go along.
- *Review responsible cooking practices with the group.* These practices include the following:
  - Wash your hands before you begin, and wash them again if you cough, sneeze, or touch hair or face.
  - Be careful with knives—even plastic knives.
  - Treat everyone with respect.
  - Cooking is most fun when everyone cooperates.
  - Listen carefully to the instructions and ask questions if you don't understand.
  - If you don't want to eat something, politely say, "No, thank you." Do not say it is gross or nasty—someone else may love the taste.

Conclude with eating together if that is possible or appropriate. Make the ambience pleasant. Some nutrition educators bring paper tablecloths, and even vases of flowers, so that the eating experience is enjoyable.

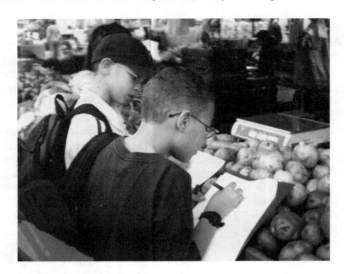

Nutrition education at the farmers' market.

Nutrition Education in Action 16-1 provides information on CookShop as an example of a program that uses cooking in the classroom as a means of nutrition education (Liquori et al. 1998; Wadsworth 2005).

Conducting Grocery Store and Farmers' Market Tours

Tours of grocery stores or farmers' markets can be a wonderful experience for all ages. As noted before, everyone loves food! Such tours can be conducted in a variety of markets, ranging from small to large, and can serve many purposes.

Getting Started

Consider the following:

- *What are your objectives?* Be clear about the purpose or objectives of the supermarket or farmers' market tour. Do you wish to enhance motivation through the activity? Is it an application of other material learned? Or is it primarily a skills-building activity for those already motivated? It is generally best to be focused. For example, will you focus on how to identify low-fat foods, or will you introduce people to the large variety of fruits and vegetables available? You should have determined these objectives in Step 4 of the Stepwise Procedure (Chapter 10).
- *Who is your audience?* Are they children or adults? This will make a difference in how the experience is structured. Are they of a particular ethnic or cultural group? Are they low in resources? Your audience assessment in Step 2 of the Stepwise Procedure can provide you with this information (Chapter 8).

Planning the Tour

Get approval if the tour is to take place in a grocery store, especially if you are bringing a group of children. This usually involves the manager. The 5-a-Day program encourages grocery stores to provide tours to children, and grocery stores are often happy to conduct them, seeing it as a good opportunity to encourage families to eat more fruits and vegetables and to generate positive community relations and media publicity. You will need to schedule a time that is convenient for the store as well as for your group. Approvals are not usually needed at most farmers' markets.

Develop an educational plan for the tour. This should be designed as part of Step 4 of the design model. Determine the specific educational objectives of the tour and design several activities to achieve them. For children and adults, develop activity sheets that they can complete while at the store or market. These may include a scavenger hunt of some sort to find specific foods, such as low-fat items or specific fruits and vegetables. Or make the participants food detectives. Make the activities humorous or brain-twisters so as to provide interest and challenge.

Map out how you will proceed inside the store or market. Make arrangements for where your group can congregate while you give them the information, and determine to what extent grocery store personnel will be involved.

Making the Experience Motivating and Effective

Make the tour a physically and mentally active experience. Do not just go from aisle to aisle talking about foods! In the store, carry out some verbal activities first. For example, a tour on fruits and vegetables can begin with questions such as "What colors do you see when you look at all these fruits and vegetables?" "Can you name a red fruit that you see? A green one?" and so forth (Dole Food Company 2001).

Provide clipboards, or the equivalent, so that participants can complete written activities. Perhaps you could have them complete some kind of self-assessment relevant to the foods of focus. Then send them on a food investigation tour with a series of questions in their activity sheets. Assign points for completing various activities. The store may be willing to provide taste testing of some fruits and vegetables or of recipes made from them. This would result in a tour that challenges all the senses.

Make the tour informative and relevant to your audience. With adults in particular, the tour should teach skills as well as enhance motivation. Perhaps you can teach preparation methods for various vegetables and supply recipes, point out lower-fat versions of food products, introduce them to whole grains of various kinds, and so forth.

Clearly, there are many options for what you can do, limited only by what your group is interested in and your creativity.

Health Fairs

Many nutrition education programs find that holding a health fair is a useful activity, particularly in worksites, colleges, and community centers. As is the case for the activities described earlier, you need to start with a clear understanding of the specific purpose of the activity and of the actions or behaviors you want the participants to take as a

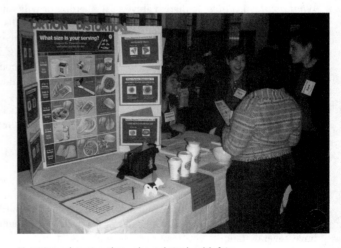

Nutrition education through worksite health fairs.

NUTRITION EDUCATION IN ACTION 16-1

CookShop

CookShop is a program of
the Food Bank For New York City

CookShop, the Food Bank For New York City's nutrition education program, provides low-income New Yorkers of all ages with the knowledge and information necessary to make healthy food choices for themselves and their families. With hands-on workshops, CookShop imparts nutrition information, teaches cooking skills, and fosters enthusiasm for fresh and affordable fruit, vegetables, legumes, and whole grains as well as offers an understanding of where food comes from, how food choices impact our bodies, and how to access healthy, affordable foods. Schools must apply to enroll in the program, and, to ensure consistent and successful implementation, teachers and peer educators receive extensive hands-on training from the Food Bank. CookShop began implementation as a classroom curriculum in New York City public schools in 1995, and now in 2010 it includes four components: CookShop Classroom, CookShop for Teens, CookShop for Adults, and CookShop Social Marketing.

CookShop Classroom is based in more than 700 elementary and after-school classrooms, reaching more than 14,000 students. The three 19-week elementary-school curricula—specifically designed for kindergarten, first-grade, and second-grade students—along with the 12-week after-school curriculum for mixed age groups, capitalize on students' natural curiosity and excitement by using sensory food exploration, cooking activities, and shared eating experiences in the classroom. Materials feature colorful illustrations of key concepts, including pictures of farmers, plant parts, and food groups. The curricula are easily incorporated into math, literacy, science, and social studies, which create stronger academic and behavioral change opportunities.

CookShop for Teens, also known as EATWISE (Educated and Aware Teens Who Inspire Smart Eating), is a peer education program specifically designed to train high-school students to become nutrition educators. With Food Bank training in nutrition and food issues plus public speaking and leadership skills, peer educators facilitate workshops about a range of nutrition topics in their own high schools and communities. Workshop topics such as healthy snacks, food access, and basic nutrition information enable participants to choose healthier options.

CookShop for Adults offers workshops to the parents/guardians of children in public schools that participate in CookShop Classroom. The Food Bank provides training, equipment, educational materials, and technical support to school staff. Workshops complement the CookShop Classroom curricula and feature simple, healthy recipes that use fresh and inexpensive foods. The program provides practical skills and knowledge that enable adults to make CookShop part of their families' daily lives.

CookShop Social Marketing launches nutrition education advertising with succinct nutrition messages delivered through various media such as radio spots, transit ads, and in-school outreach. The campaign complements the other CookShop components and aims to affect food choices through marketing strategies.

Observation and research demonstrate that the greatest impact on student dietary change comes from classroom lessons that provide cooking and eating experiences and that are complemented by related experiences outside the classroom. CookShop focuses on common, inexpensive foods that are readily available in most neighborhoods and as part of Federal School Lunch Program menus.

The CookShop program and its curriculum materials are developed and implemented by the Food Bank For New York City, a non-profit organization. More information about the program can be found on the Food Bank's website, http://www.foodbanknyc.org.

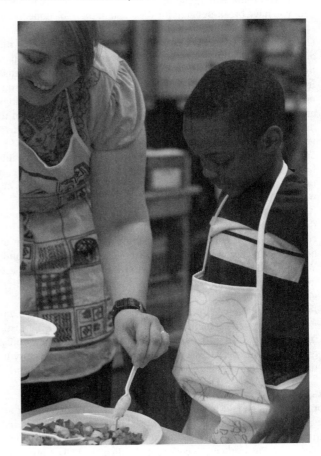

CookShop Classroom.

CookShop logo courtesy of Food Bank For New York City.

Sources: Liquori, T., P. D. Koch, I. R. Contento, and J. Castle. 1998. The CookShop program: Outcome evaluation of a nutrition education program linking lunchroom food experiences with classroom cooking experiences. *Journal of Nutrition Education* 30:302–313; and Wadsworth, K. 2005. From farm to table: The making of a classroom chef. Presented at the Society for Nutrition Education Annual Conference, Orlando, Florida.

result of participating in the health fair. Health fairs take some effort and planning, so you will have to start early. Develop a time line based on the following considerations.

Getting Started

Be clear about the purpose or objectives of the health fair. Do you want the fair to attract attention as a kickoff event to motivate people to attend other activities of the program, such as group education or physical activity sessions? Or is it a standalone event where you want to motivate individuals to take a certain action and provide some skills on how to do it?

Planning the Health Fair

Consider the following:

- *Site.* Select or find a location. This may depend on how many people you think will attend and hence the space you will need. Will you have break-out activities? Can all of these be done in the same space, or will you need additional rooms?
- *Other potential participants.* Will program staff conduct all the activities or will you invite other similar agencies or groups to participate? For example, if the focus of the health fair is to increase fruit and vegetable consumption, you may want to ask personnel from a nearby hospital to conduct blood pressure screenings as motivation. Or you may want someone from a local gym to demonstrate activities people can do in the home. This will help you decide how many tables you will need.
- *Raffles.* If you will use raffles as a motivator to attend the health fair, early on you will need to seek out local vendors who can provide items to raffle off, such as membership to a gym. This will require letters and/or phone calls.
- *Activities.* Brainstorm the topics or issues you will focus on. Limit them depending on the scope of your fair. For each, decide on the central message. Each message or topic should have a table or booth on which you will display posters using a foamcore stand. You will need to develop quizzes, activities, and handouts. These need to be motivating and informative, using theory-based strategies as appropriate.
- *Promotion and advertising.* You can promote the fair using a variety of approaches, such as posters displayed around the institution, postcards sent to various departments or to community groups, e-mail messages sent to selected audiences, or a story in the institution's newsletter or local newspaper.

Making the Experience Motivating and Effective

Staff or volunteers should have on name tags and be ready to greet attendees. Staff should be assigned to meet other vendors or participants and help them set up. The displays should look professional, attractive, and welcoming. The raffle products should be displayed all on one table so that attendees can see what they might get if they complete quizzes or other activities. Have someone take pictures so that they can be used as follow-up motivators if posted, for writeups about the event, and for evaluation or documentation purposes.

■ MASS MEDIA AND SOCIAL MARKETING ACTIVITIES

A brief discussion of social marketing and mass media activities is included here because a mass media campaign or social marketing component often accompanies in-person, in-institution activities as part of a larger program. Activities often described as social marketing are really mass media nutrition communication campaigns. Nutrition mass media campaigns involve communication strategies to disseminate messages to targeted audiences through a variety of mass channels such as newspaper articles, radio public service announcements (PSAs), or paid advertising. Social marketing, on the other hand, is a complex enterprise that often includes mass media campaigns, but may not, and involves the larger enterprise of marketing. It is described only briefly here in terms of its use in nutrition education. Whether designing mass media campaigns or developing social marketing activities, nutrition educators usually work in collaboration with mass media or social marketing experts.

Nutrition Mass Media Communication Campaigns

A mass media communication campaign is usually described as an intervention that "intends to generate specific outcomes or effects, in a relatively large number of individuals, usually within a specified period of time, and through an organized set of communication activities" (Rogers & Storey 1988; Institute of Medicine [IOM] 2002). Such campaigns are designed to reach large audiences using multiple channels. They usually require substantial resources in terms of money and effort. Campaigns seek to "influence the adoption of recommended health behaviors by influencing what the public knows about the behavior and/or by influencing actual and/or perceived social norms, and/or by changing actual skills and confidence in skills (self-efficacy), all of which are assumed to influence behavior" (IOM 2002). They are often part of social marketing programs. Such campaigns are sometimes conducted along with efforts to change the environment using a multiple-level, ecological model of health promotion.

The process of developing such campaigns involves consideration of the communication principles described in the last chapter and engagement in a process somewhat similar to that described in the six-step nutrition education design model used in this book, as follows: selecting the intended audience and specific behavioral outcomes, conducting extensive formative research (needs analysis) with the audience, choosing the message strategy and how the messages will be worded and executed, selecting the channels and settings for dissemination, and conducting ongoing monitoring and evaluation. Detailed instructions on how exactly to design and implement health communications can be found in documents such as *Making Health Communication Programs Work*, published by the National Cancer Institute (2004), and *Speaking of Health*, from the Institute of Medicine (2002).

Social Marketing

The term *social marketing* is defined in many different ways. Kotler and Zaltman (1971) first proposed that marketing principles could be applied to socially relevant programs, ideas, or behaviors. They saw social marketing as the design, implementation, and control of programs seeking to increase the acceptability of a social idea or practice of a target group. The term often refers to a systematic planning process that focuses on consumer behavior (understanding the target group's values, attitudes, barriers, and incentives to change), developing clear messages, designing interventions, implementing them, and evaluating results on a continual basis. It also refers to a particular conceptual framework about how to bring about behavior change. The definitions have in common the notion that social marketing is a set of systematic procedures to promote personal and societal welfare. The following subsections first describe the conceptual framework and then the social marketing process.

Conceptual Framework

Social marketing is based on the following set of considerations (Kotler & Zaltman 1971; Lefebvre & Flora 1988; Kotler & Roberto 1989; Andreasen 1995; Rothschild 1999; Alcay & Bell 2000; Kotler & Lee 2008):

- Social marketing is applied to causes that are considered to be beneficial to both individuals and society.
- It seeks to promote the voluntary behavior of intended audiences so as to reduce risk or enhance health, not simply to increase awareness or alter attitudes.
- It does so by offering intended audience members reinforcing incentives and/or consequences in an environment that invites voluntary change or exchange (see below).
- Social marketing is tailored to the unique perspectives, needs, and experiences of the intended audience with input from representatives of that audience.
- Social marketing strives to create conditions in the social structure that facilitate the behavioral changes promoted.
- Social marketing uses the processes and concepts of marketing.

This section focuses on some central ideas and practices that are useful for nutrition education.

Self-Interest

Individuals are assumed to act in their own self-interest. Although there are many determinants of behavior beyond self-interest (Mansbridge 1990), it has been proposed that self-interest plays some role in most contexts of human interaction. Self-interest can be seen as similar to the concept of outcome expectations (or anticipated outcomes) from social psychological theory—outcomes people can expect from engaging in healthy behaviors such as health or decreased risk of disease. The anticipated outcomes are often long term rather than immediate as in the example of urging people to increase their intake of calcium-rich foods to reduce risk of osteoporosis. Indeed, these long-term outcomes may be in conflict with more immediate outcomes based on self-interest. For example, people choose to eat the unhealthy foods they do or not to be physically active because they have evaluated their life situations and have made their decisions based on their current judgment of their self-interest. Social marketing thus seeks to promote change by offering benefits that the intended audience perceives to be in their self-interest, as identified through thorough market research or needs analyses. That is, it offers "the benefits they (intended audience members) want, reducing the barriers they are concerned about, and using persuasion to participate in program activity" (Kotler & Roberto 1989).

Exchange Theory

Central to social marketing is the notion of voluntary exchange of resources: one party gives up something in exchange for getting something from another party. In the case of nutrition education, this means that participants give up time, effort, convenience, or money in exchange for the benefits of enhanced physical health, improved psychological well-being, or a healthful, wholesome food system (Rothschild 1999; Alcay & Bell 2000). Your job as a nutrition educator is to demonstrate that the benefits outweigh the costs of taking action. In the design of strategies for enhancing benefits and encouraging action, social marketing uses other theories as tools, such as the theories described in Part I of this book: the health belief model, the theory of planned behavior, social cognitive theory, and the transtheoretical model.

Focus on Intended Audience Members' Wants and Needs

The design of social marketing activities is based on what individuals or consumers want or need. Although evidence from research studies is important and best practices can be very useful, social marketing adds a strong focus on what specific audience members in a given community want and need. Hence it invests heavily in *market research*, which is similar to the needs analysis process described in Chapter 8, to find out about the specific perspectives, values, attitudes, interests, and needs of a given audience. Social marketing also emphasizes pretesting potential materials, messages, and themes with the intended audience so as to refine the message based on their suggestions. If audience members influence the development of the program, it is more likely the intervention will be effective.

Segmentation of the Audience

To design messages and activities that are highly specific, social marketers try to segment or subdivide any broad category of individuals into more homogeneous subgroups using demographic criteria such as age, sex, income, and ethnicity; geographic criteria such as urban, suburban, and rural settings; psychological criteria such as motivations, readiness to change, or skill levels; and behavioral criteria such as the degree to which the group already practices the behavior of concern. Selection of which segment or subgroup to focus on can be based on various criteria, such as which group has the greatest need based on the size of the group and the incidence and severity of food- or nutrition-related conditions, which group is most ready to change, or which group has the most influence on others.

Tipping the Scales

Whereas education can increase awareness, promote active contemplation, enhance motivation, and teach food- and nutrition-related behavioral skills and self-regulation skills, social marketing goes beyond education by attempting to modify the relative attractiveness of the specific behavior. This is accomplished through the use of incentives and other benefits that positively reinforce the behavior and through the reduction of barriers or costs associated with the behavior, thereby tipping the scales in favor of the behavior, according to Rothschild (1999). Social marketing focuses on providing direct, immediate, and tangible benefits that are reinforcing. It also attempts to reduce both personal barriers, such as beliefs and expectations, and external barriers by making the environment favorable for the appropriate behavior. In the case of an intervention to increase the consumption of more fruits and vegetables, social marketers not only provide educational messages but also reduce barriers by such activities as increasing the availability of fruits and vegetables in schools, working with grocery stores to lower prices, or providing coupons that participants can redeem at stores.

Key Elements in Planning Social Marketing

The social marketing planning process systematically addresses the five Ps of the "marketing mix" considered by commercial marketers (Alcay & Bell 2000; Maibech, Rothschild, & Novelli 2002; Kotler & Lee 2008).

Product

Product refers to what is exchanged with the intended audience for a price. The product may not be a tangible item but a service, practice, or intangible idea such as health. For the product to be "buyable," people must first perceive that they have a problem and that the product being offered is a good solution. Here, formative research is important to unveil consumers' perceptions about the problem and how strongly they feel that they can do something to solve the problem. Thus, products are desired behaviors, benefits of these behaviors, and any tangible objects and services offered to support the behaviors.

The core product can be a health idea or behavior that is of benefit to individuals. For example, the idea can be improved health, or the action can be eating five to nine servings of fruits and vegetables daily. Supporting products can be material items, such as coupons for fruits and vegetables at farmers' markets, or a service such as a WIC clinic or nutrition education classes (but not the materials used in the classes—which are described later in this chapter in a different category). In designing a program, you have to be very clear about what exactly is your product. If it is a behavior, you need to find out from the intended audience what behaviors they see as realistic, effective, practical, or easy to do. You should also be specific: is the product the behavior of eating *more* fruits and vegetables, or eating a specific amount such as 2.5 cups a day or more?

Price

Price refers to the barriers or costs to the consumer associated with obtaining the product, such as adopting the desired behavior, and any monetary and nonmonetary incentives, recognition, and rewards used to reduce the costs. Costs can include the economic costs of eating more fruits and vegetables as well as the inconvenience and increased time involved in the preparation of healthful foods, or perhaps the psychological costs of learning new ways of eating. Social marketing recognizes that decisions to act are based on considerations of both benefits and costs. Individuals ask themselves, "What will I gain if I engage in this behavior, and what will it cost me?" Often individuals fail to take action not because they do not recognize the benefits, but because the costs are too high.

Social marketing thus seeks to increase the benefits and decrease the price or barriers of engaging in the behavior of concern (Andreasen 1995; Rothschild 1999). It does this by addressing the internal determinants of behavior discussed earlier in the book, such as perceived risk, beliefs about outcomes of taking action, knowledge, social norms, and self-confidence or self-efficacy. Social marketing also addresses external barriers such as policy, access, skills, and cultural trends by attempting to create conditions in the social structure and environment to facilitate the actions being promoted. More simply said, it attempts to make the more healthful behavior the easy behavior.

In the case of promoting fruits and vegetables to low-income mothers of young children, the benefits might be the good health of their children or wanting to enhance their children's educational opportunities and performance. Internal barriers might be lack of time and cooking skills or confusion about portion sizes for their children. External barriers might include the high cost of healthful foods such as fruits and vegetables. Food stamps and coupons for farmers' markets would be ways to reduce external barriers.

Place

Place refers to where and when the product will reach the consumer. In the case of intangible products, it is the place where the audience will receive the information. This may mean researching which media channels are most effective for reaching the intended audience. It may mean grocery stores, doctors' offices, community centers, WIC clinics, or food stamp offices. Place can also refer to where you might offer program activities (such as classes) so that they are convenient to the

intended audience. Social marketing seeks to increase the places where the product may be found, at the right times, and at the points at which audience members make their decisions. Behaviors must be easy to carry out; hence, placement must encourage the behavior. If increasing consumption of fruits and vegetables is the behavior, then the placement strategy might be to have information and messages conveniently located in the grocery store, workplace, or school lunchroom.

Promotion

The targeted audience members can be expected to voluntarily exchange their time, effort, and other resources if they are aware that the product, such as eating fruits and vegetables, offers them attractive benefits at a reasonable cost and can be practiced at convenient locations. The role of *promotion* is to create this awareness. For example, the 5-a-Day campaign complemented its efforts by placing the product (messages about fruits and vegetables) in the right places via a promotional campaign in the news media and point-of-purchase materials such as messages on grocery store bags. Promotion requires considerations such as the following:

- *What channels to use to reach the intended audience.* For fruit and vegetable consumption among low-income mothers of young children, the channels might be grocery stores, day-care centers, WIC clinics, food stamp offices, community centers, newspapers, and TV.
- *What types of messages might be effective.* The content of the messages will be based on your audience analysis or needs assessment, as described in Chapter 8. The nature of the message, such as whether to use humor, emotion, or logical reasoning, should again be based on your audience analysis. The tone of the messages should be positive, such as "We know it is hard, but we know that you want to make a change." It should also be respectful, fun, and personal.

Positioning

A fifth P often is considered in addition to the standard four Ps. The product can be positioned in such a way as to maximize benefits and minimize costs. *Positioning* is a psychological construct that involves the location of the product relative to products with which it competes. Positioning is difficult in nutrition education because it means having your product (message) outweigh the competitors. For example, it is very challenging to get teenagers to eat more fresh fruits and vegetables when they feel that the alternative products, such as high-fat snacks, taste much better. However, physical activity can be repositioned as a form of relaxation rather than as exercise (which some may view negatively). Serving fruits and vegetables can be positioned as taking care of yourself, and serving healthful meals to your family can be positioned as an act of love.

Designing Social Marketing Activities

As you have seen, social marketing programs are tailored to the unique perspectives, needs, and experiences of the target audience and also seek to create conditions in the social structure and environment that facilitate the actions being promoted (Andreasen 1999; Alcay & Bell 2000). The set of procedures for designing social marketing is similar to that described in models of health communication and the six-step nutrition education design model used in this book. In social marketing these steps are usually referred to as formative research and planning, strategy design, implementation, and evaluation. To develop the social marketing campaign or activities, nutrition educators usually work in collaboration with health communication and social marketing experts. These experts are especially important in the formative research, message development, and planning stages. Hence the design phase is only summarized briefly here.

Formative research and planning involve setting goals, selecting the audience segment or subgroup to work with, and identifying the focus of the intervention. The focus may be change in individual attitudes or behaviors, community norms, policies, or all three. The various channels are selected at this time, such as posters, classes, community events, changes in availability of the foods in the stores, or policies in schools and workplaces. An environmental analysis is conducted and community participation sought. Formative research seeks to understand the motivations, attitudes, and behaviors of the intended audience, as well as the audience's perceptions of the benefits and costs of taking the recommended action.

Strategy design includes designing the campaign message based on the formative research and pretesting the message using focus groups and surveys. The marketing mix, or five Ps, is selected at this time.

Implementation usually involves considerable collaboration with individuals and organizations in the community. This is described in greater detail in the next subsection. Funding and changes in social structures are sought so that the programs can be maintained over the long term.

Evaluation is important. There are many approaches, the simplest of which is to see whether the audience can recall campaign messages. Another measure is extent of exposure—the number of activities that audience members have attended, such as classes or workshops, live food demonstrations, or health fairs, or the amount of materials they have taken home. Other measures are surveys of mediator of behavior/change such as knowledge, beliefs, attitudes, behavioral intent, or stage of change. Behaviors can be self-reported through a survey or using monitoring data such as the increase in sales of fruits and vegetables in grocery stores or increased attendance at fitness classes and gyms.

Implementing Social Marketing Involving Mass Media and Related Activities

Social marketing often involves the mass media, but not always. This section describes the use of social marketing in a program that involves the mass media as a primary channel—the Pick a Better Snack campaign—and in a program that did not—the Food Friends program.

Social marketing that uses mass media as the primary channel usually requires the collaboration of many individuals and organizations. Such campaigns can be local, community-wide, statewide, or national. Some potential practical methods for implementing social marketing are summarized here based on the literature and best practices of those who have been involved. These methods are useful to nutrition educators who are interested in incorporating mass media and community support components into their programs. The following suggestions are based on the experience of the Pick a Better Snack campaign in Iowa (Iowa Department of Public Health n.d.).

Media Activities

1. *Develop media partnerships.* Prior to the initiation of the campaign, actively solicit print, outdoor, and broadcast media partnerships to extend the reach of the campaign to audiences that would otherwise be out of the program's reach for financial reasons.
   - Meet with local television and radio station public service directors, station promotional managers, and print advertising managers to identify opportunities for partnerships.
   - Draw up a simple joint agreement that outlines how each partner will be identified in collaborative efforts, such as whose logos will be on media events. Such agreements avoid misunderstandings later on and engender trust.

2. *Introduce the campaign to the community.* You have only one shot to introduce your campaign. The challenge here is to make as big a splash as you can with a few simple messages and to get media coverage.
   - Plan a kickoff event such as a press conference. Select a site with a compelling visual element for broadcast media where a story can be told, such as at a farmers' market, grocery store, or after-school program.
   - Carefully develop two to four key messages to serve as the focus of the news conference or event.

3. *Sustain ongoing media relationships.* Work with local media to develop periodic articles or special features on the importance of your message, as did the Pick a Better Snack campaign.
   - Identify a few key reporters and news editors who are responsible for covering food or health issues and work on building a good working relationship with them. Contact them from time to time by phone or e-mail with news about campaign events or article ideas. Follow up with information to support your story ideas. Or send them a draft of a potential article for them to modify.
   - Offer to serve as a resource for them on other food and nutrition issues.

4. *Plan an outdoor campaign if feasible.* Place your messages on billboards, bus benches, buses, or bus shelters. These can be paid for or placed as PSAs.
   - Work with outdoor media companies to identify the best locations for your intended audience and obtain cost estimates.
   - Outdoor media companies will frequently run billboards with PSAs at no charge for the space. These may not be placed in prime locations, so negotiate with them about placement and duration.

Community Outreach

1. *Develop a newsletter.* Develop a simple, inexpensive newsletter to keep key partners and targeted segments of the campaign's audience informed about your activities and progress.

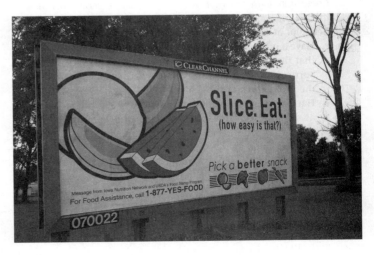

Billboards are another way to get the message out.

- The frequency of the newsletter will depend on your ability to develop a simple system for its regular development and distribution, but should be at least quarterly.
- Because it will go to a variety of stakeholders, the newsletter should also include information relevant to the campaign, such as recipes and actionable ideas for taking the action promoted by the campaign.

2. *Collaborate with community organizations.* Collaborate with community organizations regarding events that would bring benefit to your program and the organization, such as farmers' markets, local food drives, broadcast media, and health fairs.
   - Work with a local farmers' market to organize an event that would both bring people to the farmers' market and bring awareness to the campaign messages. Demonstrate simple recipes reflecting the campaign action (such as eating more fruits and vegetables), decorate with campaign posters, and wear campaign-related tee-shirts.
   - Work with other organizations at special events they may sponsor, such as community health fairs sponsored by local radio or TV stations.

3. *Place campaign literature in strategic locations.* Distribute program literature to the public in several health- and medical services–related settings throughout the community.
   - Work with your local medical society leadership to encourage them to recommend to their members that they participate by being willing to serve as distribution points for your campaign literature (such as posters, recipes, or bookmarks) to their clients.
   - Distribute your written PSAs to county medical groups for inclusion in their regular member newsletters.

Working with Schools

1. *Work with school food service staff.* Provide a campaign promotional package to food service directors for use in school cafeterias, suggests the Pick a Better Snack campaign.
   - In this package include several posters and selected samples of point-of-sale materials to allow them to dress up the lunch line.
   - Encourage food service directors to periodically focus on the campaign for a week, such as to promote fruits and vegetables or low-fat milk that week.

2. *Coordinate with parent–teacher organization (PTO) open houses and school events.* Solicit local schools' PTOs to promote your goal behavior at their social events and fundraising sales.
   - Have a booth at the PTO/school open house to raise awareness that the school is focusing on the campaign goal through its curriculum. Outline what parents can do at home to support the campaign's target goal.
   - Hand out samples of foods promoted by your campaign, as well as recipes, postcards, book markers, and so forth.
   - Seek PTO volunteers to promote imaginative after-school snacks, foods for sporting events, and school fundraisers (in place of bake sales) that support the campaign goals.

Grocery Store Activities

1. *Conduct in-store or farmers' market demonstrations.* Volunteer to conduct in-store food demonstrations in a local grocery store. (See Dole Food Company [2001] for tips on how to conduct one with students.)
   - Work with the store manager to get approval to do a demonstration.

- Demonstrate only one or two very simple ideas for the promoted foods; hand out recipes and other campaign material.

2. *Use incentive cards to persuade individuals to try promoted foods.* The campaign may develop incentives for children to eat certain foods, such as fruits and vegetables, by handing out cards (through schools, WIC clinics, or other food-related settings) with activities printed on them for the whole family to do. In the Pick a Better Snack campaign, when the family verified that the activity had been completed, they took the card to a participating grocery store or returned it to the school to redeem it for an incentive. Focus group research in several locations has shown that "unfamiliarity" and fear of wasting food are frequently barriers to trying new foods. Incentives thus can be free samples of campaign-related food items to help families overcome the barrier of fearing to purchase foods that their children will not eat.
   - Develop a system for distribution of the educational incentive items.
   - Work with store managers to develop a redemption procedure.

3. *Provide in-store signage.* Develop signs to identify the foods promoted by the campaign.
   - Set up criteria for classifying food items as qualifying as target foods. For example, if low-fat foods are a focus, define what you mean by *low-fat.* Come with a list of foods that qualify.
   - Work out with the store manager who will place the signs, who will monitor them, and who will change them as needed.

Implementing Social Marketing Involving Other Channels

Social marketing principles can be used to design and implement programs that do not involve the mass media. For example, social marketing has been used to design a variety of community-based and even school-based programs. The key approaches in design are to conduct extensive formative research to identify the potential audiences, the important nutritional issues, and the key channels to use with an intended audience.

Food Friends

The program called Food Friends provides an example of the social marketing process (Young et al. 2004; Johnson et al. 2007). This program was directed at promoting healthful food choices among low-income families.

Formative Research

Focus groups are a major method of collecting formative research data in social marketing. They can be used to identify the audience segment with which you can work. In this example, focus groups were conducted with low-income elderly individuals and with low-income parents with children. Results from focus groups usually help you narrow the target population. In the example of Food Friends, families with young children ages 3 to 7 were selected. Next, you conduct focus groups with the selected audience. Here, you can be more specific, for example, asking about the target group's eating practices, barriers to healthful eating, and preferred communication channels. Through this process, the audience identified in the Food Friends program was preschoolers, the behavior chosen was "trying new foods," and the site for delivery of the message was Head Start centers. Novel foods to include in the program were identified from a food frequency questionnaire. These steps are similar to Steps 1 and 2 of the Stepwise Procedure used in this book.

Campaign Strategy

Formative research provides the basis of campaign strategy. In the case of Food Friends, it led to the selection of an intervention involving education and marketing strategies to be distributed through Head Start programs (not through the mass media). They included nutrition activities, novel foods offered during afternoon snack time, and parental involvement through the publication of articles in the monthly Head Start newsletter. Food Friends is described in **Nutrition Education in Action 16-2**.

WIC Social Marketing Program

Table 16-2 presents a case example of the use of social marketing to plan strategies to reduce barriers for WIC participants to shop at farmers' markets. The five Ps provide the planning framework.

NUTRITION EDUCATION IN ACTION 16-2

Food Friends: A Nutrition Education Initiative for Preschool Children Using Social Marketing Principles

The Food Friends program was directed at promoting healthful food choices among low-income families in Colorado. It used social marketing as a framework for developing the program, including extensive formative research to identify key behaviors or practices that would promote health. Included in the formative research were focus groups, an extensive food frequency questionnaire to identify foods that preschoolers eat, and concept pretesting. Through this process, the audience identified was preschoolers, the behavior chosen was "trying new foods," and the selected site for delivery of the message was Head Start centers. Children are served meals and snacks in this setting, permitting the program to provide children with the opportunity to taste and become familiar with new foods. The characters have names such as Ollie Orange, Marty Milk, and Corinne Carrot, and they have magical powers. Children who try new foods acquire these magical powers.

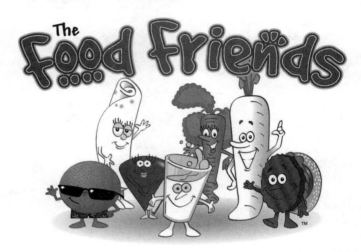

Program

Food Friends: Fun with New Foods

The 12-week program included a blend of education and marketing strategies and used social cognitive theory to support developmental learning skills such as fine and gross motor control, listening and language skills, sensory evaluations, and problem solving. Activities included the following:

- "Food Friend Memory Card game," a memory activity
- "Edible Food Faces," a tasting party
- "Fruit and Vegetable Mystery Bags"
- Reading of storybooks with a "trying new foods" theme
- New foods offered three times per week during afternoon snack time
- Parental involvement: four articles in the monthly Head Start newsletter

The social marketing process and attention to the four Ps—product, price, place, and promotion—were helpful in developing a program specifically tailored to preschoolers and their families.

Food Friends: Get Movin' with Mighty Moves

A companion 18-week physical activity program consists of 18 weeks of 15–20 minute sessions led by the teacher four days per week. Each character has *Mighty Moves* (gross motor skills) as well as magical powers. Different motor skills are introduced each week and, later, skill patterns. Children who practice these motor skills acquire magical powers.

Evaluation

Fun with New Foods

A study using two experimental and two control Head Start centers found increased preference for and willingness to try new foods in preschool children at the experimental sites. The program was positively received by Head Start staff.

Get Movin' with Mighty Moves

Data were collected from 276 children and their families before and after the program. Results showed that the program led to significant increases in gross motor skills compared to the control group. The program was very well received by teachers and parents.

The Food Friends logo is used courtesy of Department of Food Science and Nutrition, Colorado State University. http://www.foodfriends.org.

Source: Young, L., J. Anderson, L. Beckstrom, L. Bellows, and S. L. Johnson. 2004. Using social marketing principles to guide the development of a nutrition education initiative for preschool-aged children. *Journal of Nutrition Education and Behavior* 36:250–257; and Johnson, S. L., L. Bellows, L. Beckstrom, and J. Anderson. 2007. Evaluation of a social marketing campaign targeting preschool children. *American Journal of Health Behavior* 31(1):44–55

TABLE 16-2	Social Marketing Case Study Example: Farmers' Market Coupons for WIC Clients			
	Using the Four Ps to Overcome Barriers			
Barriers	**Product**	**Price**	**Place**	**Promotion**
I don't know where to park at the market.	Print places to park on map on new coupon folder.			Have staff visit the market so that they can describe where to park.
I'm embarrassed around other shoppers when using coupons, and vendors seem a little irritated with the coupons.	Use mystery shoppers (even WIC staff) to evaluate service.	Consider feasibility of a "scanning" card rather than coupons.		
It's difficult to find signs that qualify farmers for WIC coupons. Sometimes they are below the tables and can't be seen.			Provide "poles" for farmers to use to display a sign that can be seen above the crowds.	Have WIC signs be the 5 A Day sign instead of the "WIC coupons accepted here" sign.
I'm concerned about not getting change back from $2 coupons. It's such a waste.		Reduce size of coupons to $1 versus $2.		
I lose the checks or forget where I put them.	Create a folder for checks, as opposed to loose, similar to an airline ticket folder.			
I'm afraid of what WIC counselors will think if I decline the coupons.		Offer clients with hesitation or barriers "a half pack" of coupons.		
I don't know what some of the fruits and vegetables are that I saw the last time (e.g., kohlrabi).				Use dedicated whiteboard in clinic to describe what's in season.
I don't know how to cook some of the fruits and vegetables.	Offer cooking classes and provide recipes.			
I don't have transportation.			Organize car pools from the clinic office.	
I don't really like vegetables.	Offer cooking classes and recipes.	Offer "half pack" of coupons to see if individual can find things to like.		
I don't know where the market is.	Print places to park on new coupon folder.			Have staff visit the market so they can describe where to park.
I work and can't get there during the week, and on weekends I'm too busy.			Recruit interested farmers to deliver select items to the clinic.	
I don't know what's in season, so I don't know what I'll find at the market.				Use dedicated whiteboard in clinic to describe what's in season.
I'm concerned about returning checks that I didn't use, but I feel bad just keeping them when someone else could use them.		Allow return of unused checks, with no questions asked.		
I can't use all these checks in one visit, and then it takes too much to get back to the market.		Allow return of unused checks, with no questions asked.	Recruit interested farmers to deliver select items to clinic.	

Source: The Association of State Nutrition Network Administrators, Society for Nutrition Education, Division of Social Marketing. 2003. Using the 4Ps to overcome barriers to behavior change. http://www.sne.org/specialinterest.htm. Used with permission.

Comparing Social Marketing and Nutrition Education

Many years ago, an early social marketer, Richard Manoff (1985), who had achieved considerable success in improving nutrition in several developing countries, quipped at a Society for Nutrition Education meeting that "anything that works is social marketing; anything that does not is nutrition education." Others, on the other hand, criticize social marketing as too simplistic, not promoting the critical thinking and reflection that are needed in making informed choices in a complex food system (Van Den Heede & Pelican 1995). The debate continues even as many nutrition education programs incorporate social marketing activities as a component. This section compares the two endeavors on three features considered to be central to social marketing: it tailors messages and strategies to the unique perspectives, needs, and experiences of the target audience; it is a systematic audience-based planning process; and it goes beyond nutrition education by aiming to create conditions in the social structure and environment that reduce barriers and facilitate the actions being promoted.

Audience Focus

Social marketing's consumer or audience focus and emphasis on thorough formative research or audience analysis as a first step is similar to the needs assessment or audience analysis process that constitutes the first step in designing theory-based nutrition education. The contrast is in the level of importance given to this step. Social marketing spends considerable time and effort on this step to understand its audience and tailor its messages, whereas nutrition education programs often spend little time on this step. However, theory-based nutrition education also requires that a thorough needs analysis be conducted to identify the many mediators of behavior change, including motivators and reinforcers of action and barriers to change. Two chapters in this book are devoted to such assessments. In addition, social marketers also spend considerable resources in pretesting messages with potential audience members. Pilot testing is also always considered an important part of nutrition education. Still, social marketing does provide a good reminder about the importance of understanding the intended audiences.

Systematic Planning Process

As you examine the *process* of audience-based social marketing, you can see that it is not very different from the systematic process used in designing good health education or nutrition education. The steps in social marketing of formative research and planning, including a clear statement of objectives; strategy design, including strategy formation, and message and material development; pretesting; implementation; and evaluation and feedback are very similar to the steps of any systematic educational planning process, including the Stepwise Procedure for Designing Theory-Based Nutrition Education used in this book. The use of the five Ps provides an interesting way to think of the strategy design process. Yet a careful examination shows that these five Ps overlap many theory variables. Social marketers do remind nutrition educators, however, to be more systematic in their planning process.

Reducing Tangible Barriers

Finally, social marketing is described as going beyond education by attempting to modify the relative attractiveness of the specific behavior. It does so through providing tangible and immediate benefits that are reinforcing and through reducing both personal barriers, such as beliefs and expectations, and external barriers by making the environment favorable for the appropriate behavior. Theory-based nutrition education also seeks to increase the perception of benefits and decrease internal barriers, as has been described in great detail in this book. Nutrition education also increasingly incorporates environmental supports for action—including policy and system modification—as part of its programming. The use of the social-ecological approach, described earlier in the book, is an example of this trend. The two enterprises of social marketing and nutrition education thus share many characteristics.

Social Marketing and Nutrition Education

Social marketing contributes to nutrition education a reminder to involve consumers or the public intensely in developing the program, to value their input, and to offer a sense of participant empowerment. Its set of planning ideas or tools, such as the five Ps, can also be very useful to nutrition education. The channels favored by social marketing, such as the mass media, offer the potential to reach a large portion of the population and to change the informational and normative environment. (Remember, though, that social marketing is not the same as a mass media campaign.)

On the other hand, nutrition education, when conducted with groups, goes beyond social marketing by providing a set of learning opportunities for the intended audience to develop and practice food- and nutrition-related cognitive skills, including critical thinking skills, as well as affective and behavior-specific skills that can assist individuals to make choices and take action on complex behaviors and issues. Venues such as facilitated group discussion also provide for social support and reinforcement of learning. Social marketing can thus be used as a component of a multicomponent nutrition education or health promotion program.

■ USING NEW TECHNOLOGIES

Many other channels for nutrition education have been explored. A few are briefly summarized here.

Individually Tailored Messages

Individually tailored messages can enhance the effectiveness of communications through nonpersonal media such as letters, newsletters, and computers. In this approach, a targeted group—such as employees at a worksite or clients of a physician—is sent a questionnaire that asks them about their current practices with respect to the target behavior, as well as their beliefs, attitudes, social norms, perceived barriers, or state of change. They are then sent computer-generated letters that specifically address their own particular set of beliefs and practices. The tailored communication can also be a newsletter or a magazine. Evidence shows that such a tailored approach improves communication attention and satisfaction. That is, instead of reading a general mailing or newsletter containing information that may not be relevant, the person reads only information that is specifically relevant to his or her beliefs or stage in the dietary change process. Thus, this approach addresses issues that are personally relevant to the target audience and the choices they have to make. Evidence suggests that such an approach may enhance effectiveness compared with general communications (Brug, Campbell, & Van Assema 1999; Brug, Oenema, & Campbell 2003). Tailoring can also be based on the core cultural values of a given cultural group in addition to behavioral theory constructs and has been found to enhance effectiveness (Kreuter et al. 2003, 2005).

Computer-tailored personal letters, newsletters, and magazines have been used with a variety of audiences: general practitioners' clients, healthy employees, healthy volunteers, retirees, members of health maintenance organizations, and church members. Another channel that can be used is an interactive computer approach: one study used computers in the classroom (Ezendam, Oenema, et al. 2007); another study was designed to motivate and assist people to eat more fiber by using a very specific food choice strategy; another used touch-screen computers accompanied by in-person counseling and follow-up telephone counseling (Brinberg, Axelson, & Price 2000; Stevens et al. 2002). Web-based tailored messages and interactive approaches can also be used (Oenema, Brug, & Lechner 2001; Debourdeaudhuij, Stevens, Vandelanotte, & Brug 2007).

Promising New Technologies

Besides computer-tailored letters and newsletters, other nontraditional channels have been explored and show promise.

Telephone

Motivational interviewing over the telephone has shown some effectiveness. People calling in for cancer-related information to the national Cancer Information Service received a brief proactive education intervention over the telephone involving motivational and educational messages tailored to the caller's stage of readiness for eating at least five servings of fruits and vegetables daily (Marcus et al. 2001). Though brief, this interaction resulted in significant increase in fruit and vegetable consumption. Members of black churches were also reached with telephone motivational interviewing with some success (Resnicow et al. 2001).

Multimedia Soap Opera

A multimedia approach using tailored soap opera and interactive infomercials that provided individualized feedback, knowledge, and strategies for lowering fat based on stage of change was effective (Campbell et al. 1999).

The Web

The World Wide Web offers many opportunities for nutrition education and indeed many programs provide nutrition education directly to the public through this medium (Brug, Oenema, & Raat 2005; Kroeze, Werkman, & Brug 2006). Because many people already use the Web to find health information, a well-designed, attractive website that has accurate information from a credible source can be a very valuable method for getting nutrition messages out. Nutrition educators usually work with Web designers with specific skills to develop the programs, and thus this process may be expensive.

Digital Photo Receivers

Digital photo receivers (DPRs) offer a promising approach. A DPR looks like a photo in a photo frame that sits on a table, where the photos change frequently to provide a slide show. Thus, it can sit in a WIC office, senior center, or food bank for clients to view. DPRs use automated photo-sharing technology to receive, store, display, and organize digital photos. Programs can originate from one website and be sent to several facilities so that individual sites do not have to worry about setting up the programs. One study used such technology for low-income audiences that addressed the importance of breakfast and eating more fruits and vegetables to increase folic acid intake (Rifkin et al. 2006). The slides changed every 10 seconds and the entire program was 90 seconds long. Participants found the program easy to read and were positive about the medium for learning about nutrition.

Tailored Nutrition Education Through E-mail

A study used e-mail in a worksite. Batch e-mails were sent out inviting people to participate. Individuals completed a health assessment instru-ment on diet and physical activity. They received immediate feedback. If they decided to continue, they were asked to choose to increase physical activity, increase fruits and vegetables, or decrease saturated fat and trans fat and added sugar. They then received personalized small-step goals to choose to work on each week for three months. It resulted in significant improvements in diet and physical activity (Sternfeld et al. 2009).

Self-Monitoring Through Text Messages

Text messages and e-mails through smart phones, hand-held computers, or PDAs have been found to be very useful in helping individuals self-monitor their diet and activity-related behaviors (Fjeldsoe, Marshall, & Miller 2009). After counseling or group sessions where individuals receive nutrition education, they can then receive messages, reminders, and tips daily, or even several times a day, depending on their choice. Messages through this channel have been useful for helping people lose weight or regulate their blood glucose level (Patrick, Raab, Adams, et al. 2009; Newton, Wiltshire, & Elley 2009). Some have found the use of cell phones to take pictures of all foods eaten to be helpful in helping people lose weight (Zepeda 2009).

Using Portable Hand-Held Technologies

One study found that a hand-held computer (also known as a personal digital assistant [PDA]) was effective in increasing vegetable and whole grain intake in mid-life and older adults (Atienza et al. 2008). Other studies have found text messaging useful for self-monitoring of sweetened beverage intake, physical activity, and screen time in children (Shapiro et al. 2008); for adherence to dietary recommendations in women (Glanz et al. 2006); and for support for youths with diabetes (Franklin et al. 2006). Other communication modalities, such as Facebook and Twitter, are being explored.

Using the Internet with Youths

A 9-week, 5-a-Day Boy Scouts achievement badge program—which involved troop activities and an Internet intervention—resulted in increased intakes of fruits and juice (Thompson et al. 2009). Also, a home-based, 8-week Internet intervention with girls improved fruit and vegetable intakes and physical activity (Thompson et al. 2008).

Educational Computer Games

Video games provide extensive player involvement and are being explored for delivering health behavior change interventions in an engaging way (Baranowski et al. 2008). A theory-based psychoeducational game for fourth graders was highly effective in increasing fruit and vegetable intakes (Baranowski et al. 2003), and another game for middle school youths was able to teach goal-setting skills (Thompson et al. 2007). A randomized control study of a computer game with young adults found positive results on mediators and intentions to eat a healthy diet (Peng 2009).

■ SUMMARY

Nutrition education for the public can be delivered through a variety of venues. This chapter describes some of the main channels and media you can use. It is important that you carefully determine your objectives when you use each of the channels and supporting materials. Sessions with groups are enhanced with the use of visuals, which can range from real foods and food packages to flip charts and PowerPoint slide presentations. Visuals should be interesting but simple. They should be clearly visible and appropriate in size so that you never have to say, "I know you can't read this, but . . ." Written materials such as brochures, flyers, and handouts are also widely used. If they are to be effective, however, you should carefully tailor each piece to your intended audience and make the writing motivational and reader-friendly. Written materials should be designed to look interesting and be easy to read. Other supporting channels include cooking or food preparation activities, conducting grocery tours, and planning health fairs.

This chapter also describes how nutrition educators can be involved in mass media communication campaigns as well as social marketing activities. Delivering nutrition education through these channels usually involves working with experts in these fields and within coalitions and collaborations. The principles of social marketing are described as well as many of the kinds of activities that nutrition educators can participate in as part of social marketing campaigns. Several other nontraditional channels were also described. **Table 16-3** summarizes various channels and their advantages and disadvantages. It should be clear that there are numerous channels that you can use with any audience. This chapter had the space to describe only some of them. There are many more venues through which nutrition education can be delivered, limited only by your imagination!

TABLE 16-3	**Communication Channels and Activities: Pros and Cons**		
Type of Channel	**Activities**	**Pros**	**Cons**
Interpersonal channels	• Nutrition education with groups • Facilitated group discussion • Workshops • Patient counseling	• Permit two-way, personal discussion • More effective in increasing motivations; influential, supportive • Most effective for teaching nutrition-related and self-regulation skills, helping/caring	• Can be expensive • Can be time-consuming • Can have limited reach for intended audience • Can be difficult to link into interpersonal channels
Organizational and community channels	• Community meetings and other events • Organizational meetings and conferences • Workplace campaigns	• May be familiar to audience, trusted, and influential • May provide more motivation and/or support than media alone • Can sometimes be inexpensive • Can offer shared experiences • Can reach larger intended audience in one place	• Can be costly, time-consuming to establish • May not provide personalized attention • Organizational constraints may require message approval • May lose control of message if adapted to fit organizational needs
Mass media channels Newspapers	• Ads • Inserted sections on a health topic (paid) • News • Feature stories • Letters to the editor • Op-ed pieces	• Can reach broad intended audiences rapidly • Can convey health news and breakthroughs more thoroughly than TV or radio and faster than magazines • Intended audience has chance to clip, reread, contemplate, and pass along material	• Coverage demands a newsworthy item • Larger-circulation papers may take only paid ads and inserts • Exposure usually limited to one day • Article placement requires contracts and may be time-consuming
Radio	• Ads (paid or public service placement) • News • Public affairs/talk shows • Dramatic programming (entertainment, education)	• Range of formats available to reach intended audiences with known listening preferences • Paid ads or specific programming can reach intended audience when they are most receptive • Paid ads can be relatively inexpensive • Ad production costs are low relative to TV	• Reaches smaller intended audiences than TV • PSAs run infrequently and at low listening times • Many stations have limited formats that may not be conducive to health messages • Difficult for intended audiences to retain or pass on material

(continues)

TABLE 16-3	**Communication Channels and Activities: Pros and Cons** *(continued)*		
Type of Channel	**Activities**	**Pros**	**Cons**
Television	• Ads (paid or PSAs) • News • Public affairs/talk shows • Dramatic programming (entertainment, education)	• Reaches potentially the largest and widest range of intended audiences • Visual combined with audio good for emotional appeals and demonstrating behaviors • Can reach low-income intended audiences • Paid ads or specific programming can reach intended audience when most receptive • Ads allow message and its execution to be controlled	• Ads are expensive to produce • Paid advertising is expensive • PSAs run infrequently and at low viewing times • Message may be obscured by commercial clutter • Can be difficult for intended audiences to retain or pass on material
Internet	• Websites • Email mailing lists • Chat rooms • Newsgroups • Ads (paid or public service placement)	• Can reach large numbers of people rapidly • Can instantaneously update and disseminate information • Can control information provided • Can tailor information specifically for intended audiences • Can be interactive • Can provide health information in a graphically appealing way • Can combine the audiovisual benefits of TV or radio with the self-paced benefits of print media	• Can be expensive • Many intended audiences do not have access to Internet • Intended audience must be proactive—must search or sign up for information • Newsgroups and chat rooms may require monitoring • Can require maintenance over time

Note: PSA = public service announcement.

Source: Modified from National Cancer Institute. 2004. *Making health communication programs work* (NIH Publication No. 04-5145). Bethesda, MD: National Cancer Institute, U.S. Department of Health and Human Services.

Questions and Activities

1. What are the major advantages of using supporting visuals when working with groups?

2. What kinds of visuals might you use when working with groups? Describe how your choice might differ depending on your audience, such as teens in an after-school program, older adults at a senior citizen center, or a professional group at a conference.

3. List the design principles you would use to avoid having to say to a group, "I know that you cannot read this, but . . ."

4. Prepare a poster (or PowerPoint slide) for use with a group that depicts one idea or theme. Write a description of your objectives for the visual and your intended audience. Write an analysis of your visual explaining how you used art and design principles to enhance quality.

5. You have prepared well for your session, your visuals are in place, and you are now in front of the group. Describe five guidelines for presenting the visuals in an effective manner.

6. Many nutrition educators use printed materials. What purposes might they serve? Describe them.

7. Think of the last time you developed a printed piece. What objectives did you expect it to serve? Do you think it achieved your objectives? Why or why not?

8. How would you ensure that your printed materials are motivating and effective? Describe three specific ways of doing so.

9. You have decided that you will use cooking or food preparation as part of your nutrition education intervention. Based on what you have read, describe three guidelines to ensure a successful learning experience for your participants.

10. What purposes might be served by organizing nutrition education events at health fairs? Describe three tips to ensure that your purposes are met.

11. A central concept in social marketing is the concept of the "exchange." Describe this concept carefully.

12. Compare nutrition education and social marketing. How do they relate to each other?

13. Design social marketing for one of the following situations. Indicate what exactly is the exchange in this setting and how you used the five Ps in your design.

References

Alcay, R., and R. A. Bell. 2000. *Promoting nutrition and physical activity through social marketing: Current practices and recommendations*. Davis: Center of Advanced Studies in Nutrition and Social Marketing, University of California.

Andreasen, A. R. 1995. *Marketing social change: Changing behavior to promote health, social development, and the environment*. San Francisco: Jossey-Bass.

Atienza, A. A., A. C. King, B. M. Olveira. D. K. Ahn, and C. D. Gardener. 2008. Using hand-held computer technologies to improve dietary intake. *American Journal of Preventive Medicine* 34:514ñ518.

Baranowski, T., R. Buday, D. I. Thompson, and J. Baranowski. 2008. Playing for real: video games and stories for health-related behavior change. *American Journal of Preventive Medicine* 34:74ñ82.

Baranowski, T., J. Baranowski, K. W. Cullen, et al. 2003. Squirrel's Quest: Dietary outcome evaluation of a multimedia game. *American Journal of Preventive Medicine* 24:52–61.

Brinberg, D., M. L. Axelson, and S. Price. 2000. Changing food knowledge, food choice, and dietary fiber consumption by using tailored messages. *Appetite* 35:35–43.

Brown, B. J., and B. J. Hermann. 2005. Cooking classes increase fruit and vegetables intake and food safety behaviors in youth and adults. *Journal of Nutrition Education and Behavior* 37:1004–1005.

Brug, J., M. Campbell, and P. Van Assema. 1999. The application and impact of computer-generated personalized nutrition education: A review of the literature. *Patient Education and Counseling* 36:145–156.

Brug, J., A. Oenema, and M. K. Campbell. 2003. Past, present, and future of computer-tailored nutrition education. *American Journal of Clinical Nutrition* 77(Suppl):1028S–1033S.

Brug, J., A. Oenema, and H. Raat. 2005. The Internet and nutrition education: Challenges and opportunities. *European Journal of Clinical Nutrition* 59(suppl): S130–S139.

Campbell, M. K., L. Honess-Morreale, D. Farrell, E. Carbone, and M. Brasure. 1999. A tailored multimedia nutrition education pilot program for low-income women receiving food assistance. *Health Education Research* 14:257–267.

De Bourdeaudhuij, I., V. Stevens, C. Vandelanotte, and J. Brug. 2007. Evaluation of an interactive computer-tailored nutrition intervention in a real-life setting. *Annals of Behavioral Medicine* 33(1):39–48.

Dole Food Company, Inc. 2001. *5 A Day supermarket tours: A guide for retailers*. Oakland, CA: Dole Food Company, Nutrition and Health Program. http://www.dole5aday.com/Retailers/pdfs/5TourRetailerGuide.pdf.

Ezendam, N. P., A. Oenema, P. M. van de Looij-Jansen, and J. Brug. 2007. Design and evaluation protocol of "Fatant-Phat," a computer-tailored intervention to prevent weight gain in adolescents. *BMC Public Health* 12;7:324.

Fjeldsoe B. S., A. L. Marshall, and Y. D. Miller. 2009. Behavior change interventions delivered by mobile telephone short-message service. *American Journal of Preventive Medicine* 36(2):165–173.

Franklin, V. L., A. Waller, C. Pagliari, and S. A. Green. 2006. A randomized control trial of Sweet Talk, a text-messaging system to support young people with diabetes. *Diabetic Medicine* 23:1332ñ1338.

Frederisksen, L. W., L. J. Solomon, and K. A. Brehony, eds. 1984. *Marketing health behavior: Principles, techniques, and applications*. New York: Plenum Press.

Glanz, K., S. Murphy, J. Moylan, D. Evensen, and J. D. Curb. 2006. Improved self-monitoring and adherence with hand-held computers: a pilot study. *American Journal of Health Promotion* 20:165ñ170.

Institute of Medicine. 2002. *Speaking of health: Assessing health communication strategies for diverse populations*. Washington, DC: National Academies Press.

Iowa Department of Public Health. n.d. Pick a better snack. www.idph.state.ia.us/Pickabettersnack/default.asp.

Johnson, S. L., L. Bellows, L. Beckstrom, and J. Anderson. 2007. Evaluation of a social marketing campaign targeting preschool children. *American Journal of Health Behavior* 31(1):44–55.

Knight, S., and C. Probart. 1992. How to avoid saying "I know you can't read this but . . ." *Journal of Nutrition Education* 24:94B.

Kotler, P., and N. R. Lee. 2008. *Social marketing: Influencing behaviors for good*. 3rd ed. Thousand Oaks, CA: Sage.

Kotler, P., and E. L. Roberto. 1989. *Social marketing: Strategies for changing public behavior*. New York: The Free Press.

Kotler, P., and G. Zaltman. 1971, July. Social marketing: An approach to planned social change. *Journal of Marketing* 3–12.

Kreuter, M. W., S. N. Kukwago, D. C. Bucholtz, E. M. Clark, and V. Sanders-Thompson. 2003. Achieving cultural appropriateness in health promotion programs: Targeted and tailored approaches. *Health Education and Behavior* 30:133–146.

Kreuter, M. W., C. Sugg-Skinner, C. L. Holt, et al. 2005. Cultural tailoring for mammography and fruit and vegetables intake among low-income African-American women in urban public health centers. *Preventive Medicine* 41:53–62.

Kroeze, W., A. Werkman, and J. Brug. 2006. A systematic review of randomized trials on the effectiveness of computer-tailored education and physical activity and dietary behaviors. *Annals of Behavioral Medicine* 31(3):205–223.

Lefebure, C., and J. Flora. 1988. Social marketing and public health. *Health Education Quarterly* 15:299–315.

Liquori, T., P. D. Koch, I. R. Contento, and J. Castle. 1998. The CookShop program: Outcome evaluation of a nutrition education program linking lunchroom food experiences with classroom cooking experiences. *Journal of Nutrition Education* 30:302–313.

Lucas, S. E. 2004. *The art of public speaking.* 8th ed. New York: McGraw-Hill.

Maibech, E. W., M. L. Rothschild, and W. D. Novelli. 2002. Social marketing. In *Health behavior and health education: Theory, research and practice,* edited by K. Glanz, B. K. Rimer, and F. M. Lewis. San Francisco: Jossey-Bass.

Manoff, R. K. 1985. *Social marketing.* New York: Praeger.

Mansbridge, J. J. 1990. *Beyond self-interest.* Chicago: University of Chicago Press.

Marcus, A. C., J. Heimendinger, P. Wolfe, et al. 2001. A randomized trial of a brief intervention to increase fruit and vegetable intake: A replication study among callers to the CIS. *Preventive Medicine* 33:204–216.

National Cancer Institute. 2004. *Making health communication programs work* (NIH Publication No. 04-5145). Bethesda, MD: National Cancer Institute, U.S. Department of Health and Human Services.

Newton, K. H., E. J. Wiltshire, and C. R. Elley. 2009, May. Pedometers and text messaging to increase physical activity: Randomized controlled trial of adolescents with type 1 diabetes. *Diabetes Care* 32(5):813–815.

Oenema, A., J. Brug, and L. Lechner. 2001. Web-based tailored nutrition education: Results of a randomized control trial. *Health Education Research* 16:647–660.

Patrick, K., F. Raab, M. A. Adams, et al. 2009. A text-message–based intervention for weight loss: Randomized controlled trial. *Journal of Medical Internet Research* 11(1):e1.

Peng, W. 2009. Design and evaluation of a computer game to promote a healthy diet for young adults. *Health Communication* 24:115ñ127.

Raines, C., and L. Williamson. 1995. *Using visual aids: The effective use of type, color, and graphics.* Revised ed. Menlo Park, CA: Crisp Learning.

Resnicow, K., A. Jackson, T. Wang, et al. 2001. A motivational interviewing intervention to increase fruit and vegetable intake through black churches: Results of the Eat for Life trial. *American Journal of Public Health* 91:1686–1693.

Rifkin R., B. Lohse, J. Bagdonis, and J. Stotts. 2006. Digital photo receivers are a viable technology for nutrition education of low-income persons. *Journal of Nutrition Education and Behavior* 38:326–328.

Rogers, E. M., and J. D. Storey. 1988. Communications campaigns. In *Handbook of communication science,* edited by C. R. Berger and S. H. Chaffee. Newbury Park, CA: Sage.

Rothschild, M. L. 1999. Carrots, sticks, and promises: A conceptual framework for the management of public health and social issue behaviors. *Journal of Marketing* 63:24–37.

Shapiro, J. R., S. Bauer, R. M. Hamer, et al. 2008. Use of text-messaging for monitoring sugar-sweetened beverages, physical activity, and screen time in children: a pilot study. *Journal of Nutrition Education and Behavior* 40:385ñ391.

Smith, S. B., and B. J. Alford. 1989. Literate and semi-literate audiences: Tips for effective teaching. *Journal of Nutrition Education* 20:238C–D.

Sternfeld, B. C. Block, C. P. Quesenberry Jr., et al. 2009. Improving diet and physical activity with ALIVE: A worksite randomized trial. *American Journal of Preventive Medicine* 36(6):475–483.

Stevens, V. J., R. E. Glasgow, D. J. Toobert, N. Karanja, and K. S. Smith. 2002. Randomized trial of a brief dietary intervention to decrease consumption of fat and increase consumption of fruits and vegetables. *American Journal of Health Promotion* 16:129–134.

Thompson, D., T. Baranowski, R. Buday, J. Baranowski, et al. 2007. In pursuit of change: youth response to intensive goal setting embedded in a serious video game. *Journal of Diabetes Science and Technology* 1:907ñ917.

Thompson, D., T. Baranowski, K. Cullen, K. Watson, et al. 2008. Food, fun, and fitness, Internet program for girls: pilot evaluation of an e-Health youth obesity prevention program examining predictors of obesity. *Preventive Medicine* 47:494ñ497.

Thompson, D., T. Baranowski, J. Baranowski, K. Cullen, R. Jago, K. Watson, and Y. Liu. 2009. Boy Scouts 5-a-Day badge: outcome results of a troop and Internet intervention. *Preventive Medicine* 49:518ñ526.

Van Den Heede, F. A, and S. Pelican. 1995. Reflections on marketing as an inappropriate model for nutrition education. *Journal of Nutrition Education* 27:141–145.

Wadsworth, K. 2005. From farm to table: The making of a classroom chef. Presented at the Society for Nutrition Education Conference, Orlando, FL.

Young, L., J. Anderson, L. Beckstrom, L. Bellows, and S. L. Johnson. 2004. Using social marketing principles to guide the development of a nutrition education initiative for preschool-aged children. *Journal of Nutrition Education and Behavior* 36:250–257.

Zepeda, L. 2009, April. The picture of health. *O, The Oprah Magazine* 108.

CHAPTER 17

Working with Diverse Population Groups

....

OVERVIEW   This chapter provides an overview of strategies to use to deliver nutrition education to various age and population groups.

CHAPTER OUTLINE
- Introduction
- Working with children, youth, and adults
- Working with diverse cultural groups
- Low-literacy audiences
- Summary

LEARNING OBJECTIVES   At the end of the chapter, you will be able to:
- Describe key features of the cognitive and emotional development of children and adolescents
- Demonstrate understanding of ways to deliver nutrition education activities that are appropriate to the developmental level of youth
- Demonstrate understanding of ways to conduct nutrition education activities that are based on adult education principles
- Describe key features of cultural competence, cultural sensitivity, and cultural appropriateness in the nutrition education context
- Demonstrate understanding of ways to deliver nutrition education activities that are culturally appropriate
- Demonstrate understanding of ways to deliver nutrition education activities that are appropriate for low-literacy audiences
- Apply design principles for written and visual materials for use in nutrition education for low-literacy audiences

....

■ INTRODUCTION

At a nutrition education session, a group of mothers of young children sit in a circle around a room, sharing their experiences of trying to provide healthful meals for their young children. They are animated and fully engaged with each other for an hour as they share challenges and successes. The educator facilitates the discussion unobtrusively and helps the group to come to closure about what they will do about this issue during the coming week.

Try to imagine a group of preschoolers sitting in a circle and having a similar discussion for an hour, with little guidance from a nutrition educator. Totally impossible, of course! Clearly, the way nutrition education is delivered must be tailored to the group with which you are working. It is thus important to understand the differing characteristics of different population groups. Nutrition educators work in numerous settings, as you saw in Chapter 1: communities, health care settings, schools, food- and food-system-related community and advocacy organizations, and workplaces. In addition, nutrition educators work with many diverse audiences, differing by age, sex, ethnicity, developmental stages, socioeconomic status, geographic location, and so forth. They also work with many groups that have specific food- or nutrition-related issues, such as people with diabetes, pregnant and lactating women, and those who are overweight, to name a few.

This chapter focuses on audiences at different ages and stages of life, from different cultural backgrounds, and with different literacy levels. It provides some background information on each audience and makes suggestions regarding nutrition education delivery methods that are appropriate for each (Contento, Balch, et al. 1995). You should consider some of these differences in appropriate delivery methods at the time you are designing your educational plan or lesson plan.

■ WORKING WITH CHILDREN, YOUTH, AND ADULTS

Children are not little adults. Children are undergoing rapid physical, cognitive, and socioemotional development. Hence, they have their own particular set of concerns and ways of viewing the world, and these change from the preschool years through adolescence. They are in the process of developing various cognitive structures and abilities, understandings of the world, motor skills, social skills, and emotional coping strategies that most adults take for granted. They develop these through their explorations of the world (Piaget & Inhelder 1969) and through social interaction with skilled individuals embedded in a sociocultural backdrop (Vygotsky 1962; Bronfenbrenner 1979). Understanding how children develop and how they learn about food and eating is crucial for nutrition education.

The Preschool Child

The way young children view and experience the world is qualitatively different from that of adults. Child development research provides evidence that the cognitive world of preschool children is creative, fanciful, and free. However, they are becoming less dependent on their direct sensorimotor actions for direction of behavior and are increasingly able to function in a symbolic-conceptual mode in their thinking, for example, using scribbled designs to represent people, cars, houses, and other objects. They have some causal reasoning ability, but it does not lead to abstract generalizations or formation of logical concepts, as in older children or adults. Their attention span is short and they cannot distinguish between their perspective and that of another person. It is not surprising, then, that children younger than 4 years cannot consistently discern between television advertising and the informational content of programs. Children between 4 and 8 years can distinguish between television advertising and program content but do not effectively understand that the intent of television advertising is to persuade them.

Preschool children learn by manipulating the environment rather than by passive listening—that is, they learn by exploring, questioning, comparing, and labeling. Physical manipulation skills are being developed when children touch, feel, look, mix up, turn over, and throw things. Emotionally, exploration and the need to test independence are important during this time. They take on more initiative and are more purposeful. They are eager to learn, usually from other people: they observe parents, teachers, and other children, they role play, and they start to accumulate and process information.

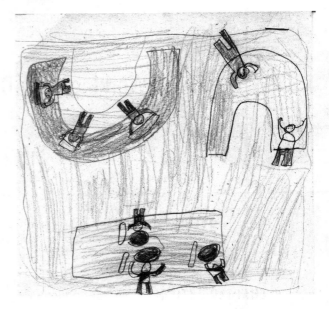

Family meals.

Young Children's Thinking About Food and Nutrition

Research on preschool children suggests that whereas 2-year-olds are only able to name or identify objects, 3- to 5-year-olds can begin to place them into categories such as size, color, and shape. In the food area, they can easily identify foods and are beginning to classify them. However, they classify foods based on observable qualities such as shape and color and on function rather than by nutrient content (Michela & Contento 1984; Matheson, Spranger, & Saxe 2002). They are beginning to be able to relate foods to health (Singleton, Achterberg, & Shannon 1992), but they do not really know what happens to food in the body to bring about its effects on health (Contento 1981).

When preschool children playing in toy kitchens were asked to make a meal for a research assistant, they demonstrated that they already had some knowledge of meal planning, food preparation, table preparation, food serving, eating, and cleaning up (Matheson et al. 2002). They also had notions about eating rules such as "You must eat a little bit of everything," "Eat it—it is good for you," and "This is mine and that's yours; you can eat whatever you want." These observations suggest that nutrition education should not focus on food group information but should instead emphasize active methods and play activities.

Children are not born with the natural ability to choose a nutritious diet: they have to learn to do so. The accumulating evidence from research suggests that early experience with food and eating has an impact on the development of food preferences and on the regulation of amount of food eaten in several ways.

- *Familiarity with the food.* Very young children show a neophobic response, or reluctance to taste new or unfamiliar foods, a natural and protective mechanism that is one of the most common reasons for food rejection. However, repeated exposures increase children's preference for a food or beverage (Birch 1999). A longitudinal study found that a large percentage of children's food preferences were formed as early as age 2 to 3 years and did not change over the five-year period of the study, at which point the children were age 8 (Skinner et al. 2002). Other studies have shown that dislike of foods can be transformed into liking when children are repeatedly exposed to foods through tasting and eating (Wardle, Cooke, et al. 2003; Wardle, Herrara, et al. 2003).

- *Association of foods with the physiological consequences of eating.* Very young children seem to be able to regulate the amount they eat based almost solely on their physiological reactions to foods (i.e., feeling full) (Birch 1987, 1999). As they get older, however, children eat substantially more when larger portions are offered, suggesting that the ability to respond solely to internal physiological cues decreases with age as external factors become more influential (Rolls, Engell, & Birch 2000; Orlet Fisher, Rolls, & Birch 2003; Rolls et al. 2002). Indeed, they often eat in the absence of hunger (Fisher & Birch 2002).

- *Association of foods with the emotional tone of the social interactions that surround feeding.* Children come to prefer foods that are eaten in a positive emotional atmosphere (Birch 1987) as well as foods eaten by their peers. A survey of Head Start parents showed that their own positive nutrition-related attitudes were related to more pleasant family mealtimes, fewer negative mealtime practices, and less troublesome child eating behaviors (Gable & Lutz 2001). Head Start program mealtime environments and practices can thus contribute importantly to young children coming to like healthful foods.

- *Learning and self-regulation.* As children develop the ability to identify which food cues are relevant in beginning, continuing, and ending eating, learning and self-regulation become extremely important. As noted previously, very young children seem to be able to regulate the amount they eat based primarily on their physiological reactions to foods, but as they get older, external factors, including parenting practices, become influential as well. For example, there is some evidence suggesting that in mainstream culture parents who have eating issues of their own or who impose strong control over their children's intake may interfere with their children's ability to regulate their intake on their own (Faith et al. 2004). The role of parental control may be more complex in children of diverse ethnic and socioeconomic backgrounds (Robinson et al. 2001; Contento, Zybert, & Williams 2005) because parents' control and restriction may be interpreted as love and responsibility in some cultures (Lin & Liang 2005). However, the studies do all support the recommended practice that it is the responsibility of the adults in families, day-care centers, and schools to provide healthful foods, and it is the responsibility of the child to choose how much of these foods to eat (Satter 1999).

From consistent practice in making choices from an array of healthful foods, children learn healthful eating patterns and develop the ability to regulate how much of these foods to eat.

Methods for Delivering Nutrition Education Appropriately to Preschool Children

What practical methods can you use, then, to increase the effectiveness of nutrition education for young children? Based on the information just discussed and on the research literature, the following methods of delivering nutrition education are likely to be useful.

Use Food-Based Activities

Food-based activities such as tasting parties, food preparation, and activities designed to engage the five senses with food are useful. Provide daily exposure to healthful meals and snacks to increase children's preferences for these foods. Nutrition educators note that meals and snacks provided at child-care centers should be seen as the centerpiece of nutrition education and should be offered in a positive eating atmosphere.

Create Developmentally Appropriate Learning Experiences

Child development theory and research suggest that no amount of "teaching" will make young children learn concepts that are beyond the capability of their cognitive structures to understand. On the other hand, preschoolers should not just be entertained because they are assumed to be unable to understand (Hertzler & DeBord 1994). Young children have certain cognitive skills that can be used in nutrition education. Programs need to be tailored to children's level of emotional and motor developmental levels. Design activities that take into account the observations that 2- to 3-year-olds can name foods eaten at home or seen in the store and describe the tastes and textures of foods, whereas older preschoolers can classify foods by color and function, identify foods seen on TV, and learn reading skills by reading food-themed storybooks. In terms of the link between food and health, 2- to 3-year-olds can name body parts and tell the location of organs, such as eyes, and what they do. Older preschoolers can compare breathing and pulse rate when doing different activities and can state general connections between food and the body, for example, that carrots are good for your eyes.

Apply Activity- and Play-Based Teaching Methods

Design activity-based teaching methods and play-based curricula that build on children's naturalistic environments and interests. These activities should have clear messages so that they are "minds-on" as well as "hands-on." Studies show that where interventions had an impact on knowledge and eating practices, active participation by children in a nonthreatening environment was most conducive to success. Employ activities such as art projects, songs, jingles, role playing, stories, puppets, and puzzles. Curricula can focus on play. Toy kitchens or grocery stores provide opportunities for nutrition education. In addition, children can role play trying new foods or practicing food safety behaviors in these contexts (Matheson et al. 2002). Children can work in school gardens, learning about how food grows.

Focus on Behaviors

Identify specific children's behaviors to focus on, such as trying new foods, eating vegetables, or eating healthful snacks. Then work with parents and preschool staff to model eating healthful meals and snacks, offer foods to children in a positive social environment, and use rewards appropriately. For example, "trying new foods" was the behavior addressed in a social marketing campaign directed at preschoolers, called Food Friends (discussed in Nutrition Education in Action 16-2). It used many of the kinds of activities described earlier: sensory activities that included "fruit and vegetable mystery bags," storybooks, opportunities to try new foods, and parental involvement (Young et al. 2004; Johnson et al. 2007).

Encourage Self-Regulation

Parents and preschools can encourage the child's ability to self-regulate. It is the responsibility of families and preschools to provide children with healthful foods in appropriate settings and at appropriate times, but children should be able to choose how much to eat from among these foods. From this practice children will learn to self-regulate the appropriate amounts of food to eat to satisfy hunger. These self-regulation skills will become increasingly cognitive, as well as biological, in nature

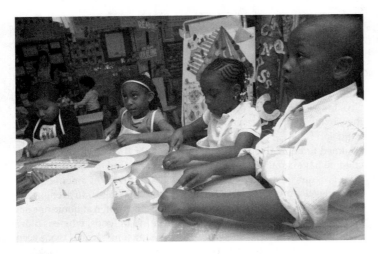

Cooking helps young children develop motor skills and increases the liking for vegetables.

as children develop cognitively and are exposed to, and have to make conscious choices from, an increasing array of foods, many of which are very attractive in a variety of nonhealthful ways. Children can be encouraged to pay attention to their hunger cues and to eat when they are hungry and to stop when they are full. These are cognitive activities, requiring conscious decisions.

Involve Parents and Families

Involving families either as major recipients of the program or in conjunction with the program offered to the preschool child is crucial for nutrition education of children this age (**Box 17-1**) (Ventura & Birch 2008). Parents and teachers working together can make more of an impact through mutual reinforcement than either can alone. Studies with Head Start found that educating and encouraging parents were effective in increasing children's knowledge and reported consumption of more nutritious foods. The Food Friends program incorporated a parent component, as discussed in Nutrition Education in Action 16-2.

Middle Childhood and Adolescence

Children grow and change rapidly during the school years. Middle childhood (ages 6–11) is a time of major cognitive development and mastery of cognitive, physical, and social skills. Children at this age are eager to understand people and the world around them. They like being physically active as their bodies grow steadily in muscle mass and strength and as they grow taller. They progress from dependence on their parents to increasing independence, with an increasing interest in developing friendships with others.

$\mathcal{B}$ox 17-1   Core Nutrition Messages for Children and Families

For Mothers of Preschoolers

Role Modeling Messages

1. They learn from watching you. Eat fruits and veggies, and your kids will, too.
2. They take their lead from you. Eat fruits and veggies, and your kids will, too.

Cooking and Eating Together Messages*

1. Cook together. Eat together. Talk together. Make mealtime a family time.
2. Make meals and memories together. It's a lesson they'll use for life.

Division of Feeding Responsibility Messages

1. Let them learn by serving themselves. Let your kids serve themselves at dinner. Teach them to take small amounts first. Tell them they can get more if they're still hungry.
2. Sometimes new foods take time. Kids don't always take to new foods right away. Offer new fruits and veggies numerous times. Give them a taste at first, and be patient.
3. Patience works better than pressure. Offer your children new foods and then let them choose how much to eat. Kids are more likely to enjoy something when eating it is their own choice. This also helps them learn to be independent.

For Mothers of Elementary School-Age Children

Availability/Accessibility Messages

1. Want your kids to reach for a healthy snack? Make sure fruits and veggies are in reach.*
2. When they come home hungry, have fruits and veggies ready to eat.*
3. Let your kids be "produce pickers." Help them pick fruits and veggies at the store.
4. They're still growing. Help your kids grow strong. Serve fat-free or low milk at meals.

For 8- to 10-Year-Old Children

Food Preference, Beliefs, and Asking Behavior Messages

1. Eat smart to play hard. Drink milk (low-fat or fat-free) at meals.
2. Fuel up with milk at meals, and soar through your day like a rocket ship.
3. Snack like a super hero. Power up with fruit and yogurt.
4. Eat smart to play hard. Eat fruits and veggies at meals and snacks.
5. Fuel up with fruits and veggies, and soar through your day like a rocket ship.

Note: *Consumer-tested supporting content (e.g. bulleted tips, stories, recipes) is available on the USDA's website.
Source: U.S. Department of Agriculture. 2009, January. Core Nutrition Messages. http://www.fns.usda.gov/fns/corenutritionmessages/default.html.

During adolescence (ages 12–19), growth accelerates, leading to dramatic physical, developmental, and social changes that can affect eating patterns. Diet quality declines as children move from childhood through adolescence. Their eating patterns put them at risk for current and future health problems, as shown in **Box 17-2**. They have considerable spending power, and they often have considerable autonomy in food choices as well. A number of these factors influence the choice of methods for delivering nutrition education.

Cognitive Development

Cognitive maturity influences what children can learn from nutrition education. The child comes to school with a host of ideas about the physical and natural world, and these are different from those of adults. Nutrition educators need to understand these differences to communicate well with them. Children are motivated to learn and acquire knowledge and are full of curiosity. In the early school years, children move beyond intuitive thinking to be able to think causally, although reasoning is likely to be limited to concrete objects and specific experiences. They tend to think like scientists, asking many "why" questions. They like to do experiments and can theorize. However, they often maintain their old theories regardless of the evidence and are more likely to be influenced by happenstance events than by overall patterns. They think of food in functional terms. One study found they classified on the basis of sweet versus nonsweet foods; meals versus more versatile foods and drinks; whole, fresh foods versus more highly processed foods; and plants versus animal foods (Michela & Contento 1984). Children's information-processing capacity also increases during the school years, but they use behavioral, concrete, and specific cues to define health, and the criteria for their food choices are specific and immediate (such as taste or cost).

Adolescents begin to think more abstractly and more logically and are able to formulate hypotheses to explain occurrences and imagine alternative explanations for what is observed. They are thus capable of more abstract concepts linking food and health. They begin to develop the ability to grasp the deeper meanings of problems and to think reflectively and critically, keeping an open mind. Becoming more idealistic, they begin to think about idealistic characteristics for themselves and others and to compare themselves and others to ideal standards. They are intrigued by social, political, and moral issues and are willing to speak out on them. In the food area, many become vegetarians or become involved in important food- and nutrition-related causes.

Emotional and Social Development

The emotional and social development of children and youth are important to consider when delivering nutrition education. During middle and late childhood, children spend an increasing amount of time with their peers. Friendships are important because they provide stimulation in the form of interesting information and excitement, a familiar playmate, support, encouragement and feedback, intimacy, affection, and a trusting relationship where aspects of the self can be shared. Friendship also provides a means of social comparison, whereby the child can find out where she or he stands with respect to others. During this period, children begin to understand the perspective of another person and develop greater self-understanding. Development of self-esteem or sense of self-worth is important and can be fostered by providing emotional support and approval and opportunities to develop real skills and a sense of achievement. Self-esteem can also be enhanced by learning to cope with problems realistically rather than avoid them.

During adolescence, pubertal changes occur, resulting in rapid growth and sexual maturation. Adolescents also become intensely interested in their body image. They worry about their sexual appearance. They also develop a special kind of egocentrism. Whereas preschoolers' egocentrism derives from the inability to distinguish between their own perspective and that of someone else, adolescent egocentrism is distinguished by belief in an imaginary audience and in a personal fable (Elkind 1978). In terms of imaginary audience, adolescents are very aware of other people and believe that others are as preoccupied with them as they are with themselves. They feel they are on stage and the rest of the world is their audience. This leads to the desire to be noticed and visible. At the same time this leads to great concerns. For example, the young woman is sure that everyone will notice and comment on the small, almost invisible spot on her sweater, or the young man imagines that all eyes will be on the tiny blemish on his face. In terms of personal fable, adolescents believe in their personal uniqueness, which results in believing that no one else can understand how they really feel. To foster this uniqueness, adolescents create stories

---

Box 17-2 Typical Eating Patterns of Adolescents in the United States and Their Implications

Patterns
- Chaotic eating patterns
- Eat rapidly and away from home
- Spend their own money
- Exposed to more than eight hours per day of various media (TV, computer, radio, magazines)
- Reliance on fast food and convenience food
- Begin to buy and prepare more food for themselves
- Influence parents' buying; do some of the family shopping
- Replacement of milk with soft drinks and other sweetened beverages

Statistics
- Less than 25% of adolescents, grades 9–12, eat at least five servings of fruits and vegetables per day.
- The average teen visits a fast food restaurant just over two times a week and spends $5 a visit, for a total of $13 billion each year in fast food restaurants.
- Teens spend $9.6 billion in food and snack stores each year.
- They spend $736 million each year on vending machines.

Why Are These Patterns a Problem?
- Fast foods tend to be high in fat, sugar, and/or salt.
- Sweetened beverages are high in calories.
- Fast foods tend to be low in iron, calcium, riboflavin, vitamin A, folic acid, and vitamin C.
- Inadequate intake of calcium in adolescence can set the stage for osteoporosis later on.
- The rate of type 2 diabetes is increasing among adolescents.

about themselves that are filled with fantasy. They believe that what is really important is what is going on with their particular circle of friends and events at school.

As they grow older, adolescents become more independent, trying to establish themselves as unique individuals. They also start developing a better understanding of their own strengths and weaknesses and think about the future. They struggle with how they should relate to their friends and family in terms of how to be close to them yet maintain their own independence.

Adolescents' Thinking, Concerns, and Behaviors with Respect to Food, Nutrition, and Health

Adolescents' eating behaviors are influenced by factors at many levels as shown in the social-ecological model: *individual factors*, both psy-

chological and biological; *interpersonal factors* such as family and peers; *community settings* such as schools or fast food outlets; and *societal factors* such as mass media, marketing, and sociocultural norms (Story, Neumark-Sztainer, & French 2002). Factors influencing food choices include hunger and food cravings, time, convenience, cost and availability of foods, perceived benefits, mood, body image, and habit. Major barriers to healthy eating include a lack of sense of urgency about personal health in relation to other more pressing concerns and preferring the taste of other foods (Neumark-Sztainer et al. 1999). **Box 17-3** notes the implications for nutrition education of the cognitive and social development characteristics of adolescents.

Focus group research has found that adolescents have a significant amount of knowledge about healthful foods and believe that healthful eating involves balance, moderation, and variety. However, they find it

---

$\mathcal{B}$ox 17-3 Cognitive and Emotional Development of Children and Adolescents: Implications for Nutrition Education

Middle Childhood

Characteristics
- Have ideas or theories of how the natural world works that are different from those of adults
- Black-and-white thinkers: causal thinking is more developed, but reasoning still limited to concrete objects and specific experiences
- Criteria for food choice are specific and immediate
- Curious and motivated to learn: they particularly like to do experiments
- Trust and respect adults
- Playmates and peer friendships are increasingly important
- Beginning to desire autonomy

Implications for Nutrition Education
- Use fantasy characters and stories in nutrition education
- Address benefits related to having more energy and/or improved performance in sports
- Use active methods
- Focus on the functional meanings of food
- Include handouts with bright pictures and direct messages
- Foster self-esteem
- Use simple goal-setting activities and foster cognitive self-regulation

Early Adolescence

Characteristics
- Causal reasoning becoming more developed
- Criteria for food choice are specific and immediate
- Relationships between food and health are becoming of interest
- Trust and respect adults
- Anxious about peer relationships
- Ambivalent about autonomy
- Preoccupied with the body and body image, and uncomfortable with the physical changes of puberty

- Willing to do or say anything that makes them look or feel better about their body image
- Interested in immediate results

Implications for Nutrition Education
- Address benefits related to looking healthy, having more energy, and/or performance in sports
- Focus on short-term goals
- Include simplified instructions, handouts with bright pictures, and direct messages
- Use active methods

Middle Adolescence

Characteristics
- Abstract thinking skills developing
- Criteria for food choice are becoming more complex, with increased reasoning about consequences
- Greatly influenced by peers
- Mistrustful of adults; recurrently challenge adult authority
- Listen to peers more than adults
- Consider independence to be very important and experience significant cognitive development
- More in charge of the food they eat
- Temporary rejection of family dietary patterns

Implications for Nutrition Education
- Design activities to analyze social influences such as television advertising, the media, what's available in neighborhood stores or stores around their schools, and what their friends eat, and their own response to these influences
- Focus on how to make healthful choices when eating out
- Use food demonstrations and taste tests
- Use simplified problem-identification techniques, role playing, and "what if" scenarios
- Guided goal setting is possible
- Foster teenagers' increasing independence while maintaining a caring, yet authoritative role

Box 17-3 Cognitive and Emotional Development of Children and Adolescents: Implications for Nutrition Education (*continued*)

Late Adolescence

Characteristics

- Abstract thinking more developed; with experience, teens become more skilled at problem solving and decision making
- Criteria for food choice are becoming more complex: understand the notion of making trade-offs
- More established body image
- Orientation toward the future and making plans
- Becoming increasingly independent; less challenging of adult authority
- More consistent in their values and beliefs
- Developing intimacy and permanent relationships
- Begin to think of long term and about improving their overall health
- Still want to make their own decisions, but are more open to information provided by health care providers

Implications for Nutrition Education

- Build educational experiences around motivations that are particularly meaningful to this age group
- Present dietary recommendations and give the rationales behind them
- Focus on behaviors that adolescents have control over
- Discussions of complex issues are now possible, and homework-type assignments are appropriate
- Foster cognitive self-regulation involving goal-setting and action plans
- Teach skills to address long-term goals
- Provide food preparation experiences if possible
- Respect their independence and encourage their decision-making skills

difficult to eat healthfully because of their perceived lack of time, the limited availability of healthful options in school, and a general lack of concern about following recommendations (Neumark-Sztainer et al. 1997; Croll, Neumark-Sztainer, & Story 2001).

The weight and body image concerns of adolescents have been of particular interest to nutrition educators. Studies have found that adolescents often attempt to make their weights conform to societal ideals by practicing many weight control behaviors. Most adolescents practice healthy weight control behaviors (85% of girls and 70% of boys in one survey). Some adolescents, particularly those who are overweight, practice some unhealthy weight control behaviors or even behaviors that are extreme (Neumark-Sztainer et al. 2002). However, those who use moderate methods of weight control have more healthful eating and exercise patterns than those who are extreme dieters or nondieters, suggesting that they might be practicing some degree of self-monitoring and self-regulation (Story et al. 1998).

Cognitive-Motivational Processes and Self-Regulation

The fact that children and adolescents are not concerned about health and nutrition issues to any major extent when they are making food choices is not surprising, given that they do not perceive any urgency to change and that the future seems so distant (Story & Resnick 1986; Neumark-Sztainer et al. 1999). In addition it has been found that nutrition knowledge alone does not ensure that children and adolescents (or adults, for that matter) will adopt healthful behaviors (Gibson & Wardle 1998).

However, studies show that cognitive-motivational processes do become increasingly important influences on food choice as children become older and more developed cognitively. That is, older children and adolescents become more able to link cause and effect and to perceive the consequences of their actions (Contento & Michela 1998). Thus, they can make food choices in light of their perceptions of anticipated consequences from eating particular foods. Adolescents can make trade-offs among their desired consequences. For example, dieting adolescents in one study were willing to forgo taste and convenience to some degree to obtain less-fattening food (Contento, Michela, & Williams 1995). In

another study, adolescents were willing to balance less nutritious items with more nutritious items within a meal, and to balance less healthful lunches with more healthful dinners (Contento et al. 2006).

Remember that adolescents are not monolithic in their food choice motivations. One study found they could be divided into several subgroups with distinct orientations to food, ranging from the hedonistic group, for whom taste and convenience were paramount; to the socially controlled group, for whom friends were most important; and to the health-oriented subgroups, who were concerned about personal health (Contento, Michela, & Goldberg 1988). Those in the health-oriented groups had better diets than those in the hedonistic and socially controlled groups. Other studies have reported similar findings that those concerned about health had better diets (Gibson & Wardle 1998; Cusatis & Shannon 1996). It should be noted that health outcomes that have meaning for this group are still short-term outcomes (e.g., that they will have more energy, better athletic performance, or better-looking skin), which should thus be emphasized in nutrition education.

From a social psychological perspective, the picture that emerges from research is that older children and adolescents want particular consequences from the food they eat and become increasingly able to align their food choice behaviors with their goals. They integrate motivations and cognitions in a process of *cognitive self-regulation* (Contento & Michela 1998). This ability makes it possible for nutrition educators to incorporate the teaching of skills in goal-setting, self-monitoring, and other self-regulatory processes to this age group.

Family Influences

What the family serves is still important. Children ages 6 to 11 obtained 76% of their calories at home, and even adolescents obtained 65% (Guthrie, Lin, & Frazao 2002). Although adolescents are increasingly independent, making food choices in an ever-widening circle of settings, most still eat some meals at home. Several surveys suggest that about a quarter of teens in the United States eat seven or more meals with their family, about 40% eat three to six meals a week with them, and 20% eat about one to two meals a week, with only about 15% never eating with their families (Neumark-Sztainer et al. 2003). Increasing frequency of eating family meals among children and adolescents is associated with more healthful dietary patterns (Gillman et al. 2000; Videon & Manning 2003; Neumark-Sztainer et al. 2003).

Most adolescents in one survey reported that they enjoyed eating meals with the family and that it is a time to bring everybody together and to talk with each other (Neumark-Sztainer et al. 2000a). Major reasons for not eating together were teen schedules, a desire for autonomy, and not liking the foods served or the family atmosphere (Neumark-Sztainer et al. 2000b). Another study found that many adolescents resolved these meal-related conflicting desires by negotiating with others in the family about what to serve at home (Contento et al. 2006). This means that nutrition education can teach youth to more effectively negotiate with their families and to use what they eat at home to balance what they eat elsewhere.

Methods for Delivering Nutrition Education Appropriately to Children and Youth

Based on the background information just discussed and on the research literature, the following are suggestions for methods of delivering nutrition education that are likely to enhance effectiveness.

Focus on Behaviors or Practices Over Which Youth Have Some Control

A behaviorally focused approach to nutrition education improves effectiveness. In the case of older children and adolescents, choose behaviors for the intervention that are of nutritional concern but are also those over which youth have some control. Examples are eating fruits and vegetables, lower-fat snacks and lunches, regular breakfasts, and calcium-rich foods.

Address Motivations That Are Meaningful and Important to Youth

Link information about why to engage in healthful behaviors to motivations that are important to youth, such as having energy, being able to perform well both physically and cognitively, being strong, or having healthy-looking hair or skin. Focus on benefits such as convenience,

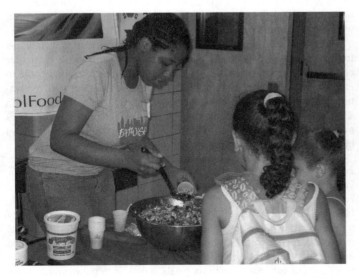

Peer education: Eatwise teens prepare food taste tests for younger children.

taste, cost, and other attributes of foods and eating patterns that are relevant to them. Explore barriers. Take into account that some are still growing and that satisfying hunger at low cost is a major motivator, whereas others, particularly girls, have made the transition through puberty and have stabilized in terms of growth.

Thus, make the case for healthful eating in terms that are meaningful for youth. For example, you can help them calculate the costs of the beverages and snacks they currently consume and show how more healthful alternatives can cost the same or less. Or show how convenient it is to prepare fruits and vegetables as snacks. This does not mean you cannot increase a sense of concern about healthful eating. You can. But rather than focusing on their own personal risk for disease, ask youth about whether they have family members who have various chronic diseases such as diabetes and how that makes them feel. This can be a useful way to address the issue of food-related disease risk.

Incorporate Self-Evaluation and Self-Assessment

Youth like self-assessments that are interesting and fun and provide a picture of themselves. A possible activity is to have the class as a group write down what they ate and drank the day before and then analyze these lists in terms of the behavior of focus for your sessions, such as eating breakfast, eating fruits and vegetables, or eating at fast food restaurants. Or you could design a checklist of actions that the group could potentially engage in and come up with a composite score to indicate how well they are doing.

Use Active Methods

Although their attention spans are now longer than those of young children, getting and holding the attention of youth still require active methods of nutrition education, perhaps alternating with mini-lectures. Food preparation or food-related demonstrations with participation of volunteers from the group can be very effective. Provide small group activities to explore issues. Be clear to yourself regarding the purpose of each activity and how it relates to your session objectives. As mentioned earlier, activities need to be minds-on as well as hands-on so as not to turn into busywork. Carefully structure such activities, with clear instructions on how to conduct the activity and accompanying worksheets or activity sheets. Grocery store or farmers' market tours, for example, are appealing to upper elementary school children. Prepare the students ahead of time and prepare activity sheets for what they will do once there.

Deliver Content Appropriately in Terms of Cognitive Developmental Level

For elementary and middle school–aged children, health outcomes are in the distant future, and hence food and nutrition content needs to be provided in formats that fit their cognitive levels. Children may respond to food and nutrition activities if they involve some kind of intrinsic reward or element of fun (Matheson & Spranger 2001). Puzzles, fantasy play, contests, quizzes, games, or computer games are engaging because they provide children with a challenge, the level of which can be set by the age of the child or group. These activities also stimulate children's curiosity if there is a meaningful objective that is part of the game or contest. Thus, fantasy, challenge, and curiosity can build on children's interest in investigations and stimulate intrinsic motivation. Nutrition content can be part of the plot or the problem to be solved by the characters involved in the fantasies and stories. One program created characters from another planet—named Hearty Heart, Dynamite Diet, Salt Sleuth, and Flash Fitness—who came to Earth to work with children and help them learn and practice health-promoting eating and exercise patterns (Leupker et al. 1996). A computer curriculum based on stories about invaders of a kingdom asked children to become squires to help the king and queen. The squires faced many challenges in their quest. The story included wizards, robots, and other fantasy creatures (Baranowski et al. 2003).

For high school students, hunger and food cravings, time, convenience, cost and availability of foods, perceived benefits, mood, body image, and habit are pressing food choice motivations. However, many issues in the field are controversial, from weight control diets, sales of sweetened beverages in schools, organic foods, and causes of world hunger to local versus global food systems. Stimulate thought and critical thinking through presentation of surprising data, interesting content, and case examples. Given that adolescents like to be challenged, design activities, such as debates or position papers, where they have an opportunity to grapple with these issues. Provide opportunities for students to propose novel or imaginative ideas to solve problems, understand and appreciate different viewpoints, and develop plans to address issues and solve problems.

Address Social Norms and Peer Influences

Help youth recognize the power of social environmental influences on their eating patterns by having them analyze television advertising, food marketing techniques, and what's available in neighborhood stores or stores around their schools. Make healthful eating desirable or cool by providing role models of importance to older children and youth. Peer educators can also be incorporated into the program, who can model healthful behaviors and address the participants' concerns.

Remember the Importance of the Affective Domain

Teens' food choices and eating practices are strongly influenced by affective and emotional factors (as is true for all people). Nutrition education can appeal to their growing sense of independence and ability to make choices for themselves as opposed to being dependent on the opinion of others. They can be encouraged to take charge of their lives. Because self-esteem is very important, activities should be respectful, build self-esteem, and never embarrass children and teens in front of others. Address body image and appearance concerns with sensitivity, being respectful of persons of all sizes.

Conduct Food-Based Activities When Possible

Everyone is interested in food, and youth are no exception. These activities can enhance motivation, overcome barriers, and provide skill development. Develop simple recipes for food preparation, particularly ones that do not require heating or complicated utensils for where facilities are limited. Be sure to test these recipes first for ease of preparation, taste, and appearance, as well as ease in transporting ingredients and utensils to the site. Unless it is designated as a cooking session, the procedures should be quick to maintain attention and motivation. The activity should also engage all the teens so that you do not have volunteers and onlookers. Set up several food preparation stations with the ingredients already measured out at each station.

Foster Cognitive Self-Regulation

Given the increasing pressure of external forces on the food choices of older children and adolescents, ranging from peer pressure, food marketing practices, and the school environment to busy schedules and time constraints that leave little time to eat healthfully, nutrition education can foster cognitive self-regulation processes that focus on mindful eating through goal setting, planning ahead, and self-monitoring. These processes are described in detail in Chapter 12. Setting specific and actionable goals is not always easy, even for adults. It is important to take the time to teach goal-setting skills, using a process of guided goal setting, which seems to work best for this age group. Guided goal setting means that you can set the *major goals* for youth to achieve through your sessions or program, such as "eating healthful snacks," and youth can set their own specific and highly individualized *action goals* to achieve these major goals, such as by stating they will "eat fruit for snacks two days next week." Help them to balance meals eaten with peers that may not be so healthful with other, more healthful meals, such as those eaten at home. They can also negotiate within the family for healthful foods they like.

The Adult Learner

Adult learners can't be threatened, coerced, or tricked into learning something new; they must want to know (Brookfield 1986; Knowles 1990; Tennant & Pogson 1995; Vella 2002). Nutrition educators thus need to focus on behaviors, practices, or issues of immediate relevance to the group.

Characteristics of Adult Learners

Adults need to know why they need to learn something before undertaking to learn it. Much of adult learning is self-initiated and conducted on their own. However, adults also often find themselves participating in learning experiences because of the requirements of workplaces or food assistance programs (such as WIC or senior meal programs), referrals by their doctors and other medical care professionals, or for other reasons. Individuals need to see the immediate usefulness of the new skills, knowledge, or attitudes they are working to acquire. Learning is a means, not an end. Most adults do not have time to waste. They may even have to arrange for child care to attend a session so that the session costs them money as well as time. Not surprisingly, they like to be convinced that the experience will be worth their time and effort.

Orientation to Learning

Adults are generally task-oriented, problem-oriented, or life-centered. Thus, they are less interested in, or enthralled by, a survey of nutrition such as provided by an overview of the food pyramid. They would rather learn about one or two key ideas and how they can be applied to a problem of relevance to them. However, there may be large differences in their preference for teaching style based on their own learning styles (see Chapter 15). For example, analytic learners may prefer that the needed information be presented to them in a straightforward but interesting presentation, whereas sociable or dynamic learners enjoy discussions. There is some agreement among adult educators that discussion is an ideal format for adult learning: it permits learners to share their own challenges and successes and to learn from the experiences of others. It reinforces their sense of self-worth and fosters their ability to make decisions. Discussions are especially useful for developing critical thinking and for creating new meaning systems out of shared experiences and collaborative interpretations of them (Brookfield 1986; Knowles 1990; Abusabha, Peacock, & Achterberg 1999; Vella 2002).

Readiness to Learn

Adults are ready to learn those things that will help them to cope effectively with their real-life situations. Thus, pregnant women and mothers of young children may become interested in nutrition education because they want to have healthy children. Other life-changing events may also increase the readiness to learn, such as beginning to live on one's own, having teenagers whose eating patterns are of concern, or being diagnosed with some health condition. They seek out a learning experience because they have a use for the knowledge or skill being sought.

Learners' Past Experience

Adults have a great quantity of prior experience with food and eating. These experiences are unique to individuals, and the differences between individuals are large. Nutrition educators may be the experts on the content, but adults are the experts on their own lives. These experiences must be honored and can greatly enrich sessions if they are built into the design of the sessions. You can find out about these past experiences through a careful and thorough needs and resources analysis. Indeed, many adults have greater experience with cooking or child-rearing than the nutrition educator. Others in the group, including the nutrition educator, can benefit from this wealth of knowledge if it is shared.

Learners as Decision Makers

Adults have a self-concept of being responsible for their own decisions and for their own lives. Healthy adults thus want respect for themselves as decision makers and resist being treated as objects and being told what to do. Indeed, quality of life increases as people are more capable of making decisions that affect their lives. Participants in nutrition education want the information you provide and are grateful for the sharing of experiences and tips from others, but they want to choose whether and how they will apply the information. This makes it imperative that sessions with adults be built on mutual respect and dialogue.

Motivation

Internal or intrinsic motivations to learn and change are more important than extrinsic motivations. Internal motivations include increased self-esteem, quality of life, job satisfaction, and health and avoidance of disease. Extrinsic motivations may include the advice of physicians or the urging of family.

Stage of Life and Roles

Adulthood is not some static state at which individuals arrive when they finish high school or get their first job. Instead, development is lifelong. Individuals grow and change throughout life. As they do, their needs, values, roles, and expectations change. These all have implications for nutrition education.

Life Stage Influences

Researchers have identified several adult life stages from in-depth interviews of individuals over time (Neugarten, Havighurst, & Tobin 1968; Gould 1978; Levinson 1978, 1996). They suggest that adults experience several main stages: leaving the family between the ages of 15 and 25; with a transition between ages 25 and 30 to becoming an adult, entering a career, and starting a family; leading to settling down and becoming one's own person between the ages of 30 and 40. At this stage, careers are usually set and individuals now have families of their own. In the middle 40s to early 50s, children have left home, and individuals begin to see that time is finite and question life's meaning. Neugarten and colleagues (1968) propose that until about this time, individuals see life in terms of "time since birth." The future stretches forth and there is time to do and see everything. The orientation is toward achievement, and death is an abstraction. After this period, individuals see life as "time left to live," where time is finite and there is time enough only to finish a few important things. Sponsoring others becomes important, and death becomes more personal. Some experience this midlife transition

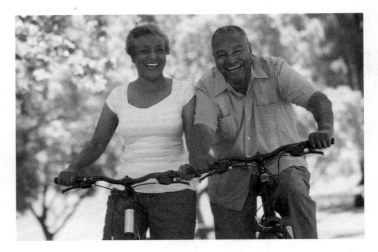

Physical activity is enjoyable at any age.

as destabilizing (the so-called midlife crisis), but most do not. This is then followed by restabilization in the 50s, where there is a renewed interest in friends and reliance on spouse or partner. This process is well illustrated in the nutrition area by the description of one woman about her changing perspective:

> When you're in your twenties you think you're not vulnerable to anything. When you're in your thirties you think you still have time. When you're in your forties you see things begin to creep up on you that have never affected you before . . . so you begin to seriously consider some of the things you've been reading about. [In your fifties] you make more conscious efforts to stick with foods and diets and meal planning that conform to better health standards. (Devine & Olson 1991)

Women's motives for preventive dietary behaviors have been found to vary with life stage because of altered perceptions of health status, body weight, and family roles and responsibilities (Devine & Olson 1991). Women with young children at home were more likely to be concerned for their children's health, resulting in a positive impact on their own diets because they prepared balanced family meals and sought to set a good example. For mothers of teenagers, there was tension between their desire to make healthful changes for their own health and the lack of acceptance of these changes by the family. The departure of grown children from the home allowed older women to make dietary changes for their own personal health, and many expressed that this stage was very satisfying.

There are also cohort effects (Neugarten et al. 1968): those who grew up in the idealistic 1960s, for example, have different values, attitudes, expectations, and behaviors than those who grew up in the baby boomer or "me" generation (see **Box 17-4**). This has been found in the nutrition area as well: those growing up between 1944 and 1954 differed from those born two decades before in their perspectives on food and gender roles in the household and the ways in which differing kinds and degrees of public information about food and nutrition affected family meals growing up (Devine & Olson 1991). The perspectives of today's generations X and Y and younger on food and nutrition issues likewise differ from those of the baby boomers. You need to be mindful of these cohort effects as you deliver nutrition education.

Box 17-4 Characteristics of Different Age Cohorts

The GI Generation, or Greatest Generation
Born between 1901 and 1924, today they are aged mid-80s and up. At 60 million strong, they were molded by the Great Depression and World War II. They won World War II and provided the nation with seven presidents. Members tend to be conservative; as a whole, they constitute the most satisfied generation.

Tips for Working with Them
- Emphasize realistic strengths, not weaknesses.
- Don't tell them they are old; just provide larger type.
- Make access easy.

The Silent Generation and Idealistic Generation
Born between 1925 and 1942, today their ages range from the late-60s to the early 80s. About 49 million strong, they were influenced by the GI generation before them. The older members of the cohort were silent in their youth, and the younger were idealistic and activist. This generation produced every major figure in the 20th-century civil rights movement, from Martin Luther King to Caesar Chavez. The Peace Corps was important to them. Members of this generation tend to be compassionate problem solvers who find strength in human relations. They are healthy and active.

Tips for Working with Them
- Emphasize expertise.
- Provide statistics and information (they are readers).
- Stress wellness.
- Emphasize willingness to help others.

Baby Boomers, or the "Me" Generation
Born between 1943 and 1964, baby boomers are now in their mid-40s to mid-60s. About 79 million strong, they were born after World War II. Many are beginning to retire. This generation tends to be focused on the individual: the "inner world," consumption, and self-gratification. They want jobs that involve individual creativity. Denial is not in their dictionary. Emphasis is on youth: a longer life means extended middle life, not old age. Nostalgia is important.

Tips for Working with Them
- Promote quickness and convenience.
- Emphasize what is in it for them to eat healthfully.

Generation X
Born between 1965 and 1981, today they are in their late 20s to mid-40s. Almost 93 million strong, they are creating new families. This generation is very group oriented. Friends have taken the place of absent parents and relatives. Group dates are common. Members are often great shoppers: going to the mall is part of their social life. The generation is diverse and entrepreneurial. Because of job insecurity, they want to control their lives. They are wired, with email addresses, laptops, and cell phones. Members tend to be interested in environmental issues.

Tips for Working with Them
- Be visual, musical, and dynamic.
- Emphasize price value.
- Stress balance in life and the impact of food behaviors on the environment.

Generation Y
Born between 1982 and 1998, today they range in age from 12 to late 20s. About 60 million strong, they are the children of baby boomers. This generation is practical and pragmatic. Members often grew up in dual-income and single-parent families, and are very involved in family purchases. They are technologically savvy: computers and other gadgets are like pens and pencils to them, and they grew up with the Web. They expect multiple options and think of time in seconds. They tend to be action oriented and socially and ecologically aware.

Tips for Working with Them
- Be visual, musical, and dynamic, but also use technologically sophisticated formats, such as CDs and PowerPoint presentations.
- Emphasize quickness and convenience.

Source: Adapted from "Who are your customers? What do they want?" *On-Site Magazine,* May 1999, pp. 21–42.

Life-Course Perspective on Food Choice
A central concept of a life-course perspective on food choice is that the development of individual food choices takes the form of stable trajectories or pathways over a person's life course. A food choice *trajectory* is a person's persistent thoughts, feelings, strategies, and actions with food and eating developed over a life course in a social and historical context (Devine et al. 1998; Devine 2005). Embedded in trajectories are transitions and turning points. *Transitions,* such as changes in roles or in health conditions, can help to shape trajectories but do not necessar-

ily change the direction of those pathways, whereas *turning points* are salient transitions, situations, or events that create long-term redirections in individuals' pathways (Devine 2005).

In the nutrition arena, these pathways are the accumulation of experiences from food upbringing, roles, ethnic traditions and identities, location, and personal health and physical well-being. Research in food choice suggests that individuals make adjustments to accommodate life-course transitions such as motherhood, menopause, midlife, and older age, but relatively few adults report major turning points (Edstrom &

Devine 2001; Devine 2005). Nutrition education activities should take into account how these past experiences may influence current beliefs, attitudes, and expectations.

Methods for Delivering Educational Strategies Appropriately to Adults: Making Learning Meaningful

What are the best ways, then, to conduct nutrition education to specifically take into consideration the special educational preferences and experiences of adults? Based on the background just discussed and on the research literature, the following methods of delivering nutrition education are likely to be effective (Contento, Balch, et al. 1995; Vella 2002; Sahyoun, Pratt, & Anderson 2004).

Provide Immediately Useful Information

At the beginning of a session, you can explain the purpose of the session and reassure participants that the session will be of immediate use to them. Provide adults with what they want and need to know—directly, clearly, and in a straightforward manner. Focus on only one or two key messages or specific behaviors, such as how to increase milk consumption or provide healthful snacks to their children. Provide realistic, not idealistic, information. Making the session relevant to any particular group of participants means that you must conduct a good assessment of the past experiences, needs, and desires of the group. If the group is ongoing, tell participants they will have an opportunity at the end of the session to suggest issues and topics to be addressed in future sessions.

Create a Safe Learning Environment

To encourage learning, ensure that the room is physically comfortable and establish ground rules about respecting the time frame of the session; confidentiality; mutual trust, respect, and helpfulness; freedom of expression; and acceptance of differences. How to create such an environment is described in great detail in Chapter 15.

Develop Respectful Relationships

Adult educator Vella (2002) emphasizes the importance of respectful relationships between the group leader and learners and among learners. Relationships of the nutrition educator to the group can involve power-over or power-with. *Power* in this context refers to providing knowledge, decision-making control, and the right to ask questions (Abusabha et al. 1999). *Power-over* is when the professional provides all the information and gives advice, expecting the group members merely to comply. Although studies show that such a means for transfer of information can result in knowledge gains, it is less likely to lead to improved problem-solving skills, reflective thinking, attitude change, or changes in behavior. In the *power-with* approach, power is shared by the expert and the participants in an active partnership. In this approach, you listen actively to what each participant is saying, you do not talk down to participants but treat them as equals, you accept them exactly as they are, and you are warm, caring, trusting, and flexible. Even where individuals may prefer presentations as a way to receive information (Olson & Kelly 1989), the attitude of respect for group participants is still crucially important.

Recognize That Adult Learners Are Decision Makers

Respect adult learners as decision makers in their lives. Also respect that they should have some say in the content of the sessions. You can achieve this in many ways. For example, when new content is introduced, you can first describe in outline form what can be included in this section, and then ask the group what they feel they need or want

to learn about the topic. Learners can thus decide what occurs for them in the learning event. This involves their taking responsibility for their own learning and not being passive listeners. There will no doubt be different viewpoints on any particular issue. The group should feel secure that their opinions will matter and that they will not be criticized. After all viewpoints have been expressed, they can then be sorted out and evaluated for their scientific merit. The role of the facilitator is crucial in keeping the group on track and ensuring that the conclusions being drawn are scientifically accurate and based on evidence. Where there are misconceptions, the nutrition educator can correct them with respect, such as saying, "I am glad it worked for you, but research suggest that . . ."

Engage Learners

Design activities that will actively engage learners. For example, design active learning tasks that can be carried out in small groups or dyads. Where appropriate, the outcome of these tasks should be open-ended and based on what the group or dyad comes up with. Provide for the opportunity to reflect on the task. These learning tasks should build on the past experience of the learners. Facilitated dialogue is another format in which all group members are fully engaged: they actively participate in learning by listening to each other and sharing with each other. Facilitated dialogue is described later in this section.

Build on Learners' Past Experience and Knowledge

Adults need to be able to integrate new ideas with what they already know if they are going to keep—and use—new information and skills. Information that conflicts sharply with what is already held to be true, and thus forces a reevaluation of the old beliefs and attitudes, should not, of course, be avoided, but recognize that it is integrated more slowly. Likewise, information that has little conceptual overlap with what is already known is acquired more slowly. So learn about the current perceptions, beliefs, or attitudes of your audience toward the issue at hand to build on what is known.

Sequence the Learning Experiences and Reinforce Them

If new how-to food and nutrition information is to be provided or new skills are to be taught, such as new food preparation methods, sequence the learning tasks from simple to complex and provide plenty of opportunities for observation and practice. Reinforce information, skills, and attitudes by repetition in diverse, engaging, and interesting ways until the knowledge and skills are learned. In group discussion, frequently summarize the key points of the discussion.

Come to Closure with Solutions

After a group of adult learners grapples with the issues that are the focus of the session and shares challenges and successes, the nutrition educator can summarize the discussion and facilitate the group coming up with common solutions. Good solutions come from full participation of the group and the shared understandings and meaning that evolve through discussion. The group feels more commitment to the solutions adopted by the group because they shared in the responsibility of arriving at final decisions about what actions to take.

Support Cognitive Self-Regulation

As with older children and adolescents, adults also have busy schedules and experience time constraints that leave little time to eat healthfully. When group participants decide individually or collectively to take action, you can support their cognitive self-regulation processes through teaching skills of goal setting, planning ahead, and self-monitoring.

These processes are described in detail in Chapter 12 of this book. Setting specific and actionable goals is important.

Example of Nutrition Education Program Based on Adult Education Principles

Choosing Healthy Options in Cooking and Eating, or the CHOICE project, was a program directed at older women that incorporated the features just discussed. The project is described in **Nutrition Education in Action 17-1**.

Facilitated Group Dialogue as an Educational Tool

Facilitated dialogue is an example of an effective tool for working with adults that incorporates all the previous strategies (Abusabha et al. 1999; Vella 2002; Sigman-Grant 2004). The word *facilitate* is derived from the Latin word meaning "to enable, to make easy." The *facilitator* is thus a person who makes it easier for people to understand (Sigman-Grant 2005). The facilitator's job is to make the group atmosphere comfortable for discussion by incorporating the actions described previously to address each of the types of learners' fears (Abusabha et al. 1999). The facilitator's role is also to move the discussion along without dominating it. The facilitator assists group members to express their ideas, helps them to think critically about issues, encourages them to talk to and listen to each other, and assists them to come to conclusions based on group input. The aim is for active participation by all of the group members and shared understandings. Use of this approach has resulted in sessions that are lively and in which group participants feel motivated and empowered.

Role of Facilitator

In the context of nutrition education, what is the role of the facilitator? What does group facilitation mean? How exactly does one function as a nutrition educator to make a group session a democratic and valuable group learning experience? How does one find the right balance between being authoritarian as a facilitator and being laissez-faire?

Some believe that the facilitator is just another member of the group, who should not direct the activities of the group. Brookfield (1986) notes that because much of adult learning is concerned with such issues as the resolution of moral difficulties, development of self-insight, reflection on experience, and reinforcement of self-worth rather than technical knowledge, there are those who argue that discussion cannot be directed, for to attempt to do so would be to close people's consciousness to alternative interpretations of the issue under discussion before these alternatives were even stated.

The facilitated dialogue reflects this approach to some extent: it is described as a method of group teaching that involves the active

---

NUTRITION EDUCATION IN ACTION 17-1

Choosing Healthy Options in Cooking and Eating (The CHOICE Project)

The Program

The major causes of death and disability among American women today include cardiovascular disease, cancer, and osteoporosis, and there is consensus that diet is related to these conditions. This program was designed to help non-at-risk, healthy older women in a free-living setting to develop eating patterns that would reduce the risk of these conditions. They were randomized into three conditions:

- A moderate-fat diet, operationalized as the American Heart Association (AHA) eating plan
- The addition of flaxseed (a good source of phytoestrogens) to the AHA eating plan, provided as a dietary supplement
- A diet high in plant foods and low in animal foods, in the form of a macrobiotic-style eating plan

During the course of 12 months, participants met for 24 nutrition education and behavioral change sessions: weekly for 14 weeks, biweekly for the next 10 weeks, and monthly for the remaining six months. The behavioral intervention strategies used to maintain subject participation and dietary adherence included:

- Seven cooking classes with hands-on experience alternating with behavioral sessions during the first 14 weeks; information provided on how to eat according to the assigned eating plan
- Cooking demonstrations with tastings at all other sessions
- Individual goal setting and development of action plans each session
- Regular feedback and encouragement based on three-day food records completed monthly by the women

- Monthly telephone calls on a random day to collect 24-hour dietary recalls, as an incentive for adherence
- Group bonding through icebreakers at start of sessions, sharing of addresses and phone numbers, facilitated discussion
- Chef's knife, apron, mug, and tote bag with CHOICE logo
- Monthly newsletter to participants during six months of monthly sessions

Evaluation Results

Results showed that women on the macrobiotic-style eating plan were able to achieve significant changes in diet, in the desired direction, for many key categories of foods targeted in the intervention. They tripled their whole-grain intakes, tripled their intake of beans and legumes, and doubled their intake of fish. They decreased their intakes of refined grain products; cut their meat, poultry and eggs, and whole milk products intake; and reduced their consumption of high-fat sweets compared to baseline values. They made these changes within the first three months and maintained them for most of the 12 months. The women in the other two eating plans, based on the AHA moderate-fat diet, made changes in their diet but these were not significant, largely because the women were already eating diets moderately low in fat.

Source: Contento, I. R., A. Persaud, E. Solomon, et al. 2004. Changes in food patterns during an intervention with women placed on eating plans with varying amounts and types of phytoestrogens. Presentation at International Society for Behavioral Nutrition and Physical Activity Annual Meeting, Washington DC.

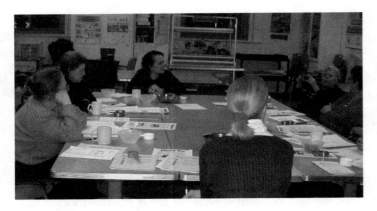

Group discussions can be helpful and supportive.

participation of all group members and the leader. Learners and facilitators are equal partners in the learning experience (Sigman-Grant 2004). The group sits in a circle, and the leader sits alongside the group members in the circle. Ideally, the group members do all the talking and in essence conduct the session. The leader talks very little as group members share with each other and learn from each other. Although the nutrition educator may be the expert on food and nutrition issues, the group members are experts on their own lives and how and whether they can incorporate the provided information into their own situations. Those who use a learner-centered approach state that "the most central point of learner-centered education is that the learner is a decision-maker. They choose *if* they learn and *if* they will change their behavior. We cannot decide for them. The learning is in the *doing* and *deciding*" (Husing & Elfant 2005).

Role of Planning: The Four As

However, it is acknowledged that open discussions about whatever topic comes to the minds of group members in laissez-faire fashion without much input from the nutrition educator are not fruitful either. Group members often express frustration with a lack of sense of progress toward any clear learning objective. In addition, as a nutrition educator working in specific programs that have specific missions, you are accountable for certain outcomes that involve addressing specific behaviors, such as recommended infant feeding practices or eating more fruits and vegetables (Sigman-Grant 2004).

In general, the sessions based on facilitated discussion are planned ahead of time, involving the preparation of an educational plan. Norris (2003) and Sigman-Grant (2004) suggest that the sequence of activities during the session can follow four *A*s as follows:

- *Anchoring:* Introduction and/or review
- *Add:* Active learning and facilitated dialogue; introduction of new concepts and new information
- *Apply:* Providing an opportunity through an interactive exercise for all participants to consider ways to use the new material and the points made within the discussion to their own lives
- *Away:* Summarizing, bringing to closure, and selection of action plans

As can be seen, the four *A*s procedure is very similar to the sequencing of learning described in Chapter 11, which is gain attention, present new material by building on prior learning, provide guidance and practice, and apply, and close. An example of a specific sequence of activities

for how such facilitated discussion can be carried out in the Women, Infants and Children (WIC) program is shown in **Box 17-5**.

Safety Versus Challenge

Facilitating a group does not mean that the group should not be challenged. Indeed, you are charged as an educator to assist group members to analyze assumptions, challenge previously accepted and internalized beliefs and values, and contemplate the validity of alternative behaviors or other ways of doing things (Brookfield 1986; Abusabha et al. 1999). All these acts can at times be uncomfortable and may even contradict the stated needs of the group. Thus, the job of the facilitator is to create learning environments that are both emotionally safe *and* challenging. In addition, in nutrition education groups, there is often much nutrition science–based motivational why-to information and how-to information and skills that need to be addressed. Thus, the educator has a role, and the group members have a role.

It can be seen, then, that facilitating groups requires considerable skill and practice to find the right balance of acceptance and challenge, of leading and being a member of the group. The nature of the facilitator's role and the degree of guidance and control will depend on the food and nutrition issue being addressed and the nature of the group.

■ WORKING WITH DIVERSE CULTURAL GROUPS

The United States is becoming increasingly multicultural, with people living in it who come from diverse ancestries and who have become part of the mainstream to varying degrees. New York City has more than 170 distinct ethnic communities. More than 130 languages and dialects are spoken by students in the Washington, D.C., school system. Los Angeles has more people of Mexican descent than any city in the world except Mexico City. Even states such as Iowa and Alabama are getting used to people speaking Spanish in their midst. Some are recent immigrants, and others have been in the country for several generations. Whereas in the past all became a part of a general "melting pot," in recent decades racial/ethnic groups have shown a wish to be acknowledged, honored, and respected for their unique heritage and contributions, resulting in more of a mosaic. Although often referred to as minorities, such subsets of the population are often a majority of the population in certain locations, and hence such a term is inaccurate and inappropriate in these cases (Bronner 1994). You thus face the challenge of providing nutrition education to a variety of people who come from a variety of cultures that are different from your own. This requires you to better understand your own culture and those of others.

Culture has been described as a set of beliefs, knowledge, traditions, values, and behavioral patterns that are developed, learned, shared, and transmitted by members of a group. It is a worldview that a group shares and hence influences perceptions about food, nutrition, and health (Sanjur 1982). Knowledge and beliefs include accepted understandings, opinions, and faith about the world. Beliefs help determine which foods are edible, appropriate preparation methods, or the meaning of a food. Traditions are customs about which foods are eaten on what occasions (e.g., weddings, birthdays), what will be eaten for health or to cure illness, or religious traditions about fasting and feasting. Values are widely held beliefs about what is worthwhile, desirable, or important for well-being. Values considered desirable in one culture may not be considered so in another culture, and these differences in value systems can influence food and nutrition practices.

Culture, then, is a learned experience, not a biologically determined one (Sanjur 1982). It is the product of interaction among generations,

$\mathcal{B}$*ox* **17-5 Specific Guidelines and Techniques for Facilitated Group Discussions in the Special Supplemental Nutrition Program for Women, Infants, and Children**

Build the Group from Within
- Assure members that the group will be structured to fit their needs and concerns.

Establish Ground Rules
- Set the time, agenda, and length of the session.
- Set rules of respecting confidentiality, sharing group responsibilities, and respecting and listening to opinions of other group members.

Begin with an Icebreaker Exercise
- Ask each group member to make a brief statement about herself, her child's needs, and anything new that happened to her during the past month.

Ask Open-Ended Questions
- Ask questions that cannot be answered by "yes" or "no."
- Involve group members in describing their own experiences.

Guide the Discussion
- Encourage others to speak.
- Keep discussion on track.
- Gently bring topics to a conclusion.

Encourage Full Participation
- Encourage quiet members to voice their ideas.
- Listen intently to each member.
- Repeat members' comments when necessary.
- Give positive feedback verbally or physically (e.g., nodding head, smiling).

Focus the Conversation
- Clarify different views.
- Restate the objectives of the session when necessary.
- Summarize the important points of the discussion.

Correct Misconceptions Artfully
- Avoid turning into the "lecturer."
- Emphasize the worth of the members' experience.
- Use responses such as, "I am glad this worked for you, but other people have found . . ."
- Ask what other group members think about the statement.

Create an Atmosphere of Acceptance
- Accept people and respect each member's feelings even when you disagree with her viewpoint.
- Do not hurt members' feelings by abruptly negating or putting down their ideas and experiences.

Summarize the Discussion
- Bring ideas together and repeat relevant information.
- Strive to make the summary the result of the members' discussion, not your own analysis.
- Repeat and clarify the solution to the nutrition problem that members agreed on.

Be Patient
- Remember, it takes time for a group to grow and develop trust.

Have Fun
- Keep a smile and enjoy sharing with and learning from the group.

Source: Abusabha, R., J. Peacock, and C. Achterberg. 1999. Facilitated group discussion. *Journal of the American Dietetic Association* 99:72–76. Used with permission of the American Dietetic Association.

always being modified over time. Consequently, it can also be unlearned. Cultures are constantly changing. Thus, you can view food habits as a dynamic process, always changing. However, every culture also resists change by self-generated mechanisms to perpetuate its cultural traits and to maintain its boundaries.

All societies have a dominant set of beliefs, values, and traditions that are shared by the majority of people. In the United States, the norms have been described as an emphasis on education, a work ethic, materialism, religion, physical appearance, cleanliness, high technology, punctuality, independence, and free enterprise. Those cultural groups whose beliefs, values, and traditions are different may not always be treated with understanding and respect (Bronner 1994).

Understanding Cultural Sensitivity and Cultural Competence

Working with a variety of cultures requires that the nutrition educator become culturally competent. This may involve several steps, according to Bronner (1994). *Cultural knowledge* is the process of learning about the worldviews of other cultures. This can be accomplished by reading books, attending workshops, watching audiovisual presentations, perusing government documents, and so forth. You can learn about the food habits and beliefs of various ethnic groups through these means. *Cultural awareness* is the process of becoming aware of your own learned biases and prejudices toward other cultures through self-assessment, while becoming aware of the beliefs, values, practices, lifestyles, and problem-solving strategies of other groups. This leads to *cultural sensitivity*, which is the awareness of your own cultural beliefs, assumptions, customs, and values as well as those of other cultural groups. You recognize that cultural differences as well as similarities exist, without assigning values to these differences as good or bad, right or wrong.

Cultural competence is a set of knowledge and interpersonal skills that allow individuals to increase their understanding and appreciation of cultural differences and similarities within, among, and between groups and to work effectively in cross-cultural situations (Bronner 1994). Being competent in cross-cultural functioning means learning new patterns of behavior and effectively applying them in the appropriate settings. Knowledge about a culture does not equal cultural competence. In fact, "book" knowledge of a culture may lead to inappropriate generalizations, such as stereotyping. Through frequent cultural encounters and engagement, nutrition educators can become aware of the heterogeneity within cultural groups. For example, although individuals from a given culture may have similar beliefs, attitudes, and practices in terms of food and nutrition, there are also many variations resulting from differences in education, age, religion, socioeconomic status, geographic location, and length of time in the country.

The goal for nutrition educators is to accompany knowledge of the culture with awareness, respect, and acceptance of the group's cultural beliefs and practices, and willingness and ability to work within the values, traditions, and customs of the participants' community (Bronner 1994).

Not only individuals but also organizations need to exhibit cultural competence. Thus, cultural competence has been defined as "a set of congruent behaviors, attitudes, and policies that come together in a system, agency, or among professionals and enables that system, agency, or those professionals to work effectively in cross-cultural situations. Operationally defined, cultural competence is the integration and transformation of knowledge about individuals and groups of people into specific standards, policies, practices, and attitudes used in appropriate cultural settings to increase the quality of services, thereby producing better outcomes" (King, Sims, & Osher 2006).

Consequently, systems and agencies, such as health systems, food and nutrition agencies, and nutrition education programs, need to become more culturally competent. Five elements have been identified as essential for contributing to a system's ability to become more culturally competent (Cross et al. 1989; Isaacs & Benjamin 1991; King et al. 2006). The system should (1) value diversity, (2) have the capacity for cultural self-assessment, (3) be conscious of the "dynamics" inherent when cultures interact, (4) institutionalize cultural knowledge, and (5) develop adaptations to service delivery reflecting an understanding of diversity between and within cultures (King et al. 2006). Further, these five elements must be manifested in every level of the service delivery system. They should be reflected in attitudes, structures, policies, and services.

Appropriate Delivery Methods for Nutrition Education for Culturally Diverse Audiences

What, then, are the implications for how nutrition education can be delivered to culturally diverse audiences? It should be noted that the psychosocial theories and models used throughout the book can provide a framework for designing the program for various cultural groups (Liou & Contento 2001). However, the theory constructs need to be operationalized to be culturally appropriate. There may also be culturally specific constructs that are important to consider in delivering nutrition education. In applying the concepts related to cultural sensitivity to health promotion and nutrition education, Resnicow and colleagues (1999) suggest that it is helpful to consider the following distinctions.

Cultural sensitivity or *cultural appropriateness* is the extent to which the design, delivery, and evaluation of nutrition education and health promotion programs incorporate the ethnic or cultural experiences, beliefs, traditions, and behaviors of a given group as well as relevant historical, social, and environmental forces. *Cultural competence,* as you have seen, is the capacity of individuals and organizations to exercise interpersonal cultural sensitivity. Thus, cultural competence refers to practitioners and agencies, whereas cultural sensitivity or appropriateness refers to the intervention messages and program materials. *Multicultural* refers to incorporating and appreciating the perspectives of multiple racial or ethnic groups without assumptions of superiority or inferiority. Thus, culturally sensitive programs are implicitly multicultural.

Cultural targeting is the process of creating culturally sensitive interventions. This often involves adapting existing materials and programs for racial/ethnic subgroups. *Culturally based* programs and messages are those that combine the culture, history, and core values of a subgroup as a medium to motivate behavior change. For example, nutrition education programs for indigenous Americans can focus on traditional foods and spiritual systems.

Surface Structure and Deep Structure

Surface Structure
Programs and materials can focus on a *surface structure* dimension, whereby materials and messages are matched to the observable social and behavioral characteristics of given cultural groups by using people, places, language, music, clothing, or food familiar to, or preferred by, the target audience (Resnicow et al. 2005). You might also use media channels that are most watched or settings uniquely used by the group to deliver the nutrition education, such as churches or ethnic community centers. Ideally, you would want to match staff ethnically to the participants. Surface structure indicates how well the intervention fits within the culture, experience, and behavioral patterns of the audience.

Deep Structure
Programs and materials that focus on *deep structure* are culturally based by building on general core values and historical, cultural, social, and environmental factors that may influence the food and nutrition behavior of the target audience (Resnicow et al. 1999). Core values that have been considered when working among some Asian groups, for example, are the importance of family, respect for older people, and the importance of maintaining balance for health, including the use of hot and cold foods to address hot and cold health conditions. Programs with African Americans have been built on the core values of commitment to family, communalism, connections to history and ancestors, and a unique sense of time, rhythm, or communication style (Resnicow et al. 1999, 2002, 2005). For the Latino culture, core values include importance of family, respect for elders, fatalism, and the importance of positive social interactions that can be the foundation for nutrition education (Bronner 1994). You need to understand and value the core values of the different groups with which you work as you deliver your program. In particular, there are differences in body image issues, such as what is an appropriate weight in the eyes of a given cultural group (Kumanyika & Morssink 1997).

Ethnic Ideals and Identities
In terms of food choice specifically, one qualitative study with three ethnic groups (African American, Latino, and white) found that ide-

als, identities, and roles interacted reciprocally and dynamically with each other and with food choices and influences on food consumption (Devine et al. 1998). *Ideals*, or deeply held beliefs about food and eating, came from multiple sources, of which ethnicity was one. For some individuals, ethnicity was dominant; for others, age or religion or other interests, such as health and fitness, were also important. *Identity* is the way people think of their own distinguishing characteristics and self-image. Ethnic identities in this study existed along with others, such as regional or family background and travel experiences, which sometimes overrode ethnic identities. Ethnic identities were most often expressed in holidays and family celebrations. Individuals also have multiple *roles*, some of which influence food choice. Women in all three cultural groups were usually the family food managers. Some African American and white men were the primary cooks for the family. *Contexts* enhanced or constrained all food choices and influenced the ability to enact cultural ideals and roles.

It is essential to remember that there are wide variations within groups in terms of ethnic/racial identity, which may be defined as the extent to which individuals identify and gravitate toward their racial/ethnic group psychologically and socially (Resnicow et al. 1999). Ethnic identity includes individuals' extent of acculturation; the degree to which they have affinity for in-group culture such as food, media, or clothes; racial/ethnic pride; attitudes toward maintaining one's culture; and involvement with those within the group and those outside the group.

Appropriate Language

There are many differences in communication styles between cultures, such as whether to speak loudly or softly; to look at the person who is speaking or avert one's gaze; to smile, nod, or interject when someone is speaking to acknowledge understanding of what the speaker says or to show little expression; and whether to rarely ask questions and provide yes/no responses or to use a direct approach and ask direct questions (Sue & Sue 1999). Rather than ask whether the group understands—which is likely to yield a yes answer in some cultures, say, "Tell me which things are not clear to you." In some cultures, it is impossible to say no to a request, so individuals may respond with "maybe" about whether the time for the session is a good time or whether they will come to the next session. In some cultures, it is acceptable to make a commitment and then to decide later to make changes to it or to decline altogether. It is assumed that one cannot predict events in one's life that may occur in the meantime. It is thus very important to learn about the specific culturally appropriate communication styles of the groups with which you will be working.

Strategies for Enhancing Cultural Appropriateness

Several strategies for making health promotion programs and materials more culturally appropriate have been proposed (Kavanagh & Kennedy 1992; Kumanyika & Morssink 1997; Resnicow et al. 1999; Kreuter et al. 2003). Those proposed by Kreuter and colleagues (2003) are briefly described in the following list. These strategies are not mutually exclusive, and most nutrition educators use several when planning programs and materials.

- *Peripheral strategies* use preferred colors, images, fonts, or pictures of group members to convey relevance to the group and to enhance acceptance. That is, the strategies match materials to the surface structure characteristics described previously. These strategies are called peripheral because they appeal to the peripheral

route to attitude change identified by Petty and Cacioppo (1986) and described earlier in the book.

- *Evidential strategies* seek to enhance the perceived relevance of the health issue for the particular group by providing scientific or epidemiological evidence for the impact of the issue on the group. For example, you can provide evidence that the group has a high incidence of heart disease or hypertension, thus raising perceived risk.
- *Linguistic strategies* strive to make the programs or materials more accessible by using the language of the group. Sometimes this just involves translating the materials into another language, or using an interpreter when you are leading groups. In some situations the interpretation may be into more than one language if the audience is multicultural.
- *Audience-involving strategies* draw directly on the experience of the intended audience by using staff members, paid or volunteer, who are drawn from the same cultural group and by involving lay community members in planning and decision making for the programs.
- *Sociocultural strategies* focus on the cultural beliefs, traditions, and behaviors, or deep structure characteristics, of the intended audience. Such strategies build upon and reinforce the group's core values to provide context and meaning for the programs and messages.

All these strategies can be used in one program (Kreuter et al. 2003). For example, a program for Latina women could use the kinds of bright colors that appeal to the women (peripheral strategy), address the increased incidence of a health condition such as diabetes experienced by Latinas compared with other groups (evidential strategy), present group sessions using straightforward words and phrases in Spanish (linguistic strategy), include stories and testimonials of other women from the community (strategy of involving the audience community), and address the belief in fatalism (sociocultural strategy).

Process for Developing Culturally Appropriate Programs and Materials

Given the wide diversity between cultural groups, it is essential that the materials and programs are appropriate to a given specific cultural group. You can do so through use of focus groups and extensive pretesting.

Focus Groups

Use focus groups to provide the basis for developing your message content and format. Using this format, you can identify both surface and deep structure elements by exploring the thoughts, feelings, language, assumptions, and practices of the group, including food preferences, shopping and cooking habits, and perceived benefits and barriers. You can also explore cultural differences by using "ethnic mapping" (Resnicow et al. 1999). Here you can ask the group whether certain foods they eat or behaviors they engage in are "mostly an ethnic thing," "equally an ethnic and white thing," or "mostly a white/American thing." Such focus groups should include individuals representing the heterogeneity within the cultural group.

Pretesting

After you have designed a draft of your materials (e.g., videos, printed materials) or program content, it is essential that you show them to a sample from your target audience for their feedback on format and content, reflecting both surface and deep structure characteristics. Some groups may like the images to portray individuals from their same racial/

ethnic group, but others may not, for example. Test the concepts being addressed and the language being used. Find out whether the group perceives any of the features to be stereotyping or insensitive.

Examples of Effective Interventions

An intervention conducted with black women illustrates how a program can be made more culturally sensitive by appropriate targeting (Kreuter et al. 2003, 2005). The study, designed to increase mammography and fruit and vegetable consumption, was based on four potentially important cultural characteristics that had been identified as being salient because they were found to be prevalent among African Americans, were associated with health-related beliefs and practices, and could be measured:

- *Religiosity*, represented by church attendance, prayer, spirituality, and beliefs about God as a causal agent in health. A message might be as follows: "The Lord has given us a powerful tool for helping find cancer before it is too late. Getting a mammogram, together with the power of prayer, will give you the best chance to live a long and healthy life" (Kreuter et al. 2003, p. 140).
- *Collectivism*, which is the belief that the basic unit of society is the community or family, not the individual, and that collective survival is a high priority. Hence, important values were cooperation, concern and responsibility for others, forgiveness, family security, friendship, and respect for tradition. A message might be as follows: "As black women, we have many important jobs. We keep our families together. We help build our communities. We work inside and outside the home. But our most important job may be to keep ourselves healthy. If we don't take care of ourselves, it is harder to take care of others" (Kreuter et al. 2003, p. 140).
- *Racial pride.* Individuals vary in a continuum in terms of the degree to which they remain immersed in their own cultural traditions, adopt the mainstream white culture, or participate in the traditions of both their own and mainstream culture. Racial pride is manifested in interest and involvement in traditional practices, preferences for African American media, belief in the importance of promoting black art and literature, or degree of practice of traditional eating practices and preferences, such as fried food. A message might be as follows: "Did you know that most cancers affect blacks more than whites? Only about 10% of blacks in our community eat five fruits and vegetables as recommended by health professionals. But you can reverse this trend by . . ." (Kreuter et al. 2003, p. 141).
- *Perception of time.* The notion of time is socially constructed, as noted in Chapter 2. The traditional Western perception of time is that it has a past, present, and future and can be divided into discrete units, which, like money or other goods, can be saved, spent, wasted, or even bought, as in "buying time" (Kreuter et al. 2003). Time well spent now can lead to a better future. People with such a future orientation are thus more likely to engage in health-promoting behaviors. In the health area, it has been found that African Americans are more present-oriented. Hence, a message can be "It is hard to think about the future when you are feeling fine today. But sometimes you can take steps today to make life better tomorrow. Getting a mammogram is another step you can take today to make life better tomorrow, since finding cancer early increases the chances of successful treatment" (Kreuter et al. 2003, p. 142).

The results showed that the program was most effective when it used both behavioral theory and cultural characteristics.

Another study, the Healthy Body/Healthy Spirit trial, examined the effect of a culturally sensitive, multicomponent self-help intervention on fruit and vegetable intake and on the physical activity of members of a set of socioeconomically diverse black churches (see **Nutrition Education in Action 17-2**).

■ LOW-LITERACY AUDIENCES

In the United States, the average reading level is at the eighth grade, with about one in five reading at the fifth-grade level, and for those older than 65 and for many cultural subgroups, about two in five reading below the fifth-grade level. This means that about 20% of the population are functionally illiterate—they can't read newspapers or physician instructions for medications. Another 30% have marginal reading skills (Doak, Doak, & Root 1996). Those with low literacy skills may not be able to read the handouts or booklets you give them or the written food and nutrition instructions you provide them.

Doak and colleagues (1996) point out that you cannot identify low-literacy individuals by their appearance or by conversation with them. They are often very good in other forms of communication and have learned to compensate so that their lack of literacy skills is not obvious. They can be poor or affluent, immigrant or native born. Sometimes those who have low literacy in English are highly literate in the language of their country of origin; others, born in this country, just never developed the skills. Low in literacy skills does not mean low in intelligence. Nutrition education can be effective if you find the appropriate format.

Poor readers, compared with skilled readers, read slowly, often one or two words at a time, so that they lose the meaning of the whole sentence. They think in terms of individual items of information rather than in categories or groups with common characteristics. They often do not understand information if it is implied; how the information is to be used must be spelled out clearly (**Figure 17-1**). Thus, they often have difficulty with analysis and synthesis of information as well as with literacy.

Comprehension is about grasping the meaning of instruction or materials and is an important aspect of literacy. Comprehension, whether verbal, written, or visual, requires that individuals pay attention to information and remember it for when they need it. Gaining the attention of the intended audience at the beginning of a session or piece of printed material is important for activating the memory system. As noted many times in this book, this can be done by vivid stories, striking visuals, or dramatic data. Getting the information into the audience's short-term memory requires you to be aware that this form of memory has a limited capacity and a short storage time. People can usually store only up to seven independent items at a time. Any more than that may mean that they will not remember *any* of the items. For those of low literacy, the number is more like three to five. Transfer from short-term to long-term memory and storage in long-term memory require that the new information links to what the audience already knows, is repeated often, and actively involves the audience.

Appropriate Delivery Methods for Low-Literacy Audiences

How can you apply these considerations to delivering nutrition education to low-literacy audiences? Many have written about this problem (e.g., Doak et al. 1996), and some key strategies are described briefly here.

General Strategies

The following strategies are applicable to all components of nutrition education.

NUTRITION EDUCATION IN ACTION 17-2

Healthy Body/Healthy Spirit: A Church-Based Nutrition and Physical Activity Intervention

The Program

The Healthy Body/Healthy Spirit program was a culturally targeted self-help intervention to increase consumption of fruits and vegetables and levels of physical activity. It was based on addressing both dimensions of surface structure, in which materials and messages are matched to observable social and behavioral characteristics of the intended audience, and deep structure, in which the intervention is based on cultural, historical, and psychological factors that are unique to the racial/ethnic identity of the audience.

The intervention built on surface structure involving food preferences, cooking practices, and exercise patterns of the audience. It also addressed deep structure issues, which included unique attitudes about body image, safety concerns, lack of time for exercise, effect of exercise on hair, religious themes, and interest in improving the health of the community (as opposed to personal health).

The study was conducted in 16 socioeconomically diverse black churches in the Atlanta area. Church members were randomized into three groups. One group received standard educational materials. The second group received culturally sensitive self-help materials, and the third received self-help materials plus motivational interviewing. The materials provided to the intervention group participants were as follows:

- *Forgotten Miracles:* An 18-minute video that centered around two families, one that tended to eat healthfully and the other that did not. Key messages were conveyed with biblical themes, such as the story of Daniel, who rejects the "kings' diet" for his own "natural diet" high in fruits and vegetables, and messages about the body being "God's temple." These culturally sensitive messages conveyed information about the health benefits of eating fruits and vegetables, analysis of costs, recipes, and cooking tips.
- *Eat for Life cookbook:* A cookbook containing recipes submitted by church members that met specified criteria. The recipes were first tested by staff.
- *Healthy Body/Healthy Spirit exercise video:* A 20-minute video hosted by African American celebrities from the Atlanta area and based on footage taped in church members' homes so as to provide real-world role models.
- *Healthy Body/Healthy Spirit guide:* A 37-page, four-color manual to accompany the video.
- *Audiocassette:* A cassette with gospel music to match a three-phase workout: warm-up, aerobic activity, and cool-down. Biblical quotes and brief excerpts from the pastors' sermons were interspersed with the music.

Evaluation Results

Slightly more than a thousand individuals were recruited from the 16 churches, of whom 906 were assessed at the end of one year. A subset of the individuals also received four culturally sensitive telephone counseling calls based on motivational interviewing techniques. Results showed that those who received the culturally sensitive intervention significantly increased their fruit and vegetable intakes and their physical activity levels compared with those who received standard educational materials.

Sources: Resnicow, K., A. Jackson, R. Braithwaite, et al. 2002. Healthy Body/Healthy Spirit: A church-based nutrition and physical activity intervention. *Health Education Research* 17:562–573; and Resnicow, K., A. Jackson, D. Blisset, et al. 2005. Results of the Healthy Body/Healthy Spirit trial. *Health Psychology* 24:339–348.

Fiber is fantastic!

There are two kinds of fiber, and they are both very good for your health. One kind of fiber is called <u>soluble</u>. The other kind of fiber is called <u>insoluble</u>.

Think of <u>soluble fiber</u> as a sponge—it soaks up water, and slows down anything going through your intestines. It also helps lower cholesterol. You can find it in fruits like bananas and apples, or vegetables like carrots and peas.

Think of <u>insoluble fiber</u> as a bristle-brush that helps clean out your tube-like intestines. It keeps things moving, which helps keep you regular! You can find it in the skins of fruits, like when you eat whole grapes or whole cherries. You can also find insoluble fiber in the skins of vegetables, like when you eat potato skins, or corn on the cob. Either way, fiber is good news for your health!

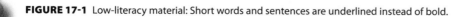

FIGURE 17-1 Low-literacy material: Short words and sentences are underlined instead of bold.

- *Know your audience.* Assess the needs and preferences of the intended audience thoroughly before designing your program, using the procedures described in Steps 1 and 2 earlier in this book. What is the group's literacy level and its readiness to learn (Figure 17-1)? Focus groups, personal interviews, or interviews with those who work closely with this audience, such as agency personnel, are all valuable means for gaining this information.

- *Pretest all materials through cognitive testing.* Use focus groups to guide you as you design your sessions. How should the issues be framed for this audience? What educational strategies do they prefer? After you have designed a draft of your sessions, pretest your message with your intended audience to determine whether the message to be delivered through educational sessions or written materials conveys the meaning you intend. This is referred to as *cognitive testing* (Alaimo, Olson, & Frongillo 1999). In particular, cognitively test any evaluation instruments that you intend to use, such as food frequency checklists or attitude items. Here, individual interviews are most helpful. Present individuals with the materials and have them complete the assignments, such as worksheets or evaluation instruments. Then use read-aloud procedures to ask them to explain to you what they think each item means. This will force you to use the language of the intended audience in your materials.

- *Limit your educational objectives.* Limit the number of educational objectives for group sessions or written materials. These objectives should state exactly what actions or behaviors the audience will be able to accomplish as a result of the educational intervention. Present the smallest amount of information possible to accomplish your goals. Three or four items of instruction are enough at any one time. This translates into one major concept—your behavioral goal—two or three motivation-related concepts on why to take action, such as perceived benefits and barriers, plus two or three examples of how to take action. Teach only "need-to-know" rather than the "nice-to-know" information.

- *Focus the content on behaviors or actions rather than on facts and principles to facilitate the ability to take action.* This entire book is based on this premise, but it is especially important for low-literacy audiences. The nutrition science information and principles presented may imply what the behaviors should be. But for a low-literacy audience, the behaviors must be spelled out clearly, not just implied. In addition, this audience usually does not need all the underlying nutrition science information to engage in the behavior.

- *Present information using a variety of ways to enhance learning.* For example, use mini-lectures, discussions, small group activities, and visuals as well as appropriate printed materials.

- *Use familiar examples and a conversational style.* Build on what they already know, and use familiar examples from their lives. For all audiences, but particularly if your audience is also a low-resources audience, refer to foods or dietary practices familiar to the audience rather than to exotic foods and national data. This helps to anchor your message in memory. Talk to them the way you would a friend.

- *Actively engage your audience.* During educational sessions, encourage people to ask questions and to share information and experiences through discussion and dialogue. Allow time for individuals to commit themselves to doing something before the next session. Then in the next session allow time for them to report

what they did on their commitment. In printed materials, engage the readers in some activity—checklists to check off, completing the blanks, circling items, and so forth.

- *Frequently repeat and review.* If the individuals are experiencing the sessions primarily through oral means, key concepts need to be repeated often so that information can move from short-term memory into long-term memory. Allow time to process information, and at the appropriate points, review what has been said or accomplished through activities. Bring the session to closure with clear conclusions. If you use handouts that require the audience to write something, be sure to have pencils ready and to allow plenty of time for them to complete the activity. For older audiences, you may need to allow time for them to find their reading glasses.

- *Treat people with respect and dignity regardless of their literacy level and, of course, regardless of socioeconomic status, race/ethnicity, religion, or country of origin.* If your audience is also a low-resources audience, note that disadvantaged groups often mistrust authority figures, so you must be willing to initiate trusting relationships. Show the group that you believe in them.

Tips for Written Materials

Many strategies for writing effective written materials are described in Chapter 16. They apply to low-literacy audiences as well. This section emphasizes those features that are additionally, or particularly, important for low-literacy audiences.

- *Write the way you speak: use the active voice.* Literacy experts such as Doak, Doak, and Root (1996) note that when you do this, your written materials become easier to read because the readability index automatically drops. They become more interesting to read. They will be easier to understand. The extra words you use when you speak help the reader to process the information.

- *Use common words.* These are words you would use when talking with a friend who was not familiar with nutrition concepts. Common words are usually short and simple words, but not always. *Doctor* is more common than *physician*, but many people are very familiar with the term *medication* even if it is a four-syllable word. If you use uncommon words, such as *hydration*, explain them. Some words are short but conceptually difficult, such as a *variety* of foods or a *balanced* diet. What exactly do you mean by *variety* or *balanced*? Explain such conceptual words.

- *Use short sentences.* Short sentences of less than 10 to 15 words are easier to understand. However, you should not sacrifice conversational style. If it is more natural to say something in a longer sentence, then do so.

- *Put the key information first.* The first part of a message is remembered best (newspapers know this). So, put the behavior or information that is key to your message up front, in the position most likely to be remembered. Assume that the reader will read just the first sentence, the first paragraph, or the first page. So, put the most important information first. For example, say, "Eating lots of fruits and vegetables [the behavioral goal of your program] each day can help lower your risk of heart disease," and then go into greater detail about the many benefits of why to eat more fruits and vegetables and how to do so.

- *Create headings, subheadings, and summaries.* Use headings to serve as guideposts or road signs. Headings and subheadings make the text look less formidable. They alert readers to what is coming up next and help them focus on the intended message. Keep the headings simple, using perhaps three to five words, and locate them right before the text that they introduce. This process also allows for delivering the written information in chunks that can be remembered.

- *Use layout and typography that make the text easier to read.* As noted in the last chapter, use short paragraphs and plenty of white space, simple fonts such as sans serif fonts, and adequate font sizes. Use short lines of 30 to 50 characters and spaces, and use bullets where appropriate, such as for lists of tips, procedures, or things to do. Highlight important information with circles, arrows, or underlining rather than all capital letters. Remember that all caps are more difficult to read. Make the page look as though it can be read in a few minutes.

Tips for Visuals

The following tips apply to the use of illustrations, charts, lists, tables, and graphs with low-literacy audiences.

- *Use visuals to enhance learning.* People remember information better when they see the message, not just hear it, as noted in earlier chapters. Visuals make information vivid and real. As Doak and colleagues note (1996), most poor readers rely on visuals and the spoken word. Visuals with a minimum of text help them to understand instructions without having to struggle with the text. Visuals, appropriately designed, can help the low-literacy reader follow step-by-step instructions for complex procedures. Visuals can also provide emotional impact that is more memorable. The written message saying that "when a mother drinks alcohol, the baby drinks alcohol" can be converted into a line drawing showing a baby inside the mother drinking from a cup when the mother does so. This can carry a more powerful and memorable message than the written word (Doak et al. 1996).
- *Use visuals to enhance motivation.* Make the cover of a booklet or the beginning of a brochure or handout appealing while clearly conveying the key message of the material. Because reading is not easy for low-literacy individuals, an appealing cover or introduction can provide the impetus to open the page or read the material. The style of artwork or the photograph needs to be appropriate to the culture so that readers can easily recognize it as familiar and can visualize themselves in the situation. Realistic line drawings are recommended over stylized or abstract images, which are often not understood. Test the style of the artwork or photograph with the intended audience for its appropriateness and motivational power.
- *Include visuals to clarify the text, but use visuals carefully.* Place the visual near the text to which it refers so that the readers' eyes do not have to go elsewhere to find the written text to understand the message. Break the information into small chunks and provide one visual for each chunk to make it easier to follow. For example, if you want to encourage walking and stair climbing, show separate drawings for walking and stair climbing. Use a simple action caption for each drawing. Or if you use a table to provide a list of foods high in fat, break up the foods into groups with a heading over each. To engage the learner, you can provide a checklist with boxes to check as a means of self-assessment.

Doak and colleagues (1996) provide many examples on how to develop effective visuals.

- *Use simple and clear illustrations.* Illustrations should include enough detail to emphasize the message but should not be so detailed as to become complex and distracting. Line drawings of people should look as real as possible and therefore should include eyes, mouth, nose, ears, and facial expressions (Doak et al. 1996). If you want to illustrate a procedure with many steps, number each of them. Photographs are also effective if they are uncluttered and the message is clearly depicted.
- *Use color appropriately.* Color can attract and hold attention and is almost expected today given the high quality of the visual media in the environment. The preference for colors varies considerably by age, gender, socioeconomic status, and ethnicity. It is thus very important to test your color choices with the intended audience to find out whether they will convey the meanings and message you intend.

■ SUMMARY

Although the key principles in designing nutrition education described in Part II of this book apply to all groups—that is, a focus on enhancing motivation and facilitating the ability to take action—the methods for delivering the educational plan for the intervention in actual practice must differ depending on the audience. Working with diverse population groups requires ensuring that your educational delivery methods are appropriate for the particular group.

In this chapter, you learned that children are not little adults—they are experiencing various stages of physical, cognitive, emotional, and social development. At each stage, they have different needs and abilities and different ways of thinking about themselves and the world that must inform the educational design and activities. Preschool children need repeated experience with tasty and healthful foods to become familiar with them, and play-based activities. As children develop, they can process more information, and cognitive motivational processes become more important. Goal-setting and cognitive self-regulation skills become more developed. At the same time emotional and social forces are important. Nutrition education needs to identify motivations that are meaningful to youth and provide opportunity to practice goal-setting and cognitive self-regulation skills.

Adults tend to engage in learning only when they see that the learning is of immediate use to them. Adults differ in life stage and roles. Nutrition education for them should build on previous experience, respect them as decision makers, and engage them actively in their own learning. Facilitated discussion or dialogue is a useful educational tool.

Given the cultural diversity in the United States, groups often differ in cultural background, which should influence how nutrition education strategies are delivered. Nutrition educators should aim to become culturally competent, which means possessing a set of knowledge and interpersonal skills that allow them to increase their understanding and appreciation of cultural differences and similarities within, among, and between groups and to work effectively in cross-cultural situations. Nutrition education programs should seek to be culturally appropriate to their intended audience. Likewise, nutrition education programs should be mindful of the literacy level of their audiences and develop oral, visual, and written communications that are appropriate to their level.

Questions and Activities

1. You have been asked to provide suggestions to a Head Start center regarding their nutrition education program for the youngsters. From what you have learned, what advice would you give?

2. You are looking over a nutrition education curriculum for grades 4 and 5. Based on what you have read in this chapter, list three features the curriculum should have that would make you conclude that the curriculum is at the appropriate developmental level.

3. You will be providing two after-school nutrition education sessions to a group of teens ages 13 to 15. Describe three educational formats you will be sure to use to gain their attention and provide skill development.

4. You plan to facilitate a group discussion and dialogue session to implement your educational plan with a group of mothers of young children. What do you see as your role as a facilitator? What challenges do you anticipate? How will you know that you are being an effective facilitator?

5. Pick a cultural group that you would like to learn about. Read about the culture of the group or talk with people from that group. For this group, what are two key nutritional concerns? Go to a grocery store that stocks foods for this cultural group. Pick two foods and learn more about them. Then identify a nutrition education material, such as a handout, pamphlet, poster, video, or healthy cookbook, that you might use with this group. In what ways is it culturally sensitive? Describe how it uses surface structure or deep structure features or both. Be specific.

References

Abusabha, R., J. Peacock, and C. Achterberg. 1999. How to make nutrition education more meaningful through facilitated group discussions. *Journal of the American Dietetic Association* 99:72–76.

Alaimo, K., C. M. Olson, and E. A. Frongillo. 1999. Importance of cognitive testing for survey items: An example from food security questionnaires. *Journal of Nutrition Education* 31:269–275.

Baranowski, T., J. Baranowski, K. W. Cullen, et al. 2003. Squire's Quest! Dietary outcome evaluation of a multimedia game. *American Journal of Preventive Medicine* 24:52–61.

Birch, L. L. 1987. The role of experience in children's food acceptance patterns. *Journal of the American Dietetic Association* 87(suppl):S36–S40.

Birch, L. L. 1999. Development of food preferences. *Annual Review of Nutrition* 19:41–62.

Bronfenbrenner, U. 1979. *The ecology of human development*. Boston: Harvard University Press.

Bronner, Y. 1994. Cultural sensitivity and nutrition counseling. *Topics in Clinical Nutrition* 9:13–19.

Brookfield, S. 1986. *Understanding and facilitating adult learning: A comprehensive analysis of principles and effective practices*. San Francisco: Jossey-Bass.

Contento, I. R. 1981. Children's thinking about food and eating: A Piagetian-based study. *Journal of Nutrition Education* 13(suppl):S86–S90.

Contento, I. R., G. I. Balch, Y. L. Bronner, et al. 1995. The effectiveness of nutrition education and implications for nutrition education policy, programs and research. A review of research. *Journal of Nutrition Education* 27:279–418.

Contento, I. R., and J. W. Michela. 1998. Nutrition and food choice behavior among children and adolescents. In *Handbook of pediatric and adolescent health psychology*, edited by R. Goreczny and C. Hensen, 249–273. Boston: Allyn & Bacon.

Contento, I. R., J. W. Michela, and C. J. Goldberg. 1988. Food choice among adolescents: Population segmentation by motivation. *Journal of Nutrition Education* 20:289–298.

Contento, I. R., J. W. Michela, and S. S. Williams. 1995. Adolescent food choice: Role of weight and dieting status. *Appetite* 25:51–76.

Contento, I. R., S. S. Williams, J. L. Michela, and A. B. Franklin. 2006. Understanding the food choice process of adolescents in the context of family and friends. *Journal of Adolescent Health* 38(5):575–582.

Contento, I. R., P. A. Zybert, and S. S. Williams. 2005. Relationship of cognitive restraint of eating and disinhibition to the quality of food choices of Latina women and their young children. *Preventive Medicine* 40:326–336.

Croll, J. K., D. Neumark-Sztainer, and M. Story. 2001. Healthy eating: What does it mean to adolescents? *Journal of Nutrition Education* 33:193–198.

Cross, T., B. Bazron, K. Dennis, and M. Isaacs. 1989. *Towards a culturally competent system of care*. Vol. 1. Washington, DC: Georgetown University Child Development Center, CASSP Technical Assistance Center.

Cusatis, D. C., and B. M. Shannon. 1996. Influences on adolescent eating behavior. *Journal of Adolescent Health* 18:27–34.

Devine, C. M. 2005. A life course perspective: Understanding food choices in time, social location, and history. *Journal of Nutrition Education and Behavior* 37:121–128.

Devine, C. M., M. Connors, C. A. Bisogni, and J. Sobal. 1998. Life-course influences on fruit and vegetables trajectories: Qualitative analysis of food choices. *Journal of Nutrition Education* 30:361–370.

Devine, C. M., and C. M. Olson. 1991. Women's dietary prevention motives: Life stage influences. *Journal of Nutrition Education* 23:269–274.

Doak, C. C., L. G. Doak, and J. H. Root. 1996. *Teaching patients with low literacy skills*. 2nd ed. Philadelphia: Lippincott.

Edstrom, K. M., and C. M. Devine. 2001. Consistency in women's orientations to food and nutrition in midlife and older age: A 10-year qualitative follow-up. *Journal of Nutrition Education* 33:215–223.

Elkind, D. 1978. Understanding the young adolescent. *Adolescence* 13:127–134.

Faith, M. S., K. S. Scanlon, L. L. Birch, L. A. Francis, and B. Sherry. 2004. Parent–child feeding strategies and their relationships to child eating and weight status. *Obesity Research* 12:1711–1722.

Fisher, J. O., and L. L. Birch. 2002. Eating in the absence of hunger and overweight in girls from 5 to 7 years of age. *American Journal of Clinical Nutrition* 76:226–231.

Gable, S., and S. Lutz. 2001. Nutrition socialization experiences of children in the Head Start program. *Journal of the American Dietetic Association* 101:572–577.

Gibson, E. L., and J. Wardle. 1998. Fruit and vegetable consumption, nutritional knowledge, and beliefs in mothers and children. *Appetite* 31:205–228.

Gillman, M. W., S. L. Rifas-Shiman, A. L. Frazier, et al. 2000. Family dinner and diet quality among older children and adolescents. *Archives of Family Medicine* 9:235–240.

Gould, R. L. 1978. *Transformations: Growth and change in adult life*. New York: Simon & Schuster.

Guthrie, J. F., B. H. Lin, and E. Frazao. 2002. Role of food prepared away from home in the American diet, 1977–1978 versus 1994–1996: Changes and consequences. *Journal of Nutrition Education and Behavior* 34:140–150.

Hertzler, A. A., and K. DeBord. 1994. Preschoolers' developmentally appropriate food and nutrition skills. *Journal of Nutrition Education* 26:166B–C.

Husing, C., and M. Elfant. 2005. Finding the teacher within: A story of learner-centered education in California WIC. *Journal of Nutrition Education and Behavior* 37(Suppl. 1):S22.

Isaacs, M., and M. Benjamin. 1991. *Towards a culturally competent system of care*. Vol. 2: *Programs which utilize culturally competent principles*. Washington, DC:

Georgetown University Child Development Center, CASSP Technical Assistance Center.

Johnson, S. L., L. Bellows, L. Beckstrom, and J. Anderson. 2007. Evaluation of a social marketing campaign targeting preschool children. *American Journal of Health Behavior* 37(1):44–55

Kavanagh, K. H., and P. H. Kennedy. 1992. *Promoting cultural diversity: Strategies for health professionals.* Newbury Park, CA: Sage.

King, M. A., A. Sims, and D. Osher. 2006. How is cultural competence integrated in education? Center for Effective Collaboration and Practice, American Institutes of Research. http://cecp.air.org.

Knowles, M. S. 1990. *The adult learner: A neglected species.* 4th ed. Houston, TX: Gulf.

Kreuter, M. W., S. N. Lukwago, R. D. Bucholtz, E. M. Clark, and V. Sanders-Thompson. 2003. Achieving cultural appropriateness in health promotion programs: Targeted and tailored approaches. *Health Education and Behavior* 30(2):133–146.

Kreuter, M. W., C. Sugg-Skinner, C. L. Holt, et al. 2005. Cultural tailoring for mammography and fruit and vegetables intake among low-income African-American women in urban public health centers. *Preventive Medicine* 41:53–62.

Kumanyika, S. K., and C. B. Morssink. 1997. Cultural appropriateness of weight management programs. In *Overweight and weight management: The health professional's guide to understanding and practice,* edited by S. Dalton. Gaithersburg, MD: Aspen.

Leupker, R. V., C. L. Perry, S. M. McKinlay, et al. 1996. Outcomes of a field trial to improve children's dietary patterns and physical activity. *Journal of the American Medical Association* 275:768–776.

Levinson, D. J. 1978. *The seasons of a man's life.* New York: Knopf.

———. 1996. *The seasons of a woman's life.* New York: Knopf.

Lin, W., and I. S. Liang. 2005. Family dining environment, parenting practices and preschoolers' food acceptance. *Journal of Nutrition Education and Behavior* 37(Suppl. 1):47.

Liou, D., and I. R. Contento. 2001. Usefulness of psychosocial theory variables in explaining fat-related dietary behavior in Chinese Americans: Association with degree of acculturation. *Journal of Nutrition Education* 33:322–331.

Matheson, D., and K. Spranger. 2001. Content analysis of the use of fantasy, challenge, and curiosity in school-based nutrition education programs. *Journal of Nutrition Education* 33:10–16.

Matheson, D., K. Spranger, and A. Saxe. 2002. Preschool children's perceptions of food and their food experiences. *Journal of Nutrition Education and Behavior* 34:85–92.

Michela, J. L., and I. R. Contento. 1984. Spontaneous classification of foods by elementary school-aged children. *Health Education Quarterly* 11:57–76.

Neugarten, B. L., R. J. Havighurst, and S. S. Tobin. 1968. Personality and patterns of aging. In *Middle age and aging,* edited by B. L. Neugarten. Chicago: University of Chicago Press.

Neumark-Sztainer, D., P. J. Hannan, M. Story, J. Croll, and C. Perry. 2003. Family meal patterns: Associations with sociodemographic characteristics and improved dietary intake among adolescents. *Journal of the American Dietetic Association* 102:317–322.

Neumark-Sztainer, D., M. Story, D. Ackard, J. Moe, and C. Perry. 2000a. The "family meal": View of adolescents. *Journal of Nutrition Education* 32:329–334.

———. 2000b. Family meals among adolescents: Findings from a pilot study. *Journal of Nutrition Education* 32:335–340.

Neumark-Sztainer, D., M. Story, P. J. Hannan, C. L. Perry, and L. M. Irving. 2002. Weight-related concerns and behaviors among overweight and nonoverweight adolescents: Implication for preventing weight-related disorders. *Archives of Pediatric Adolescent Medicine* 156:171–178.

Neumark-Sztainer, D., M. Story, C. Perry, and M. A. Casey. 1999. Factors influencing food choices of adolescents: Findings from focus-group discussions with adolescents. *Journal of the American Dietetic Association* 99:929–937.

Neumark-Sztainer, D., M. Story, E. Toporoff, J. H. Himes, M. D. Resnick, and R. W. Blum. 1997. Covariations of eating behaviors with other health-related behaviors among adolescents. *Journal of Adolescent Health* 20:450–458.

Norris, J. 2003. *From telling to teaching.* North Myrtle Beach, SC: Learning by Dialogue.

Olson, C. M., and G. L. Kelley. 1989. The challenge of implementing theory-based nutrition education. *Journal of Nutrition Education* 22:280–284.

Orlet Fisher, J., B. J. Rolls, and L. L. Birch. 2003. Children's bite size and intake of an entrée are greater with larger portions than with age-appropriate or self-selected portions. *American Journal of Clinical Nutrition* 77:1164–1170.

Petty, R. E., and J. T. Cacioppo. 1986. *Communication and persuasion: Central and peripheral routes to attitude change.* New York: Springer-Verlag.

Piaget, J., and B. Inhelder. 1969. *The psychology of the child.* New York: Basic Books.

Resnicow, K., T. Baranowski, J. S. Ahluwalia, and R. L. Braithwaite. 1999. Cultural sensitivity in public health: Defined and demystified. *Ethnicity and Disease* 9:10–21.

Resnicow, K., A. Jackson, D. Blisset, et al. 2005. Results of the Healthy Body Healthy Spirit trial. *Health Physiology* 24:339–348.

Resnicow, K., A. Jackson, R. Braithwaite, et al. 2002. Healthy Body/Healthy Spirit: A church-based nutrition and physical activity intervention. *Health Education Research* 17:562–573.

Robinson, T. N., M. Kiernan, D. M. Matheson, and K. D. Haydel. 2001. Is parental control over children's eating associated with childhood obesity? Results from a population-based sample of third graders. *Obesity Research* 9:306–312.

Rolls, B. J., D. Engell, and L. L. Birch. 2000. Serving portion size influences 5-year-old but not 3-year-old children's food intakes. *Journal of the American Dietetic Association* 180:232–234.

Sahyoun, N. R., C. A. Pratt, and A. Anderson. 2004. Evaluation of nutrition education for older adults: A proposed framework. *Journal of the American Dietetic Association* 104:58–69.

Sanjur, D. 1982. *Social and cultural perspectives in nutrition.* Englewood Cliffs, NJ: Prentice Hall.

Satter, E. 1999. *Secrets of feeding a healthy family.* Madison, WI: Kelcy Press.

Sigman-Grant, M. 2004. *Facilitated dialogue basics: A self-study guide for nutrition educators. Let's dance.* University of Nevada, Cooperative Extension. SP04-21.

Singleton, J. C., C. L. Achterberg, and B. M. Shannon. 1992. Role of food and nutrition: The health perceptions of young children. *Journal of the American Dietetic Association* 92:67–70.

Skinner, J. D., B. R. Carruth, B. Wendy, and P. J. Ziegler. 2002. Children's food preferences: A longitudinal analysis. *Journal of the American Dietetic Association* 102:1638–1647.

Story, M., D. Neumark-Sztainer, and S. I. French. 2002. Individual and environmental influences on adolescent eating behaviors. *Journal of the American Dietetic Association* 2:S40–S51.

Story, M., D. Neumark-Sztainer, N. Sherwood, J. Stang, and D. Murray. 1998. Dieting status and its relationship to eating and physical activity behaviors in a representative sample of US adolescents. *Journal of the American Dietetic Association* 98:1127–1135, 1255.

Story, M., and M. D. Resnick. 1986. Adolescents' views on food and nutrition. *Journal of Nutrition Education* 18:188–192.

Sue, D. W., and D. Sue. 1999. *Counseling the culturally different: Theory and practice.* 3rd ed. New York: Wiley.

Tennant, M., and P. Pogson. 1995. *Learning and change in the adult years: A developmental perspective.* San Francisco: Jossey-Bass.

Vella, J. 2002. *Learning to listen, learning to teach: The power of dialogue in educating adults.* Revised ed. San Francisco: Jossey-Bass.

Ventura, A. K., and L. Birch. 2008. Does parenting affect children's eating and weight status? *International Journal of Behavioral Nutrition and Physical Activity* 5:15.

Videon, T. M., and C. K. Manning. 2003. Influences on adolescent eating patterns: The importance of family meals. *Journal of Adolescent Health* 32:365–373.

Vygotsky, L. S. 1962. *Thought and language.* Cambridge, MA: MIT Press.

Wardle, J., L. J. Cooke, E. L. Gibson, M. Sapochnik, A. Sheiham, and M. Lawson. 2003. Increasing children's acceptance of vegetables: A randomized trial of parent-led exposure. *Appetite* 40:55–162.

Wardle, J., M. L. Herrera, L. J. Cooke, and E. L. Gibson. 2003. Modifying children's food preferences: The effects of exposure and rewards on acceptance of an unfamiliar vegetable. *European Journal of Clinical Nutrition* 57:341–348.

Young, L., J. J. Anderson, L. Beckstrom, L. Bellows, and S. L. Johnson. 2004. Using social marketing principles to guide the development of a nutrition education initiative for preschool-aged children. *Journal of Nutrition Education and Behavior* 36:250–257.

Nutrition Educators as Change Agents in the Environment

OVERVIEW

This chapter describes ways in which nutrition educators can help to shape the profession and to act as change agents in the larger environment by working with others to shape legislation about nutrition education and by educating policy makers in government.

CHAPTER OUTLINE

- Introduction
- Keeping up with nutrition education research and best practices
- Helping to shape the profession
- Ethics in nutrition education
- Participating in community coalitions
- Advocating for nutrition and nutrition education
- Educating policymakers in government
- You can't do everything, but you can do something

LEARNING OBJECTIVES

At the end of the chapter, you will be able to:

- State reasons why it is important to participate in professional associations relevant to nutrition education
- Identity ways you can help to shape the profession
- Understand the importance of policies regarding outside sponsorship of nutrition education professional activities and conflicts of interest
- Describe ways you can affect the larger environment by participating in community networks and coalitions
- Appreciate the importance of educating policy makers in government, such as elected officials

■ INTRODUCTION

You attend your first professional meeting of dietitians, extension nutritionists, nutrition educators, and others. You are amazed to see so many activities going on and are both excited and overwhelmed. At sessions, you hear about various programs and projects that people are involved in. They spark ideas for you to use in your professional work.

You learn new information from research. You hear about committees and task force reports. You learn about government policies at the state and national level that might affect your work and you wonder, Should I get involved? If so, how do I do that?

Providing nutrition education directly to the public is your major role as a nutrition educator. You do this through direct in-person activities with groups, indirect activities such as printed materials and media campaigns, and policy and systems change activities to foster environments supportive of the program's targeted behaviors and practices. Nutrition educators also have the opportunity to develop and grow by networking with others and being involved in professional organizations. They can make their voices heard in the organizations of which they are members and even help to shape their policies and practices by participation and actions. Nutrition educators also have the opportunity to make a difference in the world by advocating for nutrition education policies and programs in the larger environment. This chapter describes some ways in which you can be involved in the nutrition education professional community.

KEEPING UP WITH NUTRITION EDUCATION RESEARCH AND BEST PRACTICES

This book began by noting that this is a great time for nutrition education. It is needed now more than ever, and research and evidence for best practices provides the tools you need to assist the public to achieve health and well-being. You have seen that nutrition education is more likely to be effective when it focuses on behaviors and practices, uses theory and research evidence from behavioral nutrition and nutrition education to guide the strategies it uses, and addresses multiple sources of influence. Effective nutrition education is not short-term work; it takes time to facilitate the progress of individuals and communities through various stages of change: from awareness and active contemplation, through various levels of motivational readiness to change, through how-to activities to enable change, to maintenance of change. Consequently, the motivators and reinforcers of change and the environmental supports of change need to be multifaceted, continually updated, and maintained.

Research in this area is active and ongoing. New understandings of how to facilitate change and new tools are being generated. Keeping up to date on nutrition education research is important to maintain your effectiveness as a nutrition educator. You can do this by reading the relevant journals and by attending nutrition education and behavioral nutrition (not just nutrition science) workshops, meetings, and confer-

ences. **Box 18-1** lists some of the professional organizations particularly relevant to nutrition educators.

HELPING TO SHAPE THE PROFESSION

As a nutrition educator you also have the opportunity to participate in and shape the profession. There are many ways to do this. One way is to join one or more professional associations. For example, there are local and state dietetic associations to which you can belong, as well as national associations such as the Society for Nutrition Education and the American Dietetic Association. Through these organizations you will meet others just like you—individuals who are excited to be in the nutrition education profession and helping the public eat well and who are dealing with the same dilemmas and constraints. These organizations provide a forum for you to network with others and share ideas, learn about best practices, receive updates on information that may be important in your work, and learn about regulations and policy actions that affect the profession or the public at large.

You also have the opportunity to make your opinions heard. Professional associations are member organizations, made up of others just like you. Although state and national organizations may have some paid staff, all are dependent on members' volunteer participation to operate. These associations thus become whatever members want them to be. If you are a student member, many organizations have student rates that extend to the first year of "professional enrollment" or "new professionals." Many organizations have what are called sections, divisions, or affiliates. These provide opportunities to network with colleagues who have like interests or are related geographically.

Who They Are

What are some associations where you might find a professional home? For nutrition educators, some of the most relevant ones include the Society for Nutrition Education (SNE), American Dietetic Association (ADA), School Nutrition Association (SNA), American Public Health Association, International Society for Behavioral Nutrition and Physical Activity, American Association of Family and Consumer Sciences, American Diabetes Association, American Society for Nutrition, and the Society for Behavioral Medicine. Information on some of these is provided in Box 18-1. Of course, many nutrition educators belong to several professional associations.

Getting to Know Them and Vice Versa

Getting involved in an organization is key to getting to know it. Reading the organization's journal by itself will not bring about opportunities to participate fully or shape the profession. As you get to know the organization, the organization will get to know you. As you offer to serve on committees and task forces and hold offices, over time the organization will come to you asking for your involvement.

A key way to get started in the process of knowing and getting known is to attend the organization's annual meeting. Annual meetings provide opportunities for more than learning from experts. They are opportunities for meeting your colleagues, expressing your thoughts, and supporting your position in the various units that run the organization and professions. The divisions, special interest units, caucuses, and affiliates all provide opportunities for input. Although these units may meet during the year and have electronic mailing lists and bulletin boards, it is at the annual meetings that members all come together to discuss, plan, and strategize. This also applies to meetings of state or local affiliates,

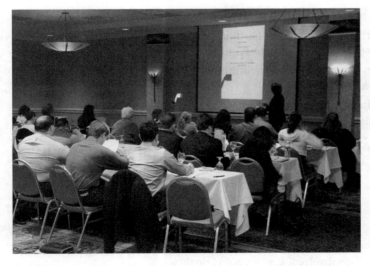

Becoming a member of a professional organization is a great way to become involved in your profession, and the level of participation is up to you.

Box 18-1 **Professional Associations of Particular Relevance to Nutrition Educators**

Society for Nutrition Education (SNE)

Mission: The Society for Nutrition Education promotes effective nutrition education and communication to support and improve healthful behaviors.

Identity statement: SNE is an international organization of nutrition education professionals who are dedicated to promoting healthful sustainable food choices and who share a vision of healthy people in healthy communities. Our members conduct research in education, behavior, and communication; develop and disseminate innovative nutrition education strategies and communicate information on food, nutrition, and health issues to students, professionals, policy makers, and the public. SNE members share ideas and resources through our journal, newsletter, annual conference, and members-only listserv. Our divisions offer networking opportunities for members with similar interests and expertise. Divisions include Healthy Aging, Children, Communications, Food and Nutrition Extension Education, Higher Education, International, Industry, Public Health, Social Marketing, Sustainable Food Systems, and Weight Realities. SNE also has some regional affiliates and an Advisory Committee on Public Policy that helps provide focus on national issues of importance to society members.

Website: http://www.sne.org

American Dietetic Association (ADA)

Mission: Empower members to be the nation's food and nutrition leaders.

Identity statement: The ADA is the world's largest organization of food and nutrition professionals. The ADA is committed to improving the nation's health and advocating the profession of dietetics through research, education, and advocacy.

Dietetic Practice Groups (DPGs) and state affiliates provide opportunities for networking based on area of practice, interest, and geography. DPGs include groups based on area of practice (e.g., Gerontological Nutritionists DPG) as well as areas of interest (e.g., the Hunger and Environmental Nutrition DPG).

Website: http://www.eatright.org

School Nutrition Association (SNA) (Formerly the American School Food Service Association, ASFSA)

Mission: To advance good nutrition for all children. The association works to ensure all children have access to healthful school meals and nutrition education by
- Providing members with education and training
- Setting standards through certification and credentialing
- Gathering and transmitting regulatory, legislative, industry, nutritional, and other types of information related to school nutrition

- Representing the nutritional interests of all children

Identity statement: SNA is dedicated solely to the support and well-being of school nutrition professionals in advancing good nutrition for all children. Since 1946, SNA has been advancing the availability and quality of school nutrition programs as an integral part of a student's education. SNA has 52 state affiliates and hundreds of local chapters.

Website: http://www.schoolnutrition.org

American Association of Family and Consumer Sciences (AAFCS)

Mission: To provide leadership and support for professionals whose work assists individuals, families, and communities in making informed decisions about their well-being and relationships as well as resources to achieve optimal quality of life.

Identity statement: AAFCS strives to improve the quality and standards of individual and family life by providing educational programs, influencing public policy, and through communication. Members work to empower individuals, strengthen families, and enable communities. Through divisions, members provide guidance and practical knowledge about the things of everyday life, including human growth and development, personal behavior, housing and environment, food and nutrition, apparel and textiles, and resource management, so that students and consumers can make sound decisions and enjoy a healthy, productive, and more fulfilling life. Professional sections and state affiliates offer other opportunities for networking.

Website: http://www.aafcs.org

International Society for Behavioral Nutrition and Physical Activity (ISBNPA)

Mission: ISBNPA stimulates, promotes, and advocates innovative research and policy in the area of behavioral nutrition and physical activity toward the betterment of human health worldwide. Its purposes are as follows:
- Conduct scientific meetings, congresses, and symposia in which current research on behavioral issues in nutrition and physical activity will be discussed by researchers in related fields
- Disseminate information on research being done in behavioral issues in nutrition and physical activity through newsletters and other communications
- Provide information to and encourage continued support by public and private bodies that support research in behavioral issues in nutrition and physical activity
- Promote and facilitate the dissemination of knowledge of behavioral issues in nutrition and physical activity to the

(continues)

> ## *Box* 18-1   Professional Associations of Particular Relevance to Nutrition Educators *(continued)*
>
> public and to educators, scholars, and health professionals through any lawful means
> - Promote and assist communication between researchers on issues of behavioral nutrition and physical activity and members of scientific and scholarly organizations whose members do research in other related health and medical fields through joint meetings, shared membership lists, joint publications, and any other lawful means
>
> **Identity statement:** ISBNPA has an international presence, with nearly 400 members representing 29 countries. Its members come together from more than 40 government agencies and industry and professional organizations, as well as close to 150 academic and medical institutions. Members bring to this organization a diversity of experience and expertise.
>
> **Website:** http://www.isbnpa.org
>
> **Association for the Study of Food and Society (ASFS)**
>
> **Mission:** The Association for the Study of Food and Society is a multidisciplinary international organization dedicated to exploring the complex relationships among food, culture, and society.
>
> **Identity statement:** The ASFS's members, who approach the study of food from numerous disciplines in the humanities, social sciences, and sciences, as well as in the world of food
>
> beyond the academy, draw on a wide range of theoretical and practical approaches and seek to promote discussions about food that transgress traditional boundaries. The association holds annual meetings with the Agriculture, Food, and Human Values Society and publishes the journal *Food, Culture & Society*.
>
> **Website:** http://www.food-culture.org
>
> **Society for Behavioral Medicine (SBM)**
>
> **Mission:** The Society of Behavioral Medicine is a multidisciplinary organization of clinicians, educators, and scientists dedicated to promoting the study of the interactions of behavior with biology and the environment, and the application of that knowledge to improve the health and well-being of individuals, families, communities, and populations.
>
> **Identity statement:** Better health through behavior change. The SBM's goals are to
> - Enhance the value of SBM as a base for networking, professional growth, and information exchange
> - Establish SBM as a visible and influential champion of behavioral medicine
> - Develop the capacity to secure resources to achieve SBM's goals and mission
>
> **Website:** http://www.sbm.org

which often focus on more regional professional issues; membership or town meetings; and gatherings to discuss specific issues.

Finding Where You Fit

Finding your home in the profession involves finding not only the organization but also the specialty units within it that are right for you. Initially it may be the specialty units, defined as divisions, sections, or practice groups, and local, state, and regional affiliates that are of more interest to you than the organization itself. They are smaller and therefore more manageable. They also provide a common ground of interest in specific issues or approaches that may feel comfortable to you. Many nutrition educators belong to more than one such unit. Over time you may change your focus or move on, but you will often find that the relationships you have developed keep you involved and, through networking, offer opportunities in other groups and locations.

Attend the business meetings of the specialty unit or division to find out the main issues facing the organization or unit, the activities completed or contemplated, and the financial situation of the organization as well as the sources of funding for the organization.

Determining your fit is based often on your relationships with the people in the unit or organization and the ability to work synergistically to have an impact, discuss common interests, and share war stories. You can join communication forums, such as listservs. Find out if there is a mentoring program. There may be a specific student unit, and often

the governing boards have student representatives. Even as a student you have an opportunity to affect the profession.

Join a Subcommittee or Task Force

Professional associations are always seeking interested members to participate. You do not have to wait to be asked! Look for notices seeking participation and input. This, too, is a way to shape the profession. If you don't feel comfortable sitting on a committee or being part of a task force, respond when the organization asks for member input or opinions. Let leadership know you're interested in an issue. Over time, as your name is recognized as an involved member, leadership will come to you. In fact, managing your time so as not to become overextended may become the more important consideration!

Write

You can participate by helping to write for, or edit, the newsletter for your specialty unit or division. You can help to write background papers or participate with others in writing position papers on some issue that is a passion of yours. You can write letters to the editor or write articles. All these actions provide opportunities to be involved and have an impact.

Participate in Program Planning Activities

Organizations and the specialty units within them always need to plan future conferences or meetings. Attend the open planning sessions and provide your suggestions for sessions, topics, or speakers. Join the planning committee if you can. Help shape the agenda for the meetings.

Participate in Member-Initiated Resolutions or Issues Management Processes

Many professional associations have a process whereby an individual, a group of members, or a division or committee can write up and submit resolutions or statements for the membership to vote on, which then go to the association for action. In most cases the resolutions advocate that the association take a position or action on some issue, or advocate that the association establish a policy. The American Dietetic Association uses an issues management process as the communication process whereby members can convey their concerns about contemporary issues to the leadership (American Dietetic Association [ADA] 2001). The Society for Nutrition Education uses a member-initiated resolutions process (SNE 2006). Such a process is a very effective way to influence the professional association as well as the larger policy environment. Past resolutions of the Society for Nutrition Education are found on its website (www.sne.org). These provide some interesting insights into membership interests and concerns. These resolutions are conveyed to the agencies and groups designated in the resolutions where they often have important impacts on food- and nutrition-related policy. The resolutions of the American Dietetic Association are also available from that organization (http://www.eatright.org).

Run for Office

Making the commitment to be a part of the process may very well lead you to run for an office. You may be nominated or you may decide to nominate yourself. Don't be shy. If you want to have an impact and be involved, let others know. This applies to running for offices at the specialty unit or division level as well as at the organizational level.

Volunteer

Whatever you do, find some way to be involved. The connections you make can be very important for you over the long term. In the process of volunteering, you get to know others, they get to know you, and the profession becomes stronger because of all the participatory voices. Also keep in mind that professional organizations cannot run on the dues they raise alone or the funds they may acquire through foundation grants. They need volunteers. Some active members have used a rule of thumb of volunteering an hour a week and found it to be very rewarding, both personally and professionally.

■ ETHICS IN NUTRITION EDUCATION: MAINTAINING CREDIBILITY

As mentioned earlier in the book, one of the most cherished assets nutrition educators have is credibility—to clients and program participants, to the professional community, to government, and to the public at large. When you lose your credibility, you lose your effectiveness. This same principle applies to the professional associations to which you belong, and indeed to the profession as a whole. Professional associations, and indeed the profession, must be seen as credible sources of information and recommendations.

What does this mean? It means that just as is the case for individuals, so also the recommendations made by the professional associations must be seen as being based on sound science. The professional associations must not stand to gain financially, or *seem* to gain financially, from their recommendations. In recent years, professional associations, as well as

private voluntary organizations, research programs using public funds, and all government and quasi-government committees, have developed sponsorship policies that apply to potential sponsors of activities of the organization, and conflict of interest policies that apply to individuals. Much of the impetus for this development came from the concern of members of organizations and of the public about undue commercial influence that might affect the credibility of the organization.

Sponsorship of Nutrition Education Programs and Professional Activities

Professional associations and organizations that provide nutrition education are always in need of funds. Membership dues, government or foundation grants, or grants from academic institutions do not always generate enough funds for these organizations to do what they need or want to do. It would appear natural to turn to the food industry for such funding. Organizations may go to individual corporations or to commodity groups. Funding can be sought for individual activities, such as a specific one-time professional meeting or a specific session or social event at the annual meeting, or for the annual meeting of an organization as a whole. Funds can also be sought for a particular fact sheet or position paper, or for a specific project or particular community outreach activity. The food industry may also contribute to the professional organization as a whole.

Members in several professional associations raised concerns about undue influence, potentially biased positions, conflict of interest, and the appearance of conflict of interest. They were concerned that corporate need for profits and nutrition professionals' interests in the health of the public may at times come into conflict (Nestle 2002). These concerns were often raised through the resolutions process or issues management process. In response to membership concerns, many professional organizations developed guidelines so that sponsorship by, and collaborations with, the food industry (or fitness industry) can be conducted in an ethical and mutually beneficial manner.

Guiding principles usually include the following (Society for Nutrition Educaton [SNE] 2002):

- The organization should secure sponsorship arrangements that further the organization's mission and vision, retain the organization's independence, maintain objectivity, promote trust, avoid conflicts of interest, and guard its professional values.
- The sponsorship should be consistent with the organization's commitment to the free exchange of ideas, opinions, research findings, and other information related to members' interests and activities.
- There should be transparency about relationships, clearly specified expectations, understanding of the value of the sponsor's contribution, and methods of accountability.
- Protection of the reputation of the organization is of utmost importance, along with full disclosure, information that is science based, and avoidance of the appearance of endorsement.

Conflicts of Interest

Members in several professional organizations were also instrumental in initiating policies about conflict of interest and disclosure. Members were concerned that speakers (whether members or invited guests) were not disclosing professional and corporate relationships they had when they spoke at conferences or sat on an organization's boards, committees, and task forces. Members felt it was important to know that a given speaker or board member, whatever his or her primary professional designations, also had paid consulting or other relationships with the food industry or some other relevant group. Because professional associations are member-run organizations, members' voices are important and are heard. The outcome has been that many organizations have developed policies and procedures that address these concerns of membership.

The American Dietetic Association, for example, has a policy that requires all persons speaking or making presentations at ADA programs to disclose any dualities of interest (conflict of interest) that might be perceived as affecting or influencing their presentations; such disclosures are made known to the attendees and audience for such programs (ADA n.d.).

Most professional associations or societies also require all those who are on the governing board, committees, policy bodies, or task forces, and those who are officers at the division or specialty unit level, to complete an annual conflict of interest form. Some associations also require that at the beginning of each committee or task force meeting, the agenda items be reviewed and an opportunity provided for members of the committee to disclose if they have a conflict of interest on any given item. If they do, they may be asked to recuse themselves altogether from that item or to participate in the discussion but not vote (SNE 2005). All would agree that transparency is good for everyone.

Notice that these policy changes were frequently initiated by members asking for change. This is another example of how you can make a difference in the profession by your actions.

Such self-disclosures of conflict of interest have become routine for all government and quasi-government committees, task forces, and other bodies. They are also required now for all government research and other grant recipients.

Tests for Conflict of Interest

How do you test yourself to determine whether you have a conflict of interest? Ask yourself, Would others trust my comments, decisions, actions, or votes if they knew about my relationships with other organizations and/or my situation? How would I feel if the roles were reversed—would I feel misled or betrayed?

Conflicts of interest involve the abuse, actual or potential, of the trust people have in professionals. Conflicts of interest thus not only injure particular clients and employers but also damage the whole profession by reducing the trust people have in professionals in general (McDonald 2004). Perception is a critical component here. If your colleagues or the public find out information after the fact and perceive a conflict of interest, the perception can do as much damage as the reality. Disclosure and transparency are key ways to address a conflict of interest, allowing others to weigh what you say. It may be appropriate not to participate in a given activity, a determination that can only occur if public acknowledgment of possible conflict is made.

■ PARTICIPATING IN COMMUNITY COALITIONS

Earlier this book discussed ways in which nutrition education intervention programs can include environmental components to promote opportunities for participants to take the actions that are advocated by the program (see Chapters 6 and 13). Even if your program does not have an environmental change component, you can, as a nutrition education professional, participate in a number of activities in the community where you can be a change agent in the larger environment.

You need to help others understand that nutrition education professionals are much more than people who offer lectures and workshops.

For the public to understand what you do, you need to be out there working with the community. Here are some examples of volunteer opportunities with community coalitions, networks, or other community groups.

Food Policy Councils

A food policy council (FPC) consists of stakeholders from various segments of a state or local food system. Councils can be officially sanctioned through a government action such as an Executive Order or can be a grassroots effort. The primary goal of many food policy councils is to examine the operation of a local food system and provide ideas or recommendations for how it can be improved (Desjardin et al. 2005).

Who better to be part of the process than the nutrition educator? It makes sense for nutrition educators to play a key role in food policy councils. Desjardin et al. (2005) point out that nutrition educators contribute food and nutrition knowledge and provide legitimacy as health professionals. Having nutrition professionals on board can broaden the scope of food policy councils, where members may be more concerned with emergency food assistance or agriculture policy in the most traditional sense. It also means a food policy council can get in-house help with proposal and report writing, research and evaluation, and media communication. Nutrition educators can also offer essential organizational and planning skills.

Local Wellness Policy

The Child Nutrition and WIC Reauthorization Act of 2004 (Section 204) required every local school district that offers the USDA school lunch program to develop and implement a local wellness policy (Fox 2005). The mandate provides that nutrition guidelines must:

- Be developed for all foods available on the school campus during the school day
- Include goals for nutrition education, physical activity, and other school-based activities to promote student wellness
- Have a plan for measuring implementation
- Involve parents, students, school food representatives, school board members, administrators, and the public in development

Strong nutrition components will make strong wellness policies, and the nutrition educator can be a facilitator of this process and/or serve as a resource. As is the case with food policy councils, school wellness councils are multidisciplinary, and assessment is important. Examples of self-assessment and planning tools include the School Health Index (SHI) from the Centers for Disease Control and Prevention (CDC 2005) and Changing the Scene from the Team Nutrition Program of the U.S. Department of Agriculture (USDA 2000).

Although most schools now have wellness policy councils not all are functioning fully. Also, most have written school policies, but again they may not be fully implemented. As a nutrition educator, you bring your skills in assessment and in facilitation of dialogue to the table; these are critical to a functional wellness policy. Wellness policies must be evaluated, and you can provide useful skills in this task as well.

Nutrition Education Networks

Nutrition education networks came into being in the mid-1990s when the Food and Nutrition Service (FNS) of the USDA approved cooperative agreements to establish nutrition education networks in 22 states (Association of State Nutrition Network Administrators 2004). The funding objective was to create self-sustaining statewide networks to implement nutrition education for food stamp–eligible adults and children, building on existing efforts, developing public–private partnerships, and using social marketing. It was envisioned that the networks would be the catalyst to integrate nutrition education messages across the food assistance programs and public–private programs (Association of State Nutrition Network Administrators 2004). This networking process would be designed to:

- Maximize public and private resources
- Identify specific client needs and relevant ways to address these needs
- Recruit and leverage community organizations to deliver appropriate messages

Such networks continue to provide considerable opportunities to network and coordinate nutrition education activities in states and local areas (ASNHA).

Community Coalitions

There are no doubt many other local or national coalitions of food and nutrition professionals concerned with a variety of issues that would welcome your participation. Issues might include food security, concerns about the sustainability of food systems, urban gardens, farmers' markets, special populations such as those with HIV/AIDS or diabetes, or childhood overweight prevention. Your insights and expertise as a nutrition educator can be very important to the effective functioning of these coalitions.

■ ADVOCATING FOR NUTRITION AND NUTRITION EDUCATION

You can be a change agent in the larger environment through advocacy activities. These include written communications, providing testimony to governmental and quasi-governmental groups, and helping to shape legislation that affects the nutritional well-being of the public and the support of nutrition education.

Written Communications

Written communications take many forms. The most notable, of course, are letters: you can make your voice heard through writing to newspapers, to legislators, and others. You can also write articles. However, you can also write other documents that can have a tremendous impact on the decision making of individuals, organizations, and government. These can include position papers, policy papers, issue fact sheets, and background papers. Although "key expert members" may write the initial background documents and subsequent papers, you usually have an opportunity to provide input into these documents if you wish and let your wish be known.

Testimony, Hearings, and Forums

Governmental bodies often seek information from professionals about a specific issue using a variety of formats. Testimony and hearings usually come about in response to an invitation or public announcement to provide evidence to a session or committee of Congress, or to other governmental or quasi-governmental bodies, such as committees of the National Academy of Sciences. Hearings are usually open to the public and are designed for committees to obtain information and opinions from professionals or the public on proposed legislation, an investigation, or other activities of government. Hearings may also be purely exploratory in nature, a forum for professionals and the public to provide testimony and data about topics of current interest.

Forums or listening sessions provide opportunities for sharing comments in person or in writing. If you feel passionate about a particular issue, you can seek to testify. Sometimes you can do this on your own, on the basis of being a professional in the field. Or you may testify through your professional group, in which case you must make sure the leadership knows you are interested in presenting testimony.

Helping to Shape Legislation

Some legislation, once passed, is permanent. However, some legislation is written so that it must be renewed after some stated period of time or it will expire. This happens typically in five-year increments, but the time period may be longer or shorter. Key examples of federal legislation that affect nutrition education include the following:

- The Child Nutrition and WIC Reauthorization Act
- The Farm Bill
- The Ryan White Act
- The Older Americans Act

See **Box 18-2** for more information.

You can help shape such legislation by becoming actively involved in the process of making recommendations. For example, the Child Nutrition and WIC Reauthorization Act was due to expire in 2004. In 2002, concerned organizations began to meet to discuss what they would advocate for at renewal time. A one-day meeting was held, sponsored by the National Alliance for Nutrition and Activity, an umbrella organization with more than 30 member organizations, and the Society for Nutrition Education. The meeting was called "The Future of Nutrition Education: Child Nutrition Reauthorization Opportunities." The purpose of this meeting was to bring together stakeholders to discuss the current state of child nutrition education, develop ideas for strengthening child nutrition education, and aid member organizations in developing policy recommendations regarding child nutrition education.

The group was made up of nearly 30 participants representing a variety of food and nutrition professional organizations and advocacy groups interested in strengthening child nutrition education. Over the course of the day and through numerous other activities over the course of the ensuing months, the group developed program recommendations such as the following (American Public Health Association n.d.):

- Allocate adequate funding to reflect nutrition education as a priority.
- Develop and implement evaluation and reporting components.
- Create key nutrition coordinators at the federal, state, and local levels and identify clear roles and responsibilities.
- Provide funding for new and existing staff.

These recommendations became the basis of a white paper on child nutrition education and of other activities that were designed to influence the shape of the legislation. Nutrition educators volunteered their time to participate in these activities. Out of this process came the mandate to set up local wellness committees in school districts to develop policy regarding food and health in schools (see Chapter 13). You can make an important contribution by adding your voice to those of other nutrition educators in activities such as these so as to make a difference in the larger environment.

A number of organizations serve as advocates of food and nutrition policy and legislation at the local, state, and federal levels. They monitor the various food and nutrition programs, alert the profession about new initiatives and changes that are being contemplated, and advocate

Box 18-2 **Legislation That Affects Nutrition Education Programs**

Child Nutrition Reauthorization

Child Nutrition Reauthorization includes legislation that covers the primary government food programs outside of the Food Stamp Program and related education components. Programs include the following:

- National School Lunch Program (NSLP)
- School Breakfast Program (SBP)
- Child and Adult Care Food Program (CACFP)
- Summer Food Service Program (SFSP)
- Special Milk Program (SMP)
- Women, Infants, and Children (WIC), which includes the WIC Farmers Market Nutrition Program (FMNP)
- Fruit and Vegetable Snack Program
- Team Nutrition Program and language for the Team Nutrition Network
- School Wellness Policy legislation
- Language for access to local foods and school gardens

The Farm Bill

The Farm Bill is a series of 10 titles; 4 in particular relate directly to nutrition education. These cover international and national nutrition education and related programs, research, and "miscellaneous" components (respectively, Titles III, IV, VII, and X). This act is also a key source of nutrition education funding and research.

- Title III, the Trade Title, includes the McGovern-Dole International Food for Education and Nutrition Program.
- Title IV, known as the Nutrition Title, covers the Food Stamp Program (FSP), Food Stamp Nutrition Education (FNSE), and Community Food Project Grants (CFPG); commodity distribution programs that are often associated with nutrition outreach, such as the Emergency Food Assistance Program (TEFAP), the Commodity Supplemental Food Program (CSFP), and the Department of Defense Fresh Program (DoD Fresh); funds for child nutrition programs such as commodities for school meals; primary funding for Senior FMNP and additional funding for the WIC FMNP program; the Nutrition Information and Awareness Pilot Program; and startup grants for some institutions participating in the National School Lunch and School Breakfast programs that purchase locally produced foods (the latter two have never received funding).
- Title VII, known as Research and Related Matters, includes the Education and Administration of Land Grant institutions, with programs such as the Cooperative State Education Research, and Extension Service (CSREES), which includes

the Community Food Projects (CFP), the Expanded Food and Nutrition Education Program (EFNEP), and Sustainable Agriculture Research and Education Grants (SARE). The title also includes the Organic Agriculture Research and Extension Initiative.

- Title X is for miscellaneous programs such as country-of-origin labeling, irradiated food/pasteurization, and biotechnology education.

The Ryan White Comprehensive AIDS Resources Emergency (CARE) Act

The Ryan White Act is federal legislation that addresses the unmet health needs of persons living with human immunodeficiency virus (HIV) by funding primary health care and support services. The CARE Act was named after Ryan White, an Indiana teenager whose courageous struggle with HIV/AIDS and against AIDS-related discrimination helped educate the nation.

Older Americans Act

The Older Americans Act was originally signed into law by President Lyndon B. Johnson. In addition to creating the Administration on Aging, it authorized grants to states for community planning and services programs, as well as for research, demonstration, and training projects in the field of aging. Later amendments to the act added grants to Area Agencies on Aging for local needs identification, planning, and funding of services, including but not limited to nutrition programs in the community as well as for those who are homebound; programs that serve Native American elders; services targeted at low-income minority elders; health promotion and disease prevention activities; in-home services for frail elders; and those services that protect the rights of older persons, such as the long-term care ombudsman program.

Sources: Administration on Aging, U.S. Department of Health and Human Services. *Older Americans Act.* http://www.aoa.gov/about/legbudg/oaa/legbudg_oaa .asp; Health Resources and Services Administration, U.S. Department of Health and Human Services. HIV/AIDS Bureau. http://hab.hrsa.gov/history.htm; National Campaign for Sustainable Agriculture. 2006, January. What's in a farm bill? http://www.sustainableagriculture.net/primer.php; U.S. Congress, House of Representatives. 2002, May. *Farm Security and Rural Investment Act of 2002 conference report to accompany HR 2646.* 107th Congress, 2nd session. Report 107-424. Washington, DC: Government Printing Office. http://www.nrcs.usda.gov/ about/legislative/pdf/2002FarmBillConferenceReport.pdf; and U.S Department of Agriculture. 2002. Farm Bill 2002. http://www.usda.gov/farmbill2002/.

for programs that benefit the public. One such organization is the Food Research and Action Center (FRAC). Located in Washington, D.C., it is a leading national organization working to improve public policies to eradicate hunger and undernutrition in the United States. FRAC de-

scribes itself as "a nonprofit and nonpartisan research and public policy center that serves as the hub of an anti-hunger network of thousands of individuals and agencies across the country" (http://www.frac.org). Its staff includes a variety of professionals, dominated by lawyers. However, nutritionists have an important role to play in organizations such as FRAC at the local, state, or national level.

■ EDUCATING POLICYMAKERS IN GOVERNMENT

Chapter 13 talked about the importance of educating and working with policymakers and decision makers so as to promote environments that are conducive to food and nutrition behaviors. These policymakers were school principals, community leaders, worksite management, local agencies, and others. This section discusses educating policymakers in government—elected officials.

Why Educate Elected Government Officials?

Elected government officials are the ones who will vote on legislation and make policy on issues that are of concern to you as a nutrition educator, such as funding for nutrition and for nutrition education through a variety of programs. Legislators are always sensitive to their constituents, so you, as an individual, *can* have an impact on them.

Who Are Your Elected Officials?

There are policy makers at many levels—local, city, county, state, and federal—and those who participate in nutrition education policy work say that it is important for you to know each one by name. Finding out who represents you should not be difficult in this age of technology. Go to the Web-based page of your local or state government; there will most likely be a tool there that will assist you in identifying your representative. Or try the Government Guide (http://votenote.aol.com/mygov/dbq/officials/). This site provides information on representatives at all levels and keeps you up to date on the activities of your legislators. At the federal level, you can also use http://www.senate.gov for senators and http://www.house.gov for members of the House of Representatives.

Get to Know Them and Let Them Get to Know You

Once you know who your elected representatives are, the next step is to find out about them. Go to their websites and find out the following:

- Their interests
- Legislation they support
- Committees they sit on

You put them there through your vote, and now you can help them work *for* you. You may think voting is not important, but it is. When you vote, you are designating the person who is ultimately going to work on your behalf. You need to let them know what you want and why it is important. If there is no funding for nutrition education at the federal level, many members of the public will not get the nutrition education they need, especially those in greatest need, such as those with few resources and those who live in low-income neighborhoods. Many issues of great importance will never be addressed, and many nutrition education jobs will not exist. You can use a variety of tools alone or in combination, but it is imperative to take action. Some methods are listed here.

- *Phone calls.* You can call your local office or, if the legislator travels between home and the state or national capitol, call that office. Either way, the legislator will get your message.
- *Meet legislators and meet with their staff.* It is great for them to know you by face; again, it can be in the district office, at the seat of government, or at both locations. Often you will not be able to meet with the legislator but can meet with the staff. The administrative assistant (AA) often acts as chief of staff and is

involved in policy decisions. The legislative director (LD) is in charge of the work of the legislative aides (LAs), who focus on a specific issue, such as health, transportation, or education. In fact, asking to meet and work with the legislative aide who works on your area of interest in the case of federal representatives can be most productive. They are the ones who do the research, provide the recommendations, and often write the legislation that is very important to nutrition education.

When it comes to making an appointment, do not wait until the last minute. Be sure you are registered to vote. Be prepared to tell the scheduler (an actual position) what you intend to talk about. In fact, it is very likely you will be asked to put your request in writing before it will even be considered. Faxing and e-mail are common since the terrorist events of 2001, but each office is different, so you need to determine what works best for the particular office. Confirm your appointment the day before.

Prepare in advance, know your key points, and bring your business card. Stay on topic. You are paying them, but be realistic and expect the meeting to last only 15 minutes. Come with a brief handout, and if there is a visual to share, bring it. A picture can say volumes, as can a graph. If you are asked a question and don't know the answer, don't guess. Tell them you will find out the answer and be sure to follow up with whatever you promise and with a thank-you note.

Inviting your legislator to your place of work or your local agency can also be a great opportunity for you and for the legislator. Make the offer and be sincere. Although they might not take you up on it, knowing you want them there can help. Photo ops are very important for them in the communication age.

- *Letters.* Letters can be sent to express your perspective, offer your help on an issue, ask for a meeting, or as a thank-you note. Today letters are not as easy a way to communicate with many government offices, especially in Washington, D.C., so you can use

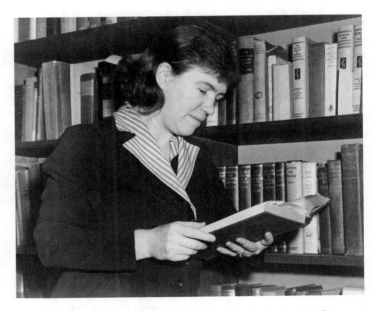

As anthropologist Margaret Mead once said, "Never doubt that a small group of thoughtful committed people can change the world. Indeed, it is the only thing that ever has."

e-mail. If you do use e-mail, stay formal in your letter composition. A resource for writing a letter is the Government Guide (http://votenote.aol.com).

- *Contribute to them.* Although legislators work for you, they still need funds to support their campaigns. There are a number of options, and finding the one that works for you is important. You can give them money directly, go through a political action committee (PAC), attend functions they have, or a combination of these. Contributions do have value and are recognized.

- *Stay in touch with them.* Meeting with legislators is not a one-shot deal. You want to know them, and they need to know you and the nutrition education issues you are most concerned about. If you stay in touch, they will be more ready to meet with you when you want their support for some policy or legislation that is important to you and the nutrition education community.

- *Become a legislative aide yourself.* A great way to influence food and nutrition policy through the legislative process is to become a legislative aide yourself. Several nutritionists or nutrition educators have gone to work on the staffs of elected officials. They add expertise to the office, advocate for food and nutrition policy, and help legislators write policy that is needed and sound. One such person is described in **Nutrition Education in Action 18-1**. Some nutritionists and dietitians have even run for office themselves.

■ YOU CAN'T DO EVERYTHING, BUT YOU CAN DO SOMETHING

This book has sought to provide you with the motivation, conceptual understanding, and skills for you to develop, implement, and evaluate nutrition education that is behavior focused and evidence based and that links theory, research, and practice. This final chapter has sought to stimulate you to become actively involved in the profession of nutrition education and to participate in actions that will have an impact on the larger environment. These actions can increase the ability of the nutrition education profession to advance the health of the nation's citizens.

As you have seen, you have many opportunities to make a difference in the world. Although you don't need to do everything, you can do something. And, doing something with others can help us achieve the goal of healthy people in healthy communities.

NUTRITION EDUCATION IN ACTION 18-1

A Nutritionist Working in Legislation

After he completed his undergraduate degree in psychology, Robert Stern realized that he was interested in community food issues and wanted to make a difference in the world. He returned to school and received a master's degree in nutrition education. While working in a community health center near the capital of New York, Albany, he had occasion to interact with regional organizations concerned with food issues that worked with the state legislature. He also worked on the campaign of a friend who was elected to state office. When his federally funded job ended, he sent his resumé to his elected friend, who thought he was a good match with the New York State Assembly Task Force on Food, Farm, and Nutrition Policy. The task force had an opening, and he got the job. Over the years he worked his way up to program manager for the task force.

Mission of the Task Force

- To develop programs, legislation, and budget initiatives that mutually benefit New York consumers, producers, and marketers of food in urban, suburban, and rural communities
- To provide oversight of implementation of state and federal food, nutrition, and agricultural programs
- To provide information and support concerning food policy issues to the task force chair, Speaker, assembly, and the public

Task Force Issue Areas

- Federal, state, and local food assistance programs (e.g., food stamps, WIC, school meals, senior meals, emergency food programs)
- Improving the marketing of New York farm and food products (e.g., government, school, and institutional purchasing; sales in supermarkets; farmers' market expansion; small-scale food processing; farm product distribution)
- Nutrition and health; nutrition education (e.g., childhood obesity prevention, concern for foods of minimal nutritional value, and increased fresh fruits and vegetables in schools); food allergies; insurance coverage for nutrition therapy
- Consumer concerns (e.g., labeling of food, contamination of food, genetic engineering, effectiveness of herbal supplements)
- Food-related community and economic development (e.g., farmers' markets, kitchen incubators, food entrepreneurs, restaurants featuring local products)
- Environmental and community impact of farming and food production (e.g., farmland protection, watersheds and farming, farm labor)
- Food policy councils

As program manager, Stern manages the legislative work related to these activities: he responds to and translates policy issues into legislation and budget recommendations; he initiates, develops, and manages public hearings and meetings around the state as needed; he negotiates; and he writes letters, newsletters, and press releases. The work changes over time and is always dependent on the direction the chair of the task force wants to take. Although the politicians make the final decision, he is pleased that he has the opportunity to help shape legislation on issues that are of concern to nutritionists and the public.

Questions and Activities

1. Identify two professional associations, local or national, that you think will be a good home for your interests as a nutrition educator. List their addresses and membership criteria. Make a plan to join.
2. List some of the strengths that you bring to the profession. Based on these, describe two ways in which you can help shape the profession.
3. Why is it important for nutrition education professional organizations to maintain or increase their credibility? Describe policy actions they can take to ensure ethical practices.
4. Define what is meant by "conflict of interest." Why is it important for individuals and organizations to disclose potential conflicts of interest?
5. Describe at least two ways in which member-initiated actions have had an impact on professional association policy changes.
6. In what ways can nutrition educators help to shape legislation that will have an impact on nutrition education?
7. Where would you like to be a year from now? Five years from now? Describe ways that will help you get from here to there.
8. Do you know who your legislators are at the federal, state, and local levels? Complete the following table. For each of your elected officials, list his or her address or email address and phone number. Make a date to contact these officials.

Your Elected Official to	Contact Information: Address, Email, Phone	Committee That Person Is On: Special Interests	Date You Contacted or Will Contact Person
City/town council			
State senate			
State assembly			
U.S. Senate			
U.S. House of Representatives			

References

American Dietetics Association. n.d. *HOD backgrounder: Dietetics professionals and ADA organizational units relations with industry.* http://www.eatright.org/ada/files/Industrybackgrounder.doc.

———. 2001. The issues management process: An evolving process, focused on member value. http://www.eatright.org/cps/rde/xchg/ada/hs.xsl/home_531_ENU_HTML.htm.

American Public Health Association. n.d. National Alliance for Nutrition and Activity: Child Nutrition Program reauthorization recommendations. http://www.apha.org/legislative/factsheets/ChildNutrition.pdf.

Association of State Nutrition Network Administrators. 2004. *Food Stamp Nutrition Education Networks: Partners for better health.* http://www.ces-fsne.org/pdfs/04ASNNAsummary.pdf.

———. 2010. *Professional tools and conference proceedings: SNAP–Ed connection.* http://snap.nal.usda.gov.

Centers for Disease Control and Prevention. 2005. *Welcome to the School Health Index (SHI): A self-assessment and planning guide.* http://apps.nccd.cdc.gov/shi/default.aspx.

Desjardin, E., L. Drake, F. Estrow, and S. Roberts. 2005, July. Food policy councils and the role nutritionists play. Presented at the annual conference of the Society for Nutrition Education, Orlando, FL.

Food Research and Action Center (FRAC). 2006. http://www.frac.org.

Fox, T. 2005, July. Local wellness policies. PowerPoint presentation at the annual conference of the Society for Nutrition Education, Orlando, FL.

McDonald, M. 2004. Ethics and conflict of interest. Vancouver, BC: The W. Maurice Young Centre for Applied Ethics. http://www.ethics.ubc.ca/people/mcdonald/conflict.htm.

Nestle, M. 2002. *Food politics: How the food industry influences nutrition and health.* Berkeley: University of California Press.

Society for Nutrition Education. 2002, January. *Society for Nutrition Education sponsorship guidelines.* http://www.sne.org/sponsorshipguidelines.pdf.

———. 2005. Conflict of interest. In *Society for Nutrition Education policies and procedures manual*, Section 6.9. Approved by the SNE Board April 11, 2005.

———. 2006. *Society for Nutrition Education resolutions process.* http://www.sne.org/documents/FinalResolutionprocess51305amendedJuly2006.doc.

U.S. Department of Agriculture. 2000. *Changing the scene: Improving the school nutrition environment.* Alexandria, VA: U.S. Department of Agriculture, Food and Nutrition Service. http://www.fns.usda.gov/tn/Healthy/changing.html.

Index

Problem solving skills, 273–274
Procedural knowledge, 98
Processed foods, 5, 7, 34
Process evaluation, 323
ProChildren study, 125
Product, defined, 381–382
Professional development, 418–421
Project LEAN, 70, 71
Promotional activities, 136, 382
Prostate cancer, 38
Psychological processes, 45, 65–66, 82–84, 146, 174
Psychomotor domain, 225, 227, 229
Public health nutrition, 20–21
Public policies, 121

Q

Qualitative data, program evaluation, 327, 333–334
Qualitative evaluation methods, 335
Qualitative studies, 47
Quality of life years (QALY), 17
Quasi-experimental designs, 334
Questionnaires, 100, 327, 328–329
Questions, program evaluation, 324–325, 327
Quiet members, group dynamics, 359

R

Randomized control trial (RCT), 334
Readability, 333
Reading level, written materials, 374
Reading skills, audience, 410–413
Recipes, 372–375
Reinforcement, 96, 98, 103, 272
Relapse prevention, 98, 103, 280–283
Reliability, program evaluation, 333
Religious beliefs, 175
Reproducibility, 333
Research
    health action process approach model, 106
    health belief model, 69
    health issues, identification of, 151–152
    keeping current, 418
    literature review, 153, 155
    nutrition education as, 17
    precaution adoption process model, 70, 72–73
    self-determination theory, 82–84
    social cognitive theory, 100–102
    theory and practice, 49
    theory of planned behavior, 77–82
    transtheoretical model, 111–112
Resistance, resolving, 254
Resistors, group dynamics, 360
Resources, food choice and, 182

Rewards, food as, 30
Rewards, goal setting, 280
Rewards, managing, 110
Risk appraisals, 68, 69–70, 84–85, 245–248
Rite Bite, 252–253
Rock on Café, 308
Role playing, 243
Routines, 79, 87, 252, 283
Ryan White Comprehensive AIDS Resources Emergency (CARE) Act, 424

S

Safe learning environments, 358
Safety concerns, 406
Salt, preference for, 28
Satiety, 7, 28, 30
School-based interventions
    case study, 231, 309, 311–315
    empowerment projects, 129
    environmental change, 125–126, 302–305
    family involvement, 123
    food choices and, 33
    gardens, 304
    guidelines for, 213
    overview, 18
    policies, 133
    program components, 211–212
    Rock on Café, 308
    social marketing, 384
School children, research studies, 84
School Lunch Program, 33
School Nutrition Association (SNA), 418, 419
Scoring, program evaluation data, 327
Self-assessments
    adolescents, 400
    educational strategies using, 252
    goal setting, 278
    health belief model, 84
    risk perception, 245–248
    social cognitive theory, 97
    theory of planned behavior, 78, 87
Self-commitment, 110
Self-determination theory (SDT), 82–84, 89, 206, 277
Self-efficacy
    action phase, program design, 201
    activities, designing, 250, 274–275
    coping, self-efficacy, 283
    health action process approach model, 102, 104–106
    health belief model, 68
    motivation and, 51
    perception of, 77, 87, 177
    social cognitive theory, 96, 97, 114–115
    strategies for improving, 272
    transtheoretical model, 110

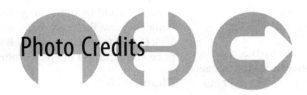

Photo Credits

University; **page 327** Courtesy of Linking Food and the Environment, Teachers College Columbia University

Chapter 15

Page 354 Courtesy of John and Karen Hollingsworth/U.S. Fish & Wildlife Services; **page 355** © Doctor Kan/ShutterStock, Inc.; **page 356** Courtesy of Food Bank For New York City; **page 363** © Photo-Create/ShutterStock, Inc.

Chapter 16

Page 369 © WoodyStock/Alamy Images; **16-2** © Edyta Powlowska/ShutterStock, Inc.; **page 378 (left)** Courtesy of Linking Food and the Environment, Teachers College Columbia University; **page 378 (right)** Courtesy of Teachers College Columbia University; **page 379** Courtesy of Food Bank For New York City; **page 383** Courtesy of Iowa Nutrition Network, Iowa Department of Public Health, and Iowa Department of Education

Chapter 17

Page 394 Courtesy of Cooking with Kids; **page 396** Courtesy of Food Bank For New York City; **page 400** Courtesy of Food Bank For New York City; **page 402** © Monkey Business Images/ShutterStock, Inc.; **page 406** Courtesy of Fredi Kronenberg; **page 411** © Photodisc

Chapter 18

Page 418 © Igor Karon/ShutterStock, Inc.; **page 425** Courtesy of Library of Congress, Prints & Photographs Division [reproduction number LC-USZ62-120226]

Unless otherwise indicated, all photographs and illustrations are under copyright of Jones and Bartlett Publishers, LLC, or have been provided by the author.